Veterinary Bacteriology

Veterinary Bacteriology

Editor: Evelyn Webb

STATES
ACADEMIC PRESS
www.statesacademicpress.com

States Academic Press,
109 South 5th Street,
Brooklyn, NY 11249, USA

Visit us on the World Wide Web at:
www.statesacademicpress.com

ISBN: 978-1-63989-556-4 (Hardback)

Cataloging-in-Publication Data

Veterinary bacteriology / edited by Evelyn Webb.
p. cm.
Includes bibliographical references and index.
ISBN 978-1-63989-556-4
1. Veterinary bacteriology. 2. Bacterial diseases in animals. 3. Veterinary microbiology.
4. Medical bacteriology. I. Webb, Evelyn.

SF780.3 .V48 2022
636.089 601 4--dc23

Table of Contents

Preface IX

Chapter 1 **Characterization of common carp (*Cyprinus carpio* L.) interferon regulatory factor 5 (IRF5) and its expression in response to viral and bacterial challenges** 1
Yaoyao Zhu, Chenchen Qi, Shijuan Shan, Fumiao Zhang, Hua Li, Liguo An and Guiwen Yang

Chapter 2 **A 10-day vacancy period after cleaning and disinfection has no effect on the bacterial load in pig nursery units** 13
K. Luyckx, S. Millet, S. Van Weyenberg, L. Herman, M. Heyndrickx, J. Dewulf and K. De Reu

Chapter 3 **Sero-prevalence of specific *Leptospira* serovars in fattening pigs from 5 provinces** 19
Hu Suk Lee, Nguyen Viet Khong, Huyen Nguyen Xuan, Vuong Bui Nghia, Hung Nguyen-Viet and Delia Grace

Chapter 4 **Prediction of marbofloxacin dosage for the pig pneumonia pathogens *Actinobacillus pleuropneumoniae* and *Pasteurella multocida* by pharmacokinetic/pharmacodynamic modelling** 26
Lucy Dorey, Ludovic Pelligand and Peter Lees

Chapter 5 **Changes in serum proteins after endotoxin administration in healthy and choline-treated calves** 36
Z. Yilmaz, O. Eralp Inan, M. Kocaturk, A. T. Baykal, O. Hacariz, I. Hatipoglu, A. Tvarijonaviciute, M. Cansev, J. Ceron and I. H. Ulus

Chapter 6 **Quadruplex PCR assay for identification of *Corynebacterium pseudotuberculosis* differentiating biovar Ovis and Equi** 44
Sintia Almeida, Elaine M. S. Dorneles, Carlos Diniz, Vinícius Abreu, Cassiana Sousa, Jorianne Alves, Adriana Carneiro, Priscilla Bagano, Sharon Spier, Debmalya Barh, Andrey P. Lage, Henrique Figueiredo and Vasco Azevedo

Chapter 7 **Comparison of the fecal bacterial microbiota of healthy and diarrheic foals at two and four weeks of life** 52
A. Schoster, H. R. Staemp li, L. G. Guardabassi, M. Jalali and J. S. Weese

Chapter 8 **Case definition terminology for paratuberculosis (Johne's disease)** 62
R. J. Whittington, D. J. Begg, K. de Silva, A. C. Purdie, N. K. Dhand and K. M. Plain

Chapter 9 **Comparison of competitive exclusion with classical cleaning and disinfection on bacterial load in pig nursery units** 75
K. Luyckx, S. Millet, S. Van Weyenberg, L. Herman, M. Heyndrickx, J. Dewulf and K. De Reu

Chapter 10 **Prevalence, antimicrobial susceptibility and risk factors associated with non-typhoidal *Salmonella* on Ugandan layer hen farms**......85
Terence Odoch, Yngvild Wasteson, Trine L'Abée-Lund, Adrian Muwonge, Clovice Kankya, Luke Nyakarahuka, Sarah Tegule and Eystein Skjerve

Chapter 11 **A robust PCR for the differentiation of potential virulent strains of *Haemophilus parasuis***......95
N. Galofré-Milà, F. Correa-Fiz, S. Lacouture, M. Gottschalk, K. Strutzberg-Minder, A. Bensaid, S. Pina-Pedrero and V. Aragon

Chapter 12 **European multicenter study on antimicrobial resistance in bacteria isolated from companion animal urinary tract infections**......100
Cátia Marques, Luís Telo Gama, Adriana Belas, Karin Bergström, Stéphanie Beurlet, Alexandra Briend-Marchal, Els M. Broens, Marta Costa, Delphine Criel, Peter Damborg, Marloes A. M. van Dijk, Astrid M. van Dongen, Roswitha Dorsch, Carmen Martin Espada, Bernhard Gerber, Maria Kritsepi-Konstantinou, Igor Loncaric, Domenico Mion, Dusan Misic, Rebeca Movilla, Gudrun Overesch, Vincent Perreten, Xavier Roura, Joachim Steenbergen, Dorina Timofte, Georg Wolf, Renato Giulio Zanoni, Sarah Schmitt, Luca Guardabassi and Constança Pomba

Chapter 13 **OmpA protein sequence-based typing and virulence-associated gene profiles of *Pasteurella multocida* isolates associated with bovine haemorrhagic septicaemia and porcine pneumonic pasteurellosis**......117
Teerasak E-kobon, Ratiporn Leeanan, Saengtian Pannoi, Pornchai Anuntasomboon, Pacharee Thongkamkoon and Arinthip Thamchaipenet

Chapter 14 **Determination of N-acylhomoserine lactones of *Pseudomonas aeruginosa* in clinical samples from dogs with otitis externa**......130
Darja Kušar, Karin Šrimpf, Petra Isaković, Lina Kalšek, Javid Hosseini, Irena Zdovc, Tina Kotnik, Modest Vengušt and Gabrijela Tavčar-Kalcher

Chapter 15 **Tick- and fly-borne bacteria in ungulates: the prevalence of *Anaplasma phagocytophilum*, haemoplasmas and rickettsiae in water buffalo and deer species**......141
Sándor Hornok, László Sugár, Isabel G. Fernández de Mera, José de la Fuente, Gábor Horváth, Tibor Kovács, Attila Micsutka, Enikő Gönczi, Barbara Flaisz, Nóra Takács, Róbert Farkas, Marina L. Meli and Regina Hofmann-Lehmann

Chapter 16 ***Coxiella* and *Bartonella* spp. in bats (Chiroptera) captured in the Brazilian Atlantic Forest biome**......148
Michelle Santos Ferreira, Alexandro Guterres, Tatiana Rozental, Roberto Leonan Morim Novaes, Emmanuel Messias Vilar, Renata Carvalho de Oliveira, Jorlan Fernandes, Danielle Forneas, Adonai Alvino Junior, Martha Lima Brandão, José Luis Passos Cordeiro, Martín Roberto Del Valle Alvarez, Sergio Luiz Althoff, Ricardo Moratelli, Pedro Cordeiro-Estrela, Rui Cerqueira da Silva and Elba Regina Sampaio de Lemos

Chapter 17 **Diagnostic tools of caprine and ovine anaplasmosis**......158
I. I. Shabana, N. M. Alhadlag and H. Zaraket

Chapter 18 **Molecular characterization of fluoroquinolone and/or cephalosporin resistance in *Shigella sonnei* isolates from yaks** 166
Zhen Zhu, Yuxiang Shi, Xuzheng Zhou, Bing Li and Jiyu Zhang

Chapter 19 **A novel approach to identifying and quantifying neutrophil extracellular trap formation in septic dogs using immunofluorescence microscopy** 175
Ronald H. L. Li, Lynelle R. Johnson, Casey Kohen and Fern Tablin

Chapter 20 **Invasion and replication of *Yersinia ruckeri* in fish cell cultures** 182
Simon Menanteau-Ledouble, Mark L. Lawrence and Mansour El-Matbouli

Chapter 21 **Bacteria and parasites in *Podarcis sicula* and *P. sicula klemmerii*** 193
Ludovico Dipineto, Pasquale Raia, Lorena Varriale, Luca Borrelli, Vittorio Botta, Carmela Serio, Michele Capasso and Laura Rinaldi

Chapter 22 **Vector-borne and zoonotic diseases of dogs in North-west New South Wales and the Northern Territory** 199
Amanda J. Shapiro, Graeme Brown, Jacqueline M. Norris, Katrina L. Bosward, Debbie J. Marriot, Nandhakumar Balakrishnan, Edward B. Breitschwerdt and Richard Malik

Chapter 23 **Characterization of the bacterial gut microbiota of piglets suffering from new neonatal porcine diarrhoea** 212
Marie Louise Hermann-Bank, Kerstin Skovgaard, Anders Stockmarr, Mikael Lenz Strube, Niels Larsen, Hanne Kongsted, Hans-Christian Ingerslev, Lars Mølbak and Mette Boye

Permissions

List of Contributors

Index

Preface

Over the recent decade, advancements and applications have progressed exponentially. This has led to the increased interest in this field and projects are being conducted to enhance knowledge. The main objective of this book is to present some of the critical challenges and provide insights into possible solutions. This book will answer the varied questions that arise in the field and also provide an increased scope for furthering studies.

The field of veterinary bacteriology plays an important role in veterinary medicine and human health. Veterinary bacteriology is the study of bacteria found in animal species. These bacteria can either be pathogenic or non-pathogenic and can cause infectious diseases in animals. Bacteria are classified into different categories on the basis of their nature and uniqueness. The use of biochemical tests for characterization and identification of bacteria is very helpful to understand their nature and characteristics. An infectious bacterial disease could be specific to an organ. Mastitis, collibacillosis in cattle, enterotoxaemia, infectious necrotic hepatitis and para tuberculosis in sheep, greasy pig disease and pneumonia in pigs are some of the common bacterial diseases. The book studies, analyses and upholds the pillars of veterinary bacteriology and its utmost significance in modern times. It also brings forth some of the most innovative concepts and elucidates the unexplored aspects of this field. This book will help new researchers by foregrounding their knowledge in veterinary bacteriology.

I hope that this book, with its visionary approach, will be a valuable addition and will promote interest among readers. Each of the authors has provided their extraordinary competence in their specific fields by providing different perspectives as they come from diverse nations and regions. I thank them for their contributions.

Editor

1

Characterization of common carp (*Cyprinus carpio* L.) interferon regulatory factor 5 (IRF5) and its expression in response to viral and bacterial challenges

Yaoyao Zhu, Chenchen Qi, Shijuan Shan, Fumiao Zhang, Hua Li, Liguo An* and Guiwen Yang*

Abstract

Background: Common carp (*Cyprinus carpio* L.), one of the most economically valuable commercial farming fish species in China, is often infected by a variety of viruses. As the first line of defence against microbial pathogens, the innate immune system plays a crucial role in teleost fish, which are lower vertebrates. Interferon (IFN) regulatory factor 5 (IRF5) is a key molecule in antiviral immunity that regulating the expression of IFN and other pro-inflammatory cytokines. It is necessary to gain more insight into the common carp IFN system and the function of fish IRF5 in the antiviral and antibacterial response.

Results: In the present study, we characterized the cDNA and genomic sequence of the IRF5 gene in common carp, and analysed tissue distribution and expression profile of this gene in response to polyinosinic:polycytidylic acid (poly I:C) and lipopolysaccharides (LPS) treatment. The common carp IRF5 (ccIRF5) gene is 5790 bp in length and is composed of 9 exons and 8 introns. The open reading frame (ORF) of ccIRF5 is 1554 bp, and encodes 517 amino acid protein. The putative ccIRF5 protein shares identity (65.4–90.0 %) with other fish IRF5s and contains a DNA binding domain (DBD), a middle region (MR), an IRF-associated domain (IAD), a virus activated domain (VAD) and two nuclear localization signals (NLSs) similar to those found in vertebrate IRF5. Phylogenetic analysis clustered ccIRF5 into the IRF5 subfamily with other vertebrate IRF5 and IRF6 genes. Real-time PCR analysis revealed that ccIRF5 mRNA was expressed in all examined tissues of healthy carps, with high levels observed in the gills and the brain. After poly I:C challenge, expression levels of ccIRF5, tumour-necrosis factor α (ccTNFα) and two IFN stimulated genes [ISGs (ccISG5 and ccPKR)] were up-regulated in seven immune-related tissues (liver, spleen, head kidney, foregut, hindgut, skin and gills). Furthermore, all four genes were up-regulated *in vitro* upon poly I:C and LPS challenges.

Conclusions: Our findings suggest that IRF5 might play an important role in regulating the antiviral and antibacterial response in fish. These results could provide a clue for preventing common carp infection by pathogenic microorganisms present in the aquatic environment.

Keywords: IRF5, Common carp (*Cyprinus carpio* L.), Poly I:C, LPS, Gene expression

* Correspondence: an.liguo58@gmail.com; yanggw@sdnu.edu.cn
Shandong Provincial Key Laboratory of Animal Resistance Biology, College of Life Science, Shandong Normal University, No. 88 East Wenhua Road, Jinan 250014, People's Republic of China

Background

Interferon (IFN) regulatory factors (IRFs) are key transcriptional mediators of virus-, bacteria- and IFN-induced signalling pathways, and they play an important role in antiviral defence, immune response, cell growth regulation, apoptosis and oncogenesis [1–3]. IRFs were originally identified as participating in the transcriptional regulators of IFN and IFN stimulated genes (ISGs) [4]. To date, eleven IRF family members have been identified in vertebrate, including IRF1, IRF2, IRF3, IRF4 [also known as PU.1 interaction partner (PIP), lymphoid-specific IRF (LSIRF) or consensus sequence-binding protein in adult T-cell leukemia cell line or activated T cells (ICSAT)], IRF5, IRF6, IRF7, IRF8 [also known as IFN consensus sequence binding protein (ICSBP)], IRF9 [also called as ISG factor 3 gamma (ISGF3γ)], IRF10 and IRF11. However, IRF10 and 11 have been identified in fish but in mammalians [5]. IRFs used to be classified into three groups according to differences in the C-terminal region: activators (IRF1, 3, 5, 7, 9 and 10), repressors (IRF2 and 8) and multifunctional factors that both activate and repress gene transcription (IRF2, 4, 5 and 7) [3, 4]. All members share a well-conserved N-terminal DNA-binding domain (DBD), and the conserved tryptophan repeat cluster in the first 120 amino acids of the DBD is responsible for binding the promoters of target genes [6]. IRF-associated domain (IAD) in the C-terminal of IRF3-11 mediates the interactions between IRFs and other protein to form transcriptional complexes [7].

Human IRF5 plays a crucial role in regulating the expression of IFN-α and IFN-β, mediating the virus- and cell type-specific immune response. IRF5 is also critical for the retinoic acid-inducible gene I (RIG-I) and Toll-like receptors immune pathways [8–12]. Other reports have also indicated that IRF5 may promote lymphocyte differentiation and apoptosis [9]. IRF5 knockout mice were reported to be susceptible to viral infections, while, the expression levels of type I IFNs and other pro-inflammatory cytokines including tumour-necrosis factor (TNF)-α, interleukin (IL)-6 and IL-12, were reduced in response to viral infections [12, 13].

IRF5 have been previously identified in several fish species, including grass carp (*Ctenopharyngodon idella*) [14], zebrafish (*Danio rerio*) [15], Atlantic salmon (*Salmo salar*) [16], Japanese flounder (*Paralichthys olivaceus*) [17], rock bream (*Oplegnathus fasciatus*) [18], half-smooth tongue sole (*Cynoglossus semilaevis*) [19], channel catfish (*Ictalurus Punctatus*) [20], Mi-iuy croaker (*Miichthys miiuy*) (unpublished data) and paddlefish (*Polyodon spathula*) [21]. Common carp (*Cyprinus carpio* L.), one of the most economically valuable commercial farming fish species, is often infected by a wide variety of viruses [22, 23]. To date, among the IRFs, only IRF3 and IRF7 have been identified in common carp [22]. Additional studies are needed to gain a better insight into the IFN system in common carp and the function of fish IRF5 in the antiviral and antibacterial immune response. In the present study, we characterized the cDNA sequence and genomic structure of IRF5 from common carp. We reported the evolutionary relationship of common carp IRF5 (ccIRF5) gene with other IRF genes. What's more, we analysed its tissue-specific distribution in twelve tissues and expression profiles upon polyinosinic:polycytidylic acid (poly I:C) and lipopolysaccharides (LPS) stimulation both in vivo and in vitro by using real-time PCR.

Methods

Fish and poly I:C challenge

Common carp (body weight approximately 200 g) were obtained from the Fresh Water Fishery Research Institute of Shandong Province, China. Fish were reared in aerated freshwater tanks at 24–26 °C and were fed twice per day with commercial carp pellets (Shandong Tianshen Fishing Feedstuff Co., Ltd). After acclimatization for 1 week, the fish were used for the experiments.

Poly I:C (Sigma, USA) was re-suspended in phosphate-buffered saline (PBS) for the immune challenge experiments. Fish were intraperitoneally injected with 500 μl of a poly I:C solution (2.6 mg/ml) per fish, while un-challenged fish served as controls (indicated as 0 h). After injection, all fish were placed into a rectangular tank containing fresh water. At 0, 3, 6, 12, 24, 48 and 72 h post-injection (hpi), three fish in each group were euthanized and seven tissues including liver, spleen, head kidney, skin, gills, foregut and hindgut were sampled for total RNA extraction.

RNA and genomic DNA extraction

Total RNA was extracted from different tissues of common carp using an RNA simple Total RNA Kit (TIANGEN) according to the manufacturer's instructions. Total RNA quality and concentration were determined by 1 % gel electrophoresis and ultraviolet spectrophotometry, respectively. RNA samples had an OD260:OD280 ratio between 1.8 and 2.0. Genomic DNA was then removed and first-strand cDNA was synthesized by using the FastQuant RT Kit (containing gDNase) (TIANGEN) following the manufacturer's protocol. Genomic DNA was extracted from the spleen of healthy fish using a TIANamp Genomic DNA Kit (TIANGEN).

Cloning of cDNA and genomic sequences

A pair of primers, IRF5-F and IRF5-R (shown in Table 1), designed based on the conserved regions of different IRF5 genes, was used to amplify the corresponding ccIRF5 sequence from spleen cDNA of healthy fish. The PCR cycling parameters were 94 °C for 5 min, followed by 30 cycles of 94 °C for 30 s, 54 °C for 30 s, 72 °C for

Table 1 Primers used in this study

Primer	Sequence (5′-3′)	Application	GenBank No.
IRF5-F	GCAAGTACCAGGAAGGAG	Homologous amplification	
IRF5-R	AAATCAGTTAAGGGCAACA		
IRF5-3 F1	GTCACTCATTCTGTAGGCCCT	First round 3′-RACE PCR	
IRF5-3 F2	GCAGAGAACCAGGTTCATCC	Nested 3′-RACE PCR	
IRF5-5R1	TGTCCTTCGTGCCATCGTAGTG	First round 5′-RACE PCR	
IRF5-5R2	GTTTAGGGCACAGCGGAGATT	Nested 5′-RACE PCR	
IRF5g1-F	CAGCACCATGAGTGGTCAACCACG	For the first intron	
IRF5g1-R	AATATAGAGTTCTCCTCCTCCAG		
IRF5g2-F	AGGACTGCACTGGCTCAATCAAGA	For the second intron	
IRF5g2-R	ATCTACTCCTTCCTGATACTTGCCT		
IRF5g3-F	ATGGAAAGCCAATCTCCGCTGTG	For the third, fourth and fifth intron	
IRF5g3-R	GTAACATGAGCGGACTGCTCAGC		
IRF5g4-F	AGTGCAATCAAAGTTGAGCAGGCA	For the sixth intron	
IRF5g4-R	ATGATCGGTATAGAACCTCTGCTT		
IRF5g5-F	ACGCCATCAGGCTGTGCCAGTGTA	For the seventh intron	
IRF5g5-R	CAATGATGAGCTTTTTCTCCTTG		
IRF5g6-F	GCTTCGGTGAGGACTGGCCAGACA	For the eighth intron	
IRF5g6-R	ACTCTGCAGAAGTCTGTGGAGCT		
IRF5-rF	CCTGGGCTCAGAACATCCACTAAC	Real-time PCR	
IRF5-rR	AGTATGGCATCATAGAGGGCACCT		
TNFα-F	ACAGGTGATGGTGTCGAGGAGGA	Real-time PCR	JF957372
TNFα-R	TCTGAGACTTGTTGAGCGTGAAG		
S11-F	CCGTGGGTGACATCGTTACA	Real-time PCR	AB012087
S11-R	TCAGGACATTGAACCTCACTGTCT		
ISG15-F	GTGAGCGGTGAAGCCACAGTTG	Real-time PCR	KP115358
ISG15-R	GCGAACCGTTATCGGCAGACAG		
PKR-F	AGGCTTGATCCACAGAGACCTGAA	Real-time PCR	JX516101
PKR-R	CGTTCCAGAAGTTGCACGTCATTG		

50 s, and a final extension step of 72 °C for 10 min. Then, the full-length cDNA of ccIRF5 was obtained by the rapid amplification of the cDNA ends (RACE) method using a 3′-Full RACE and 5′-Full RACE Core Set Kit (TaKaRa). The detailed procedure was performed as described in the user manual, and two primers pairs (IRF5-3 F1/-3 F2 and IRF5-5R1/5R2) were used in the RACE-PCR (shown in Table 1).

PCR products were analysed by electrophoresis on a 1 % agarose gel and the anticipated fragments were purified from agarose gels. These fragments were ligated into the pMD18-T vector (TaKaRa) and transformed into competent *Escherichia coli* DH-5α competent cells, and recombinants were identified and sequenced (Invitrogen).

Sequence and phylogenetic analysis

The full-length cDNA sequence of ccIRF5 was compared with other corresponding IRF5 sequences by using the BLAST program from the National Center for Biotechnology Information (NCBI) [24] and the MegAlign program DNASTAR. The putative ORF and the protein prediction were analysed with Editseq within DNASTAR. The protein domains were predicted with simple modular architecture research tool (SMART) [25]. Phylogenetic analysis was performed with MEGA 5.0, using the neighbor-joining method. Homologous sequences were searched using the NCBI BLAST server.

Leukocyte isolation and in vitro challenges

The methods for isolating common carp leukocytes from peripheral blood (PBLs) and head kidney (HKLs) have been described by Rymuszka et al. [26]. Peripheral blood was diluted 1:1 with Leibovitz's L-15 medium (supplemented with 10 U/ml of heparin, 10 mM HEPES, 60 mM NaCl, 5 % FBS, 100 U/ml penicillin, 100 μg/ml streptomycin, and 250 ng/ml amphotericin B) and layered on a 65 % Percoll (Sigma) solution, and centrifuged at 2500 rpm for 30 min at 4 °C. The cells were washed by centrifugation in PBS and re-suspended in cold Leibovitz's L-15 medium.

Head kidney cell suspensions were obtained by gently pressing the tissue with a plunger through a 100-μm sterile nylon mesh with Leibovitz's L-15 medium. Percoll layers of 51 and 34 % were used and centrifuged at 1500 rpm for 30 min at 4 °C. The cell layers at the interphase were collected and washed twice with Leibovitz's L-15 medium.

For stimulation experiments, 1×10^6 cells were maintained at 25 °C in a 24-well tissue culture plate with 0.5 mg/ml poly I:C and 1 mg/ml LPS (suspended in PBS), while un-challenged cells served as controls (indicated as 0 h). The cells were harvested at 0, 3, 6, 9, 12 and 24 hpi and RNA was extracted and reverse transcribed.

Real-time quantitative PCR

The inducible expression profiles of ccIRF5, ccTNFα and two ISG genes [ccISG15 and ccPKR (protein kinase R)] upon poly I:C and LPS challenges were analysed by real-time PCR using gene-specific primers (Table 1) on an iQ5 Real-time PCR instrument (Bio-Rad). Reactions were performed in a 20 μl volume using SYBR Green RealMasterMix (TIANGEN). Cycling conditions were one cycle of 94 °C for 5 min, followed by 40 cycles of 94 °C for 20 s, 60 °C for 30 s and 72 °C for 20 s. The 40S ribosomal protein S11 gene was amplified in parallel as a housekeeping control for normalization [27]. The amplification efficiency of the primers used in the real-time PCR was between 0.80 and 0.86. All samples were analysed in triplicate. Standard curves were run on the same plate. The real-time PCR data were analysed with the $2^{-\Delta\Delta CT}$ method.

Statistical analysis

Differences in relative gene expression between the challenged group and the control group were tested using one-way analysis of variance (ANOVA) in Graphpad Prism 5. P values < 0.05 were considered statistically significant.

Results

Characterization of the cDNA sequence of ccIRF5

The full-length cDNA of ccIRF5 (GenBank Accession No.: KP979609) was 2042 bp, consisting of a 5'-untranslated region (UTR) of 266 bp, a 3'-UTR of 222 bp with a polyadenylation signal (AATAAA) starting 30 bp upstream of the poly (A) tail and an ORF of 1554 bp encoding a peptide of 517 amino acids. The predicted molecular weight of ccIRF5 is 58.5 kDa, and the isoelectric point is 5.8. The deduced amino acid sequence of ccIRF5 shares higher identities with the fish IRF5s (65.4 % of *P. spathula* to 90.0 % of *C. idella*) than with IRF5s of other species (51.6 % of *G. gallus* to 56.7 % of *M. musculus*) (Table 2) and contains a DBD, a middle region (MR), an IAD and a virus activated domain (VAD) (Fig. 1).

Genomic structure of ccIRF5

The ccIRF5 gene is 5798 bp and is composed of 9 exons and 8 introns (Fig. 2). The exon-intron splice junctions follow the AG/GT rule (Table 3). The ccIRF5 gene has the same size exons as the grass carp IRF5, while, the introns sizes are different, which are 495, 804, 225, 131, 88, 761, 518, and 766 bp (listed in Additional file 1).

Phylogenetic analysis

The phylogenetic tree was constructed based on a Clustal W alignment using MEGA 5.0 by the neighbor-joining method. All IRF members were divided into four subfamilies: IRF1, IRF2, and zebrafish IRF11 belonged to the IRF1 subfamily, IRF3 and IRF7 belonging to the IRF3 subfamily; IRF4, 8, 9, and 10 belonging to the IRF4 subfamily; IRF5 and IRF6 belonging to the IRF5 subfamily. In the phylogenetic tree, ccIRF5 showed a closer relationship with genes from other cyprinid fish, including grass carp and zebrafish IRF5s, and clustered into the fish IRF5 subgroup (Fig. 3).

Table 2 Amino acid identities (%) of ccIRF5 to other vertebrate IRF5 proteins

Species	Protein length (aa)	GeneBank No.	Full-length identities	DBD identities
Ctenopharyngodon idella	519	ACT83675	90.0	96.5
Danio rerio	498	ABY91289	87.9	93.9
Ictalurus Punctatus	478	AHH37262	76.8	85.1
Paralichthys olivaceus	472	AEY55357	68.9	75.4
Scophthalmus maximus	487	AEG76960	69.7	75.4
Salmo salar	532	NP_001133324	69.6	82.5
Oplegnathus fasciatus	498	AFZ93894	69.7	80.7
Miichthys miiuy	492	AHB59743	70.1	80.7
Polyodon spathula	496	AEW27153	65.4	74.6
Xenopus laevis	517	NP_001088065	56.9	73.7
Gallus gallus	472	NP_001026758	51.6	58.8
Mus musculus	497	AAB81997	56.7	67.5
Homo sapiens	498	AAH04201	55.3	67.5

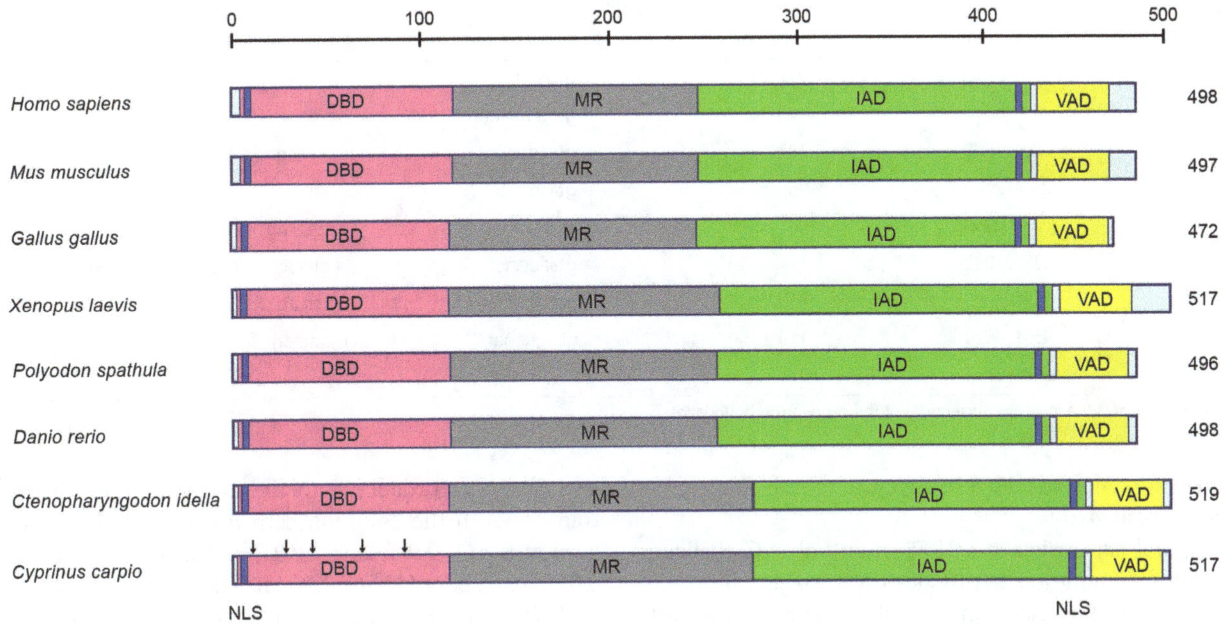

Fig. 1 Domain organization of ccIRF5 and other vertebrate IRF5 proteins. The DBD (*pink*), MR (*grey*), IAD (*green*) and VAD (*yellow*) are depicted in different colours. The two NLSs are boxed in blue and the conserved tryptophan residues are indicated by downward arrowheads. Numbers refer to the length of the amino acid sequences. The accession numbers are listed in Table 2

Tissue distribution of ccIRF5 mRNA in healthy carps

Constitutive expression of ccIRF5 mRNA in various tissues (gills, brain, skin, spleen, gonad, head kidney, buccal epithelium, hindgut, foregut, muscle, liver and blood) of healthy carps was examined by real-time PCR. The highest expression levels were in the gills and the brain, followed by the skin, the spleen, the gonad, the head kidney, the buccal epithelium, the hindgut, the foregut and the muscle, while low expression was observed in the liver and the blood (Fig. 4).

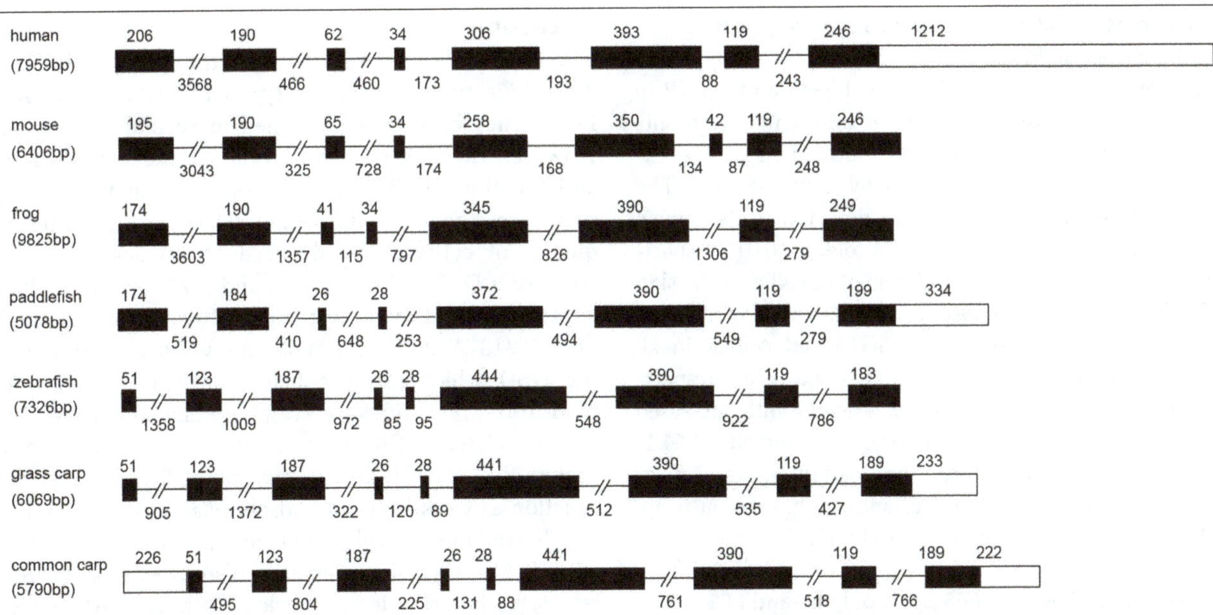

Fig. 2 Schematic diagram of exon-intron arrangement of IRF5 genes from various vertebrates. Exons are indicated by boxes and introns by straight or interrupted lines (>200 bp). The numbers above the boxes and below the lines indicate the lengths of exons and introns, respectively. Sequences selected are the following IRF5s: Human (Gene ID 3663), Mouse (Gene ID 27056), Paddlefish (Gene ID JF511655), Zebrafish (Gene ID 405811), Grass carp (GenBank: FJ556995) and Common carp (GenBank: KP979609)

Table 3 Intron-exon junctions and flanking sequences of the ccIRF5 gene

Exon no.	Position in DNA	Exon size (bp)	Splice donor	Splice acceptor	Intron size (bp)
1	1–277	277	**gt**gaattgtg	accctgcc**ag**	495
2	773–896	123	**gt**gagtaata	tgctcttc**ag**	804
3	1701–1888	187	**gt**aaggaccg	ttgatttt**ag**	225
4	2114–2140	26	**gt**aagttctg	tgcctttc**ag**	131
5	2272–2300	28	**gt**aagatttt	tgcttgac**ag**	88
6	2389–2830	441	**gt**aagcctct	tcttctct**ag**	761
7	3592–3982	390	**gt**aagaggaa	ttcttctc**ag**	518
8	4501–4620	119	**gt**ttggagat	cgttatct**ag**	766
9	5487–5798	411			

Bold text indicates the invariant nucleotides of the exon-intron boundaries

Gene expression of ccIRF5 in response to poly I:C challenge in vivo

Temporal expression of ccIRF5 upon poly I:C challenge in seven immune-related tissues (liver, spleen, head kidney, foregut, hindgut, skin and gills) was examined at 0, 3, 6, 12, 24, 48 and 72 hpi using real-time PCR. The highest expression levels in different tissues were reached at different time points. The maximum induction of ccIRF5 in mucosa-associated tissues including the foregut, the hindgut, the skin and the gills, occurred within 24 hpi. In contrast, the expression levels in the spleen, the head kidney and the liver were up-regulated at later time points (48 and 72 hpi). The expression of ccIRF5 was weakly up-regulated in all tested tissues (1.7- to 4.2-fold, $p < 0.01$ or $p < 0.05$) except in the foregut (22.8-fold increase, $p < 0.01$) (Fig. 5).

Gene expression of ccTNFα and ccISGs in response to poly I:C challenge in vivo

The expression levels of ccTNFα, ccISG15 and ccPKR in all tested tissues were increased at different time points upon stimulation with poly I:C. Subsequently, the expression levels decreased gradually until 48 hpi. The highest induction of ccTNFα was detected in the spleen (42.3- fold, $p < 0.01$) and liver (20.4-fold, $p < 0.01$), respectively. Whereas, the expression levels of ccTNFα in the skin (2.8-fold) and the gills (5.8-fold, $p < 0.05$) were weakly up-regulated. The expression of ccISG15 and ccPKR in all tested tissues reached peak levels at 3 and 6 hpi, respectively. Fold induction of ccISG15 was significantly increased in the foregut (3464.8-fold, $p < 0.05$) and hindgut (1364.1-fold, $p < 0.05$). Furthermore, the highest expression of ccPKR was observed in the liver and the hindgut at 6 hpi by 95.9-fold and 88.1-fold, respectively (Fig. 6).

Expression profiles of ccIRF5 upon poly I:C and LPS challenges in vitro

To further investigate the antiviral and antibacterial response of ccIRF5 in vitro, common carp PBLs and HKLs were isolated and challenged them with poly I:C or LPS. In accordance with the in vivo studies, ccIRF5 transcripts in the common carp PBLs reached the peak level at 3 hpi (2.9-fold, $p < 0.05$) and 6 hpi (2.0-fold $p < 0.05$), upon poly I:C and LPS challenges, respectively. As well as in the HKLs, expression of ccIRF5 reached the peak level at 24 hpi by 5.2-fold and 3.3-fold upon poly I:C and LPS challenges, respectively (Fig. 7).

Expression profiles of ccTNFα and ccISGs in poly I:C- and LPS- stimulated PBLs

All three genes were up-regulated at 3 hpi by both poly I:C and LPS challenges in the PBLs. However, compared to the challenge by poly I:C (4.1- to 29.1-fold), expression levels of the three genes were weakly induced upon LPS challenge (1.8- to 3.2-fold) (Fig. 8).

Discussion

The IRF family of transcription factors plays an important role in the regulation of type I IFN genes and ISGs. IRF5 genes have been identified in several vertebrates. However, there is no evidence about the identification and function of IRF5 in common carp. In the present study, we cloned the full-length cDNA and genomic sequence of ccIRF5. The deduced amino acid sequence contains a DBD, a MR, an IAD and a VAD (Fig. 1). Similar to other IRF5s in vertebrates, five tryptophan residues (W13, W28, W40, W60 and W79) are present in the DBD which forms a helix-turn-helix structure to bind to the IFN stimulated response element (IRSE)/IRF binding element (IRF-E) consensus in the target promoters [28]. The VAD that comprises all serine residues function as virus-induced phosphorylation sites. The MR which contains a proline-rich domain and is less conserved. Although this domain is also present in IRF3, 4 and 6, its function is still unclear [29]. The IAD, which was originally identified in IRF8, can form transcriptional complexes with other IRFs or transcriptional co-modulators to initiate the transcription of target genes [7]. Chen W et al. reported that the dimerization

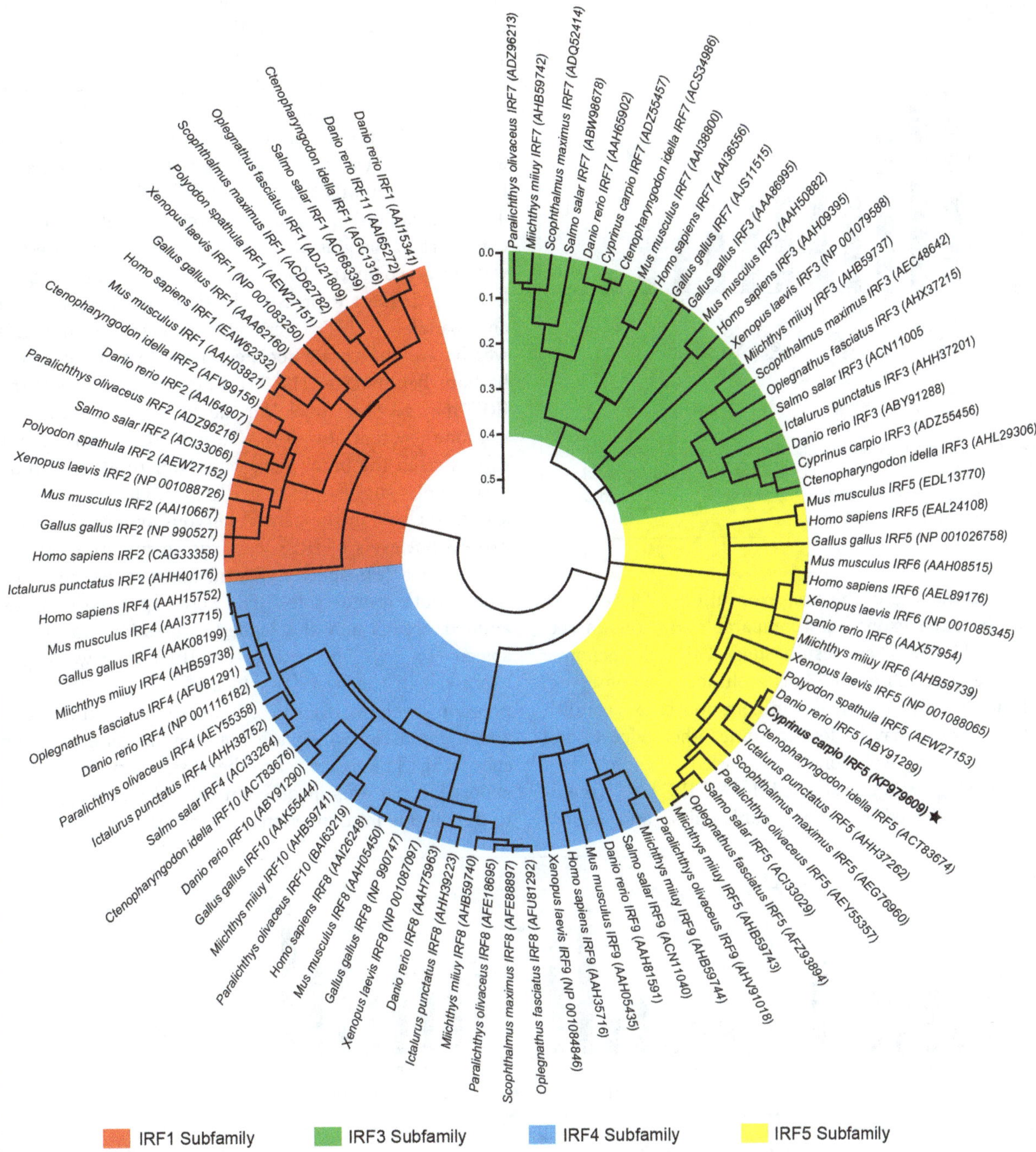

Fig. 3 Phylogenetic tree of ccIRF5 with known IRFs in vertebrates. The tree was constructed using the neighbor-joining method within the MEGA 5.0. Numbers above the nodes are bootstrap values on 1000 replicates. The GenBank accession numbers for the IRF sequences are shown within the brackets next to each species

between hydrophobic and ionic interactions in the IAD played a crucial role in the high basal activity of IRFs [30]. Similar to other IRF5s, two nuclear localization signals (NLSs) are found in the N- and C-termini of the predicted ccIRF5 protein, and these NLRs play an important role in IRF nuclear translocation and retention in virus-infected cells [11, 14, 17].

Similar to IRF5 genes of other Cypriniformes (zebrafish and grass carp), the genomic sequence of ccIRF5 is also composed of 9 exons and 8 introns. However, the IRF5 genes in human and several other vertebrates contain 8 exons and 7 introns. Interestingly, the sizes of the first and second exons, which encode the DBD of IRF5s in common carp, zebrafish and grass carp, are

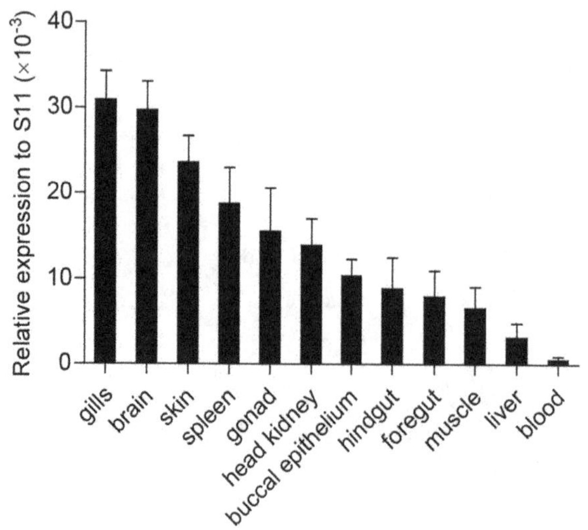

Fig. 4 Tissue distribution analysis of ccIRF5 mRNA by real-time PCR. Total RNA was isolated from various tissues of healthy carps. Gene expression levels were normalized to 40S ribosomal protein S11 mRNA. The data are presented as the mean ± S.D. ($n = 3$)

similar to the size of the first exon in other vertebrates, while the other exons sizes comparable to exons in vertebrates (Fig. 2). These results suggest that the genomic structure of vertebrate IRF5s is evolutionarily conserved, and the first intron of IRF5s in common carp, zebrafish and grass carp may be lost in some other teleosts and tetrapods during evolution.

The phylogenetic tree showed that all IRF family members were divided into four subfamilies, and ccIRF5 showed a closer relationship with other cyprinids, including grass carp and zebrafish IRF5s, which were well clustered into the fish IRF5 subgroup (Fig. 3). This result matches the evolutionary relationship observed at the genomic structure level for the IRF5s in all species (Fig. 2).

The ccIRF5 transcripts were ubiquitously expressed in all tested tissues of healthy carp, which was similar to the expression of other known fish IRFs [14, 31–35]. The highest ccIRF5 expression levels in healthy common carp were in the gills and the brain, while low expression was observed in the liver and the blood (Fig. 4). Similarly, the highest expression levels of Japanese flounder and paddlefish IRF5 were also detected in the gills, which are mucosa-associated lymphoid tissues that harbour lymphocytes [17, 21]. These results suggest that IRF5 may be crucial role for the activity of the mucosal immune system in fish. Turbot IRF5 was highly expressed in the brain, with which our result is in more agreement, suggesting that IRF5 might also play a significant role in the central nervous system [36]. High expression levels of IRF5 were shown in various tissues of different fish species. For instance, grass carp and half-smooth tongue sole IRF5s were expressed in all examined organs and the highest expression was in the spleen [14, 19]. The rock bream IRF5 gene was highly expressed in the liver [18]. In contrast, the highest expression levels of IRF5 in zebrafish were in the ovaries and the muscle, which are not immune-associated tissues [15]. The reason for the dissimilarities in IRF5 expression patterns in different fish species may be due to the diverse immune systems of fishes.

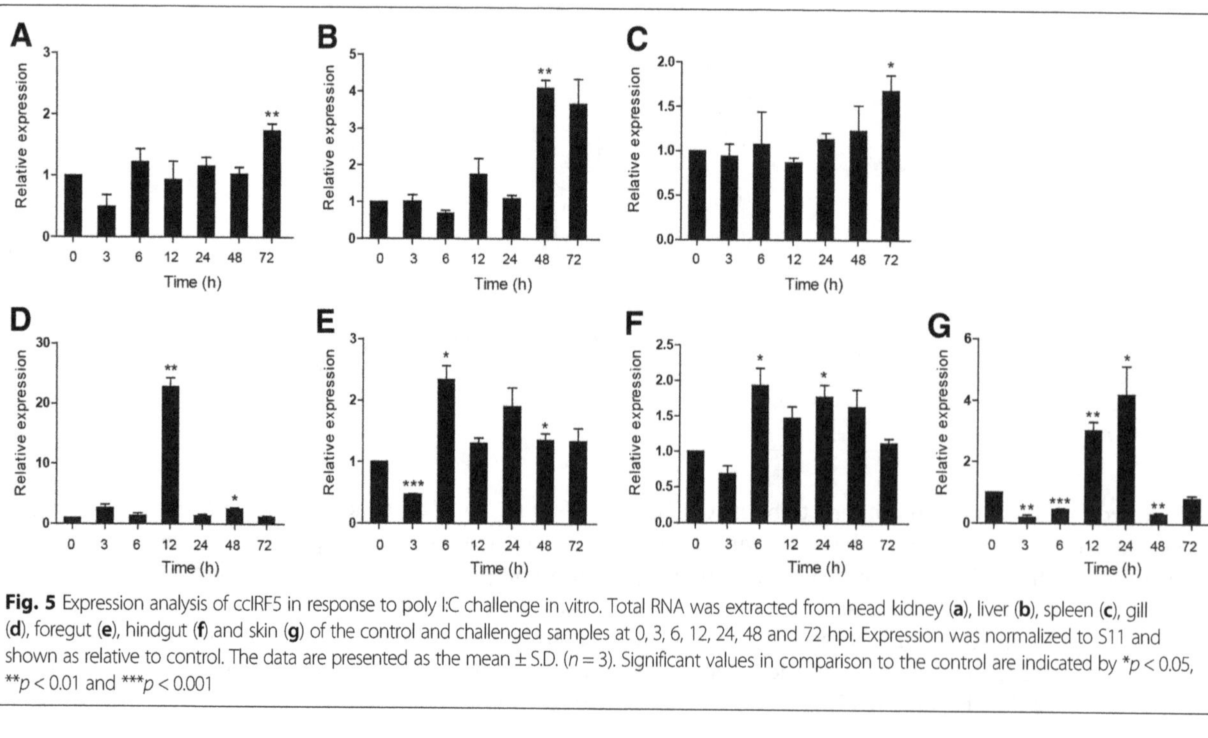

Fig. 5 Expression analysis of ccIRF5 in response to poly I:C challenge in vitro. Total RNA was extracted from head kidney (**a**), liver (**b**), spleen (**c**), gill (**d**), foregut (**e**), hindgut (**f**) and skin (**g**) of the control and challenged samples at 0, 3, 6, 12, 24, 48 and 72 hpi. Expression was normalized to S11 and shown as relative to control. The data are presented as the mean ± S.D. ($n = 3$). Significant values in comparison to the control are indicated by *$p < 0.05$, **$p < 0.01$ and ***$p < 0.001$

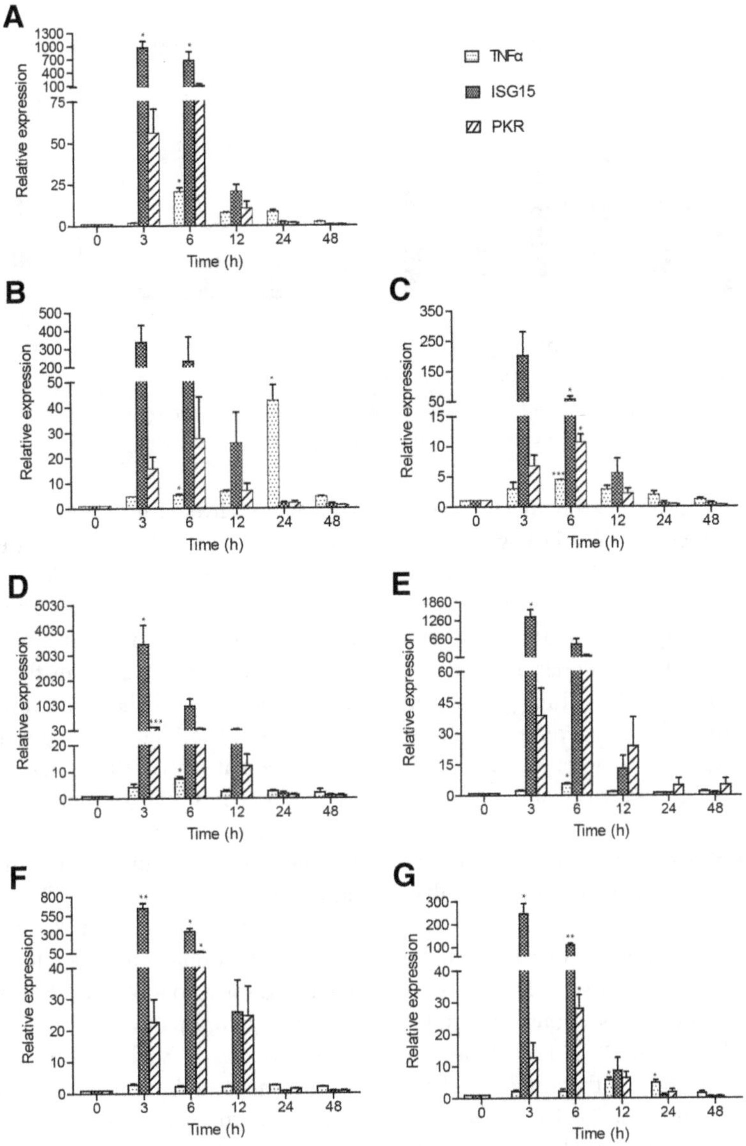

Fig. 6 Expression analysis of ccTNFα and ccISGs in response to poly I:C challenge *in vitro*. Total RNA was extracted from head kidney (**a**), liver (**b**), spleen (**c**), gill (**d**), foregut (**e**), hindgut (**f**) and skin (**g**) of the control and challenged samples (shown in Fig. 5). The expression was normalized to S11 and shown as relative to control. The data are presented as the mean ± S.D. ($n = 3$). Significant values in comparison to the control are indicated by $*p < 0.05$, $**p < 0.01$ and $***p < 0.001$

Previous studies have highlighted the important role of IRF5 in regulating the expression of IFN and other pro-inflammatory cytokines in TLR7 and 8 antiviral responses [13]. To gain insight into the role of ccIRF5 in response to the treatment with poly I:C, which is a synthetic double-stranded RNA, the temporal expression of ccIRF5 in seven immune-related tissues was examined. As shown in Fig. 5, the expression levels of ccIRF5 in different tissues reached peak levels at different time points. The maximum induction of ccIRF5 in mucosa-associated tissues including the foregut, the hindgut, the skin and the gills, occurred within 24 hpi compared to the expression levels in the spleen, the head kidney and the liver (at 48 and 72 hpi). This phenomenon may be because the fish mucosal immune system is the first line of defence against the invading pathogens. The expression of ccIRF5 was slightly up-regulated in all tested tissues (1.7- to 4.2-fold), with the exception of the foregut (22.8-fold). Similarly, the expression levels of IRF3 and IRF7 mRNA were highly up-regulated in the intestine of spring viraemia of carp virus (SVCV)-infected common carps [22]. These results may indicate that the IRF family plays a key role in the intestinal immune system. The expression levels of IRF5 in the immune and

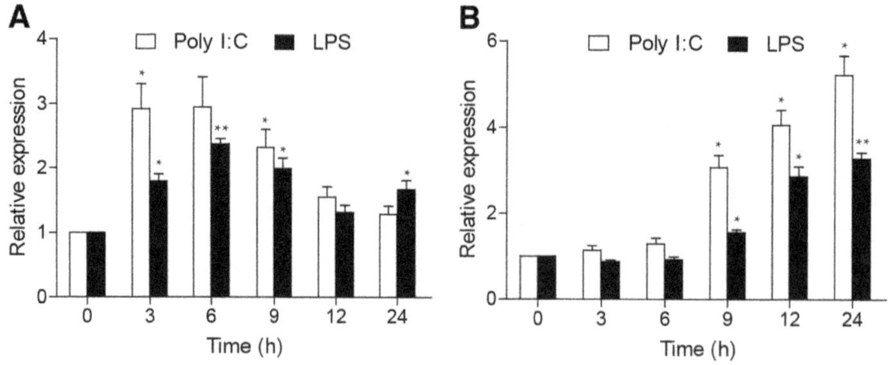

Fig. 7 Expression levels of ccIRF5 in the PBLs (**a**) and HKLs (**b**) induced by ploy I:C and LPS in vivo. Total RNA was extracted from control and challenged samples at 0, 3, 6, 9, 12 and 24 hpi. The expression was normalized to S11 and shown relative to control. The data are presented as the mean ± S.D. ($n = 3$). Significant values in comparison to the control are indicated by $^{*}p < 0.05$ and * $^{*}p < 0.01$

non-immune tissues of zebrafish, rock bream and turbot were weakly affected by infectious poly I:C, which is in accordance with our study [15, 18, 36]. In contrast, the induction magnitude of IRF5 was much stronger in the tissues of poly I:C-injected Japanese flounder [17]. In addition, fish (grass carp, Japanese flounder, rock bream, turbot and half-smooth tongue soles) IRF5 genes were reported to be significantly induced by different pathogens (grass carp reovirus, lymphocystis disease virus, iridovirus, turbot reddish body iridovirus and megalocytivirus) [14, 15, 17–19, 36]. These results indicate that fish IRF5 may respond to different pathogens in a tissue- or virus-specific manner, but the mechanism involved require further investigation.

TNFα, a potent proinflammatory cytokine produced following PAMP recognition by PRRs, and ISGs were also observed at different time points upon the stimulation of poly I:C in vivo by real-time PCR. The highest induction of ccTNFα was detected in the spleen and the liver at 24 hpi (42.3- fold) and 6 hpi (20.4-fold), respectively (Fig. 6). This finding is potentially because the spleen and liver are key innate immune tissues in fish that have a rich resident population of macrophages and lymphocytes, which secrete large quantity of TNFα upon stimulation with pathogens. The Skin, the gills and the intestine (including foregut and hindgut) are important mucosal lymphoid tissues in fish [37]. In this study, following poly I:C challenge, ccISG15 and ccPKR in the foregut and the hindgut were significantly induced. This result indicates that IRF5 might play an important role in mucosal immune system. Further, in our preliminary studies, gene expression of ccIFN and ccMx in all tested tissues was also significantly induced by poly I:C stimulation (unpublished data). In Japanese flounder and turbot, Mx expression was strongly induced by poly I:C in the head kidney and the gills [38, 39]. Thus, these results suggest a role of ccIRF5 in the activation of downstream antiviral pathways.

In accordance with the in vivo study, ccIRF5 transcripts in common carp PBLs and HKLs were induced upon the stimulation of poly I:C and LPS (Fig. 7). The reason for this phenomenon might because of the

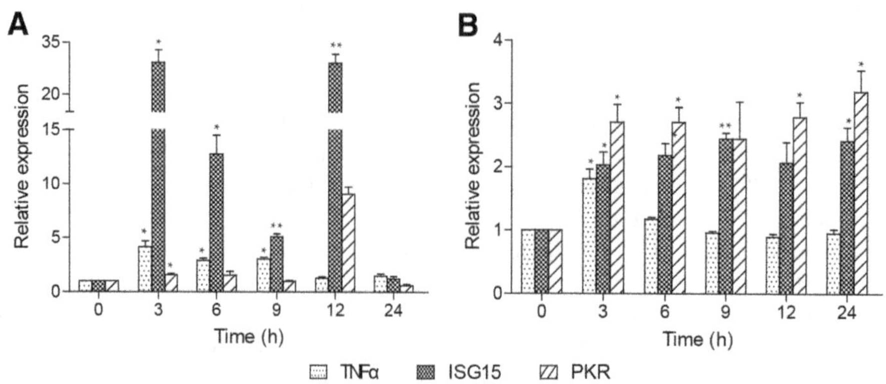

Fig. 8 Expression analysis of ccTNFα and ccISGs in common carp PBLs upon poly I:C (**a**) and LPS (**b**) challenges. Total RNA was extracted from the challenged samples at each time point (shown in Fig. 7). The expression was normalized to S11 and shown relative to control. The data are presented as the mean ± S.D. ($n = 3$). Significant values in comparison to the control are indicated by $^{*}p < 0.05$ and $^{**}p < 0.01$

presence of immune cells, including monocytes, granulocytes and lymphocytes [40, 41]. Notably, the highest induction of ccIRF5 in the PBLs (3 to 6 hpi) was earlier than the induction in the HKLs (24 hpi). This might be due to that IRF family members perform different cellular activities in a cell type-specific way [42].

Mx and TNFα were induced upon transfection of IRF5 in rock bream heart cells [18]. In this study, ccTNFα, ccISG15 and ccPKR transcripts in common carp PBLs were significantly up-regulated upon the two stimuli (Fig. 8). Intriguingly, following LPS stimulation, ccISG15 and ccPKR expression reached the highest level at 24 hpi, which was later than the stimulation by poly I:C. And the fold change of the three genes induced by poly I:C (4.1- to 29.1-fold) was stronger than that induced by LPS (1.8- to 3.2-fold). This phenomenon may be due to that IRF5 mediates immune response in a pathogen-specific way. In accordance with our study, expression of IRF5 in half-smooth tongue sole was significantly increased post bacterial infection in vivo [19]. Therefore, these results are signifying ccIRF5 may be not only play an the important role in regulating the antiviral immune response, as reported for mammalian IRF5, but also can respond to bacterial challenge [12, 43].

Conclusions

In summary, we report the cloning and characterization of an IRF5 gene from common carp at transcriptional and genomic DNA levels. Furthermore, we describe tissue distribution and in vivo and in vitro induction of ccIRF5, ccTNFα and ccISGs upon stimulation with poly I:C and LPS. Our findings suggest that IRF5 might play an important role in regulating the antiviral and antibacterial response in fish, and these results could provide a clue for preventing common carp infection by pathogenic microorganisms present in the aquatic environment.

Abbreviations

ANOVA, analysis of variance; cc, common carp; DBD, DNA binding domain; HKLs, leukocytes from head kidney; hpi, hours post-injection; IAD, interferon regulatory factor-associated domain; ICSAT, interferon consensus sequence-binding protein in adult T-cell leukemia cell line or activated T cells; ICSBP, interferon consensus sequence binding protein; IFN, interferon; IL, interleukin; IRF, interferon regulatory factor; IRF-E, interferon regulatory factor binding element; IRSE, interferon stimulated response element; ISG, interferon stimulated gene; ISGF3γ, interferon stimulated gene factor 3 gamma; LPS, lipopolysaccharides; LSIRF, lymphoid-specific interferon regulatory factor; MR, middle region; NCBI, National Center for Biotechnology Information; NLSs, nuclear localization signals; ORF, open reading frame; PBLs, leukocytes from peripheral blood; PBS, phosphate-buffered saline; PIP, PU.1 interaction partner; PKR, protein kinase R; poly I:C, polyinosinic:polycytidylic acid; RACE, rapid amplification of the cDNA ends; RIG-I, retinoic acid-inducible gene I; SMART, simple modular architecture research tool; SVCV, spring viraemia of carp virus; TNFα, tumour-necrosis factor α; UTR, untranslated region; VAD, virus activated domain

Acknowledgements

Not applicable.

Funding

This research was supported by the Shandong Provincial Natural Foundation of China (ZR2014CZ004 and ZR2014CQ051) and the University Independent Innovation Project of Jinan (200906020).

Authors' contributions

YYZ and LGA participated in the design of the study, performed the experiments, collected and analysed data, and drafted the manuscript. CCQ cloned and sequenced the ccIRF5 gene. SJS and HL helped with the animal experiments. FMZ participated in the acquisition of preliminary data and performed the statistical analysis. GWY conceived the study and participated in its design and coordination. All authors read and approved the final manuscript.

Competing interests

The authors declare that they have no competing interests.

Consent for publication

Not applicable.

References

1. Nguyen H, Hiscott J, Pitha PM. The growing family of interferon regulatory factors. Cytokine Growth Factor Rev. 1997;8(4):293–312.
2. Harada H, Taniguchi T, Tanaka N. The role of interferon regulatory factors in the interferon system and cell growth control. Biochimie. 1998;80(8-9):641–50.
3. Barnes B, Lubyova B, Pitha PM. On the role of IRF in host defense. J Interferon Cytokine Res. 2002;22(1):59–71.
4. Mamane Y, Heylbroeck C, Genin P, Algarte M, Servant MJ, LePage C, et al. Interferon regulatory factors: the next generation. Gene. 1999;237(1):1–14.
5. Huang B, Qi ZT, Xu Z, Nie P. Global characterization of interferon regulatory factor (IRF) genes in vertebrates: glimpse of the diversification in evolution. BMC Immunol. 2010;11:22.
6. Paun A, Pitha PM. The IRF family, revisited. Biochimie. 2007;89(6-7):744–53.
7. Eroshkin A, Mushegian A. Conserved transactivation domain shared by interferon regulatory factors and Smad morphogens. J Mol Med (Berl). 1999;77(5):403–5.
8. Barnes BJ, Moore PA, Pitha PM. Virus-specific activation of a novel interferon regulatory factor, IRF-5, results in the induction of distinct interferon alpha genes. J Biol Chem. 2001;276(26):23382–90.
9. Tamura T, Yanai H, Savitsky D, Taniguchi T. The IRF family transcription factors in immunity and oncogenesis. Annu Rev Immunol. 2008;26:535–84.
10. Honda K, Taniguchi T. IRFs: master regulators of signalling by Toll-like receptors and cytosolic pattern-recognition receptors. Nat Rev Immunol. 2006;6(9):644–58.
11. Barnes BJ, Kellum MJ, Field AE, Pitha PM. Multiple regulatory domains of IRF-5 control activation, cellular localization, and induction of chemokines that mediate recruitment of T lymphocytes. Mol Cell Biol. 2002;22(16):5721–40.
12. Paun A, Reinert JT, Jiang Z, Medin C, Balkhi MY, Fitzgerald KA, et al. Functional characterization of murine interferon regulatory factor 5 (IRF-5) and its role in the innate antiviral response. J Biol Chem. 2008;283(21):14295–308.
13. Takaoka A, Yanai H, Kondo S, Duncan G, Negishi H, Mizutani T, et al. Integral role of IRF-5 in the gene induction programme activated by Toll-like receptors. Nature. 2005;434(7030):243–9.
14. Xu QQ, Chang MX, Xiao FS, Huang B, Nie P. The gene and virus-induced expression of IRF-5 in grass carp Ctenopharyngodon idella. Vet Immunol Immunopathol. 2010;134(3-4):269–78.
15. Xiang Z, Dong C, Qi L, Chen W, Huang L, Li Z, et al. Characteristics of the interferon regulatory factor pairs zfIRF5/7 and their stimulation expression by ISKNV Infection in zebrafish (Danio rerio). Dev Comp Immunol. 2010;34(12):1263–73.

16. Leong JS, Jantzen SG, von Schalburg KR, Cooper GA, Messmer AM, Liao NY, et al. Salmo salar and Esox lucius full-length cDNA sequences reveal changes in evolutionary pressures on a post-tetraploidization genome. BMC Genomics. 2010;11:279.
17. Hu GB, Lou HM, Dong XZ, Liu QM, Zhang SC. Characteristics of the interferon regulatory factor 5 (IRF5) and its expression in response to LCDV and poly I:C challenges in Japanese flounder, Paralichthys olivaceus. Dev Comp Immunol. 2012;38(2):377–82.
18. Wickramaarachchi WD, Wan Q, Lim BS, Jung HB, De Zoysa M, Park MA, et al. Genomic characterization of interferon regulatory factor 5 from rock bream (Oplegnathus fasciatus) and its role in antiviral defense. Fish Shellfish Immunol. 2014;37(2):256–67.
19. Zhang J, Li YX, Hu YH. Molecular characterization and expression analysis of eleven interferon regulatory factors in half-smooth tongue sole, Cynoglossus semilaevis. Fish Shellfish Immunol. 2015;44(1):272–82.
20. Liu S, Zhang Y, Zhou Z, Waldbieser G, Sun F, Lu J, et al. Efficient assembly and annotation of the transcriptome of catfish by RNA-Seq analysis of a doubled haploid homozygote. BMC Genomics. 2012;13:595.
21. Xiaoni G, Zhuo C, Xuzhen W, Dengqiang W, Xinwen C. Molecular cloning and characterization of interferon regulatory factor 1 (IRF-1), IRF-2 and IRF-5 in the chondrostean paddlefish Polyodon spathula and their phylogenetic importance in the Osteichthyes. Dev Comp Immunol. 2012;36(1):74–84.
22. Feng H, Liu H, Kong R, Wang L, Wang Y, Hu W, et al. Expression profiles of carp IRF-3/-7 correlate with the up-regulation of RIG-I/MAVS/TRAF3/TBK1, four pivotal molecules in RIG-I signaling pathway. Fish Shellfish Immunol. 2011;30(4-5):1159–69.
23. Fournier G, Boutier M, Stalin Raj V, Mast J, Parmentier E, Vanderwalle P, et al. Feeding Cyprinus carpio with infectious materials mediates cyprinid herpesvirus 3 entry through infection of pharyngeal periodontal mucosa. Vet Res. 2012;43:6.
24. NCBI [http://www.ncbi.nlm.nih.gov/blast].
25. SMART [http://smart.embl-heidelberg.de/].
26. Rymuszka A, Sieroslawska A. Effects of neurotoxin - anatoxin-a on common carp (Cyprinus carpio L.) innate immune cells in vitro. Neuro endocrinology letters. 2011;32 Suppl 1:84–8.
27. Engelsma MY, Stet RJ, Schipper H, Verburg-van Kemenade BM. Regulation of interleukin 1 beta RNA expression in the common carp, Cyprinus carpio L. Dev Comp Immunol. 2001;25(3):195–203.
28. Escalante CR, Yie J, Thanos D, Aggarwal AK. Structure of IRF-1 with bound DNA reveals determinants of interferon regulation. Nature. 1998; 391(6662):103–6.
29. Lin R, Mamane Y, Hiscott J. Structural and functional analysis of interferon regulatory factor 3: localization of the transactivation and autoinhibitory domains. Mol Cell Biol. 1999;19(4):2465–74.
30. Chen W, Lam SS, Srinath H, Jiang Z, Correia JJ, Schiffer CA, et al. Insights into interferon regulatory factor activation from the crystal structure of dimeric IRF5. Nat Struct Mol Biol. 2008;15(11):1213–20.
31. Yabu T, Hirose H, Hirono I, Katagiri T, Aoki T, Yamamoto E. Molecular cloning of a novel interferon regulatory factor in Japanese flounder, Paralichthys olivaceus. Mol Mar Biol Biotechnol. 1998;7(2):138–44.
32. Richardson MP, Tay BH, Goh BY, Venkatesh B, Brenner S. Molecular cloning and genomic structure of a gene encoding interferon regulatory factor in the pufferfish (Fugu rubripes). Mar Biotechnol (NY). 2001;3(2):145–51.
33. Sun B, Chang M, Chen D, Nie P. Gene structure and transcription of IRF-2 in the mandarin fish Siniperca chuatsi with the finding of alternative transcripts and microsatellite in the coding region. Immunogenetics. 2006;58(9):774–84.
34. Shi Y, Zhang YB, Zhao Z, Jiang J, Zhang QY, Gui JF. Molecular characterization and subcellular localization of Carassius auratus interferon regulatory factor-1. Dev Comp Immunol. 2008;32(2):134–46.
35. Holland JW, Karim A, Wang T, Alnabulsi A, Scott J, Collet B, et al. Molecular cloning and characterization of interferon regulatory factors 4 and 8 (IRF-4 and IRF-8) in rainbow trout, Oncorhynchus mykiss. Fish Shellfish Immunol. 2010;29(1):157–66.
36. Xia J, Hu GB, Dong XZ, Liu QM, Zhang SC. Molecular characterization and expression analysis of interferon regulatory factor 5 (IRF-5) in turbot, Scophthalmus maximus. Fish Shellfish Immunol. 2012;32(1):211–8.
37. Magnadottir B. Innate immunity of fish (overview). Fish Shellfish Immunol. 2006;20(2):137–51.
38. Hu G, Yin X, Xia J, Dong X, Zhang J, Liu Q. Molecular cloning and characterization of interferon regulatory factor 7 (IRF-7) in Japanese flounder, Paralichthys olivaceus. Fish Shellfish Immunol. 2010;29(6):963–71.
39. Hu GB, Xia J, Lou HM, Chen XL, Li J, Liu QM. An IRF-3 homolog that is up-regulated by DNA virus and poly I:C in turbot, Scophthalmus maximus. Fish Shellfish Immunol. 2011;31(6):1224–31.
40. Neumann NF, Stafford JL, Barreda D, Ainsworth AJ, Belosevic M. Antimicrobial mechanisms of fish phagocytes and their role in host defense. Dev Comp Immunol. 2001;25(8-9):807–25.
41. Li J, Barreda DR, Zhang YA, Boshra H, Gelman AE, Lapatra S, et al. B lymphocytes from early vertebrates have potent phagocytic and microbicidal abilities. Nat Immunol. 2006;7(10):1116–24.
42. Hu G, Barnes BJ. IRF-5 is a mediator of the death receptor-induced apoptotic signaling pathway. J Biol Chem. 2009;284(5):2767–77.
43. Barnes BJ, Kellum MJ, Pinder KE, Frisancho JA, Pitha PM. Interferon regulatory factor 5, a novel mediator of cell cycle arrest and cell death. Cancer Res. 2003;63(19):6424–31.

2

A 10-day vacancy period after cleaning and disinfection has no effect on the bacterial load in pig nursery units

K. Luyckx[1], S. Millet[1], S. Van Weyenberg[1], L. Herman[1], M. Heyndrickx[1,2], J. Dewulf[3] and K. De Reu[1*]

Abstract

Background: Biosecurity measures such as cleaning, disinfection and a vacancy period between production cycles on pig farms are essential to prevent disease outbreaks. No studies have tested the effect of a longer vacancy period on bacterial load in nursery units.

Methods: The present study evaluated the effect of a 10-day vacancy period in pig nursery units on total aerobic flora, *Enterococcus* spp., *Escherichia coli*, faecal coliforms and methicillin resistant *Staphylococcus aureus* (MRSA). Three vacancy periods of 10 days were monitored, each time applied in 3 units. The microbiological load was measured before disinfection and at 1, 4, 7 and 10 days after disinfection.

Results: No significant decrease or increase in *E. coli*, faecal coliforms, MRSA and *Enterococcus* spp. was noticed. Total aerobic flora counts were the lowest on day 4 after disinfection (i.e. 4.07 log CFU/625 cm^2) ($P < 0.05$), but the difference with other sampling moments was limited (i.e. 0.6 log CFU/625 cm^2) and therefore negligible. Furthermore, this observation on day 4 was not confirmed for the other microbiological parameters. After disinfection, drinking nipples were still mostly contaminated with total aerobic flora (i.e. 5.32 log CFU/625 cm^2) and *Enterococcus* spp. (i.e. 95 % of the samples were positive) ($P < 0.01$); the feeding troughs were the cleanest location (total aerobic flora: 3.53 log CFU/625 cm^2 and *Enterococcus* spp.: 50 % positive samples) ($P < 0.01$).

Conclusions: This study indicates that prolonging the vacancy period in nursery units to 10 days after disinfection with no extra biosecurity measures has no impact on the environmental load of total aerobic flora, *E. coli*, faecal coliforms, MRSA and *Enterococcus* spp..

Keywords: Nursery pigs, Between batch vacancy, Cleaning and disinfection, Bacterial load

Background

Weaned piglets are subjected to many environmental, behavioural and dietary stresses. Moreover, the intestinal gut flora is still precarious, which makes them highly susceptible to enteric diseases [1]. Disease outbreaks in animal houses can lead to animal mortality and higher condemnation rates at slaughterhouses. The resulting economic damage can be severe [2] together with preventive measures (e.g. quarantine in case of epidemics) and even destruction of farm animals [3]. In addition, foodborne zoonotic diseases are a significant and widespread global public health threat.

In nursery units, diarrhoea is one of the most important causes of economic losses in the pig industry. Post-weaning diarrhoea is multifactorial but the proliferation of pathogenic *Escherichia coli* strains throughout the intestinal tract of piglets after weaning has been shown to play a significant role [4, 5]. Another important pathogen for the pig industry is *Salmonella*. In 2011, most of the reported food-borne outbreaks (69 553 human cases) in the European Union were associated with food originating from animals. *Salmonella* was the most frequently detected causative agent (26.6 % of outbreaks) [6].

Methicillin resistant *Staphylococcus aureus* sequence type 398 (MRSA ST398) is an emerging opportunistic pathogen among farm animals, especially pigs [7–9]. Epidemiological studies have shown that they not only

* Correspondence: koen.dereu@ilvo.vlaanderen.be
[1]Institute for Agricultural and Fisheries Research (ILVO), Merelbeke, Belgium
Full list of author information is available at the end of the article

colonise pigs, but can also be transmitted to persons with direct livestock exposure. Moreover, it is indicated that MRSA ST6398 represents an increasing cause of infections in humans [10].

It is of great importance to prevent disease outbreaks through biosecurity measures rather than cure them [3]. Biosecurity includes all measures that prevent pathogens from entering a herd (external biosecurity) as well as reducing the spread of pathogens within the herd (internal biosecurity) [11]. Between production cycles, internal biosecurity measures such as cleaning, disinfection and a vacancy period are applied. Every biosecurity measure can influence the degree of infection pressure before new animals arrive.

Luyckx et al. [12] showed that a cleaning step in broiler houses caused a reduction of total aerobic flora by 2 log CFU/625 cm^2 and that a disinfection step caused a further reduction of 1.5 log CFU. In piglet nursery units, the importance of a prolonged vacancy period is unknown. The aim of the present study was to assess the evolution of the bacterial load of total aerobic flora, *Enterococcus* spp., *E. coli*, faecal coliforms and MRSA during a 10-day vacancy period in piglet nursery units. *Enterococcus* spp. and faecal coliforms are suggested to be adequate hygiene-indicator organisms for faecal contamination of surfaces. In addition, *E. coli* have been shown to be suitable index organisms for monitoring the possible presence of *Salmonella* [13–15].

Results

Before disinfection, the mean enumeration of total aerobic flora was 5.64 log CFU/625 cm^2 (Fig. 1a). The proportion of positive samples for *E. coli*, faecal coliforms and MRSA (after enrichment) and *Enterococcus* spp. was 49, 65 and 16 % (Fig. 2a) and 95 % (Fig. 3a), respectively.

On day 1 after disinfection, mean enumeration of total aerobic flora was significantly reduced to 4.44 log CFU/625 cm^2 ($P < 0.01$) (Fig. 1a). Of the 135 samples taken on day 1, 13, 23 and 7 % were positive for *E. coli*, faecal coliforms and MRSA detection, respectively (Fig. 2a). In addition, 69 % of the samples gave countable results for *Enterococcus* spp. (Fig. 3a). The proportion of positive samples for *E. coli*, faecal coliforms and *Enterococcus* spp. was significantly lower compared to the proportions found before disinfection ($P < 0.01$).

Three days later (day 4), total aerobic flora were significantly reduced to 4.07 log CFU/cm^2 ($P < 0.05$). Only 7 % of the samples were positive for *E. coli*, but the number of positive samples found for faecal coliforms and MRSA were higher (25 and 14 %, respectively). Countable results for *Enterococcus* spp. also increased to 77 %.

On day 7 after disinfection, mean enumeration of total aerobic flora was 4.24 log CFU/625 cm^2. Of all samples, 15, 29 and 13 % were positive for *E. coli*, faecal coliforms and MRSA detection, respectively and comparable to day 1, 70 % of the samples gave countable results for *Enterococcus* spp..

On day 10, total aerobic flora increased further to 4.67 log CFU/625 cm^2, which was 0.6 log CFU more than 4 days after disinfection ($P < 0.01$), but not significantly different from day 1. Proportion of positive samples for *E. coli*, faecal coliforms and MRSA were 12, 24 and 8 %, respectively. In addition, 79 % of the samples were countable for *Enterococcus* spp..

Overall, no significant differences were noticed between sampling moments after disinfection for *E. coli*, faecal coliforms, MRSA and *Enterococcus* spp..

During the entire 10-day vacancy period, the overall contamination level (total aerobic flora) was the highest

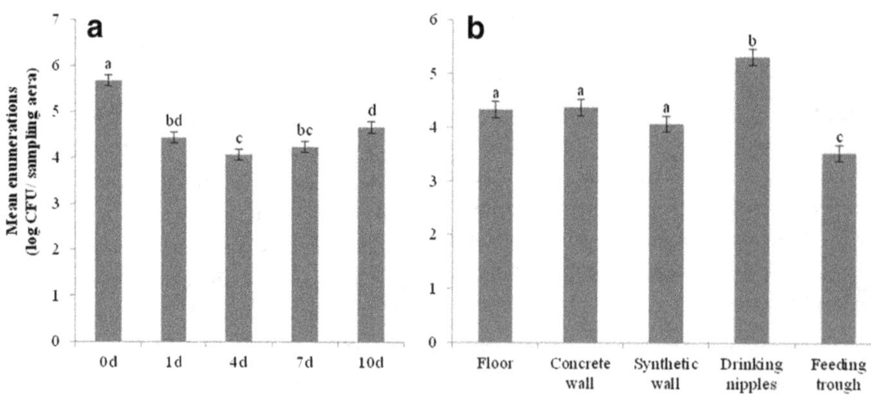

Fig. 1 Mean enumeration of total aerobic flora with standard errors. Mean enumerations are given for each sampling moment (**a**) and location after disinfection (**b**). Samples ($n = 135$) were taken before disinfection (0d) and 1 day (1d), 4 days (4d), 7 days (7d) and 10 days (10d) after disinfection. Samples ($n = 108$) were taken from each location. Significant differences between sampling moments/ locations are indicated by different letters above bars

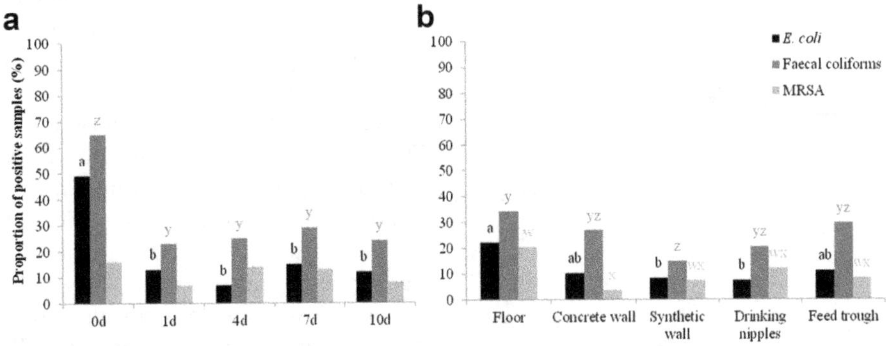

Fig. 2 Proportion of positive samples given for detection of *E. coli*, faecal coliforms and MRSA, respectively. Proportions are given for each sampling moment (**a**) and location after disinfection (**b**), in percentage. Samples ($n = 135$) were taken before disinfection (0d) and 1 day (1d), 4 days (4d), 7 days (7d) and 10 days (10d) after disinfection. Samples ($n = 108$) were taken from each location. Significant differences between sampling moments/ locations per bacteriological parameter are indicated by different letters above bars

for drinking nipples (i.e. 5.32 log CFU/625 cm^2) ($P < 0.01$) and the lowest for feeding troughs (i.e. 3.53 log CFU/ 625 cm^2) ($P < 0.01$) (Fig. 1b). Results of *Enterococcus* spp. confirmed these observations ($P < 0.01$) and also showed that the floors were still highly contaminated (i.e. still 84 % of the samples were positive) ($P < 0.01$) (Fig. 3b). Results for *E. coli*, faecal coliforms and MRSA did not indicate the most critical locations after cleaning and disinfection (C&D) (Fig. 2b).

During the vacancy period, mean temperature ranged from 15 °C to 16 °C and relative humidity (RH) from 57 to 67 % (Fig. 4). These two parameters did not have a significant effect on the different bacteriological parameters.

Discussion

Biosecurity measures, such as cleaning and disinfection (C&D) and a prolonged vacancy period of the animal houses are an essential part of the hygiene management on the farm to prevent disease outbreaks. The effect of a vacancy period of 10 days after disinfection on several bacteriological parameters was examined during this study.

Disinfection reduced the total aerobic flora by 1.2 log CFU/ sampling surface. During the following 10 day vacancy, only a small reduction was observed on day 4, though this seemed microbiological negligible (maximum difference of 0.6 log CFU/625 cm^2). One possible explanation for the observed small fluctuations and the decline of total aerobic flora on day 4 is that some bacteria can survive stressful conditions by entering a viable but nonculturable state [14]. These nonculturable bacteria were not enumerated nor detected by the methods used in this study. Another possible explanation is that residual flora could proliferate again after disinfection, due to lack of niche and nutrient competition with other bacteria. These residual bacteria could have survived the disinfection step

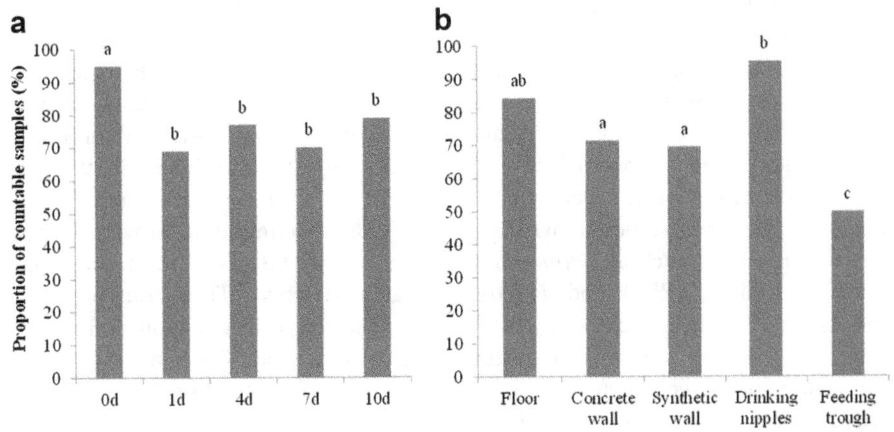

Fig. 3 Proportion of countable samples given in percentage for *Enterococcus* spp.. Proportions are given for each sampling moment (**a**) and location after disinfection (**b**). Samples ($n = 135$) were taken before disinfection (0d) and 1 day (1d), 4 days (4d), 7 days (7d) and 10 days (10d) after disinfection. Samples (n =108) were taken from each location. Significant differences between sampling moments are indicated by different letters above bars

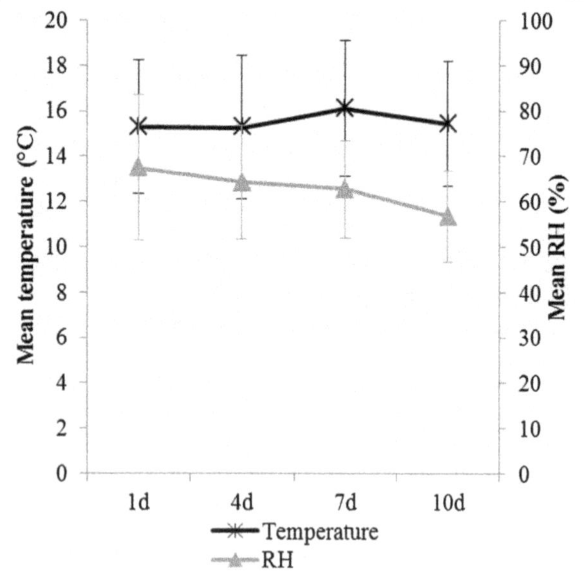

Fig. 4 Mean temperature (°C) and relative humidity (RH, %) with standard deviations given per sampling moment. Sampling moments: day 1 (1d), 4 (4d), 7 (7d), 10 (10d) after disinfection

by the presence of a resistance mechanism [16–19] or by detrimental factors present during disinfection, such as residual organic material.

Moreover, a longer vacancy period can even have a negative effect, not only financially because of a lower number of production cycles (i.e. lower income) but also bacteriologically. For example, recontamination could occur by vectors such as vermin and rodents in case of biosecurity breaches [20–22], especially when other compartments in the same building are still filled with animals or if residual organic material (e.g. faeces and feed) is present after C&D. Flies may be reservoirs and vectors of several bacteria such as *Salmonella* [20, 23, 24], *E. coli* O157:H7 [25], *Staphylococcus aureus* [26] and *Streptococcus suis* type 2 [27]. Wild rodents can also carry pathogens such as *Salmonella, Campylobacter, Yersinia* and MRSA ST398 [28–31]. As biosecurity measures are very well implemented on the pilot farm, it can be assumed that on other farms, the bacteriological load and infection pressure may even increase during vacancy.

Some bacteria can survive for long periods under various conditions in the environment, such as *Salmonella, Staphylococcus aureus* (including MRSA) and *Enterococcus* spp. [32]. The results from the present study indicate that a prolonged vacancy period without extra biosecurity measures creates no reduction in these bacteria. Extra biosecurity measures such as specific pathogen control programs and pest control during the vacancy period could therefore be beneficial.

Finally, the contamination levels of several locations were analysed during the vacancy period. Drinking nipples were still mostly contaminated with total aerobic flora and *Enterococcus* spp.. Luyckx et al. [33] showed that drinking cups are critical locations for C&D in broiler houses. Drinking water from these contaminated sources could be a possible cause for disease in animals. Therefore extra attention should be given to these locations during C&D and during the vacancy period. In addition, also disinfection of drinking lines is recommended as they can be contaminated with biofilms, including pathogenic bacteria [34]. As this study is carried out on an experimental farm, also other locations can be identified as critical locations for C&D, due to their different specific structural design or composition compared to the studied farm.

Conclusion

This study indicates that a vacancy period up to 10 days after cleaning and disinfection with no extra biosecurity measures has no beneficial effect on the bacterial load of total aerobic flora, *E. coli*, faecal coliforms, MRSA and *Enterococcus* spp. in piglet nursery units.

Methods

Sampling plan

This study was carried out in 6 identical nursery units (A1 to A3 and B1 to B3) on the experimental pig farm at the Institute for Agricultural and Fisheries Research (ILVO, Merelbeke, Belgium). Each unit consists of 8 pens of 1.8 m^2. Piglets were moved to these units immediately after weaning (4 weeks of age) and stayed there for 6 weeks. Each pen housed 6 piglets. Pen flooring was a synthetic grid, under which a board slopes towards a centrally-located slurry pit. Units A1 to A3 were monitored during 2 successive vacancy periods in February and April 2015 and units B1 to B3 during 1 vacancy period in March 2015. After pig removal, units were soaked with water. The day after, units were cleaned with hot water (80 °C), then disinfected with 1 % (v/v) MS Megades (Schippers, Bladel, The Netherlands) on the same day. The disinfection product consists of glutaraldehyde and quaternary ammonium compounds. After cleaning and disinfection, the pen remained vacant for 10 days. During this vacancy period, temperature and relative humidity (RH) were monitored hourly using thermo-hygrometers (Ilog EI-HS-D-32-L, ESCORT data logging systems). Three random pens per unit were sampled before disinfection and at 1, 4, 7 and 10 days after disinfection. Per sampling moment, 135 samples were taken, for a total of 675 samples.

Sample processing

Sponge swab samples (3 M, SSL100, St. Paul, MN, USA), pre-moistened with 10 mL Ringers solution (Oxoid, BR0052G, Basingstoke, Hampshire, England), were taken at 5 locations per pen: floor, concrete wall, synthetic wall, drinking nipples and feeding trough. Sampling of 3 pens per unit resulted in triplicates per type of location or 15 swab samples per unit at each time point. To neutralise the residual action of the disinfectants on the microbiological growth, 10 mL Dey Engley neutralising broth (Sigma Aldrich, Fluka, D3435, St-Louis, MO, USA) was used to pre-moisten the sponge swab samples that were used on day 1 after disinfection. A surface of 625 cm^2 (A4 paper format) was sampled whenever possible. Because the surface of the drinking nipples was smaller than 625 cm^2, 2 drinking nipples per pen were sampled. Samples were transported to the lab under refrigeration and were processed immediately. For all measured pathogens, selected relevant parameters and enumeration or detection techniques were based on Luyckx et al. [12]. Swab samples were first diluted with 30 mL of Buffered Peptone Water (BPW, Oxoid, CM0509) and then homogenised by placing them in a Masticator (IUL instruments, S.A., Barcelona, Spain). Prior to plating, swab samples were further diluted in dilution series in saline peptone water (Bio Trading, K110B009AA, Mijdrecht, The Netherlands) to produce countable results on the selected agar media: Plate Count Agar (Oxoid, CM0325) for total aerobic flora and Slanetz and Bartley (Oxoid, CM0377) for *Enterococcus* spp. (lower enumeration limit 30 CFU/625 cm^2). Plate Count Agar and Slanetz and Bartley plates were incubated at 30 and 37 °C during 72 and 48 h, respectively. A 10 mL BPW fraction was also transferred to a Stomacher® bag and mixed with 10 mL double concentrated Mueller Hinton Broth (Oxoid, CM0405) and 13 % (w/v) sodium chloride (Merck, 1.06404.500, Darmstadt, Germany). After overnight incubation of this solution at 37 °C, 100 µl was plated on chromID® MRSA SMART (MRSM, bioMérieux, Marcy l'Etoile, France) for the detection of MRSA. ChromID® MRSA SMART were incubated at 37 °C for 24–48 h. The remaining BPW fraction (original sample) was also incubated overnight at 37 °C for additional analyses: for detection of *E. coli* and faecal coliforms, 10 µl of the enrichment broth was plated onto Rapid *E. coli* medium (Biorad, 356–4024, Marnes-la-Coquettes, France) and incubated for 24 h at 44 °C.

Statistical analysis

The distribution of the log-transformed enumerations of total aerobic flora and *Enterococcus* spp. was analysed via graphs (Q-Q plot and histogram). The log-transformed enumerations of total aerobic flora followed a normal distribution. A linear regression model was conducted to evaluate the effect of a vacancy period and location on the log-transformed total aerobic flora enumerations (dependent variable). To assess the effect of predictor variables (vacancy period and location) on the non-normally distributed outcome variables, variables describing the enumeration and detection of the different bacteria (*Enterococcus* spp., *E.* coli, faecal coliforms and MRSA) were transformed into binary variables (absent or below the detection limit = 0, present = 1). Subsequently a logistic regression analysis was carried out. Temperature and RH were added as covariates in both models. Variable "unit" was included as a random effect in both models to correct for measurements within one unit.

Post-hoc comparison was performed with a Tukey-Kramer test. *P*-values ≤ 0.05 were considered as significant. All statistical analyses were carried out using Statistical Analysis System software (SAS®, version 9.4, SAS Institute Inc., Cary, NC, USA).

Abbreviations

0d: Day before disinfection; 10d: 10 days after disinfection; 1d: 1 day after disinfection; 4d: 4 days after disinfection; 7d: 7 days after disinfection; BPW: Buffered peptone water; C&D: Cleaning and disinfection; CFU: Colony forming units; *E. coli*: *Escherichia coli*; MRSA: Methicillin resistant *Staphylococcus aureus*; RH: Relative humidity

Acknowledgements

Many thanks go to Kristof Dierkens and Eline Dumoleijn for their practical support. We also thank Miriam Levenson for English-language editing of this manuscript.

Funding

This research is funded by the Belgian Federal Public Service for Health, Food Chain Safety and Environment (RT 11/8 Cleandesopt).

Authors' contributions

KL was involved in the sample collection, laboratory analyses, analyses, interpretation of the data and drafting the manuscript. JD, SM and KD coordinated the study. SVW evaluated the statistical analyses. KL, SM, SVW, LH, MH, JD and KD contributed to development and writing of the paper. All authors read and approved the final manuscript.

Competing interest

The authors declare that they have no competing interests.

Consent for publication

Not applicable.

Author details

[1]Institute for Agricultural and Fisheries Research (ILVO), Merelbeke, Belgium. [2]Department of Pathology, Bacteriology and Poultry Diseases, Ghent University, Faculty of Veterinary Medicine, Merelbeke, Belgium. [3]Veterinary Epidemiology Unit, Department of Reproduction, Obstetrics and Herd Health, Faculty of Veterinary Medicine, Ghent University, Merelbeke, Belgium.

References

1. Hopwood DE, Hampson DJ. Interactions between the intestinal microflora, diet and diarrhoea, and their influences on piglet health in the immediate post-weaning period. In: Pluske JR, Dividich J, Verstegen MWA, editors. Weaning the pig: concept and consequences. Wageningen: Wageningen Academic Publishers; 2003.

2. Jung A, Rautenschlein S. Comprehensive report of an Enterococcus cecorum infection in a broiler flock in Northern Germany. BMC Vet Res. 2014;10:1. Available from: http://www.biomedcentral.com/1746-6148/10/311.
3. Gelaude P, Schlepers M, Verlinden M, Laanen M, Dewulf J. Biocheck. UGent: a quantitative tool to measure biosecurity at broiler farms and the relationship with technical performances and antimicrobial use. Poult Sci. 2014;93:2740–51. [cited 2015 Mar 13]. Available from: https://biblio.ugent.be/record/5790918.
4. Hampson DJ. Postweining Escherichia coli *diarrhoea in pigs in* Escherichia coli. In: Hampson DJ, editor. Domestic animals and humans. Wallingford: CAB International; 1994.
5. Richards WPC, Fraser CM. Coliform enteritis of weaned pigs. A description of the disease and its association with haemolytic *Escherichia coli*. Cornell Vet. 1961;51:245–57.
6. European Food Safety Authority (EFSA). The European Union summary report on trens and sources of zoonoses, zoonotic agents and food-borne outbreaks in 2011. EFSA J. 2014;12:3547.
7. Vanderhaeghen W, Hermans K, Haesebrouck F, Butaye P. Methicillin-resistant *Staphylococcus aureus* (MRSA) in food production animals. Epidemiol Infect. 2010;138:606–25. 2010/02/04 ed. Available from: http://journals.cambridge.org/download.php?file=%2FHYG%2FHYG138_05%2FS0950268809991567a.pdf&code=16772c8a999fa94b13924f0d065b8fde.
8. Weese JS. Methicillin-resistant *Staphylococcus aureus* in animals. ILAR J. 2010; 51:233–44. 2010/12/07 ed. Available from: http://ilarjournal.oxfordjournals.org/content/51/3/233.full.pdf.
9. Smith TC, Pearson N. The emergence of *Staphylococcus aureus* ST398. Vector Borne Zoonotic Dis. 2011;11:327–39.
10. Köck R, Schaumburg F, Mellmann A, Köksal M, Jurke A, Becker K, et al. Livestock-associated methicillin-resistant *Staphylococcus aureus* (MRSA) as causes of human infection and colonization in Germany. PLoS One. 2013;8:e55040.
11. Sarrazin S, Cay AB, Laureyns J, Dewulf J. A survey on biosecurity and management practices in selected Belgian cattle farms. Prev Vet Med. 2014; 117:129–39. [cited 2015 Apr 28]. Available from: http://www.ncbi.nlm.nih.gov/pubmed/25156945.
12. Luyckx K, Dewulf J, Van Weyenberg S, Herman L, Zoons J, Vervaet E, et al. Comparison of sampling procedures and microbiological and non-microbiological parameters to evaluate cleaning and disinfection in broiler houses. Poult Sci. 2015;94:740–9. 2015/02/15 ed. Available from: http://ps.oxfordjournals.org/content/94/4/740.full.pdf.
13. Dewaele I, Ducatelle R, Herman L, Heyndrickx M, De Reu K. Sensitivity to disinfection of bacterial indicator organisms for monitoring the *Salmonella* Enteritidis status of layer farms after cleaning and disinfection. Poult Sci. 2011;90:1185–90.
14. Winfield MD, Groisman EA. Role of nonhost environments in the lifestyles of Salmonella and Escherichia coli. Appl Environ Microbiol. 2003;69:3687–94. Available from: http://aem.asm.org/content/67/7/3687.full.
15. Gradel KO, Jørgensen JC, Andersen JS, Corry JEL. Monitoring the efficacy of steam and formaldehyde treatment of naturally *Salmonella*-infected layer houses. J Appl Microbiol. 2004;96:613–22.
16. Russell AD. Mechanisms of bacterial resistance to antibiotics and biocides. Prog Med Chem. 1998;35:133–97. 2000/05/05 ed.
17. Mateu E, Martin M. Why is anti-microbial resistance a veterinary problem as well? J Vet Med B Infect Dis Vet Public Health. 2001;48:569–81. 2001/11/16 ed. Available from: http://onlinelibrary.wiley.com/store/10.1111/j.1439-0450.2001.00475.x/asset/j.1439-0450.2001.00475.x.pdf?v=1&t=i8u4961r&s=2d0e01a74bfb566ed1ff925d23959c110a903188.
18. Soumet C, Fourreau E, Legrandois P, Maris P. Resistance to phenicol compounds following adaptation to quaternary ammonium compounds in *Escherichia coli*. Vet Microbiol. 2012;14:147–52.
19. Callens BF, Haesebrouck F, Maes D, Butaye P, Dewulf J, Boyen F. Clinical resistance and decreased susceptibility in *Streptococcus suis* isolates from clinically healthy fattening pigs. Microb Drug Resist. 2013;19:146–51. [cited 2015 Jun 10]. Available from: http://www.ncbi.nlm.nih.gov/pubmed/23249177.
20. Dewaele I, Van Meirhaeghe H, Rasschaert G, Vanrobaeys M, De Graef E, Herman L, et al. Persistent *Salmonella* Enteritidis environmental contamination on layer farms in the context of an implemented national control program with obligatory vaccination. Poult Sci. 2012;91:282–91.
21. Hald B, Skovgård H, Bang DD, Pedersen K, Dybdahl J, Jespersen JB, et al. Flies and *Campylobacter* infection of broiler flocks. Emerg Infect Dis. 2004;10: 1490–2. [cited 2015 Apr 29]. Available from: http://www.pubmedcentral.nih.gov/articlerender.fcgi?artid=3320412&tool=pmcentrez&rendertype=abstract.
22. Meerburg BG, Vermeer HM, Kijlstra A. Controlling risks of pathogen transmission by flies on organic pig farms: a review. Outlook Agric. 2007;36: 193–7. IP Publishing Ltd; 2007 [cited 2015 Apr 29]. Available from: http://www.ingentaconnect.com/content/ip/ooa/2007/00000036/00000003/art00006.
23. Holt PS, Geden CJ, Moore RW, Gast RK. Isolation of *Salmonella enterica* serovar Enteritidis from houseflies (Musca domestica) found in rooms containing *Salmonella* serovar Enteritidis-challenged hens. Appl Environ Microbiol. 2007;73:6030–5. [cited 2015 Apr 29];73:6030–5. Available from: http://www.pubmedcentral.nih.gov/articlerender.fcgi?artid=2075029&tool=pmcentrez&rendertype=abstract.
24. Olsen AR, Hammack TS. Isolation of *Salmonella* spp. from the housefly, Musca domestica L., and the dump fly, Hydrotaea aenescens (Wiedemann) (Diptera: Muscidae), at caged-layer houses. J Food Prot. 2000;63:958–60. [cited 2015 Apr 29]. Available from: http://www.ncbi.nlm.nih.gov/pubmed/10914668.
25. Szalanski AL, Owens CB, McKay T, Steelman CD. Detection of *Campylobacter* and *Escherichia coli* O157:H7 from filth flies by polymerase chain reaction. Med Vet Entomol. 2004;18:241–6. [cited 2015 Apr 24]. Available from: http://www.ncbi.nlm.nih.gov/pubmed/15347391.
26. Owens WE, Oliver SP, Gillespie BE, Ray CH, Nickerson SC. Role of horn flies (Haematobia irritans) in *Staphylococcus aureus*-induced mastitis in dairy heifers. Am J Vet Res. 1998;59:1122–4. [cited 2015 Apr 29]. Available from: http://europepmc.org/abstract/med/9736388.
27. Marois C, Le Devendec L, Gottschalk M, Kobisch M. Detection and molecular typing of *Streptococcus suis*in tonsils from live pigs in France. Can J Vet Res. 2007;71:14–22. [cited 2015 Oct 2]. Available from: /pmc/articles/PMC1635993/?report=abstract.
28. Backhans A, Fellström C. Rodents on pig and chicken farms - a potential threat to human and animal health. Infect Ecol Epidemiol. 2012 [cited 2015 Apr 29];2. Available from: http://www.pubmedcentral.nih.gov/articlerender.fcgi?artid=3426328&tool=pmcentrez&rendertype=abstract
29. Pletinckx LJ, Dewulf J, De Bleecker Y, Rasschaert G, Goddeeris BM, De Man I. Effect of a disinfection strategy on the methicillin-resistant *Staphylococcus aureus* CC398 prevalence of sows, their piglets and the barn environment. J Appl Microbiol. 2013;114:1634–41. 2013/04/05 ed. Available from: http://onlinelibrary.wiley.com/store/10.1111/jam.12201/asset/jam12201.pdf?v=1&t=i8u49xuk&s=d66db3229e37a9c36dabf54f1cdf3da2d7b397e8.
30. van de Giessen AW, van Santen-Verheuvel MG, Hengeveld PD, Bosch T, Broens EM, Reusken CBEM. Occurrence of methicillin-resistant *Staphylococcus aureus* in rats living on pig farms. Prev Vet Med. 2009;91: 270–3. [cited 2015 May 8]. Available from: http://www.ncbi.nlm.nih.gov/pubmed/19523703.
31. Dewaele I, Rasschaert G, Wildemauwe C, Van Meirhaeghe H, Vanrobaeys M, De Graef E, et al. Polyphasic characterization of *Salmonella* Enteritidis isolates on persistently contaminated layer farms during the implementation of a national control program with obligatory vaccination: a longitudinal study. Poult Sci. 2012;91:2727–35. [cited 2015 Dec 1]. Available from: http://www.ncbi.nlm.nih.gov/pubmed/23091125.
32. Kramer A, Schwebke I, Kampf G. How long do nosocomial pathogens persist on inanimate surfaces? A systematic review. BMC Infect Dis. 2006;6: 130. [cited 2015 May 7]. Available from: http://www.biomedcentral.com/1471-2334/6/130.
33. Luyckx K, VanWeyenberg S, Dewulf J, Herman L, Zoons J, Vervaet E, et al. On-farm comparisons of different cleaning protocols in broiler houses. Poult Sci. 2015;94:1986–93.
34. Gannon V, Grace D, Atwill ER. Zoonotic waterborne pathogens in livestock and their excreta-interventions. In: Dufour A, Bartram J, Bos R, Gannon V, editors. Animal waste, water quality and human health. London: IWA Publishing; 2012.

3

Sero-prevalence of specific *Leptospira* serovars in fattening pigs from 5 provinces in Vietnam

Hu Suk Lee[1*], Nguyen Viet Khong[2], Huyen Nguyen Xuan[2], Vuong Bui Nghia[2], Hung Nguyen-Viet[1] and Delia Grace[3]

Abstract

Background: Leptospirosis is a zoonotic bacterial disease with a worldwide distribution. In Vietnam, leptospirosis is considered endemic. In pigs, leptospirosis can result in reproductive problems (such as abortion and infertility) which lead to economic loss. In addition, transmission to people presents a public health risk. In Vietnam, few national studies have been conducted on sero-prevalence of leptospirosis in pigs. The main objective of this study was to evaluate the sero-prevalence and incidence of presumptive infective *leptospira* serovars in fattening pigs from 5 provinces in Vietnam.

Results: Blood samples from fattening pigs were randomly collected at slaughterhouses. We collected 1959 sera samples from 5 provinces (Son La, Hanoi, Nghe An, Dak Lak and An Giang) between January and early June 2016. The microscopic agglutination test (MAT) was used to identify the serogroups/serovars. Overall, the sero-prevalence was 8.17% (95% CI: 6.99–9.47) and serovar Tarassovi Mitis (2.19%) had the highest prevalence followed by Australis (1. 94%), Javanica (1.68%) and Autumnalis (1.17%) using a cutoff (≥ 1:100). The sero-prevalence among female pigs (5.28%, 95% CI: 3.94–6.93) was slightly higher than among male pigs (4.88%, 95% CI: 3.51–6.58), but this difference was not statistically significant.

Conclusions: Leptospirosis in pigs may be a useful indicator of the human/animal burden in Vietnam and a risk assessment tool. The presence of some of the identified serovars suggests that wildlife may play an important role in the transmission of leptospirosis to domesticated pigs in Vietnam. Therefore, strengthened monitoring and surveillance systems are needed to better understand the epidemiology of the disease and prevent or reduce infection in humans and animals.

Keywords: Leptospirosis, Vietnam, Pig, Serovar, Microscopic agglutination test (MAT)

Background

Leptospirosis is a zoonotic bacterial disease with a worldwide distribution [1–4]. It is caused by more than 250 pathogenic serovars of the genus *Leptospira* [5]. More than 150 mammals can be infected with *Leptospira* spp. Reservoir hosts include rodents, wild animals and domestic animals (such as cattle, pigs and dogs) [6–10]. *Leptospira interrogans* serovar Bratislava has been associated with reproductive problems in pigs (such as abortion, infertility and birth of weak piglets), which lead to economic loss [11, 12]. In addition, pigs are considered to be reservoir hosts for serovars Muenchen, Pomona and Tarassovi Mitis and can also be infected with Icterohaemorrhagiae from rats, Canicola from dogs and Hardjo from cattle [13–19].

In Vietnam, leptospirosis was first identified in 1930, and the country is considered endemic with a peak during the rainy season [5, 20–22]. In 2012, a total of 241 rats were collected in the Mekong delta in Vietnam and of those, 18.3% tested positive for *Leptospira* serovars [19]. The identified serovars with the highest prevalence were *Rattus norvegicus* (33.0%), *Bandicota indica* (26.5%) and *Rattus tanezumi* (24.6%). It is assumed that rats are important reservoirs of the disease. In 2002, a study conducted in the Mekong Delta found that the seroprevalence

* Correspondence: H.S.Lee@cgiar.org
[1]International Livestock Research Institute, Regional Office for East and Southeast Asia, Room 301-302, B1 Building, Van Phuc Diplomatic Compound, 298 Kim Ma Street, Ba Dinh District, Hanoi, Vietnam
Full list of author information is available at the end of the article

in sows was 73% using a cut-off of 1:100. The serovar with the highest prevalence was Braitsalva (52%). Although leptospirosis is a notifiable disease in humans in Vietnam, only a few cases have been reported to the centralized system. However, previous studies show that leptospirosis is a public health concern and is often responsible for 20% of acute fevers of unknown origin [22–25]. A study conducted among healthy people in the Mekong Delta identified the following positive serovars: Bataviae (21.7%), Panama (15.2%), Icterohaemorrhagiae (13.7%) and Australis (8.7%) [24].

To our knowledge, few studies have been conducted to evaluate the sero-prevalence of leptospirosis in pigs in Vietnam. Therefore, the main objective of this study was to evaluate the sero-prevalence and incidence of presumptive infective *Leptospira* serovars in fattening pigs from 5 provinces in Vietnam.

Methods

Blood samples from fattening pigs (6–9 months old and weighing 60–120 kg) were randomly collected from the jugular vein at slaughterhouses from 5 provinces (Son La, Hanoi, Nghe An, Dak Lak and An Giang) between January and early June 2016. The selected provinces were representative of the different ecological and climatic zones in Vietnam. To evaluate the sero-prevalence of serovars in each province, the research team confirmed that all pigs sampled were raised in the respective province and not imported from other provinces.

All blood samples were immediately placed in cool boxes at slaughterhouses. Sera were extracted after centrifugation and stored at −20 °C at local laboratories until they were transported to the National Institute of Veterinary Research (NIVR) in Hanoi for analysis. The sample size was calculated based on 50% prevalence, a precision level of 5 and 95% confidence interval using STATA. This indicated at least 385 samples per province were to be collected using multi-stage sampling [province (5), district (25), commune (125)]. For each province, a total of 25 communes (5 communes per district) were selected from 5 districts, based on the availability of pig slaughterhouses. Within each commune, 15–16 samples were randomly collected from more than one slaughterhouse. However, we were not able to achieve the sample size in some communes due to lack of time and resources. Additional information (date of collection, sampling area and sex) was collected using a check-list.

The microscopic agglutination test (MAT) was used to identify the serogroups/serovars using two-fold serial dilutions of serum in testing, starting with 1:100 up to 1:800. Each serovar result was recorded as the highest dilution of the serum which showed at least 50% agglutination of live leptospires compared to the control sample. Positive tests were defined as MAT results ≥1:100 for at least one of the 15 serovars (Table 1). A logistic regression model was constructed with the cluster effect (by having commune as a random effect) to evaluate the association between the sex and positivity when controlling for age (6–9 months old). The logistic regression model was assessed for goodness-of-fit using the Hosmer-Lemeshow test [26]. The results were expressed as Odds ratio (OR) and 95% confidence interval (CI). An alpha level of <0.05

Table 1 List of *Leptospira* antigens used in the MAT

No.	Genomospecies	Serogroup	Serovar	Strain
1	*L. interrogans*	Australis	Australis	Ballico
2	L. interrogans	Autumnalis	Autumnaliss	Akiyami A
3	L. interrogans	Bataviae	Bataviae	Van Tienen
4	L. interrogans	Canicola	Canicola	Hond Utrech IV
5	L. kirschneri	Grippotyphosa	Grippotyphosa	Moskva V
6	L. interrogans	Hebdomadis	Hebdomadis	Hebdomadis
7	L. interrogans	Icterohaemorrhagiae	Icterohaemorrhagiae	Verdun
8	L. borgpetersenii	Javanica	Javanica	Veldrat Batavia 46
9	L. noguchii	Panama	Panama	CZ214K
10	L. interrogans	Pomona	Pomona	Pomona
11	L. interrogans	Pyrogenes	Pyrogenes	Salinem
12	L. borgpetersenii	Sejroe	Hardjo	Hardjo Bovis
13	L. borgpetersenii	Sejroe	Saxkoebing	Mus 24
14	*L. biflexa*	Semaranga	Patoc	Patoc I
15	L. borgpetersenii	Tarassovi	Tarassovi	Mitis Johnson

Reference: http://www.kit.nl/biomedical-research/product-category/leptospira-strains/

was set for statistical significance. All data were recorded in Microsoft Excel 2010 and analyzed using STATA (version 14.0, StataCorp, College Station, TX, USA). ArcGIS version 10.3.1 (ESRI, Redlands, CA, USA) was used to generate the map (Fig. 1).

Results

We collected 1959 sera samples from 5 provinces. However, seven samples from Nghe An and three samples from Son La showed hemolysis and, were discarded from the study. We detected reactions against nine different serovars. Overall, the sero-prevalence was 8.17% (95% CI: 6.99–9.47). Yen Chau district in Son La province had the highest sero-prevalence. Hanoi province (9.49%) had the highest sero-prevalence whereas Dak Lak province (7.01%) had the lowest sero-prevalence, but the differences were not statistically significant (Table 2). The most frequently detected presumptive infective serogroup was Tarassovi Mitis (2.19%), followed by Australis (1.94%), Javanica (1.68%), Autumnalis (1.17%) and Grippotyphosa (1.07%) using a cutoff titer of ≥1:100 (Table 3). Considering province and serovars Autumnalis, Australis, Grippotyphosa, Javanica and Australis had the highest sero-prevalences in Hanoi, Son La, Nghe An, Dak Lak and An Giang, respectively (Fig. 2). By using a low cutoff titer (≥ 1:100), the percentage of positive MAT results for Leptospira serovars was highest for Tarassovi Mitis (2.20%) and Australis (1.94%) (Table 3). A total of 6 samples were positive for two or more serovars: one sample with three serovars (Australis, Grippotyphosa and Javanica) and five samples with two serovars.

The sero-prevalence among female pigs (5.28%, 95% CI: 3.94–6.93) was slightly higher than among male pigs (4.88%, 95% CI: 3.51–6.58). The logistic regression model showed that there was no statistically significant difference between male and female (Table 4). The Hosmer-Lemeshow goodness of fit test showed that there was evidence of poor fit.

Among positive serovars using a different cutoff [1:100 (no. 167), 1:200 (no. 57), 1:400 (no. 21) and 1:800 (no. 13)], the proportion of serovars Australis (except for 1:800 titer), Grippotyphosa and Icterohaemorrhagiae increased as the cutoff titer increased, whereas it decreased for Autumnalis, Javanica and Tarassovi (Fig. 3).

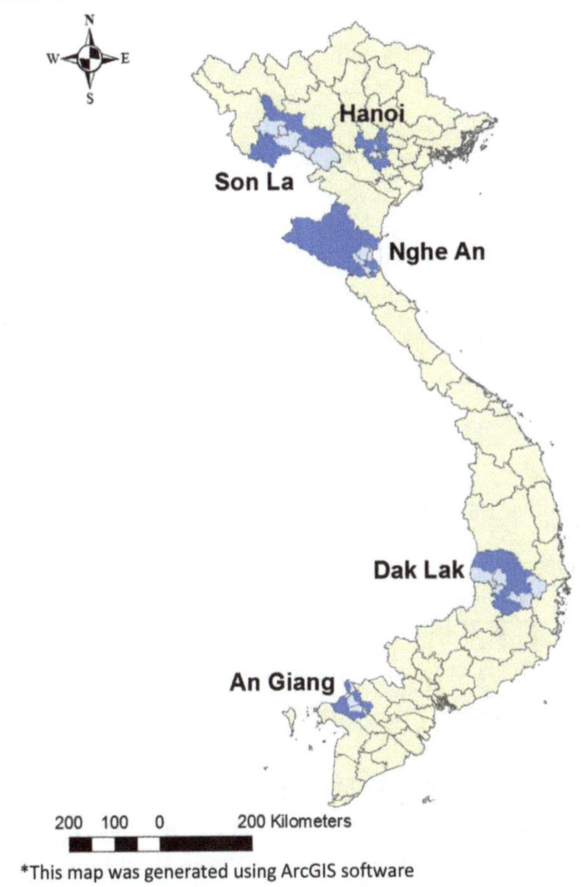

Fig. 1 Selected sampling districts (*light blue*) within each province (*dark blue*). *This map was generated using ArcGIS software

Discussion

This large, national study was conducted to assess the sero-prevalence of specific *Leptospira* serovars in pigs across the country. Overall, the sero-prevalence was lower than reported in previous studies (ranging from 13 to 79%) [27–30]. This may be because our samples were collected during the dry and early wet seasons when sero-prevalence is likely to be lower than in the rainy season [31]. Also, most of the previous studies were conducted in the Mekong delta in southern Vietnam that is relatively close to river areas, which might provide more opportunities to come into contact with contaminated water. In addition, samples were collected from slaughterhouses and so represent relatively young animals (pigs age: 6–9 months). One study suggested that older pigs were more likely to be exposed to *Leptospira* [28]. Moreover, animals sent for slaughter may be less likely to be visibly ill. We found that Tarassovi Mitis, Australis, Javanica, Autumnalis and Grippotyphosa had relatively high positive rates which were similar to those reported by the previous studies [27, 28]. Pigs are considered a reservoir for serovar Tarassovi Mitis which had the highest positive rate in our study, but one study showed that Pomona had the highest rate [32]. Another study found that Bratislava had the highest sero-prevalence among sows in the Mekong Delta of Vietnam, but it was not included in our analysis [28]. Serovars Australis, Grippotyphosa, Tarassovi Mitis were

Table 2 Sero-prevalence (%) with 95% CI for *Leptospira* serovars in fattening pigs in Vietnam using MAT

Province (no.)	District (no.)	Sero-positive samples (a titer ≥ 1:100 for any serovars)	Sero-positive (%) with 95% CI (each district)	Sero-positive (%) with 95% CI (each province)
Hanoi (390)	Chuong My (57)	4	7.01 (1.94–17.00)	9.49 (6.77–12.84)
	Hoai Duc (56)	9	16.07 (7.62–28.33)	
	Thanh Oai (106)	7	6.60 (2.70–13.13)	
	Thanh Tri (90)	6	6.67 (2.49–13.95)	
	Dan Phuong (81)	11	13.58 (6.98–23.00)	
Son La (384)	Mai Son (77)	4	5.19 (1.43–12.77)	7.03 (4.68–10.07)
	Moc Chau (77)	1	1.30 (0.03–7.02)	
	Son La (76)	2	2.63 (0.332–9.18)	
	Thuan Chau (76)	2	2.63 (0.332–9.18)	
	Yen Chau (77)	18	23.38 (14.48–34.41)	
Nghe An (380)	Dien Chau (73)	7	9.59 (3.94–18.76)	8.68 (6.05–11.98)
	Nam Dan (68)	8	11.76 (5.22–21.87)	
	TP. Vinh (95)	8	8.42 (3.71–15.92)	
	Yen Thanh (67)	3	4.48 (0.93–12.53)	
	Do Luong (77)	7	9.09 (3.73–17.84)	
Dak Lak (385)	Buon Don (81)	5	6.17 (2.03–13.82)	7.01 (4.67–10.04)
	Cu Mgar (77)	3	3.90 (0.81–10.97)	
	Krong Bong (67)	4	5.97 (1.65–14.59)	
	M'Drak (79)	11	13.92 (7.16–23.55)	
	Buon Me Thuot (81)	4	4.94 (1.36–12.16)	
An Giang (384)	Chau Phu (80)	9	11.25 (5.28–20.28)	9.38 (6.65–12.74)
	Chau Thanh (85)	8	9.41 (4.15–17.71)	
	Chau Doc (84)	3	3.57 (0.74–10.08)	
	Long Xuyen (83)	8	9.64 (4.25–18.11)	
	Tan Chau (88)	8	9.09 (4.01–17.13)	
Total	1959	160	8.17 (6.99–9.47)	8.17 (6.99–9.47)

Table 3 MAT results for *Leptospira* serovars in pigs by using 4 cutoff titers during the study period

Sero-positive results Serovar	Total tested samples (n)	≥ 1:100		≥ 1:200		≥ 1:400		≥ 1:800	
		n	% (95% CI)	*n*	% (95% CI)	*n*	% (95% CI)	*n*	% (95% CI)
Tarassovi Mitis	1959	43	2.20 (1.55–2.84)	11	0.56 (0.23–0.89)	3	0.15 (0–0.33)	1	0.05 (0–0.15)
Australis	1959	38	1.94 (1.37–2.65)	16	0.82 (0.42–1.22)	7	0.36 (0.09–0.62)	4	0.20 (0.001–0.40)
Javanica	1959	33	1.68 (1.11–2.25)	8	0.41 (0.13–0.69)	3	0.15 (0–0.33)	1	0.05 (0–0.15)
Autumnalis	1959	23	1.17 (0.75–1.76)	7	0.36 (0.09–0.62)	2	0.10 (0–0.24)	1	0.05 (0–0.15)
Grippotyphosa	1959	21	1.07 (0.62–1.53)	9	0.46 (0.16–0.76)	4	0.20 (0.001–0.40)	4	0.20 (0.001–0.40)
Canicola	1959	2	0.10 (0–0.24)	1	0.05 (0–0.15)	0	Null	0	Null
Hebdomadis	1959	2	0.10 (0–0.24)	1	0.05 (0–0.15)	0	Null	0	Null
Icterohaemorrhagiae	1959	2	0.10 (0–0.24)	2	0.10 (0–0.24)	2	0.10 (0–0.24)	1	0.05 (0–0.15)
Hardjo	1959	1	0.05 (0–0.15)	1	0.05 (0–0.15)	0	Null	0	Null

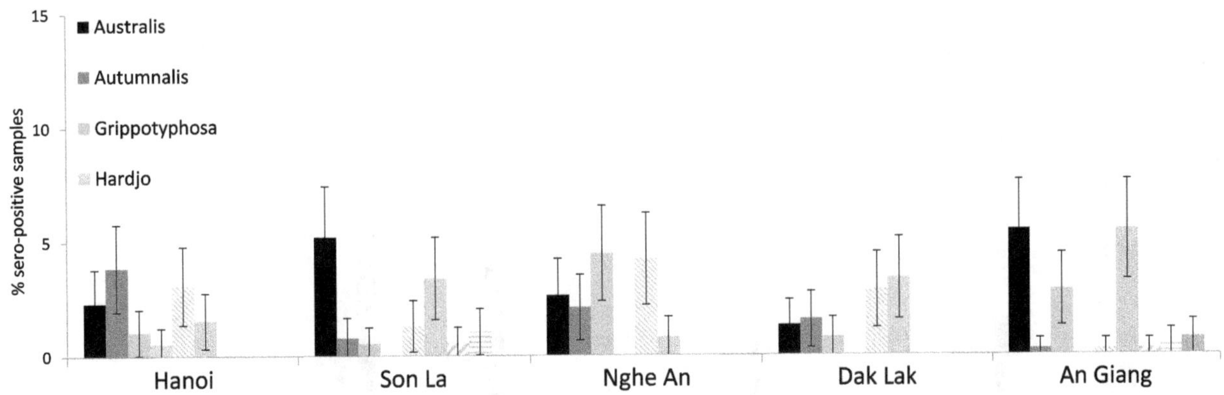

Fig. 2 Percentage with 95% confidence interval of sero-positive samples by serovar in each province using cutoff titer ≥1:100

detected in our study, and other studies also found these serovars in wild boars [33–35]. In France, a re-emergence of brucellosis in outdoor pigs was linked to contact with wild boars [36]. It is possible that wild boars may play an important role in the transmission of leptospirosis to domesticated pigs in Vietnam. In addition, we detected serovars Javanica and Icterohaemorrhagiae, implying that rats may have infected pigs [19]. Other studies found that increased movement of wild animals during fall and early winter, associated with seeking shelter and food for the winter season, increases contact with domestic animals or organisms shed by wild animals [35, 37]. Further investigations are required to better understand the role of wildlife in transmission of leptospirosis in Vietnam.

Leptospirosis in humans is a notifiable disease in Vietnam (one of 28 notifiable diseases) that should be reported to the preventive medicine networks. However, due to lack of medical facilities and public awareness, few human cases have been reported in Vietnam. Only 48 cases were officially reported between 2008 and 2013 (annual incidence rate: 0.011 per 100,000). Surveys typically find higher levels; one study conducted in Tien Giang (Mekong Delta region) found a sero-prevalence of 18.8% among 1400 and the most prevalent serovars were Bataviae, Panama, Icterohaemorrhagiae and Australis [24]. A serological study conducted among children in southern Vietnam in 2003 reported a sero-prevalence of 12.8% [25].

Leptospirosis is considered an occupational risk for agriculture workers, mining workers, sewer maintenance workers, veterinarians and other individuals who are likely to come into contact with contaminated water or soil and infected animals [4].

Serovars Autumnalis, Australis, Grippotyphosa and Javanica have been recognized as major causes of human leptospirosis in Asian countries, and were detected in our study. It is possible that the disease could be transmitted from pigs to humans [20, 38, 39]. In Vietnam, small-scale pig production accounts for 80% of the total production, providing opportunities for transmission from pigs to farmers and their families [40]. In the United States of America, an epidemiological study showed that swine producers and slaughterhouse workers had relatively higher sero-prevalence of leptospirosis in comparison with other occupational groups [41]. In Mexico, keeping domestic livestock (cattle and pigs) significantly increased the odds of disease in a rural community [42]. Therefore, swine sero-prevalence may be useful as a surrogate marker of the human/animal leptospirosis incidence in Vietnam. Additional studies could evaluate the sero-prevalence in agricultural farmers and butchers as well as identifying the modes of transmission and potential risk factors through surveys of farm workers.

In particular, potential environmental risk factors (such as climate factors, rural or urban status and proximity to lakes and rivers) should be evaluated. Previous studies showed a seasonal pattern and a positive association with the amount of rainfall [31, 36, 43]. In Vietnam, there are two distinct seasons: dry (from January to May) and wet (from June to December). It could be possible that outbreaks of leptospirosis are more likely to occur during the wet season in Vietnam. Therefore, strengthened monitoring and surveillance systems are needed to better understand the epidemiology of leptospirosis and prevent or reduce infection in humans and animals.

Table 4 Logistic regression model of leptospirosis with random effect (positive was considered if cutoff titer ≥1:100)

Variable	Category	Adjusted Odds ratio	95% CI	*P*-value
Sex	Female	Reference	N/A	N/A
	Male	1.09	0.77–1.55	0.624

CI confidence interval, *NA* not applicable as reference group

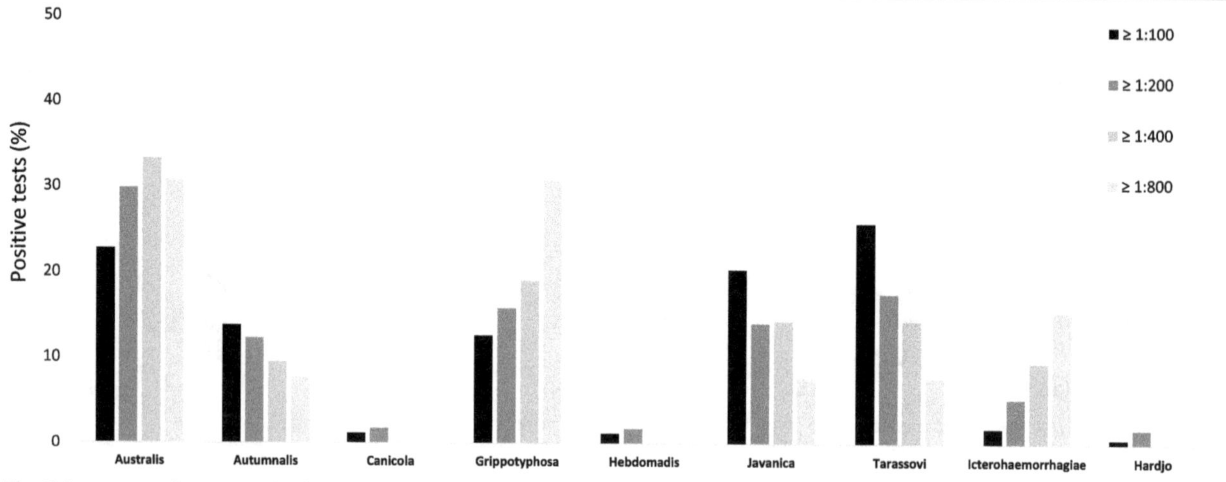

Fig. 3 Percentage of positive MATs by Leptospira serovar using 4 different cutoff titers during the study period

Conclusion

Leptospirosis in pigs may be a useful indicator of the human/animal burden in Vietnam and a risk assessment tool. These studies are a way of providing evidence to veterinarians on diagnosis, vaccination and control of zoonotic pathogens. In addition, the presence of some of the identified serovars suggests that wildlife may play an important role in the transmission of leptospirosis to domesticated pigs in Vietnam. Further investigation is needed in each region into the possible role of different wildlife species or environmental conditions in contributing to infection.

Abbreviations

CI: Confidence interval; MAT: Microscopic agglutination test; NIVR: National institute of veterinary research

Acknowledgments

We would like to thank the National Institute of Veterinary Research under the Ministry of Agriculture and Rural Development in Vietnam for supporting sample collection and analysis on leptospirosis.

Funding

We acknowledge the CGIAR Fund Council, the Australian Centre for International Agricultural Research, Irish Aid, the European Union, the International Fund for Agricultural Development, Netherlands, New Zealand, Switzerland, the United Kingdom, the United States Agency for International Development and Thailand for funding to the CGIAR Research Program on Climate Change, Agriculture and Food Security.

Authors' contributions

Conceived and designed the experiments: HSL, HNV and DG. Performed the experiments: HSL, NVK, HNX and VBN Analyzed the data: HSL, HNX and VBN. Wrote the paper: HSL, HNV and DG. All authors read and approved the final manuscript.

Competing interests

The authors declare that they have no competing interests.

Consent for publication

Not applicable.

Author details

[1]International Livestock Research Institute, Regional Office for East and Southeast Asia, Room 301-302, B1 Building, Van Phuc Diplomatic Compound, 298 Kim Ma Street, Ba Dinh District, Hanoi, Vietnam. [2]National Institute of Veterinary Research, 86 Truong Chinh, Phuong Mai, Dong Da, Hanoi, Vietnam. [3]International Livestock Research Institute, Nairobi, Kenya.

References

1. Alston JM, Broom JC, Doughty C. Leptospirosis in men and animals. Edinburgh: E&S Livingstone; 1958.
2. Faine S. *Leptospira* and leptospirosis. Boca Raton: CRC Press Inc; 1994.
3. Pappas G, Papadimitriou P, Siozopoulou V, Christou L, Akritidis N. The globalization of leptospirosis: worldwide incidence trends. Int J Infect Dis. 2008;12:351–7.
4. Bharti AR, Nally JE, Ricaldi JN, Matthias MA, Diaz MM, Lovett MA, Levett PN, Gilman RH, Willig MR, Gotuzzo E. Leptospirosis: a zoonotic disease of global importance. Lancet Infect Dis. 2003;3:757–71.
5. Levett PN, Haake DA. *Leptospira* species (leptospirosis), Mandell, Douglas and Bennett's principles and practice of infectious diseases. 7th ed. Philadelphia: Churchill-Livingstone; 2010. p. 3059–4005.
6. Hanson L. Leptospirosis in domestic animals: the public health perspective. J Am Vet Med Assoc. 1982;181:1505–9.
7. Heisey G, Nimmanitya S, Karnchanachetanee C, Tingpalapong M, Samransamruajkit S, Hansukjariya P, Elwell M, Ward G. Epidemiology and characterization of leptospirosis at an urban and provincial site in Thailand. Southeast Asian J Trop Med Public Health. 1988;19:317–22.
8. Bolin CA (1996) Diagnosis of leptospirosis: a reemerging disease of companion animals, Seminars in veterinary medicine and surgery (small animal).
9. Brown CA, Roberts AW, Miller M, Davis D, Brown SA, Bolin CA, Jarecki-Black J, Greene C, Miller-Liebl D. *Leptospira interrogans* serovar grippotyphosa infection in dogs. J Am Vet Med Assoc. 1996;209:1265–7.
10. Ayanegui-Alcerreca M, Wilson P, Mackintosh C, Collins-Emerson J, Heuer C, Midwinter A, Castillo-Alcala F. Leptospirosis in farmed deer in New Zealand: a review. N Z Vet J. 2007;55:102–8.
11. Ellis WA. Leptospirosis as a cause of reproductive failure. Vet Clin North Am Food Anim Pract. 1994;10:463–78.
12. Van Til LD, Dohoo IR. A serological survey of leptospirosis in Prince Edward Island swine herds and its association with infertility. Can J Vet Res. 1991;55: 352–5.
13. Baker TF, McEwen SA, Prescott JF, Meek AH. The prevalence of leptospirosis and its association with multifocal interstitial nephritis in swine at slaughter. Can J Vet Res. 1989;53:290–4.
14. Hathaway S, Little T. Prevalence and clinical significance of leptospiral antibodies in pigs in England. Vet Rec. 1981;108:224–8.

15. Ellis WA, Montgomery JM, Thiermann AB. Restriction endonuclease analysis as a taxonomic tool in the study of pig isolates belonging to the Australis serogroup of *Leptospira interrogans*. J Clin Microbiol. 1991;29:957–61.
16. Bolin CA, Cassells JA, Hill HT, Frantz JC, Nielsen JN. Reproductive failure associated with *Leptospira interrogans* serovar bratislava infection of swine. J Vet Diagn Investig. 1991;3:152–4.
17. Ellis W, McParland P, Bryson D, Cassells J. Prevalence of *Leptospira* infection in aborted pigs in Northern Ireland. Vet Rec. 1986;118:63–5.
18. Ryan T, Marshall R. Isolation of a leptospire belonging to serogroup tarassovi. N Z Vet J. 1976;24:212–3.
19. Loan HK, Van Cuong N, Takhampunya R, Kiet BT, Campbell J, Them LN, Bryant JE, Tippayachai B, Van Hoang N, Morand S. How important are rats as vectors of leptospirosis in the Mekong Delta of Vietnam? Vector Borne Zoonotic Dis. 2015;15:56–64.
20. Vaucel M. Le serodiagnostic de Martin et Pettit au Tonkin. Resultats de 800 sero-agglutinations. Bull Soc Patholog Exot. 1936;29:251–7.
21. Sejvar J, Tangkanakul W, Ratanasang P, Dowell SF. An outbreak of leptospirosis, Thailand-the importance of the laboratory. Southeast Asian J Trop Med Public Health. 2005;36:289–95.
22. Laras K, Cao BV, Bounlu K, Nguyen TK, Olson JG, Thongchanh S, Tran NV, Hoang KL, Punjabi N, Ha BK, Ung SA, Insisiengmay S, Watts DM, Beecham HJ, Corwin AL. The importance of leptospirosis in Southeast Asia. AmJTrop Med Hyg. 2002;67:278–86.
23. Berman SJ, Tsai CC, Holmes K, Fresh JW, Watten RH. Sporadic anicteric leptospirosis in South Vietnam: a study in 150 patients. Ann Intern Med. 1973;79:167–73.
24. Van CT, Thuy NT, San NH, Hien TT, Baranton G, Perolat P. Human leptospirosis in the Mekong delta, Viet Nam. Trans R Soc Trop Med Hyg. 1998;92:625–28.
25. Thai KT, Binh TQ, Giao PT, Phuong HL, Hungle Q, Van Nam N, Nga TT, Goris MG, de Vries PJ. Seroepidemiology of leptospirosis in southern Vietnamese children. Tropical Med Int Health. 2006;11:738–45.
26. Hosmer DW, Hosmer T, Le Cessie S, Lemeshow S. A comparison of goodness-of-fit tests for the logistic regression model. Stat Med. 1997;16:965–80.
27. Boqvist S, Montgomery JM, Hurst M, Thu HT, Engvall EO, Gunnarsson A, Magnusson U. Leptospira in slaughtered fattening pigs in southern Vietnam: presence of the bacteria in the kidneys and association with morphological findings. Vet Microbiol. 2003;93:361–8.
28. Boqvist S, Chau BL, Gunnarsson A, Olsson Engvall E, Vågsholm I, Magnusson U. Animal-and herd-level risk factors for leptospiral seropositivity among sows in the Mekong delta, Vietnam. Prev Vet Med. 2002;53:233–45.
29. Thu HTV, Hieu TC (2002) Prevalence of *Leptospira* in pigs in Tan Phu Thanh village. Research topics of livestock production.
30. Cao V, Dang-Trinh MA, Alonso S, Gilbert J, Lapar M, Khang DN, Van Hiep M (2014) *Leptospira* spp. serogroups identification in human and pig serum samples from two provinces in Vietnam. *Poster.*
31. Sethi S, Sharma N, Kakkar N, Taneja J, Chatterjee SS, Banga SS, Sharma M. Increasing trends of leptospirosis in northern India: a clinico-epidemiological study. PLoS Negl Trop Dis. 2010;4:e579.
32. Mason RJ, Fleming PJS, Smythe LD, Dohnt MF, Norris MA, Symonds ML. *Leptospira interrogans* antibodies in feral pigs from New South Wales. J Wilddi Dis. 1998;34:738–43.
33. Hartskeerl PA, Terpstra WJ. Leptospirosis in wild animals. Vet Q. 1996;18:149–50.
34. Kmety E. Leptospirosenherde in der Slowakei. Zentralbl Bakt. 1955;163:464–76.
35. Feldhamer GA, Thompson BC, Chapman JA. Wild mammals of North America: biology, management, and conservation. USA: JHU Press; 2003.
36. Kim SH, Jang JY. Correlations between climate change-related infectious diseases and meteorological factors in Korea. J Prev Med Public Health. 2010;43:436–44.
37. Bixler A, Gittleman JL. Variation in home range and use of habitat in the striped skunk (*Mephitis mephitis*). J Zool. 2000;251:525–33.
38. Seng H, Sok T, Tangkanakul W, Petkanchanapong W, Kositanont U, Sareth H, Hor B, Jiraphongsa C. Leptospirosis in Takeo Province, Kingdom of Cambodia. J Med Assoc Thail. 2007;90:546–51.
39. Victoriano AF, Smythe LD, Gloriani-Barzaga N, Cavinta LL, Kasai T, Limpakarnjanarat K, Ong BL, Gongal G, Hall J, Coulombe CA. Leptospirosis in the Asia Pacific region. BMC Infect Dis. 2009;9:147.
40. MLA Lapar, Vu TB, Ehui S 2003 Identifying barriers to entry to livestock input and output markets in South-East Asia: the case of Vietnam, ILRI (aka ILCA and ILRAD).
41. Campagnolo ER, Warwick MC, Marx HL Jr, Cowart RP, Donnell HD Jr, Bajani MD, Bragg SL, Esteban JE, Alt DP, Tappero JW, Bolin CA, Ashford DA. Analysis of the 1998 outbreak of leptospirosis in Missouri in humans exposed to infected swine. J Am Vet Med Assoc. 2000;216:676–82.
42. Leal-Castellanos CB, García-Suárez R, González-Figueroa E, Fuentes-Allen JL, Escobedo-de la Peñal J. Risk factors and the prevalence of leptospirosis infection in a rural community of Chiapas, Mexico. Epidemiol Infect. 2003; 131:1149–56.
43. Romero EC, Bernardo CC, Yasuda PH. Human leptospirosis: a twenty-nine-year serological study in São Paulo, Brazil. Rev Inst Med Trop Sao Paulo. 2003;45:245–8.

4

Prediction of marbofloxacin dosage for the pig pneumonia pathogens *Actinobacillus pleuropneumoniae* and *Pasteurella multocida* by pharmacokinetic/pharmacodynamic modelling

Lucy Dorey*, Ludovic Pelligand and Peter Lees

Abstract

Background: Bacterial pneumonia in pigs occurs widely and requires antimicrobial therapy. It is commonly caused by the pathogens *Actinobacillus pleuropneumoniae* and *Pasteurella multocida*. Marbofloxacin is an antimicrobial drug of the fluoroquinolone class, licensed for use against these organisms in the pig. In recent years there have been major developments in dosage schedule design, based on integration and modelling of pharmacokinetic (PK) and pharmacodynamic (PD) data, with the objective of optimising efficacy and minimising the emergence of resistance. From in vitro time-kill curves in pig serum, PK/PD breakpoint Area under the curve (AUC) $_{24h}$ /minimum inhibitory concentration (MIC) values were determined and used in conjunction with published PK, serum protein binding data and MIC distributions to predict dosages based on Monte Carlo simulation (MCS).

Results: For three levels of inhibition of growth, bacteriostasis and 3 and $4\log_{10}$ reductions in bacterial count, mean AUC_{24h}/MIC values were 20.9, 45.2 and 71.7 h, respectively, for *P. multocida* and 32.4, 48.7 and 55.5 h for *A. pleuropneumoniae*. Based on these breakpoint values, doses for each pathogen were predicted for several clinical scenarios: (1) bacteriostatic and bactericidal levels of kill; (2) 50 and 90% target attainment rates (TAR); and (3) single dosing and daily dosing at steady state. MCS for 90% TAR predicted single doses to achieve bacteriostatic and bactericidal actions over 48 h of 0.44 and 0.95 mg/kg (*P. multocida*) and 0.28 and 0.66 mg/kg (*A. pleuropneumoniae*). For daily doses at steady state, and 90% TAR bacteriostatic and bactericidal actions, dosages of 0.28 and 0.59 mg/kg (*P. multocida*) and 0.22 and 0.39 mg/kg (*A. pleuropneumoniae*) were required for pigs aged 12 weeks. Doses were also predicted for pigs aged 16 and 27 weeks.

Conclusions: PK/PD modelling with MCS approaches to dose determination demonstrates the possibility of tailoring clinical dose rates to a range of bacterial kill end-points.

Keywords: Marbofloxacin, Pharmacokinetic/Pharmacodynamic, *A. Pleuropneumoniae*, *P. Multocida*, Pig, Monte Carlo simulation, Time-kill curves

* Correspondence: ldorey@rvc.ac.uk
Comparative Biological Sciences, Royal Veterinary College, London University, London, UK

Background

Marbofloxacin is a synthetic third-generation fluoroquinolone, developed for sole veterinary use. It has high bioavailability when administered to pigs by intramuscular injection [1]. It accumulates in the cytosol of macrophages, leucocytes, neutrophils, epithelial lining fluid and plasma [2, 3]. Marbofloxacin, as a lipid-soluble organic acid and low to moderate plasma protein binding, achieves good tissue penetration and a high volume of distribution [4]. Concentrations in the lung, liver and kidney exceed those in plasma. However, concentrations in the biophase, the pulmonary epithelial lining fluid in pigs with pneumonia, at steady state will be determined by free drug concentration in plasma. This has been shown to be 50.6% of total concentration in pigs [4].

Lees and Aliabadi [4] reported that marbofloxacin exerts a prolonged post-antibiotic (PAE) and sub-minimum inhibitory concentration (MIC) PAE effects. It has a broad spectrum of antibacterial activity, is bactericidal and exerts a concentration-dependent killing action [5]. The antimicrobial spectrum includes Brucella spp. and Mycoplasma spp. Marbofloxacin is licensed for treatment of pneumonia caused by the pig pneumonia pathogens, *Actinobacillus pleuropneumoniae, Pasteurella multocida* and *Streptococcus suis* [6]. Bacterial pneumonia in pigs is also caused by other organisms, including *Bordetella bronchiseptica* and *Mycoplasma hyopneumoniae.*

Over the last two decades, there have been major advances in designing dosage schedules of antimicrobial drugs, based on integration and modelling of pharmacodynamic (PD) and pharmacokinetic (PK) data. These approaches have provided novel strategies for predicting drug dosages that optimise efficacy and minimise opportunities for the emergence and subsequent spread of resistance [6–15]. Optimising dosage may involve reducing doses which may be too high as well as increasing doses when they are too low.

Many authors have proposed that, for fluoroquinolones as a group, the integrated PK/PD indices correlating with successful therapeutic outcome are maximum plasma concentration (C_{max})/MIC and area under plasma concentration-time curve (AUC_{24h})/MIC ratios [5, 7, 8, 11, 16, 17].

The PD parameter most commonly used in establishing the potency of antimicrobial drugs is MIC, the lowest concentration based on two-fold dilutions, inhibiting visible bacterial growth after 24 h incubation under standard conditions (Clinical and Laboratory Standards Institute (CLSI) M31-A3) [18]. Most laboratories use the internationally recommended CLSI guidelines to ensure standardisation [13]. However, these guidelines have limitations regarding accuracy, because they involve the use of doubling dilutions, giving potential for up to 100% error on single isolate estimates. For many purposes, this is acceptable, and indeed is necessary, when large numbers of isolates are to be examined. However, it may not always be appropriate when MIC is correlated with PK data as a basis for PK/PD breakpoint determination. Therefore, based on methods previously described [19–21] five overlapping sets of two-fold dilutions were used in this study to reduce inaccuracy from up to 100% to no more than 20%. The mutant prevention concentration (MPC) was used as an additional indicator of potency to MIC; it is defined as the lowest drug concentration required for preventing the growth of the least susceptible cells present in high density bacterial populations.

A second consideration is that CLSI and European Union Committee on Antimicrobial Testing (EUCAST) methods of MIC determination require the use of broths formulated to optimize the growth of each species of bacteria. Therefore, there is almost universal use of internationally recognised guidelines, methods and standards for MIC determination. However, when the objective of potency determination is prediction of dosage for clinical efficacy, based on PK/PD breakpoints, conditions should be representative of in vivo pathological circumstances. Zeitlinger et al. [22] commented that "bacteria with appropriate and well-defined growth in the selected medium should be employed" and "in order to be able to extrapolate data from various models to in vivo situations, models should always attempt to mimic physiological conditions as closely as possible".

Whilst serum is not identical to extravascular infection site fluids, it is likely to be closer in chemical composition to the biophase than broths, and indeed in immunological constituents also [22, 23]. A comparison of broth MICs with potency determined in biological fluids is therefore relevant to PK/PD breakpoint estimation. For some drugs and pathogens, calculation of a scaling factor to bridge between broth and serum MICs may be warranted [7, 15, 23, 24]. In this investigation MICs and time-kill data were generated for marbofloxacin in pig serum. They were thus determined with reasonable accuracy and in a biological matrix.

With the objectives of: extending the therapeutic life of older antimicrobial drugs; ensuring their prudent use and; minimising the emergence of resistance, there have been many proposals to re-evaluate dose schedules that were set, in many instances, prior to the application of PK/PD breakpoints [8–11, 13–15, 19]. For example, Mouton et al. [9] have described the EUCAST approach to dosage re-evaluation. In summary, these authors have proposed that a sound approach to setting dose schedules is to link PK parameters and variables with appropriate indices of potency, applying the general equation for systemically acting drugs (Fig. 1) [19, 25, 26].

The aims of this study were: (1) to integrate published PK variables for the pig with MIC data for pig pathogens

$$DO = \frac{Cl \times Breakpoint\ Index \times Targeted\ plasma\ concentration}{F\ \%}$$

DO:	Daily dose (mg/kg per day)
Cl:	Body Clearance (per h)
Breakpoint index:	Index for required effect (AUC_{24h}/MIC) (h)
Targeted plasma concentration:	MIC_{90} (μg/mL)
F%:	Bioavailability (from 0 to 1)

Fig. 1 Formula for calculation of the daily antimicrobial drug dose based on PK and PD variables

obtained in our laboratory in order to generate values of the three PK/PD parameters, C_{max}/MIC, C_{av}/MIC and T > MIC, for *A. pleuropneumoniae* and *P. multocida*; (2) to model data from time-kill studies of *A. pleuropneumoniae* and *P. multocida*, using multiples of MIC over the range 0.25–8.0 MIC, in order to generate PK/PD breakpoint values of AUC_{24h}/MIC for three levels of bacterial kill, bacteriostasis, bactericidal and $4\log_{10}$ reduction in inoculum count; (3) to use published PK data and PK/PD breakpoints, with serum protein binding data and literature MIC distributions, in Monte Carlo simulations (MCS) to predict dose schedules required for: (a) bacteriostatic and bactericidal levels of kill; (b) for 50 and 90% Target Attainment rate (TAR); and (c) for single dosing and daily dosing at steady state.

Methods

Minimum inhibitory concentration

Twenty isolates each of *A. pleuropneumoniae* and *P. multocida* were obtained from EU cases of pig pneumonia. These were screened for ability to grow logarithmically in broths and pig serum. Of those exhibiting logarithmic growth in both matrices, MICs in broth were determined by microdilution using two-fold dilutions. From the sensitive isolates, six of each species were selected and MICs re-determined, using artificial broths (Cation Adjusted Mueller Hinton broth for *P. multocida* and Columbia broth for *A. pleuropneumoniae*) in accordance with CLSI guidelines, except that five sets of overlapping 2-fold serial dilutions of marbofloxacin were prepared, as described by Dorey et al. [27]. In addition, the guidelines were adapted to additionally use pig serum in place of broth to enable comparison of the two matrices.

PK/PD breakpoint determination

For the six isolates each of *A. pleuropneumoniae* and *P. multocida*, eight marbofloxacin concentrations, as multiples of MIC, ranging from 0.25 to 8xMIC, were used in time-kill studies over 24 h incubation periods. Determinations were made separately in serum and broth (CB for *A. pleuropneumoniae* and CAMHB for *P. multocida*), as previously described [27, 28]. Each test was repeated in triplicate for the six isolates of each species in both growth matrices. The time-kill curves established bacteriostatic, bactericidal and $4\log_{10}$ reductions in count at 24 h; based on the sigmoidal E_{max} equation (Fig. 2) the

$$E = E_0 + \frac{E_{max} \times C_e^N}{EC_{50}^N + C_e^N} X\ 100$$

E	Effect
E_0	Bacterial growth after 24 h incubation in the absence of drug (control samples), expressed as $\log_{10}$ CFU/mL subtracted from the initial inoculum expressed as $\log_{10}$ CFU/mL after 24 h
E_{max}	The maximum obtainable effect in $\log_{10}$ CFU/mL over 24 h
EC_{50}	AUC_{24h}/MIC producing 50% of maximum response (h)
C_e	AUC_{24h}/MIC (h)
N	The Hill coefficient which describes the gradient of the AUC_{24h}/MIC-effect curve

Fig. 2 The sigmoidal Emax equation used to model time-kill data by non-linear regression [27]

data were modelled to provide AUC_{24h}/MIC breakpoint values for these three levels of growth inhibition.: E = 0, bacteriostatic, that is $0\log_{10}$ reduction in CFU/mL after 24 h incubation; E = −3, bactericidal, $3\log_{10}$ reduction in CFU/mL; and E = −4, $4\log_{10}$ reduction in bacterial count.

Dose prediction

Deterministic approach

For dose prediction using the deterministic approach, mean PK values were obtained from Schneider et al. [1] and PK/PD breakpoint values were used from the present study, together with MIC_{90} values for *P. multocida* and *A. pleuropneumoniae* for marbofloxacin obtained from de Jong et al. [29] (Fig. 3).

Monte Carlo simulation

As the PK/PD index that best predicts efficacy for marbofloxacin is the ratio AUC_{24h}/MIC, the equation used to calculate dose was:

$$Dose_{(per\ day)} = \frac{Cl \times \frac{AUC_{(24h)}}{MIC_e} \times MIC_{distribution}}{f_u \times F}$$

where Cl = body clearance per h, $AUC_{(24h)}/MIC_e$ (in h) = ratio of experimentally determined area under the serum concentration-time curve over 24 h to the MIC (MIC_e) of the experimental isolates – six per species - (i.e. the PK/PD breakpoint), $MIC_{distribution}$ = distribution of MICs from epidemiological literature [29], f_u (from 0 to 1) = fraction of drug not bound to serum protein and F = bioavailability (from 0 to 1). Thus, calculation of dose depends on: (1) assessment of both PK (Cl, F, $f_{u,}$) and PD (MIC) properties; and (2) determination of an appropriate breakpoint value of the $AUC_{(24h)}/MIC$ ratio. This Equation is appropriate for determining daily dosage once steady state has been reached. However, the calculated dose when the initial drug concentration in serum is zero, is very likely to be higher than the dose determined for maintaining the steady state concentration.

Loading doses were calculated for three time periods, 0–24, 0–48 and 0–72 h [7]; the formulae for calculation of dosage for a 48 h period are presented in Fig. 4.

All dosages were computed using Monte Carlo simulation in Oracle Crystal Ball (Oracle Corporation, Redwood Shores, CA, USA), for TAR of 50 and 90%. The probabilities of distribution for the dosage estimation were run for 50,000 simulated trials. Data input comprised: 1) marbofloxacin whole body clearance scaled by bioavailability; clearance data were obtained from the equation Clearance = Dose/AUC, for pigs of three ages [27, 16 and 2 weeks]; 2) drug binding to serum protein [27]; 3) AUC_{24h}/MIC breakpoints derived from time-kill curves; and 4) MIC field distribution data [1] (Fig.3). For the MIC field distributions, values were corrected using the serum:broth MIC ratio, as the reported MIC literature values were determined in broth.

Results

Minimum inhibitory concentrations

Geometric mean MIC serum:broth ratios for *P. multocida* and *A. pleuropneumoniae* (six isolates of each species) were 1.12:1 and 0.79:1, respectively. For MPC, the ratios were 1.32:1 and 0.99:1, respectively. These did not differ significantly from unity. However, as free drug concentration in pig serum was previously shown to be 50.6% (Dorey et al. 2016b) [28] and as protein bound drug is microbiologically inactive, the corrected ratios, fraction unbound (fu) serum:broth MIC were 0.50:1 and 0.40:1, and 0.67:1 and 0.50:1 for MPC, indicating small (in microbiological terms) but significantly greater potency of marbofloxacin in serum than in broth.

PK/PD breakpoint values

For each isolate of each organism, growth inhibition curves were generated in the time-kill studies in broth and pig serum. Examples are presented in Fig. 5.

From the time-kill curves, PK/PD breakpoints were derived and are presented in Tables 1 (*P. multocida*) and 2 (*A. pleuropneumoniae*). For three levels of inhibition of growth, bacteriostasis and 3 and $4\log_{10}$ reductions in bacterial count, mean AUC_{24h}/MIC values were 20.9, 45.2 and 71.7 h, respectively, for *P. multocida* for serum. Corresponding broth values were 26.5, 41.8 and 48.9 h. For *A. pleuropneumoniae* in serum, breakpoints were

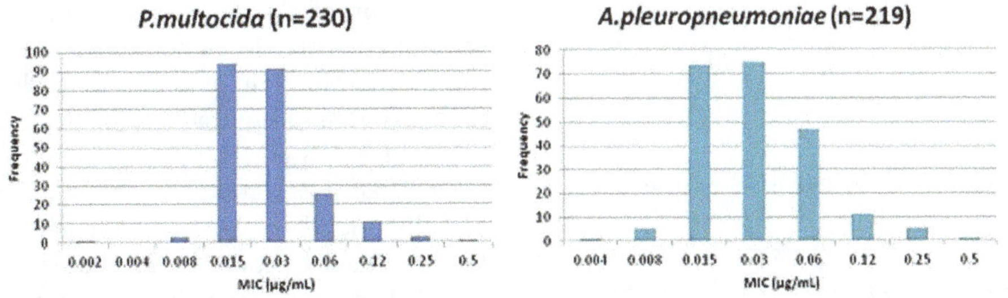

Fig. 3 Marbofloxacin MIC distributions of *P. multocida* (*n* = 230) and *A. pleuropneumoniae* (*n* = 219) indicating frequency of MICs. MIC data were generated using CLSI guidelines by de Jong et al. [29]). All isolates were from European countries

$$A. \quad Dose_{Loading\ dose\ 48h} = \frac{1}{1 - exp^{-(k_{10}\ x\ \tau)}} x\ Dose_{Maintenance\ per\ 48h}$$

$$B. \quad Dose_{Loading\ dose\ 48h} = \frac{1}{1 - exp^{-(k_{10}\ x\ 48)}} x\ Cl_{48h}\ x\ \frac{K_{PD}\ x\ MIC_{Distribution}}{F\ x\ f_u}$$

$$C. \quad Dose_{Loading\ dose\ 48h} = \frac{\left(Accumulation\ ratio\ x \frac{Cl}{F}\right) x\ 48h\ x\ K_{PD}\ x\ MIC_{Distribution}}{(f_u\ x\ F)}$$

Fig. 4 Formulae for calculation of the loading dose for 48 h duration of action, where eq. **a** can be expressed as eq. **b** and simplified as eq. **c**. K_{10} = elimination rate constant; τ = dosing interval in h; Cl_{48} = body clearance over 48 h; K_{PD} breakpoint = AUC divided by 24; $MIC_{Distribution}$ = MICs determined from epidemiological surveys; F = bioavailability (from 0 to 1); f_u = fraction of drug not bound to protein binding

32.4, 48.7 and 55.5 h. and for broth values were 24.8, 42.0 and 54.0 h. Differences between broth and serum, at each level of kill, were relatively small, despite differences between broth MICs and serum MICs corrected for drug binding to serum protein. This is not unexpected, as each inhibition curve was derived using MIC multiples for each fluid.

As a measure of inter-isolate variability, coefficients of variation were determined. These were small to moderate in magnitude (Tables 1 and 2).

Dividing the AUC_{24h}/MIC ratios by 24 yields concentrations, as MIC multiples, producing bacteriostatic, bactericidal and $4\log_{10}$ reductions in count; these are the K_{PD} values. Numerical values were, respectively, 1.10, 1.74 and 2.04 for *P. multocida* in broth and 0.87, 1.88 and 2.99 for this organism in serum. Corresponding values for *A. pleuropneumoniae* were 1.03, 1.75 and 2.25 (broth) and 1.35, 2.03 and 2.31 (serum).

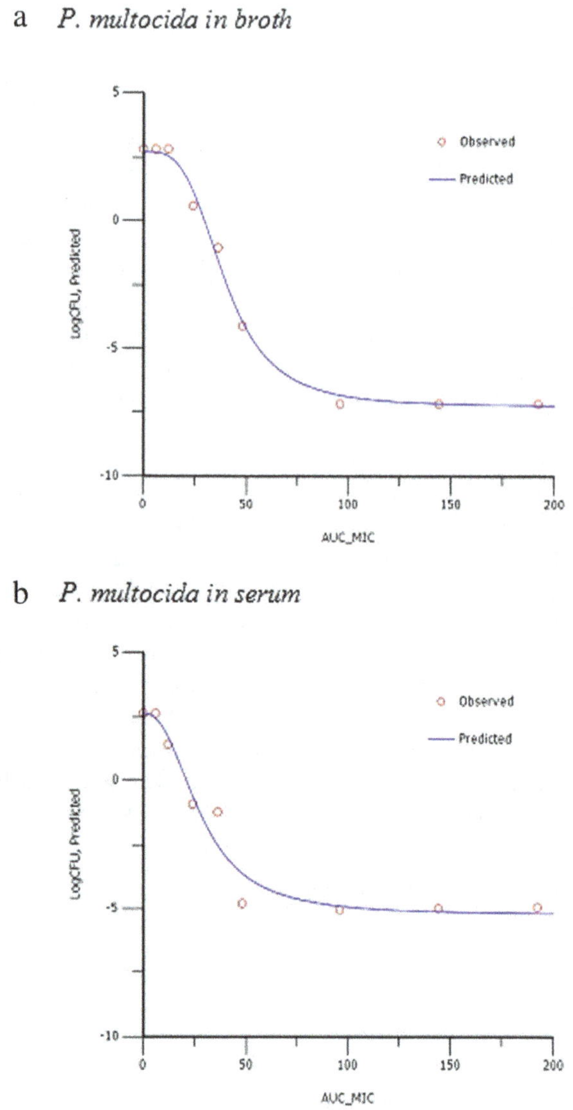

Fig. 5 Example plots of AUC_{24h}/MIC (h) versus change in bacterial count ($\log_{10}$ CFU/mL) for *P. multocida* in (**a**) broth and (**b**) serum. The points represent observed values and the curves are lines of best fit

Dose determination at steady state (deterministic approach)

Clearance and bioavailability data for healthy pigs were obtained from the literature [1]. Table 3 indicates predicted doses required, at steady state, to achieve three levels of kill. Bactericidal levels of kill were obtained with doses 0.41 mg/kg/day for *P. multocida* and 0.26 mg/kg/day for *A. pleuropneumoniae*.

Dose determination by Monte Carlo simulation

Monte Carlo simulations were conducted using: (1) the distribution of clearance around the standard deviation, assuming normal distribution (Schneider et al. 2014) [1]; (2) the distribution of MICs for wild type organisms [29]; (3) free drug fraction in serum; (4) breakpoint values of AUC_{24h}/MIC from time-kill studies.

Predicted doses at steady state for 50% and 90% TAR and three levels of kill are presented in Table 4. Doses for bactericidal action for *P. multocida* were 0.43, 0.45 and 0.59 mg/kg, respectively, for pigs aged 27, 16 and 2 weeks. Corresponding values for *A. pleuropneumoniae* were somewhat lower, 0.29, 0.30 and 0.39 mg/kg. The

Table 1 *P. multocida* PK/PD modelling of *in vitro* marbofloxacin time-kill curves (mean, standard deviation, $n = 6$)

Parameter (units)	Broth		Serum	
	Mean	SD (CV%)	Mean	SD (CV%)
Log E_0 (CFU/mL)	2.66	0.26	2.70	0.32
Log E_{max} (CFU/mL)	−7.28	0.37	−5.65	1.43
Log E_{max} - Log E_0 (CFU/mL)	−9.95	0.11	−8.35	1.11
Gamma	3.26	1.48	1.95	0.23
AUC_{24h}/MIC for bacteriostatic action (h)	26.5	4.65 (17.5)	20.9	2.31(11.1)
AUC_{24h}/MIC_{50}(h)	38.0	8.05 (21.2)	30.5	5.39 (17.7)
AUC_{24h}/MIC for bactericidal action (h)	41.8	7.79 (18.7)	45.2	5.58 (12.3)
AUC_{24h}/MIC for 4 log10 reduction (h)	48.9	10.8 (22.0)	71.7	34.0 (47.4)

E0 = difference in number of organisms (CFU/mL) in control sample in absence of drug between time 0 and 24 h; E_{max} = difference in number of organisms (CFU/mL) in presence of marbofloxacin between time 0 and 24 h; AUC_{24}/MIC_{50} = concentration producing reduction in count to 50% of the E_{max}; Gamma = slope of the curve; detection limit = 33 CFU/mL

small numerical differences with age of pigs reflect small differences in their PK profiles. Differences in predicted dose for the two bacterial species reflect the differing distributions of MIC of wild type organisms.

Table 5 indicates calculated doses for single doses of marbofloxacin administered intramuscularly with three durations of effect, three levels of kill and TARs of 50 and 90%. For a bacteriostatic action of 24 h duration and 50% TAR, predicted doses were 0.12 and 0.03 mg/kg for *P. multocida* and *A. pleuropneumoniae*, respectively. For a TAR of 90%, a bactericidal level of kill and an action over 72 h, the predicted doses were 1.31 and 0.92 mg/kg, respectively, for *P. multocida* and *A. pleuropneumoniae*. Even for a $4\log_{10}$ reduction in count and 90% TAR, predicted doses were relatively low, 2.08 mg/kg (*P. multocida*) and 1.14 mg/kg (*A. pleuropneumoniae*).

Discussion

Pharmacokinetics, pharmacodynamics and PK/PD integration

Integration of in vitro generated potency estimates with in vivo PK data has been used extensively to generate three indices to predict clinical outcome, namely the ratios, C_{max}/MIC and AUC_{24h}/MIC and T > MIC, the time for which concentration exceeds MIC. Integration of pharmacokinetic and pharmacodynamic data for MPC are presented in the Additional file 1. All MPC ratios were much lower than the MIC ratios. From previous marbofloxacin studies, C_{max}/MIC and AUC_{24h}/MIC ratios provided good correlation with bacteriological cure in human patients [30, 31]. For fluoroquinolones used in veterinary medicine, a C_{max}/MIC of 8–10 and an AUC_{24h}/MIC greater than 100–125 h have been proposed [13]. However, other studies have suggested that a ratio of AUC_{24h}/MIC of 35–50 is effective for Gram-positive bacteria [32]. Many authors have proposed achieving numerical values of AUC_{24h}/MIC of 125:1 or 250:1 for gram negative organisms, corresponding to average concentrations over the dosing interval of 5.2 to 10.4, respectively, as a multiple of MIC.

For marbofloxacin, de Jong et al. [29] reported identical MIC_{50} values for both *A. pleuropneumoniae* and *P. multocida* of European pig origin of 0.03 μg/mL and identical MIC_{90} values of 0.06 μg/mL. Schneider et al. [1] reported

Table 2 *A. pleuropneumoniae* PK/PD modelling of in vitro marbofloxacin time-kill curves (mean, standard deviation, $n = 6$)

Parameter (units)	Broth		Serum	
	Mean	SD (CV%)	Mean	SD (CV%)
Log E_0 (CFU/mL)	2.65	0.42	1.79	0.64
Log E_{max} (CFU/mL)	−5.57	0.80	−6.71	0.65
Log E_{max} - Log E_0 (CFU/mL)	−8.23	0.38	−8.50	0.01
Gamma	3.18	1.20	4.07	0.77
AUC_{24h}/MIC for bacteriostatic action (h)	24.8	1.79 (7.2)	32.4	5.30 (16.4)
AUC_{24h}/MIC_{50}(h)	31.8	4.09 (12.9)	45.6	9.45 (20.7)
AUC_{24h}/MIC for bactericidal action (h)	42.0	4.34 (10.3)	48.7	6.58 (13.5)
AUC_{24h}/MIC for 4 log10 reduction (h)	54.0	7.04 (13.0)	55.5	6.43 (11.6)

E0 = difference in number of organisms (CFU/mL) in control sample in absence of drug between time 0 and 24 h; E_{max} = difference in number of organisms (CFU/mL) in presence of marbofloxacin between time 0 and 24 h; AUC_{24}/MIC_{50} = concentration producing reduction in count to 50% of the E_{max}; Gamma = slope of the curve; detection limit = 33 CFU/mL

Table 3 Predicted once daily doses calculated by deterministic approach

Level of kill	Predicted daily doses (mg/kg)	
	P. multocida	*A. pleuropneumoniae*
Bacteriostatic	0.19	0.15
Bactericidal	0.41	0.26
$4log_{10}$ count reduction	0.65	0.32

on marbofloxacin PK in healthy pigs, aged 12, 16 and 27 weeks, administered intramuscularly at three dose rates of 4, 8 and 16 mg/kg. PK/PD integration of data from these studies is presented in a Additional file 1 to this paper. Briefly, for both bacterial species and pigs aged 27 weeks, C_{max}/MIC_{90} ratios were 56, 105 and 258, respectively, for marbofloxacin doses of 4, 8 and 16 mg/kg. Even average concentrations over the 92 h period after dosing provided $C_{average}/MIC_{90}$ ratios of 9.6, 19.7 and 39.1 for these dose rates. Therefore, a preliminary prediction of likely successful clinical outcome for doses of marbofloxacin in the range 4–16 mg/kg can be made for pig pneumonia caused by the pathogens, *A. pleuropneumoniae* and *P. multocida.*

Table 4 Predicted once daily doses of marbofloxacin at steady state in pigs of three ages (weeks): 27 (A), 16 (B) and 12 (C)[a]

	Predicted daily doses (mg/kg)	Target Attainment Rate	
		50%	90%
A.			
P. multocida	Bacteriostatic	0.08	0.19
	Bactericidal	0.18	0.43
	Virtual eradication	0.28	0.67
A. Pleuropneumoniae	Bacteriostatic	0.07	0.17
	Bactericidal	0.12	0.29
	$4log_{10}$ reduction	0.15	0.36
B.			
P. multocida	Bacteriostatic	0.09	0.21
	Bactericidal	0.20	0.45
	Virtual eradication	0.32	0.72
A. pleuropneumoniae	Bacteriostatic	0.08	0.17
	Bactericidal	0.13	0.30
	$4log_{10}$ reduction	0.17	0.37
C.			
P. multocida	Bacteriostatic	0.13	0.28
	Bactericidal	0.28	0.59
	Virtual eradication	0.45	0.94
A. pleuropneumoniae	Bacteriostatic	0.10	0.22
	Bactericidal	0.18	0.39
	$4log_{10}$ reduction	0.22	0.48

[a]Monte Carlo simulation to achieve 50 and 90% target attainment rates at steady state for three levels of bacterial kill

Table 5 Predicted doses of marbofloxacin for three durations of activity (24, 48 and 72 h)[a]

		Target Attainment Rate			
		P.multocida		*A.pleuropneumoniae*	
Dose duration	Level of bacterial kill	50%	90%	50%	90%
0-24 h	Bacteriostatic	0.12	0.29	0.03	0.07
	Bactericidal	0.27	0.64	0.05	0.12
	4 log10 reduction	0.43	1.01	0.06	0.14
0-48 h	Bacteriostatic	0.19	0.44	0.16	0.39
	Bactericidal	0.40	0.95	0.28	0.66
	4 log10 reduction	0.64	1.51	0.34	0.82
0-72 h	Bacteriostatic	0.26	0.60	0.22	0.53
	Bactericidal	0.56	1.31	0.38	0.92
	4 log10 reduction	0.88	2.08	0.47	1.14

[a]Monte Carlo Simulation to achieve 50 and 90% target attainment rates for two levels of bacterial kill and three action durations

PK/PD modelling and breakpoint determination

PK/PD integration is not a precise tool; it should be regarded as a first initial step in predicting efficacy in clinical use. It is especially useful when correlated with outcome in clinical trials. However, the next essential step is to define PK/PD breakpoints for each antimicrobial drug acting against representative isolates of each pathogenic species. PK/PD modelling describes the whole sweep of the concentration-effect relationship. Therefore, any pre-determined level of activity, ranging from bacteriostasis to virtual eradication, indicated by the breakpoint AUC_{24h}/MIC index, can be determined. Applying PK/PD breakpoints for indices such as AUC_{24h}/MIC, derived from PK/PD modelling, with MCS provides an approach to dose prediction, which takes account of animal species based PK, wild-type MIC distributions, protein binding and breakpoints for specific bacterial species. From such time-kill studies, numerical values of PK/PD breakpoints have been determined by PK/PD modelling by previous workers [7–10, 12, 13, 21, 25, 33].

In this study, breakpoint values for each level of growth inhibition, $0log_{10}$, $3log_{10}$ and $4log_{10}$ reductions in count, were broadly similar for the two growth matrices. This is not unexpected because, although MICs in broth and serum differed, the breakpoint values are based on MIC multiples. AUC_{24h}/MIC ratios were similar for broth and serum for each level of kill, being based on MIC values separately for each matrix. Moreover, inter-isolate variability in PK/PD breakpoint values was small to moderate.

Dosage prediction

PK/PD breakpoints were used with wild type MIC distributions of susceptible pathogens and literature PK data, to conduct MCS to predict doses providing a range of pre-determined levels of kill. The deterministic approach provided an estimate of once daily doses at steady state. It is based on MIC_{90} for each pathogen and average values for other variables. It provides an initial indication of likely effective dosage, but does not take account either of variability or incidence of each input variable and in this study. Predicted daily doses were less than 0.5 mg/kg for a bactericidal kill against both pathogens. Nevertheless, the deterministic approach comprises an initial indication, prior to estimation of population doses for each selected TAR. The latter is a dose encompassing a given percentile of the target population, for example, 50 or 90% and for three pre-determined levels of bacterial kill and for both a single dose and a daily dose at steady state. Monte Carlo simulations predict doses which allow for incidence within MIC distributions and encompass best, worst and all intermediate values for distributions of Cl/F and breakpoint AUC_{24h}/MIC ratios. Furthermore, basing potency estimates on serum as a growth matrix, as in this study, has greater relevance to disease conditions than MICs determined in broths. Nevertheless, it is recognised that serum, although preferred to broth for MIC determination, is similar but not identical in composition to the biophase at infection sites, for example pulmonary epithelial lining fluid.

As discussed by Martinez et al. [8] it is the exposure achieved after the first dose, which is most relevant in determining therapeutic outcome. In this study, low marbofloxacin doses were predicted for a greater than bactericidal action, with 90% TAR in both species; for 72 h and a $4\log_{10}$ reduction in count, the predicted doses were 2.08 and 1.14 mg/kg, respectively, for *P. multocida* and *A. pleuropneumoniae.* Both dosages are less than the dosages of 4, 8 and 16 mg/kg studied by Schneider et al. [1]. To achieve a bactericidal action ($3\log_{10}$ reduction in count) for *P. multocida* for 90% TAR, once daily doses at steady state were even lower, 0.43 mg/kg for *P. multocida* and for *A. pleuropneumoniae* 0.29 mg/kg for pigs aged 27 weeks.

These predicted doses are lower than those of 2.5 mg/kg and 8 mg/kg investigated by Ding et al. [3] and Ferran et al. [34] as well as the 2 mg/kg recommended dose for several licensed marbofloxacin products. Ferren et al. [34] suggested that even lower doses of marbofloxacin could potentially eradicate low counts (10^5 CFU/mL) in the lung, while having a minimal impact on the microbiota of the large intestine. On the other hand, Vallé et al. [35] validated for the bovine pneumonia pathogens, *P. multocida* and *Mannheimia haemolytica,* the concept of a single high dose of marbofloxacin compared to a daily dose of 2 mg/kg for 3–5 days. A bactericidal effect against bovine *P. multocida* was achieved within one hour, when marbofloxacin was administered at five times the recommended daily dose (10 mg/kg).

The present study illustrates the principles of using MCS to predict dosages of marbofloxacin for the treatment of pneumonia in the young pig. The proposed dosage regimen is for *A. pleuropneumoniae* and *P.multocida* induced pneumonias only. For other organisms, independent PK/PD studies will be required. However, in future studies it will be important to extend the present findings for *A. pleuropneumoniae* and *P.multocida* also. Whilst the inter-isolate variability in PK/PD breakpoint values for bacteriostatic and bactericidal levels of kill was small in the present study, estimates were based on only six isolates for each species. Moreover, the time-kill studies generating the PK/PD breakpoints used fixed drug concentrations (eight multiples of MIC) for a fixed time period. In clinical use, on the other hand, plasma drug concentrations first increase and then decrease after intramuscular dosing, exposing organisms to a continuously variable concentration. A third consideration is the relatively small number of isolates in the report of de Jong et al. [29].

In future studies, these concerns could be addressed by increasing numbers of isolates in field distribution studies and in PK/PD breakpoint estimation studies. Moreover, exposure of organisms to varying drug concentrations could be addressed by use for example of hollow fibre methods to simulate in vivo patterns of change in concentration with time. Furthermore, marbofloxacin PK data were used as mean and standard deviation values from the literature. In future studies, it will be useful to incorporate individual animal PK data in the MCSs, and, in particular it will be helpful to use population PK data obtained in clinically ill pigs. Finally, the methodology in this study did not consider the contribution to pathogen elimination by the body's natural defence mechanisms, which are known to be important in immune competent clinical subjects. In addition, potentially beneficial properties of antimicrobial drugs, such as immunomodulatory and anti-inflammatory actions are of importance for some drug classes. Finally, dose prediction studies, as reported in this manuscript, should always be correlated with clinical and bacteriological outcomes in animal disease models and clinical trials [7, 11–13].

Conclusions

Predicted doses for marbofloxacin for treatment of respiratory tract infections in the pig, caused by *P. multocida* or *A. pleuropneumoniae,* were determined by generating PK/PD breakpoints for several levels of kill, based on modelling PK and PD data. These breakpoint values were used with published MIC distribution data [29] and PK data [1] to determine dosages for three levels of kill, and for once daily doses at steady state and for single doses with both 50% and 90% target Attainment Rates. The findings illustrate the value and principle of using Monte Carlo simulation for determination of optimal doses for a range of outcomes.

Abbreviations

CAMHB: Cation-adjusted Mueller Hinton Broth; CLSI: Clinical and Laboratory Standards Institute; EUCAST: Committee on Antimicrobial Susceptibility Testing; MCS: Monte Carlo Simulation; MHB: Mueller Hinton Broth; MIC: Minimum inhibitory concentration; PD: Pharmacodynamics; PK: Pharmacokinetics; TAR: Target Attainment Rate

Acknowledgements

Lucy Dorey was a BBSRC CASE AWARD Scholar. A Pridmore, Don Whitley Scientific, and A Rycroft, Royal Veterinary College, supplied bacterial isolates.

Funding

This project has been funded by BBSRC and Norbrook Laboratories Ltd.; grant number BB/101649X1. The funding body had no participation in the design of the study, collection, analysis, and interpretation of data, and in writing the manuscript.

Authors' contributions

LD and PL were responsible for the study design and co-ordination, data analysis and were involved in writing the manuscript. LD conducted the experiments. LP was involved in data analysis and in writing the manuscript. All authors approved the final manuscript.

Consent for publication

Not applicable.

Competing interests

The authors declare that they have no competing interests.

References

1. Schneider M, Paulin A, Dron F, Woehrle F. Pharmacokinetic of marbofloxacin in pigs after intravenous and intramuscular administration of a single dose of 8 mg/kg: dose proportionality, influence of the age of the animals and urinary elimination. J Vet Pharmacol and Ther. 2014;37(6):p523–30.
2. Boothe HW, Jones SA, Wilkie WS, Boeckh A, Stenstrom KK, Boothe DM. Evaluation of the concentration of marbofloxacin in alveolar macrophages and pulmonary epithelial lining fluid after administration in dogs. Am J Vet Res. 2005;66(10):1770–4.
3. Ding H, Li Y, Chen Z, Rizwan-ul-Haq M, Zeng Z. Plasma and tissue cage fluid pharmacokinetics of marbofloxacin after intravenous, intramuscular, and oral single-dose application in pigs. J Vet Pharmacol Ther. 2010;33(5):507–10.
4. Lees P, Aliabadi FS. Rational dosing of antimicrobial drugs: animals versus humans. Int J Antimicrob Agents. 2002;19(4):269–84.
5. Wang YC, Chan JP, Yeh KS, Chang CC, Hsuan SL, et al. Molecular characterization of enrofloxacin resistant Actinobacillus pleuropneumoniae isolates. Vet micro. 2010;142(3):309–12.
6. Vilalta C, Giboin H, Schneider M, El Garch F, Fraile L. Pharmacokinetic/pharmacodynamic evaluation of marbofloxacin in the treatment of Haemophilus parasuis and Actinobacillus pleuropneumoniae infections in nursery and fattener pigs using Monte Carlo simulations. J Vet Pharmacol Ther. 2014;37(6):542–9.
7. Lees P, Pelligand L, Illambas J, Potter T, Lacroix M, Rycroft A, et al. Pharmacokinetic/pharmacodynamic integration and modelling of amoxicillin for the calf pathogens Mannheimia haemolytica and Pasteurella multocida. J Vet Pharmacol Ther. 2015;38(5):457–70.
8. Martinez MN, Papich MG, Drusano GL. Dosing regimen matters: the importance of early intervention and rapid attainment of the pharmacokinetic/pharmacodynamic target. Antimicrob Agents Chemother. 2012;56(6):2795–805.
9. Mouton JW, Brown DF, Apfalter P, Cantón R, Giske CG, Ivanova M, et al. The role of pharmacokinetics/pharmacodynamics in setting clinical MIC breakpoints: the EUCAST approach. Clin Microbiol Infect. 2012;18(3):E37–45.
10. Mouton JW, Ambrose PG, Canton R, Drusano GL, Harbarth S, MacGowan A, et al. Conserving antibiotics for the future: new ways to use old and new drugs from a pharmacokinetic and pharmacodynamic perspective. Drug Resist Update. 2011;14(2):107–17.
11. Nielsen EI, Cars O, Friberg LE. Pharmacokinetic/pharmacodynamic (PK/PD) indices of antibiotics predicted by a semimechanistic PKPD model: a step toward model-based dose optimization. Antimicrob Agents Chemother. 2011;55(10):4619–30.
12. Nielsen EI, Friberg LE. Pharmacokinetic-pharmacodynamic modeling of antibacterial drugs. Pharmacol Rev. 2013;65(3):1053–90.
13. Papich MG. Pharmacokinetic–pharmacodynamic (PK–PD) modeling and the rational selection of dosage regimes for the prudent use of antimicrobial drugs. Vet micro. 2014;171(3):480–6.
14. Rey JF, Laffont CM, Croubels S, De Backer P, Zemirline C, Bousquet E, et al. Use of Monte Carlo simulation to determine pharmacodynamic cutoffs of amoxicillin to establish a breakpoint for antimicrobial susceptibility testing in pigs. Am J Vet Res. 2014;75(2):124–31.
15. Toutain PL, Potter T, Pelligand L, Lacroix M, Illambas J, Lees P. Standard PK/PD concepts can be applied to determine a dosage regimen for a macrolide: the case of tulathromycin in the calf. Journal of veterinary pharmacology and therapeutics. 2017;40(1):16–27.
16. Rybak MJ. Pharmacodynamics: relation to antimicrobial resistance. Am J infec control. 2006;34(5):S38–45.
17. Levison ME, Levison JH. Pharmacokinetics and pharmacodynamics of antibacterial agents. Infect Dis Clin N Am. 2009;23(4):791–815.
18. CLSI (2013) Performance Standards for Antimicrobial Disk and Dilution Susceptibility Tests for Bacteria Isolated from Animals: Approved Standard - Fourth Edition. CLSI document VET01-A4 (formerly M31-A3, 2008) Supplementary information VET01-S, 2015. ISBN 1–56238–877-0 [print]; ISBN 1–56238–878-9 [electronic]. Clinical and Laboratory Standards Institute, 950 West Valley Road, Suite 2500, Wayne, Pennsylvania 19087 USA, 2013.
19. Aliabadi FS, Lees P. Pharmacokinetics and pharmacodynamics of danofloxacin in serum and tissue fluids of goats following intravenous and intramuscular administration. Am J Vet Res. 2001 Dec 1;62(12): 1979–89.
20. Sidhu PK, Landoni MF, AliAbadi FS, Lees P. Pharmacokinetic and pharmacodynamic modelling of marbofloxacin administered alone and in combination with tolfenamic acid in goats. Vet J. 2010;184(2):219–29.
21. Sidhu P, Rassouli A, Illambas J, Potter T, Pelligand L, Rycroft A, et al. Pharmacokinetic–pharmacodynamic integration and modelling of florfenicol in calves. J Vet Pharmacol Ther. 2014;37(3):231–42.
22. Zeitlinger MA, Derendorf H, Mouton JW, Cars O, Craig WA, et al. Protein Binding: Do We Ever Learn? Antimicrob Agents Chemother. 2011;55(7):3067–74.
23. Brentnall C, Cheng Z, McKellar QA, Lees P. Pharmacodynamics of oxytetracycline administered alone and in combination with carprofen in calves. Vet Rec. 2012;171(11):273–7.
24. Dorey L, Hobson S, Lees P. What is the true in vitro potency of oxytetracycline for the pig pneumonia pathogens A. pleuropneumoniae and P. multocida? J Vet Pharmacol Ther. 2016; Doi: 10.1111/jvp.12386
25. Aliabadi FS, Lees P. Pharmacokinetics and pharmacokinetic/pharmacodynamic integration of marbofloxacin in calf serum, exudate and transudate. J Vet Pharmacol Ther. 2002;25(3):161–74.
26. Lees P, Pelligand L, Ferran A, Bousquest-Melou A, Toutain P. Application of pharmacological principles to dosage design of antimicrobial drugs. Pharmacol mat. 2015;8:22.
27. Dorey L, Hobson S, Lees P. Potency of marbofloxacin for pig pneumonia pathogens Actinobacillus pleuropneumoniae and Pasteurella multocida: comparison of growth media. Res Vet Sci. 2016. Doi: 10.1016/j.rvsc.2016.11.001.
28. Dorey L, Hobson S, Lees P. Part 2: Factors influencing the potency of marbofloxacin for pig pneumonia pathogens Actinobacillus pleuropneumoniae and Pasteurella multocida. Res Vet Sci 2016; Doi: 10. 1016/j.rvsc.2016.11.001.
29. de Jong A, Thomas V, Simjee S, Moyaert H, El Garch F, Maher K, et al. Antimicrobial susceptibility monitoring of respiratory tract pathogens isolated from diseased cattle and pigs across Europe: the VetPath study. Vet Microbiol. 2014;172(1):202–15.
30. Drusano G, Labro MT, Cars O, Mendes P, Shah P, Sörgel F, et al. Pharmacokinetics and pharmacodynamics of fluoroquinolones. Clin Microbiol Infect. 1998;4(s2):2S27–41.

31. Lode H, Borner K, Koeppe P. Pharmacodynamics of fluoroquinolones. Clin Infect Dis. 1998;27(1):33–9.
32. Drusano GL. Pharmacokinetics and pharmacodynamics of antimicrobials. Clin Infect Dis. 2007;45(Supplement 1):S89–95.
33. Toutain PL, Lees P. Integration and modelling of pharmacokinetic and pharmacodynamic data to optimize dosage regimens in veterinary medicine. J Vet Pharmacol Ther. 2004;27(6):467–77.
34. Ferran AA, Bibbal D, Pellet T, Laurentie M, Gicquel-Bruneau M, Sanders P, et al. Pharmacokinetic/pharmacodynamic assessment of the effects of parenteral administration of a fluoroquinolone on the intestinal microbiota: comparison of bactericidal activity at the gut versus the systemic level in a pig model. Int J Antimicrob Agents. 2013;42(5):429–35.
35. Vallé M, Schneider M, Galland D, Giboin H, Woehrle F. Pharmacokinetic and pharmacodynamic testing of marbofloxacin administered as a single injection for the treatment of bovine respiratory disease. J Vet Pharmacol Ther. 2012;35(6):519–28.

5

Changes in serum proteins after endotoxin administration in healthy and choline-treated calves

Z. Yilmaz[1*], O. Eralp Inan[2], M. Kocaturk[1], A. T. Baykal[3], O. Hacariz[4], I. Hatipoglu[5], A. Tvarijonaviciute[6,8], M. Cansev[7], J. Ceron[8] and I. H. Ulus[9]

Abstract

Background: This study aimed to investigate the possible serum protein changes after endotoxin administration in healthy and choline-treated calves using proteomics. These results are expected to contribute to the understanding of the pathophysiological mechanisms of endotoxemia and the beneficial effect of choline administration in this clinical situation.

Methods: Healthy-calves ($n = 20$) were divided into 4 groups: Control, Choline treated (C), Lipopolysaccharide administered (LPS), and LPS + C. Control calves received 0.9 % NaCl injection. Calves in C and LPS + C groups received choline chloride (1 mg/kg/iv). Endotoxin (LPS) was injected (2 μg/kg/iv) to the calves in LPS and LPS + C groups. Serum samples were collected before and after the treatments. Differentially expressed proteins (> 1.5 fold-change relative to controls) were identified by LC-MS/MS.

Results: After LPS administration, 14 proteins increased, and 13 proteins decreased within 48 h as compared to controls. In the LPS group, there were significant increases in serum levels of ragulator complex protein (189-fold) and galectin-3-binding protein (10-fold), but transcription factor MafF and corticosteroid binding globulin were down regulated (≥ 5 fold). As compared with the LPS group, in LPS + C group, fibrinogen gamma-B-chain and antithrombin were up-regulated, while hemopexin and histone H4 were down-regulated. Choline treatment attenuated actin alpha cardiac muscle-1 overexpression after LPS.

Conclusions: LPS administration produces changes in serum proteins associated with lipid metabolism, immune and inflammatory response, protein binding/transport, cell adhesion, venous thrombosis, cardiac contractility and blood coagulation. The administration of choline is associated with changes in proteins which can be related with its beneficial effect in this clinical situation.

Keywords: Calves, Choline, Endotoxemia, Proteomic, Sepsis

Background

Endotoxemia is defined as the presence of endotoxins in blood. This situation can occur by Gram-negative bacterial infections which liberate endotoxin (lipopolysaccharides; LPS) during rapid growth. This results in the fact that Gram-negative sepsis is associated with high mortality rates, despite comprehensive treatment in intensive care patients [1]. Studies are underway with regards to understanding the complex pathophysiological mechanism of endotoxemia, describing criteria for early diagnosis and developing new treatment approaches in order to decrease mortality [2, 3].

Intravenous choline administration show beneficial effects in the treatment of endotoxemia [4–7] in various species such as dogs and rats. Beneficial effects of intravenous choline treatment are reported in association with the activation of the efferent vagus nerve-based cholinergic anti-inflammatory pathway by the increase in nicotinic cholinergic neuro-transmission [5, 8] following enhanced acetylcholine release by choline [9]. However

* Correspondence: zyilmaz@uludag.edu.tr
[1]Department of Internal Medicine, Faculty of Veterinary Medicine, Uludag University, 16059 Bursa, Turkey
Full list of author information is available at the end of the article

the possible changes in serum proteins that choline treatment can produce has not been studied.

Proteomics analysis allows the simultaneous analysis of thousands of proteins in a sample. This could facilitate the identification of new biomarkers of use for diagnosis and prognosis of sepsis/endotoxemia [10, 11]. Thus, proteomic analyses are a growing trend in human [12] and veterinary medicine [13]. In particular proteomic studies allow identifying new proteins that change in endotoxemia, and by knowing the function of these new proteins, new mechanisms involved in endotoxemia could be elucidated and therefore increase the knowledge about its pathophysiology [14].

In the light of our previous findings [4–7], we hypothesize that the beneficial effect of choline administration in endotoxemic patients could be mediated by changes in concentrations of selected serum proteins. Therefore the objective of this study was to evaluate the possible changes that can occur in serum proteins, by a proteomic analysis, after endotoxin administration in healthy and choline-treated calves.

Methods

Experimental set up

Healthy Holstein calves (4 weeks of age; 40 kg mean weight; $n = 20$) were used in the present study. Their health status was evaluated by clinical, haematological and serum biochemical analyses. Calves were negative for bovine herpes virus, bovine leucosis virus, brucellosis, bovine viral diarrhea, foot and mouth disease, infectious bovine rhinotracheitis, paratuberculosis, and tuberculosis when tested by commercial ELISA kits (IDVet Diagnostics, Grabels, France).

Calves were randomized equally into 4 groups: Control, Choline treated (C), Lipopolysaccharide administered (LPS), and LPS + C. Calves in the Control group were injected with 0.9 % NaCl (saline; 5 ml, i.v.) twice at an interval of 5 min while those in C group received choline chloride (1 mg/kg, dissolved in 5 ml of saline, i.v., once), 5 min after 0.9 % NaCl administration (5 ml, i.v.). In the LPS group, endotoxin (LPS) was injected (2 μg/kg, dissolved in 5 ml of normal saline, i.v., once) to the calves, followed 5 min later by intravenous injection of normal saline. In LPS + C group, endotoxin injection was followed 5 min later by choline chloride injection at the doses described in the LPS and C groups, respectively [15, 16].

Clinical data

Routine clinical examinations were performed before (baseline) and 0.5–48 h after the treatments. A scoring system adapted from a previous paper [17] was used to evaluate clinical status in the study. Each parameter was scored by minimum 0 point (means normal) to maximum 6 points (means severely affected).

Serum proteomic analysis

In order to analyse differences in protein expression in the course of the study, three serum samples at each time point for each treatment were obtained and the protein profiles of the serum samples were analysed by LC-MS/MS method [18–20]. Albumin depletion from serum samples was done with albumin depletion spin columns (Pierce, Thermo Scientific). IgGs from the albumin-depleted serum samples were also depleted with an Albumin/IgG Removal Kit (Pierce, Thermo scientific). The remaining serum proteins (at same concentration for all samples) were extracted and enzymatically digested into peptides, and the resulting peptides were subjected to the nanoUPLC-ESI-qTOF-MS system (nano-ultra-performance LC and ESI quadrupole TOF MS) (Waters) with the application of data independent acquisition method also known as the MS^E as previously described in detail [20]. Minimum 3 technical replicates for each sample were used for the analysis. The proteomic data was searched against a reviewed database [including protein sequences of *Bos taurus* and an internal standard (enolase, *Saccharomyces cerevisiae*; #P00924), obtained from UniProt (htpp://www.uniprot.org)] with previously described *in silico* parameters [19]. Quantitative differences of proteins at different time points were calculated using Progenesis LC-MS software V4.0 (Nonlinear Dynamics) [20].

Chemicals

Choline chloride and endotoxin (*E. coli* lipopolysaccharide, LPS, serotype 055:B5) were purchased from Sigma Chemical Co. (St. Louis, Missouri, USA).

Statistical analysis

Results were expressed as mean ± SEM. Data were evaluated by one-way analysis of variance by repeated measures, followed by Tukey test for pairwise comparisons. Clinical scores were compared by a non-parametric test (Friedman Repeated Measure ANOVA on Ranks). *P* values less than 0.05 were considered significant.

Results

Clinical data

Clinical findings are presented as Additional file 1 (Fig. 1). Briefly, choline induced a decrease in heart and respiratory rates compared with the control animals. LPS administration increased body temperature and heart and respiratory rates as compared to their baselines. The severities of these changes in LPS + C treatment were lower ($p < 0.01$) than those of calves treated with LPS.

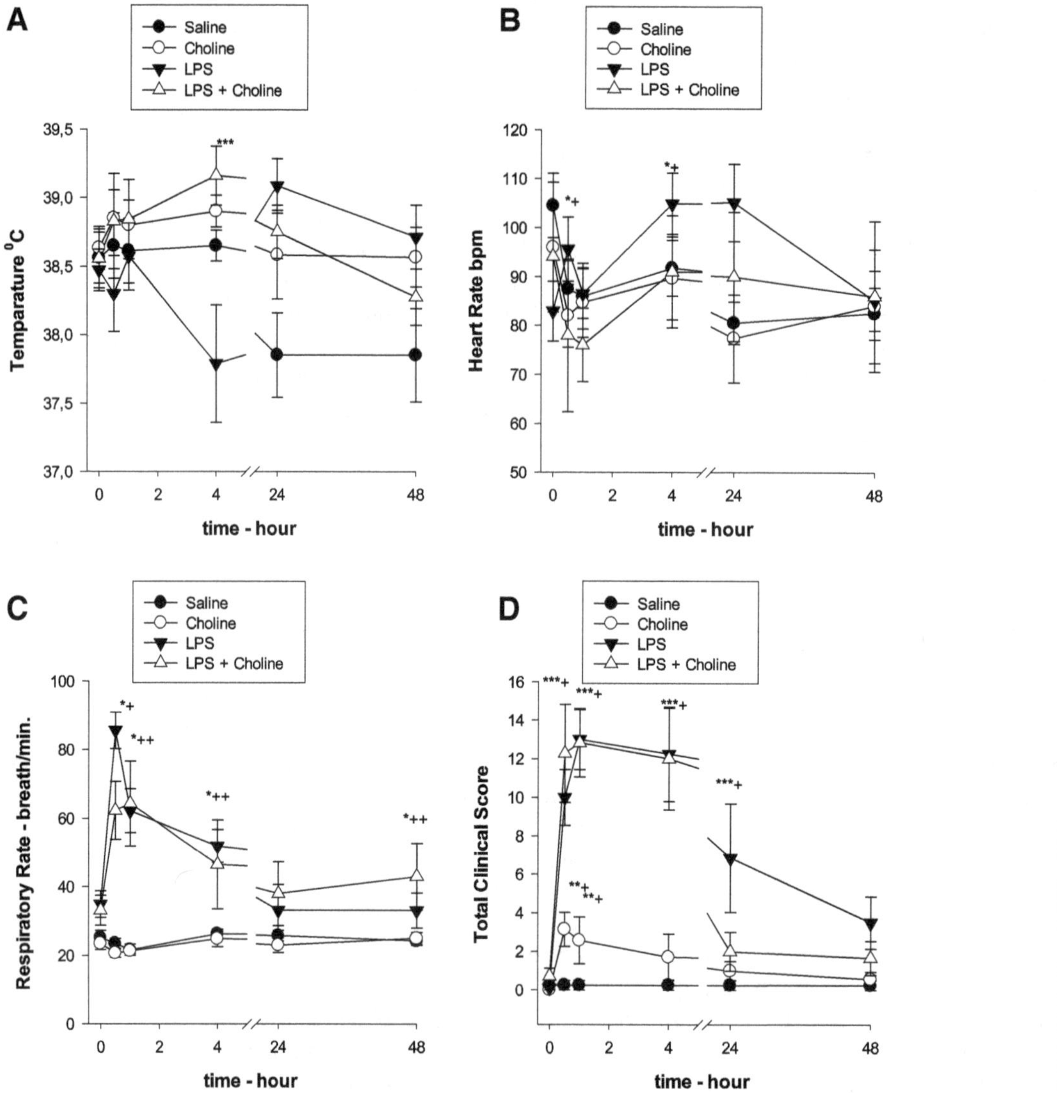

Fig. 1 Clinical parameters (**a**, temperature; **b-c**, heart and respiratory rates; and **d**, total clinical score) in saline, choline, LPS and LPS + choline groups. Calves were injected i.v. once with saline (5 ml) or saline containing choline chloride (1 mg/kg). Five minutes after the first i.v. treatment, calves received endotoxin (LPS, 2 μg/kg) in 5 ml normal saline. Measurements were performed immediately before first i.v. treatment (0 h) and 1 – 48 h after saline, choline, LPS or LPS + choline treatments. Each point represents to Mean ± SEM of six determinations. * $p < 0.05$, ** $p < 0.001$, *** $p < 0.001$ as compared to baseline + $p < 0.05$, ++ $p < 0.01$ as compared to saline group

Two calves died at 4 and 24 h after LPS and one at 48 h after LPS + C. Calves in control and choline groups survived until the end of the study.

Serum proteins

Protein expression differences among experimental groups at different time points (30 min, 1, 4 and 48 h) are shown in Table 1. Details including numerical values for the quantitative analysis obtained from the Progenesis LC-MS software are shown in Additional file 1.

A total of 76 proteins were identified across the serum samples by the proteomic analysis. After LPS administration, 14 proteins increased, whereas 13 proteins decreased within 48 h as compared to controls (Table 1). In LPS group, there was a dramatic increase (189 fold, at 24 h) in ragulator complex protein LAMTOR2 which was followed by other proteins showing changes ranging from 6 to 13 fold such as negative elongation factor E (at 4 h), galectin-3 binding protein (Gal-3BP), argininosuccinate lyase and membrane primary amine-oxidase (at 48 h). Following LPS administration, moderate decreases (< 5 fold changes) were observed in some proteins such as serpin A3-4 (at 30 min.), vitamin D binding protein (VDBP), inter alpha trypsin inhibitor heavy chain H3 (ITIH, at 4 h), apolipoprotein A IV (Apo-AIV), alpha-1B glycoprotein and serotransferrin

Table 1 Protein expression differences among experimental groups at different time points (30 min, 1 h, 4 h and 48 h)

LPS_Choline	P02081; Hemoglobin fetal subunit beta/1.52 Q9QAQ7; Non structural protein of 4 9 kDa/3.42 P02676; Fibrinogen beta chain/3.83 A2I7N1; Serpin A3 5/1.44 Q3ZC07*; Actin alpha cardiac muscle 1/15.21 Q32L76; Serum amyloid A 4 protein/1.70 A2I7N3; Serpin A3 7/1.44 *Q3ZC07*; Actin alpha cardiac muscle 1/187.33* *P0CH28*; Polyubiquitin C/1.59* *P12799; Fibrinogen gamma B chain/8.44* *Q2M2T2; U-p-C19orf71-h/2.17* *P02676; Fibrinogen beta chain/64.53*	A2I7N1; Serpin A3 5/1.44 Q9TTK6; Membrane primary amine oxidase/Infinity P01966; Hemoglobin subunit alpha/1.50 P19034; Apolipoprotein C II/2.82 Q9MYP6; beta hydroxysteroid dehydrogenase 14/26.44 Q1JQ97; Bardet Biedl syndrome 4 protein homolog/2.30 *Q9TTK6; Membrane primary amine oxidase/11.79* *P81644; Apolipoprotein A II/1.45* *P19035; Apolipoprotein C III/2.34* *Q32L76; Serum amyloid A 4 protein/2.20* *Q5E9E3; Complement C1q subcomponent subunit A/3.01* *P34955; Alpha 1 antiproteinase/1.60* *P28800; Alpha 2 antiplasmin/1.43* *P80012; von Willebrand factor Fragment/2.98*	Q9TTE1; Serpin A3 1/2.09 Q80E01; Glutaredoxin 1/2.21 Q3SZJ0; Argininosuccinate lyase/1.81 Q17QL1; Glucosamine 6 phosphate isomerase 2/2.96 Q3T0Z5; Leukocyte receptor cluster m-1-h/2.22 Q9TTE1; Serpin A3 1/1.74 Q9TTK6; Membrane primary amine oxidase/64.58 *A2I7N0; Serpin A3 4/1.47* *P41361; Antithrombin III/2.67* *P00735; Prothrombin/2.287* *P12799; Fibrinogen gamma B chain/5.92*	
LPS	P17697; Clusterin/1.43 *Q0V898; Negative elongation factor E/1.68* *Q9TTK6; Membrane primary amine oxidase/7.17* *A6QPQ2; Serpin A3 8/1.67* *O46406; Primary amine oxidase lung isozyme/3.74* *P01044; Kininogen 1/2.13* *A7E3W2; Galectin 3 binding protein/13.09* *P41356; Fusion glycoprotein F0/1.82* *O62830-2; Isoform Beta 2 of Protein phosphatase 1B/6.78* *Q3T132; Ragulator complex protein LAMTOR2/189.56* *Q3SZJ0; Argininosuccinate lyase/9.22* *Q9QAQ7; Bovine coronavirus strain OK 0514 GN 4a/4.93* *Q0V898; Negative elongation factor E/10.86* *Q28901;6-p-2-k-f-2-6-b-f/Infinity*	A2I7N2; Serpin A3 6/1.64 P81644; Apolipoprotein A II/1.62 P19035; Apolipoprotein C III/2.80 Q5E9E3; Complement C1q subcomponent subunit A/2.66 Q28901; 6-p-2-k-f-2-6-b-f/infinity *P01966; Hemoglobin subunit alpha/1.81* *P02081; Hemoglobin fetal subunit beta/1.55* *P80109; P-g-s-p-d/1.50* *Q5E9F5; Transgelin 2/2.90* *P22226; Cathelicidin 1/13.17* *Q7SIH1; Alpha 2 macroglobulin/1.41* *A2I7M9; Serpin A3 2/9.68* *P00924; ENO1 YEAST Enolase 1/1.46* *Q3MHN5; Vitamin D binding protein/1.67* *Q3ZC07*; Actin alpha cardiac muscle 1/25.52* *P80109; Phosphatidylinositol glycan specific phospholipase D/3.11* *O02659; Mannose binding protein C/5.76* *P0CH28*; Polyubiquitin C/4.09* *A8YXX7; Trefoil factor 3/4.93* *Q2TBS3; Uncharacterized protein C20orf79 homolog/4.76* *Q96629; Adenain/2.23* *P19034; Apolipoprotein C II/4.21* *Q1JP73; UPF0553 protein C9orf64 homolog/12.57*		Q9TTK6-2; Isoform 2 of Membrane primary amine oxidase/2.30 Q1JP73; UPF0553 protein C9orf64 homolog/1.95 Q56K14; 60S acidic ribosomal protein P1/Infinity *Q3SZV7; Hemopexin/2.10* *Q1JQ97; Bardet Biedl syndrome 4 protein homolog/1.48* *Q56K14;60S acidic ribosomal protein P1/Infinity* *Q96629; Adenain/1.74* *Q2KIT0; Protein HP 20 homolog/1.93* *Q5E9F5; Transgelin 2/Infinity* *P62803; Histone H4/11.67*

Table 1 Protein expression differences among experimental groups at different time points (30 min, 1 h, 4 h and 48 h) *(Continued)*

	Control	Choline	LPS	LPS_Choline
Choline	O46406; Primary amine oxidase lung isozyme/1.74 Q28901; 6-p-2-k-f-2-6-b-f/Infinity *Q2M2T2; Uncharacterized protein C19orf71/1.78* *A2I7N3; Serpin A3 7/1.56* *Q17QL1; Glucosamine 6 phosphate isomerase 2/1.48*		*A5PJC4; Ubiquitin ISG15 c. e. E2 L6/1.45* *Q80E01; Glutaredoxin 1/1.40* *Q0VCI2; Syntaxin 19/3.81*	Q0V898; Negative elongation factor E/2.4 Q05204; Lysosome associated membrane glycoprotein 1/4.03 Q56K14; 60S acidic ribosomal protein P1/8968.4 *P34955; Alpha 1 antiproteinase/1.47* *A2I7N2; Serpin A3 6/1.72* *Q3SZJ0; Argininosuccinate lyase/1.41* *Q17QL1; Glucosamine 6 phosphate isomerase 2/8.44*
Control		P80012; von Willebrand factor Fragment/2.08	A2I7N0; Serpin A3 4/1.60	P21752; Thymosin beta 10/1.45
		Q3SZK0; Solute carrier family 25 member 34/1.72	Q2TBS3; Uncharacterized protein C20orf79/2.01	Q3T132; Ragulator complex protein LAMTOR2/2.04
		Q05204; Lysosome associated membrane glycoprotein 1/2.34		P01044-2*; Isoform LMW of Kininogen 1/2.87
			Q9TTK6-2; Isoform 2 of Membrane primary amine oxidase/2.82	
		Q80E01; Glutaredoxin 1/3.37		Q58CQ9; Pantetheinase/1.58
		Q05204; Lysosome associated membrane glycoprotein 1/10.89	*Q3MHN5; Vitamin D binding protein/1.48*	
				Q96629; Adenain/1.69
		Q2KIU3; Protein HP 25 homolog 2/1.70	*P56652; Inter alpha trypsin inhibitor heavy chain H3/1.58*	
		P02081; Hemoglobin fetal subunit beta/1.72	*Q29443; Serotransferrin/1.57*	*P01044-2*; Isoform LMW of Kininogen 1/1.62*
			Q32PJ2; Apolipoprotein A IV/1.45	*Q58CQ9; Pantetheinase/1.84*
			A2I7N2; Serpin A3 6/4.57	*P21752; Thymosin beta 10/1.46*
			Q2KJF1; Alpha 1B glycoprotein/1.46	*Q9MYP6;17 beta hydroxysteroid dehydrogenase 14/2.24*
			P01966; Hemoglobin subunit alpha/1.63	
			P02070; Hemoglobin subunit beta/1.98	
			A7YY73; Transcription factor MafF/5.00	
			E1BF81; Corticosteroid binding globulin/5.27	
	Control	Choline	LPS	LPS_Choline

This table shows the identified proteins with highest mean condition (left) and lowest mean condition (bottom) among experimental groups at different time points at statistically significant level ($P < 0.05$). Relative abundance levels of the proteins with highest mean condition, compared to the proteins with lowest mean condition, are indicated after the slash (/). Time points are indicated with underline, italic and italic + underline, for 1 h, 4 h and 48 h time points, respectively. Asterisk (*) indicates the proteins, of which, isoforms are detectable (see Additional file for the accession numbers of the isoforms). Abbreviations; c. e.: conjugating enzyme, 6-p-2-k-f-2-6-b-f; 6 phosphofructo 2 kinase fructose 2 6 bisphosphatase 3 Fragment, m-1-h; member 1 homolog, U-p-C19orf71-h; Uncharacterized protein C19orf71 homolog, P-g-s-p-d; Phosphatidylinositol glycan specific phospholipase D (at 48 h). In addition more prominent decreases (≥ 5 fold changes, at 48 h) were observed in transcription factor MafF and corticosteroid binding globulin (CBG).

When compared with LPS group, in LPS + C group, glucosamine-6-phosphate isomerase-2, membrane primary amine oxidase, fibrinogen gamma B chain, antithrombin and prothrombin were markedly up-regulated, while isoform 2 of membrane primary amine oxidase, hemopexin and histone-H4 were markedly down-regulated. Actin alpha cardiac muscle-1 expression increased at 1–48 h (15–187 fold) in LPS and LPS + C groups, as compared to controls. The magnitude of increase in actin alpha cardiac muscle-1 was lower at 48 h in LPS + C group than that of LPS group. As compared to controls, following choline administration, a number of proteins (primary amine oxidase, serpin A3-7 and glucosamine-6-phosphate isomerase-2) were up-regulated while others (lysosome associated membrane glycoprotein-1 and glutaredoxin-1) were more down-regulated at different time points of the study.

Discussion

In this study, an experimental model consisting in the induction of endotoxemia by LPS administration in calves was chosen, because calves are very sensitive to LPS. Therefore is expected that the changes associated with LPS as well as its treatment will be easier to detect than with other animal models. The clinical changes occurred after LPS treatment in our experimental model in calves showed similarities with the results of experimental human [21] and animal studies of sepsis/endotoxemia [4–7, 15–17].

To our knowledge, our study describes for the first time 14 proteins that are up-regulated, and 13 proteins that are down-regulated in endotoxemia in calves. The roles of some of these altered proteins are highlighted below.

One of the proteins that were dramatically up-regulated was ragulator complex protein LAMTOR2. This protein is known to be involved in amino acid sensing and activation of mTORC1 [22], a signalling complex promoting cell growth in response to growth factors, energy levels, and amino acids. A previous study reported that severe immunological defects affecting the immunity in human primary immunodeficiency syndrome was associated with reduced levels of LAMTOR2 [22]. Hence, the elevated serum levels of ragulator complex in our study may be associated with host's response by increasing macrophage activity and enhancing adaptive immunity in response to LPS. Thus, ragulator complex may represent a new early diagnostic marker for the detection of inflammation in calves, due to its dramatic overexpression shortly after LPS treatment.

Another protein, which significantly increased in calves after LPS administration, was Gal-3BP. This protein has stimulatory activity on lymphokine-activated and natural killer cells, and also stimulates the secretion of many cytokines and interleukins in peripheral blood mononuclear cells that all play a contributory role in inflammation [23]. In this study, up-regulated expression of Gal-3BP may be associated with limiting an on-going inflammation in response to LPS, because of its immune modulatory activity [23]. In addition, overexpressed Gal-3BP may be considered as a host response to neutralize harmful effects of Galectin-3 which is released from LPS-stimulated cells to produce heightened levels of inflammatory mediators, resulting in further tissue damage and, ultimately, organ failure, characteristics of sepsis. On the other hand, Gal-3BP has a critical role in the development of venous thrombosis [24] and to increase the survival of cancer cells in the bloodstream [25], indicating that probably is involved in the pathophysiological responses of different pathological conditions.

Transcription factor MafF and CBG are associated with interleukin regulation [26], and have a protective effect in situations of cell stress, coagulation cascade activation and severe illness [27]. A possible reason for the down regulations of these proteins found in our study may be excessive use of them to neutralize detrimental effects of LPS during acute phase reaction.

Proteases from LPS-activated leukocytes can trigger tissue and organ damage and enhance the nonspecific proteolysis of plasma clotting factors in patients with severe sepsis. One example is the leukocyte elastase that is involved in the progress of complications in patients with sepsis [28]. In the present study, down regulation of ITIH-H3 in calves with LPS was most probably due to extended secretion of elastase [28], thereby this protein may be a part of the regulatory system that controls acute inflammation [29] in calves. Similar to our finding, circulating ITIH protein level was found lower in patients with severe sepsis than in healthy volunteers [28].

Confirming our previous findings in dogs and rats [4–7], we found in the present study that choline treatment improved the clinical signs associated to LPS. Further studies including larger number of calves are needed to evaluate if choline treatment could reduce mortality rate in this clinical condition. Endotoxemia studies in dogs showed that these beneficial effects of choline treatment might be related with inhibition of TNF-α synthesis [4], prevention of hepato-renal injury [4], and attenuation of the changes of serum butyrylcholinesterase and paraoxonase-1 activities [30].

Most of the down-regulated proteins after choline treatment such as kininogen-1, prothrombin, and ragulator complex are involved in coagulation and the development of DIC. Therefore the decrease of these proteins could be associated with the preventive effects of choline treatment on the development of coagulopathy, as described previously in dogs [7]. In addition the down-regulation of histones after choline treatment would be related with the protective effect of choline. Histone proteins, mainly the histones-H3 and H4, have been reported to exhibit cytotoxicity when released to the extracellular fluid in response to severe stress or inflammatory challenges like sepsis and to mediate excessive and overwhelming cell damage and death [31]. Hemopexin (Hx) is mainly expressed as an APP from liver after inflammation [32]. In this study, Hx overexpression may be related with its antioxidant role [32] to facilitate tissue repair in response to LPS [33]. Choline treatment decreased Hx overexpression in calves with LPS, probably related with the reduction in body's antioxidant needs [32, 34] due to the reduction in tissue damage produced by choline [3].

The increase found in SAA4 after choline administration could be related with the protective effect that has been described for SAA by inhibiting TNF and LPS as well as platelet aggregation [35]. In addition a correlation between SAA4 and cholinesterase has been found, therefore a link between SAA4 response and choline administration could be hypothesized [36].

Choline treatment attenuated overexpression of contractile protein actin alpha cardiac muscle-1 (ACTC1) at 48 h after LPS, indicating a protective effect of choline treatment on sepsis-induced myocardial dysfunction (SIMD). SIMD is a well-recognized manifestation of organ dysfunction in patient with sepsis [37] and calves with endotoxemia [38]. LPS-induced overexpression of ACTC1 may contribute to myocardial dysfunction during endotoxemia [39], most probably due to impaired sarcomere integrity [40]. The observed overexpression of ACTC1 may be due to decreased thymosin beta-10 expression since thymosin beta-10 plays an important role in the organization of the cytoskeleton by binding to and sequestering actin monomers resulting with an inhibition in actin polymerization [41].

Conclusion

Although this is a pilot study made with a small sample size and therefore the results should be taken with caution. It could be concluded that based on our experimental model, following LPS administration, there are changes in selected serum proteins which are associated with various biological processes such as lipid metabolism, immune and inflammatory response, protein binding and transport, cell adhesion, venous thrombosis, cardiac contraction and blood coagulation. In addition choline administration is associated with changes in serum concentrations of selected serum proteins that would be related with its beneficial effect in this clinical situation. These findings would reinforce the effectiveness of choline administration in the treatment of endotoxemia. However further studies are needed to confirm our results due to small sample size of this study, and in addition it would be interesting to evaluate the effectiveness of choline treatment in combination with other drugs such as steroidal or non-steroidal anti-inflammatory drugs.

Acknowledgement
This study (TOVAG-1110026) was supported by The Scientific and Technological Research Council of Turkey (TUBITAK).

Authors' contributions
ZY Research idea, study design, write up, corresponding author. OEI Experimental procedures. MK Experimental procedures. ATB Proteomic analysis and its validation for calves. OH Proteomic analysis and expression of proteomic results in a Table. IH Proteomic analysis. AT Biochemical analysis, and review. MC free choline measurements. JC Review and write up. IHU Statistical analysis, grammatical correction, and adviser for the study. All authors read and approved the final manuscript.

Competing interests
None of the authors has any financial or personal relationships that could inappropriately influence or bias the content of the paper.

Consent for publication
Not applicable.

Author details
[1]Department of Internal Medicine, Faculty of Veterinary Medicine, Uludag University, 16059 Bursa, Turkey. [2]Medical and Surgical Experimental Animal Practice and Research Center, Eskisehir Osmangazi University, 26480 Eskisehir, Turkey. [3]Department of Medical Biochemistry, Acibadem University School of Medicine, Istanbul, Turkey. [4]TÜBİTAK Marmara Research Center, Genetic Engineering and Biotechnology Institute, Kocaeli, Turkey. [5]Arthritis & Clinical Immunology Research Program, Oklahoma Medical Research Foundation, Oklahoma, USA. [6]Departament de Medicina i Cirurgia Animals, Universitat Autònoma de Barcelona, 08193 Bellaterra, Barcelona, Spain. [7]Department of Pharmacology, Uludag University School of Medicine, Bursa, Turkey. [8]Interdisciplinary Laboratory of Clinical Analysis, Interlab-UMU, Regional Campus of International Excellence "Campus Mare Nostrum", University of Murcia, Espinardo, Murcia 30100 , Spain. [9]Department of Pharmacology, Acibadem University School of Medicine, Istanbul, Turkey.

References
1. Morris DD. Endotoxemia in horses: a review of cellular and humoral mediators involved in its pathogenesis. J Vet Inter Med. 1991;5:167–81.
2. Adams JL, Semrad SD, Czuprynskil CJ. Administration of bacterial lipopolysaccharide elicits circulating Tumor necrosis factor-alpha in neonatal calves. J Clin Microb. 1990;8:998–1001.
3. Bistrian BR. Acute phase proteins and the systemic inflammatory response. Crit Care Med. 1999;27:452–3.
4. Ilcol YO, Yilmaz Z, Ulus IH. Endotoxin alters serum free choline and phospholipid-bound choline concentrations and choline administration attenuates endotoxin-induced organ injury in dog. Shock. 2005;24:288–93.
5. Ilcol YO, Yilmaz Z, Cansev M, Ulus IH. Choline or CDP-choline alters serum lipid responses to endotoxin in dogs and rats: involvement of the peripheral nicotinic acetylcholine receptors. Shock. 2009;32:286–94.
6. Yilmaz Z, IlcoL YO, Torun S, Ulus IH. Intravenous administration of choline or CDP-choline improves platelet count and platelet closure times in endotoxin-treated dogs. Shock. 2006;25:73–9.

7. Yilmaz Z, Ozarda Y, Cansev M, Eralp O, Kocaturk M, Ulus IH. Choline or CDP-choline attenuates coagulation abnormalities and prevents the development of acute disseminated intravascular coagulation in dogs during endotoxemia. Blood Coagul Fibrin. 2010;21:339–48.
8. Parrish WR, Rosas-Ballina M, Gallowitsch-Puerta Ochani M, Ochani K, Yang L, et al. Modulation of TNF release by choline requires alpha7 subunit nicotinic acetylcholinemediated signaling. Mol Med. 2008;14:567–74.
9. Ilcol YO, Gurun MS, Taga Y, Ulus IH. Choline increases serum insulin in rat when injected intraperitoneally and augments basal and stimulated acetylcholine release from the rat minced pancreas in vitro. Eur J Biochem. 2003;270:991–9.
10. Cao Z, Robinson RA. The role of proteomics in understanding biological mechanisms of sepsis. Proteomics-Clin Appl. 2014;8:35–52.
11. Soares AJ, Santos MF, Trugilho MR, Neves-Ferreira AG, Perales J, Domont GB. Differential proteomics of the plasma of individuals with sepsis caused by Acinetobacter baumannii. J Proteomics. 2009;73:267–78.
12. Stewart CJ, Nelson A, Treumann A, Skeath T, Cummings SP, Embleton ND, Berrington JE: Metabolomic and proteomic analysis of serum from preterm infants with necrotising entercolitis and late onset sepsis. Ped Res 2015, doi: 10.1038/pr.2015.235. (Epub ahead of print).
13. Ceciliani F, Eckersall D, Burchmore R, Lecchi C. Proteomics in veterinary medicine: applications and trends in disease pathogenesis and diagnostics. Vet Pathol. 2014;5:351–62.
14. Camprubí-Rimblas M, Artigas A, Guillamat-Prats R. An overview of proteomics on sepsis. J Phys Chem Biophys. 2015;5:183–9.
15. Semrad SD. Comparative efficacy of flunixin, ketoprofen, and ketorolac for treating endotoxemic neonatal calves. Am J Vet Res. 1993;54:1511–6.
16. Gerros TC, Semrad SD, Proctor RA, LaBorde A. Effect of dose and method of administration of endotoxin on cell mediator release in neonatal calves. Am J Vet Res. 1993;54:2121–7.
17. Coskun A, Sen I. Acute phase response and clinical changes in calves with lipopolysaccharide induced endotoxemia. Eurasian J Vet Sci. 2012;28:21–6.
18. Haçarız O, Sayers G, Baykal AT. A proteomic approach to investigate the distribution and abundance of surface and internal Fasciola hepatica proteins during the chronic stage of natural liver fluke infection in cattle. J Proteome Res. 2012;11:3592–604.
19. Haçarız O, Baykal AT, Akgün M, Kavak P, Sağıroğlu MŞ, Sayers GP. Generating a detailed protein profile of Fasciola hepatica during the chronic stage of infection in cattle. Proteomics. 2014;14:1519–30.
20. Haçarız O, Baykal AT. Investigation of the abundance of proteins secreted by Fasciola hepatica, which is exposed to environmental change inexperimental studies, with an advanced proteomic approach. Turkiye Parazitol Derg. 2014;38:106–10.
21. Calvano SE, Coyle SM. Experimental human endotoxemia: a model of the systemic inflammatory response syndrome? Surg Infect (Larchmt). 2012;13:293–9.
22. Scheffler JM, Sparber F, Tripp CH, Herrmann C, Humenberger A, Blitz J, Romani N, Stoitzner P, Huber LA. LAMTOR2 regulates dendritic cell homeostasis through FLT3-dependent mTOR signalling. Nat Commun. 2014;5:5138.
23. Fukaya Y, Shimada H, Wang LC, Zandi E, DeClerck YA. Identification of galectin-3-binding protein as a factor secreted by tumor cells that stimulates interleukin-6 expression in the bone marrow stroma. J Biol Chem. 2008;283:18573–81.
24. DeRoo EP, Wrobleski SK, Shea EM, Al-Khalil RK, Hawley AE, Henke PK, Myers Jr DD, Wakefield TW, Diaz JA. The role of galectin-3 and galectin-3-binding protein in venous thrombosis. Blood. 2015;125:1813–21.
25. Lin TW, Chang HT, Chen CH, Chen CH, Lin SW, Hsu TL, Wong CH. Galectin-3 binding protein and galectin-1 interaction in breast cancer cell aggregation and metastasis. J Am Chem Soc. 2015;137:9685–93.
26. Kim JI, Ho IC, Grusby MJ, Glimcher LH. The transcription factor c-Maf controls the production of interleukin-4 but Not other Th2 cytokines. Immunity. 1999;10(6):745–51.
27. Nenke MA, Rankin W, Chapman MJ, Stevens NE, Diener KR, Hayball JD, Lewis JG, Torpy DJ. Depletion of high-affinity corticosteroid-binding globulin corresponds to illness severity in sepsis and septic shock; clinical implications. Clin Endocrinol (Oxf). 2015;82:801–7.
28. Lim YP, Bendelja K, Opal SM, Siryaporn E, Hixson DC, Palardy JE. Correlation between mortality and the levels of inter-alpha inhibitors in the plasma of patients with severe sepsis. J Infect Dis. 2003;188:919–26.
29. Fries E, Kaczmarczyk A. Inter-alpha-inhibitor, hyaluronan and inflammation. Acta Biochim Pol. 2003;50:735–42.
30. Tvarijonaviciute A, Kocaturk M, Cansev M, Tecles F, Ceron JJ, Yilmaz Z. Serum butyrylcholinesterase and paraoxonase 1 in a canine model of endotoxemia: effects of choline administration. Res Vet Sci. 2012;93:668–74.
31. Xu J, Zhang X, Pelayo R, Monestier M, Ammollo CT, Semeraro F, Taylor FB, Esmon NL, Lupu F, Esmon CT. Extracellular histones are major mediators of death in sepsis. Nat Med. 2009;15:1318–21.
32. Tolosano E, Altruda F. Hemopexin: structure, function, and regulation DNA. J Cell Biol. 2002;21(4):297–306.
33. Schaer DJ, Vinchi F, Ingoglia G, Tolosano E, Buehler PW. Haptoglobin, hemopexin, and related defense pathways—basic science, clinical perspectives, and drug development. Front Phys. 2014;5:415.
34. Janz DR, Bastarache JA, Sills G, Wickersham N, May AK, Bernard GR, Ware LB. Association between haptoglobin, hemopexin and mortality in adults with sepsis. Crit Care. 2013;17:R272.
35. Shainkin-Kestenbaum R, Zimlichman S, Lis M, Lidor C, Pomerantz M, Knyszynski A, Preciado-Patt L, Fridkin M: Effect of serum amyloid A, HDL-apolipoprotein, on endothelial cell proliferation. Implication of an enigmatic protein to atherosclerosis. Biomed Pep Prot Nuc Acids 1996–1997, 2: 79–84.
36. Yamada T, Miyake N, Itoh K, Igari J. Further characterization of serum amyloid A4 as a minor acute phase reactant and a possible nutritional marker. Clin Chem LabMed. 2001;39:7–10.
37. Rudiger A, Singer M. Mechanisms of sepsis-induced cardiac dysfunction. Crit Care Med. 2007;35:1599–608.
38. Peek SF, Apple FS, Murakami MA, Crump PM, Semrad SD. Cardiac isoenzymes in healthy Holstein calves and calves with experimentally induced endotoxemia. Can J Vet Res. 2008;72(4):356–61.
39. Amid A, Samah NA, Yusof F. Identification of troponin I and actin, alpha cardiac muscle 1 as potential biomarkers for hearts of electrically stimulated chickens. Proteome Sci. 2012;10:1.
40. Frade AF, Teixeira PC, Ianni BM, Pissetti CW, Saba B, Wang LHT, et al. Polymorphism in the alpha cardiac muscle actin 1 gene is associated to susceptibility to chronic inflammatory cardiomyopathy. PLoS One. 2013;8:e83446.
41. Haoyuan W, Shanshan J, Yaojun Z, Ke P, Jianchuan X, Minshan C. High expression of thymosin beta 10 predicts poor prognosis for hepatocellular carcinoma after hepatectomy. World J Surg Oncol. 2014;12:226.

6

Quadruplex PCR assay for identification of *Corynebacterium pseudotuberculosis* differentiating biovar Ovis and Equi

Sintia Almeida[1*], Elaine M. S. Dorneles[2], Carlos Diniz[1,3], Vinícius Abreu[4], Cassiana Sousa[1], Jorianne Alves[5], Adriana Carneiro[5], Priscilla Bagano[1], Sharon Spier[6], Debmalya Barh[1,7], Andrey P. Lage[2], Henrique Figueiredo[8] and Vasco Azevedo[1*]

Abstract

Background: *Corynebacterium pseudotuberculosis* is classified into two biovars, nitrate-negative biovar Ovis which is the etiologic agent of caseous lymphadenitis in small ruminants and nitrate-positive biovar Equi, which causes abscesses and ulcerative lymphangitis in equines. The aim of this study was to develop a quadruplex PCR assay that would allow simultaneous detection and biovar-typing of *C. pseudotuberculosis*.

Methods: In the present study, genomes of *C. pseudotuberculosis* strains were used to identify the genes involved in the nitrate reduction pathway to improve a species identification three-primer multiplex PCR assay. The nitrate reductase gene (*narG*) was included in the PCR assay along with the *16S*, *rpoB* and *pld* genes to enhance the diagnosis of the multiplex PCR at biovar level.

Results: A novel quadruplex PCR assay for *C. pseudotuberculosis* species and biovar identification was developed. The results of the quadruplex PCR of 348 strains, 346 previously well-characterized clinical isolates of *C. pseudotuberculosis* from different hosts (goats, sheep, horse, cattle, buffalo, llamas and humans), the vaccine strain 1002 and the type strain ATCC 19410^T, were compared to the results of nitrate reductase identification by biochemical test. The McNemar's Chi-squared test used to compare the two methods used for *C. pseudotuberculosis* biovar identification showed no significant difference ($P = 0.75$) [95% CI for odds ratio (0.16–6.14)] between the quadruplex PCR and the nitrate biochemical test. Concordant results were observed for 97.13% (338 / 348) of the tested strains and the kappa value was 0.94 [95% CI (0.90–0.98)].

Conclusions: The ability of the quadruplex assay to discriminate between *C. pseudotuberculosis* biovar Ovis and Equi strains enhances its usefulness in the clinical microbiology laboratory.

Keywords: Caseous lymphadenitis, Diagnosis, Nitrate reductase, Horse, Sheep, Goats

Background

Corynebacterium pseudotuberculosis is a facultative intracellular bacterium that is the causative agent of caseous lymphadenitis (CLA) in goats and sheep, abscesses and ulcerative lymphangitis in horses and oedematous skin disease (OSD) in Buffalo. It also causes sporadic infections in other species including cattle, camels, llamas, and humans [1–4]. *C. pseudotuberculosis* can be classified in two biovars, based on their ability to convert nitrate to nitrite, nitrate-positive strains are classified as biovar Equi and the nitrate negative ones as biovar Ovis [5]. In sheep and goats, CLA is predominantly caused by biovar Ovis strains, whereas horses and buffalos are mostly infected by biovar Equi strains [6–8]. Infection by *C. pseudotuberculosis* is distributed worldwide, causing significant disease in horse, sheep and goat herds [8, 9]. The main economic losses attributed to *C. pseudotuberculosis* infection include decreased milk production, decreased weight gain, reduced value of hides due to scarring, and the cost of the drugs and labor needed to treat disease [9].

* Correspondence: sintiaalmeida@gmail.com; vasco@icb.ufmg.br
[1]Instituto de Ciências Biológicas, Federal University of Minas Gerais, Belo Horizonte, MG, Brazil
Full list of author information is available at the end of the article

Direct and indirect tests to detect *C. pseudotuberculosis* have already been proposed, such as complement fixation test [10], synergistic hemolysis inhibition test [11], microagglutination assay [12], phospholipase D (PLD) antigen-based ELISA [13] and a multiplex PCR developed by our research group [14]. While these tests are useful for clinical diagnosis in diseased animals, none can differentiate the two biovars of *C. pseudotuberculosis*, which is currently only accomplished by biochemical tests. Differences between biovars are relevant for host and tissue specificity and appear to be associated with virulence [15, 16].

Disease caused by *C. pseudotuberculosis* biovars has different clinical manifestations in the susceptible hosts [6, 8, 17, 18], and biovar identification is important for understanding the epidemiology of infection, and consequently for disease control. Moreover, biovar identification can also have clinical implications. Since cattle can be infected by strains of both biovars, which may have different tissue preferences: biovar Ovis infects chiefly the mammary gland [17] and skin [18] and biovar Equi causes ulcerative lymphangitis and coronet lesions [9, 19, 20].

A dominant genetic characteristic that differentiates the biovars of *C. pseudotuberculosis* is the presence of the nitrate reduction operon in the biovar Equi strains [21]. Additionally, biovar Equi strains have 15 genes that are absent in biovar Ovis strains, including the *narKGHJI* operon, and a gene cluster encoding the molybdopterins *moeB, moaE, molB, molA, moeY, moaC, moeA,* and *moaA* and two hypothetical proteins [21].

Currently, only nitrate reduction test distinguishes *C. pseudotuberculosis* biovars Ovis and Equi [5, 9]. The available phenotypic tests, performed in a laboratory or commercially available, for *C. pseudotuberculosis* identification are usually effective. However, the phenotypic tests can be expensive and unavailable for some laboratories that prefer to use molecular techniques. Currently, clinical microbiology laboratories are experiencing a change from classical to new diagnostic tools as PCR, real-time PCR, sequencing and MALDI-TOF mass spectrometry [22, 23], which, due to the decrease in costs, may prefer to use molecular over biochemical tests. Moreover, the molecular tests are usually faster, easier and have less subjectivity in interpretation [24].

Our collaborative group has sequenced more than 60 *C. pseudotuberculosis* strains isolated from different hosts around the world, performing genomic, proteomic and clinical studies to not only to understand the pathogen but also try to find a way to control the spread of bacteria. Thus, the aim of this study was to develop a quadruplex PCR assay that would allow simultaneous detection and biovar-typing of *C. pseudotuberculosis* strains.

Methods

Nitrate reductase genes

Presence or absence of nitrate reductase genes were analyzed in nineteen *C. pseudotuberculosis* genomes (Table 1) in our previous work [21].

Bacterial strains and culture conditions

A total of 348 *C. pseudotuberculosis* strains, 346 field isolates [25–27], *C. pseudotuberculosis* ATCC 19410^T type strain, and *C. pseudotuberculosis* 1002 vaccine strain, were used in this study. These strains were obtained from the repository of the Laboratório de Genética Celular e Molecular, Instituto de Ciências Biológicas and of the Laboratório de Bacteriologia Aplicada, Escola de Veterinária of the Universidade Federal de Minas Gerais. *C. pseudotuberculosis* biovars Ovis and Equi were aerobically grown in brain heart infusion (BHI) (Acumedia Manufacturers, Baltimore, USA) agar plates at 37 °C for 48 h. The *C. pseudotuberculosis* isolates were identified by standard biochemical tests [9, 28, 29]. Nitrate reduction was assessed using nitrate broth (Merck, Billerica, USA) and further reduction beyond nitrite was tested by addition of zinc dust (Sigma-Aldrich, St Louis, USA) [28].

Genomic DNA extraction, primers, and quadruplex PCR

Genomic DNA extraction were performed according to the previously described protocol [30]. The oligonucleotide primers used in this study are listed in Table 2. Primers used to target *16S* rRNA, *rpoB*, and *pld* genes of *C. pseudotuberculosis* were previously described [14, 31, 32]. Primers targeting the *narG* gene were designed by aligning the *narG* nucleotide sequences of *C. pseudotuberculosis* biovar Equi strains available from the whole genome sequenced strains (Table 1). Quadruplex PCR were carried out in a final volume of 50 μL, containing 20 ng of genomic DNA, 1 μM of each primer, 0.25 mM dNTPs, 1 units of *Taq* DNA polymerase (Life Technologies, Carlsbad, USA), 2 mM $MgCl_2$, and 1X buffer (200 mM Tris-HCl pH 8.4, 500 mM KCl) (Life Technologies, Carlsbad, USA). Amplification was performed using the thermal cycler (PTC-100, MJ Research, Hercules, USA) as follows: the first denaturation at 95 °C for 4 min; followed by 30 cycles of denaturation at 95 °C for 30 s, annealing at 58 °C for the 30s, and extension at 72 °C for 1.5 min. The amplified products were submitted to electrophoresis in 1.0% agarose gel (*w*/*v*) in Tris-borate-EDTA (TBE) buffer (89 mM Tris Base, 89 mM Boric Acid and 2 mM EDTA pH 8.0), stained with 0.5 mg / mL ethidium bromide and visualized under UV light.

Table 1 *Corynebacterium pseudotuberculosis* strains with the whole genome sequenced available in the NCBI GenBank (www.ncbi.nlm.nih.gov/genbank) in 2015

Strain	Biovar	Host	Country	Genome size (MB)	Sequencing status	NCBI access	Reference
1002	Ovis	Goat	Brazil,	2.33511	Complete	NC_017300.1	(37)
C231	Ovis	Sheep	Australia	2.32821	Complete	NC_017301.1	(37)
FRC41	Ovis	Human	France	2.33791	Complete	NC_014329.1	(38)
I19	Ovis	Cow	Israel	2.33773	Complete	NC_017303.1	(39)
PAT10	Ovis	Sheep	Argentine	2.33532	Complete	NC_017305.1	(40)
42/02-A	Ovis	Sheep	Australia	2.33761	Complete	NC_017306.1	(41)
3/99–5	Ovis	Sheep	Scotland	2.33794	Complete	NC_016781.1	(41)
267	Ovis	Llama	USA	2.33763	Complete	NC_017462.1	(6)
P54B96	Ovis	Antelope	South Africa	2.33794	Complete	NC_017031.1	(42)
CIP5297	Equi	Horse	Kenya	2.32059	Complete	NC_017307.1	(43)
1/06-A	Equi	Horse	USA	2.27912	Complete	NC_017308.1	(44)
316	Equi	Horse	USA	2.31041	Complete	NC_016932.1	(45)
258	Equi	Horse	Belgium	2.36982	Complete	NC_017945.1	(46)
162	Equi	Camel	UK	2.29346	Complete	NC_018019.1	(42)
31	Equi	Buffalo	Egypt	2.38969	Complete	NC_017730.1	(47)
262	Equi	Cattle	Belgium	2.32575	Complete	NZ_CP012022.1	–
MB20	Equi	Horse	USA	2.36309	Draft	JPUV01	(48)
E19	Equi	Horse	Unknow	2.36796	Complete	NZ_CP012136.1	–
CCUG27541	Equi	Horse	Unknow	2.37942	Draft	JPJB01	(49)

Table 2 List of oligonucleotide primers used in this study

Target gene	Primers	Sequence (5′ → 3′)	Amplicom size (bp)	Multiplex PCR assay	Reference
16S rRNA[a]	Forward	ACCGCACTTTAGTGTGTGTG	816	Yes	(25)
	Reverse	TCTCTACGCCGATCTTGTAT			
rpoB[a]	Forward	CGTATGAACATCGGCCAGGT	446	Yes	(26)
	Reverse	TCCATTTCGCCGAAGCGCTG			
pld[a]	Forward	ATAAGCGTAAGCAGGGAGCA	203	Yes	(14)
	Reverse	ATCAGCGGTGATTGTCTTCCAGG			
narG[a]	Forward	ACCCGTACTTGCACTCTTTC	612	Yes	Present Study
	Reverse	AGTCAGTACTTCCGCAGGTC			
narT	Forward	GCTGAAGCAAGTTCGTGTCT	202	No	Present Study
	Reverse	GTAACGGTCAGAGAACCATCC			
narK	Forward	GCTGAAGCAAGTTCGTGTCT	202	No	Present Study
	Reverse	GTAACGGTCAGAGAACCATCC			
narG2	Forward	CAACGTGGTACCTGGTATCTG	200	No	Present Study
	Reverse	CATAGGGAGAGCGAGAACAA			
narH	Forward	GATTCTACTGACCGCCATCTC	196	No	Present Study
	Reverse	ATCAGTACCTGTCATGCCTACC			
narJ	Forward	CGTGATGGTATAGAGGTGCTG	198	No	Present Study
	Reverse	GTTGGAAGCAGTAGGGAAGGGAG			
narI	Forward	CTGTATCCACACAGGTGTTCG	215	No	Present Study
	Reverse	GTATCCTACAGGCGCTGAGA			

[a]Primers used to quadriplex PCR assay

Sequencing of singleplex PCR products

In order to confirm the quadruplex PCR results, ten randomly chosen isolates were tested further in singleplex PCR assays with the four *C. pseudotuberculosis*-specific primer pairs. PCR products were purified using Agencourt AMPure XP (Beckman Coulter Company, Beverly, Massachusetts, USA) according to the manufacturer's instructions, and each product was sequenced in both directions using primers targeting the 16S rRNA, *rpoB*, *pld* and *narG* gene and the Big Dye V3.1 Terminator Kit (Applied Biosystems, USA) using an ABI 3500 DNA analyzer (Applied Biosystems, California, USA). Sequences were analyzed on the Geneious suite of molecular biology (http://www.geneious.com) with 16S rRNA (GenBank accession nos X81916, X81907, and X84255), *rpoB* (GenBank accession no. AY492239), *pld* (GenBank accession nos L16586 and L16587) and *narG* (GenBank accession no AJF93840.1) as the reference genes.

Statistical analysis

Comparison between nitrate reduction test and quadruplex PCR was performed by McNemar's Chi-squared test, and the agreement was calculated using the kappa statistic. Statistical analysis were performed using the packages psych [33] and epibasix [34] on R software version 3.2.3 [35].

Results

Comparative genome analysis showed that *C. pseudotuberculosis* biovar Equi strains (258, 31, 262, MB20, E19 and CCUG27541) had *narKGHJI* gene clusters, however strains 1/06-A, 316, 162, and CIP52.97, although showing positive results in the nitrate reduction test, did not exhibit *narKGHJI* operon in their genome. On the other hand, genomic sequence analysis identified partial genes *molB, narJ, moeA,* and *moeB* in the strains 1/06-A, 162 and CIP52.97.

Since the strains 1/06-A, 316, 162, and CIP52.97 were nitrate reductase positive in biochemical test and the genes were not identified in their genomes, primers to target *narKGHJI* cluster and *narT* gene were designed (Table 2). The PCR tests (Additional file 1: Figure S1), sequencing and the optical map showed that the genes for *narKGHJI* and *narT* are present in the genomes of those strains (data not shown).

The multiplex PCR assay that targets *16S rRNA*, *rpoB* and *pld* genes [14] was improved by the inclusion of *C. pseudotuberculosis* biovar-specific primers for the *narG* gene (*narG* – Table 2), in a novel quadruplex PCR assay (Fig. 1). The assessment of our quadruplex PCR assay was performed in a double-blind fashion. The results of the quadruplex PCR of the 348 previously well-characterized strains of *C. pseudotuberculosis* from different hosts (goats, sheep, horse, cattle, buffalo, llamas and humans) [21, 25–27] were compared to the results of nitrate reductase identification by biochemical test, and are shown in Table 3. The McNemar's Chi-squared test used to compare the two methods employed for *C. pseudotuberculosis* biovar identification showed no significant difference ($P = 0.75$), with an odds ratio of 1 (95% CI for the odds ratio: 0.16–6.14) between the quadruplex PCR and the nitrate biochemical test. Concordant results were observed for 97.13% (338/348) of the strains (Table 3), and the kappa statistic value was 0.94 [95% CI (0.90–0.98)], denoting excellent concordance between biochemical and molecular tests for nitrate reductase identification. The limit of detection of the new quadruplex PCR was 200 ng of DNA from *C. pseudotuberculosis* biovar Equi, which corresponds to approximately 100 bacteria.

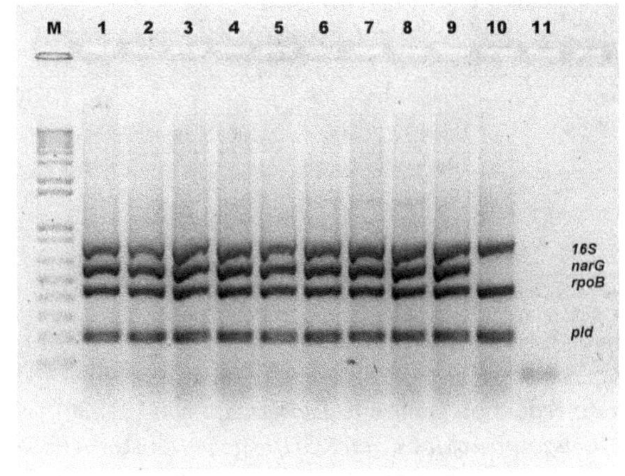

Fig. 1 Four-primer quadruplex PCR for *C. pseudotuberculosis* species and biovar identification.Agarose gel 1.5% showing the PCR amplification of quadruplex PCR assay stained with ethidium bromide (0.5 mg / mL).L: GeneRuler DNA Ladder (Fermentas, Vilnius, Lithuania); Lanes 1–9:*C. pseudotuberculosis* biovar Equi strains C31, 258, 262, 162, 5297, 1/06A, EG-37, EG-42 and I-37; Lane 10:*C. pseudotuberculosis* biovar Ovis strain 1002

Discussion

Previously, identification of *C. pseudotuberculosis* biovars was only possible only through the established procedures that included isolation and identification of the agent using biochemical tests such as the nitrate reduction test, which separates the nitrate-positive biovar Equi from nitrate negative biovar Ovis strains [5]. Herein, we developed, by the addition of a new oligonucleotide primer pair targeting the *nar*G gene to the former multiplex PCR assay [14], a robust new assay for identification of *C. pseudotuberculosis* at species and biovar levels.

The comparative genome analysis showed in *C. pseudotuberculosis* biovar Equi strains (258, 31, 262, MB20, E19 and CCUG27541) *narKGHJI* gene clusters that participate via the respiratory anaerobic process of the

Table 3 Comparison of biochemical test and a multiplex PCR assay employed for *Corynebacterium pseudotuberculosis* biovar identification

Multiplex PCR assay	Biochemical test		TOTAL
	Nitrate positive	Nitrate negative	
Nitrate positive	133	5	138
Nitrate negative	5	205	210
Total	138	210	348

McNemar's Chi-squared test = P = 0.75, Odds Ratio: 1 (95% CI for the odds ratio: 0.16–6.14)
Kappa coefficient = 0.94 (95% CI: 0.91–0.98)

nitrate reduction similar to *Escherichia coli* [21, 36]. The *C. pseudotuberculosis narKGHJI* gene cluster showed significant similarity with the protein sequences found in other Actinomycetes, such as *C. diphtheriae*, *C. glutamicum*, and *Mycobacterium tuberculosis.* All *C. pseudotuberculosis* biovar Ovis strains do not present any gene of the *narKGHJI* operon in their genomes [21].

The nitrate *locus* in *C. pseudotuberculosis* is composed of the *narKGHJI* operon and by a cluster of genes encoding the molybdopterin *moeB, moaE, molB, molA, moeY, moaC, moeA,* and *moaA* (Fig. 2) [21]. Molybdopterin is a cofactor that is indispensable for the activity of nitrate reductase. In the *narGHI* complex, the *narG* gene is a member of a superfamily of enzymes that use a Molybdopterin-guanine-dinucleotide (Mo-bisMGD) cofactor (bisMGD) for their catalytic activity.

Our results showed that among the 348 *C. pseudotuberculosis* tested, only 10 strains (2.87%) showed differences between the biovar classification provided by molecular and biochemical tests (Table 3), which was observed even after repeating the assays. Furthermore, the kappa coefficient, which is a robust statistic that measures inter-rater agreement for qualitative items, confirms that regardless of the technique used for biovar classification the results obtained were very similar. It is also important to consider that kappa values range from −1 to +1, where 1 represents a perfect agreement between the raters, and 0.81 to 1.00 represents almost perfect agreement, such as the observed in our data (0.94) [28, 37]. Discordance between both phenotypic and genotypic methods can be explained by the effect of environmental factors on gene expression [29, 38] amino-acid substitution, the genetic background of the strain (that can vary according to geographical locations) and mutations. Considering discordances due to mutations genotypic tests have proven to be more reliable and sensitive as diagnostic tool than phenotypic tests [30–32, 39–42]. Others studies also showed discordant results between genotypic versus phenotypic methods [30–32, 39–41, 43, 44].

To our acknowledgement, this is the first molecular approach able to clearly differentiate between *C. pseudotuberculosis* biovar Ovis and Equi, although different restriction patterns, ribotypes and ERIC-PCR clustering pattern have been associated to biovars [26, 36, 45–47]. The advantages of multiplex PCR assay over biochemical tests are the speed, performance and reproducibility, and the ability to test large numbers of isolates simultaneously [26, 45, 46]. Identification is based upon the number and sizes of four products amplified by PCR. Moreover, the use of molecular techniques reduces the manipulation of viable bacteria in the laboratory and consequently the risk of accidental infection, as *C. pseudotuberculosis* can eventually be a zoonotic agent [2]. Moreover, this new diagnostic tool, the quadruplex PCR assay for identification and

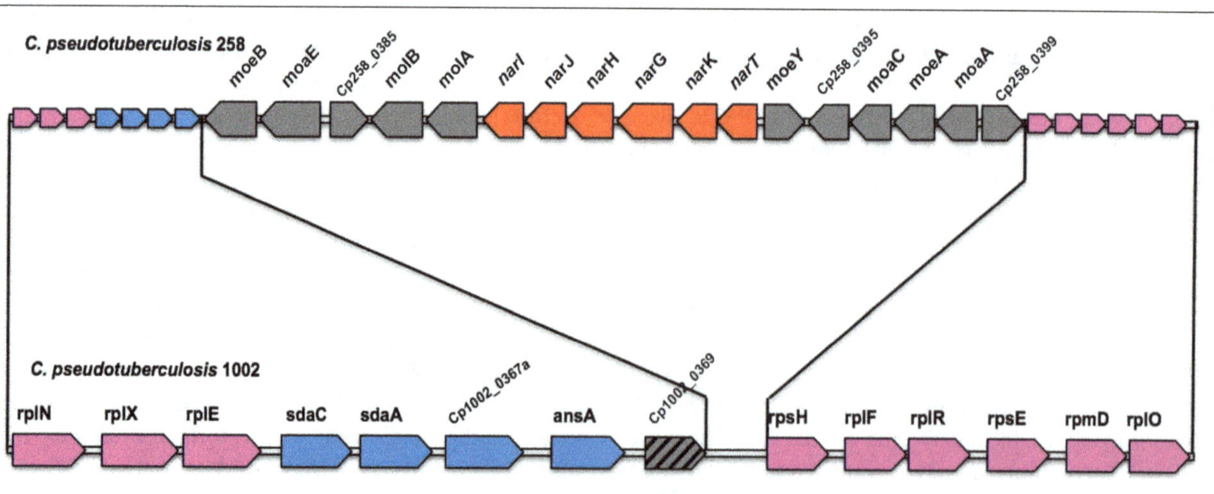

Fig. 2 Nitrate *locus* from *C. pseudotuberculosis* biovar Equi.This *locus* contains: the genes encoding the molybdopterin *moeB, moaE, molB, molA, moeY, moaC, moeA* and *moaA* and the genes encoding the nitrate reductase *narK, narG, narH, narJ, narI.* Insertion show between *ansA* and *rpsH* genes is lacking in nitrate negative *C. pseudotuberculosis* biovar Ovis strains. Arrows represent open reading frames and their orientations. Blue and pink: common genes shared between *C. pseudotuberculosis* biovar Ovis and biovar Equi strains. Pink: ribosomal proteins. Hatched: additional or different genes. Red: *narKGHJI* operon and grey: genes encoding the molybdopterin *moeB, moaE, molB, molA, moeY, moaC, moeA* and *moaA*

biotyping of *C. pseudotuberculosis* follows the new trends on clinical microbiology laboratory that is currently incorporating more molecular biology tools in its routine [23, 48]. In addition, despite not having been tested in the present study, due to its analytical sensitivity of 100 bacteria. |It is likely that this quadruplex PCR can also be applied to direct testing from clinical samples, as it has been done successfully for the three-primer (*16S* rRNA, *rpoB*, and *pld*) multiplex PCR [14].

The quadruplex PCR proposed in this study facilitates and deepens the level of identification of *C. pseudotuberculosis* strains at clinical microbiology laboratory, and thereby improves the diagnosis of infection by providing more information for decision making. These results are especially significant considering that *C. pseudotuberculosis* infects a wide range of hosts and produce different clinical manifestations. Furthermore, it was recently suggested that *C. pseudotuberculosis* biovars have differences at the molecular phylogenetic level, indicating an anagenesis process within the species [37, 49]. The evolutionary analysis of conserved genes (*rpoB, gapA, fusA,* and *rsmE*) suggesting a gradual anagenesis of *C. pseudotuberculosis* in that study [49] substantially increases the importance of a molecular technique capable of efficiently separating the biovars Ovis and Equi. In fact, a pan-genome analysis of fifteen *C. pseudotuberculosis* strains showed a significant number of genes not shared by both biovars, including remarkable differences in the 16 detected pathogenicity islands [50].

In this study, it was also observed that some *C. pseudotuberculosis* strains (1/06-A, 316, 162 and CIP52.97) were able to reduce nitrate when tested by the biochemical approach and were also positive in the quadruplex PCR assay, albeit did not show in their genomes genes associated with nitrate reduction. The genomic analysis of nitrate *locus* identified that partial genes encoding the molybdopterin and *narKGHJI* operon of these strains was absent [21]. These results may have been due to low overall coverage, poor capture efficiency of certain regions, genomic regions that were previously not assembled or poorly assembled, including unambiguously aligning repetitive regions, such as transposons, and difficulty in unambiguously aligning repetitive regions [41, 51]. Then, after resequencing of the *narKGHJI* operon region and optical mapping of these strains, it was observed that these strains have the nitrate *locus* in their genome and corrections on their information on GenBank are under way.

Conclusions

A novel quadruplex PCR assay for *C. pseudotuberculosis* species and biovar identification was developed. The nitrate reductase gene *narG* was included in the assay along with the *16S, rpoB* and *pld* genes to improve the diagnosis of the multiplex PCR at biovar level. There was a significant concordance between the biovar classification provided by the molecular and biochemical test. The ability of the expanded quadruplex PCR assay to discriminate between *C. pseudotuberculosis* biovar Ovis and Equi strains enhances its value.

Abbreviations

CLA: Caseous Lymphadenitis; Mo-bisMGD: Molybdopterin-guanine-dinucleotide; NAR: Nitrate Reductase; OSD: Oedematous Skin Disease

Acknowledgements

This study was supported by the Conselho Nacional de Desenvolvimento Científico e Tecnológico (CNPq) and the Fundação de Amparo à Pesquisa do Estado de Minas Gerais (Fapemig). APL and VA thanks CNPq for their fellowships. APL is also indebted to Programa Pesquisador Mineiro (PPM 00923-15) - Fapemig.

Funding

APL was supported by the Programa Pesquisador Mineiro – PPM (00923–15) from Fapemig and SA was supported by the Universal (481,792/2013–9) from Conselho Nacional de Desenvolvimento Científico e Tecnológico (CNPq).

Authors' contributions

SA: drafted and wrote the manuscript, and analyzed the data. ED: drafted the manuscript and performed biochemistry tests. CD: performed biochemistry tests. VACA: development of scripts and computational analysis. CS, JA and PB performed laboratory experiments. VA, DB and AL: wrote the manuscript. VA, AC, SS, AL and HF: contributed to conception and design. All authors read and approved the final manuscript.

Competing interests

The authors declare that they have no competing interests.

Author details

[1]Instituto de Ciências Biológicas, Federal University of Minas Gerais, Belo Horizonte, MG, Brazil. [2]Escola de Veterinária, Federal University of Minas Gerais, Belo Horizonte, MG, Brazil. [3]Departamento de Medicina Veterinária, Federal University of Lavras, Lavras, MG, Brazil. [4]Centro de Energia Nuclear na Agricultura, University of Sao Paulo, Piracicaba, SP, Brazil. [5]Instituto de Ciências Biológicas, Federal University of Para, Belém, PA, Brazil. [6]Department of Medicine and Epidemiology, UC Davis School of Veterinary Medicine, Davis, CA, USA. [7]Centre for Genomics and Applied Gene Technology, Institute of Integrative Omics and Applied Biotechnology (IIOAB), Nonakuri, Purba Medinipur, WB, India. [8]Aquacen - National Reference Laboratory for Aquatic Animal Diseases, Federal University of Minas Gerais, Belo Horizonte, MG, Brazil.

References

1. Shpigel NY, Elad D, Yeruham I, Winkler M, Saran A. An outbreak of Corynebacterium pseudotuberculosis infection in an Israeli dairy herd. Vet. Rec. 1993;133:89–94.
2. Peel MM, Palmer GG, Stacpoole AM, Kerr TG. Human lymphadenitis due to Corynebacterium pseudotuberculosis: report of ten cases from Australia and review. Clin. Infect. Dis. Off. Publ. Infect. Dis. Soc. Am. 1997;24:185–91.
3. Lopes T, Silva A, Thiago R, Carneiro A, Dorella FA, Rocha FS, et al. Complete genome sequence of Corynebacterium pseudotuberculosis strain Cp267, isolated from a llama. J Bacteriol. 2012;194:3567–8.
4. Tejedor-Junco MT, Lupiola P, Schulz U, Gutierrez C. Isolation of nitrate-reductase positive Corynebacterium pseudotuberculosis from dromedary camels. Trop Anim Health Prod. 2008;40:165–7.

References

1. Shpigel NY, Elad D, Yeruham I, Winkler M, Saran A. An outbreak of Corynebacterium pseudotuberculosis infection in an Israeli dairy herd. Vet. Rec. 1993;133:89–94.
2. Peel MM, Palmer GG, Stacpoole AM, Kerr TG. Human lymphadenitis due to Corynebacterium pseudotuberculosis: report of ten cases from Australia and review. Clin. Infect. Dis. Off. Publ. Infect. Dis. Soc. Am. 1997;24:185–91.
3. Lopes T, Silva A, Thiago R, Carneiro A, Dorella FA, Rocha FS, et al. Complete genome sequence of Corynebacterium pseudotuberculosis strain Cp267, isolated from a llama. J Bacteriol. 2012;194:3567–8.
4. Tejedor-Junco MT, Lupiola P, Schulz U, Gutierrez C. Isolation of nitrate-reductase positive Corynebacterium pseudotuberculosis from dromedary camels. Trop Anim Health Prod. 2008;40:165–7.
5. Biberstein EL, Knight HD, Jang S. Two biotypes of Corynebacterium pseudotuberculosis. Vet. Rec. 1971;89:691–2.
6. Selim SA. Oedematous skin disease of buffalo in Egypt. J. Vet. Med. B infect. Dis. Vet. Public Health. 2001;48:241–58.
7. Pratt SM, Spier SJ, Carroll SP, Vaughan B, Whitcomb MB, Wilson WD. Evaluation of clinical characteristics, diagnostic test results, and outcome in horses with internal infection caused by Corynebacterium pseudotuberculosis: 30 cases (1995-2003). J Am Vet Med Assoc. 2005;227:441–8.
8. Baird GJ, Fontaine MC. Corynebacterium pseudotuberculosis and its role in ovine caseous lymphadenitis. J Comp Pathol. 2007;137:179–210.
9. Guimarães, Alessandro de Sá, Carmo, Filipe Borges, Pauletti, Rebeca Barbosa, Seyffert, Núbia, Ribeiro, Dayana, Lage, Andrey Pereira, et al. Caseous lymphadenitis: epidemiology, diagnosis, and control. IIOAB J. 2011;2:33–43.
10. Shigidi MT. A comparison of five serological tests for the diagnosis of experimental Corynebacterium Ovis infection in sheep. Br Vet J. 1979;135:172–7.
11. Brown CC, Olander HJ, Alves SF. Synergistic hemolysis-inhibition titers associated with caseous lymphadenitis in a slaughterhouse survey of goats and sheep in northeastern Brazil. Can. J. Vet. Res. Rev. Can. Rech. Vét. 1987;51:46–9.
12. Menzies PI, Muckle CA. The use of a microagglutination assay for the detection of antibodies to Corynebacterium pseudotuberculosis in naturally infected sheep and goat flocks. Can J Vet Res Rev Can Rech Vét. 1989;53:313–8.
13. Dercksen DP, Brinkhof JM, Dekker-Nooren T, Maanen K, Bode CF, Baird G, et al. A comparison of four serological tests for the diagnosis of caseous lymphadenitis in sheep and goats. Vet Microbiol. 2000;75:167–75.
14. Pacheco LGC, Pena RR, Castro TLP, Dorella FA, Bahia RC, Carminati R, et al. Multiplex PCR assay for identification of Corynebacterium pseudotuberculosis from pure cultures and for rapid detection of this pathogen in clinical samples. J Med Microbiol. 2007;56:480–6.
15. Williams RA, Sadler SA. Electrophoresis of glucose-6-phosphate dehydrogenase, cell wall composition and the taxonomy of heterofermentative lactobacilli. J Gen Microbiol. 1971;65:351–8.
16. Sankarasubramanian J, Vishnu US, Gunasekaran P, Rajendhran J. A genome-wide SNP-based phylogenetic analysis distinguishes different biovars of Brucella suis. Infect Genet Evol. 2016;41:213–7.
17. Yeruham I, Braverman Y, Shpigel NY, Chizov-Ginzburg A, Saran A, Winkler M. Mastitis in dairy cattle caused by Corynebacterium pseudotuberculosis and the feasibility of transmission by houseflies. I Vet Q. 1996;18:87–9.
18. Yeruham I, Elad D, Van-Ham M, Shpigel NY, Perl S. Corynebacterium pseudotuberculosis infection in Israeli cattle: clinical and epidemiological studies. Vet. Rec. 1997;140:423–7.
19. Steinman A, Elad D, Shpigel NY. Ulcerative lymphangitis and coronet lesions in an Israeli dairy herd infected with Corynebacterium pseudotuberculosis. Vet. Rec. 1999;145:604–6.
20. Yeruham I, Elad D, Perl S, Ram A. Necrotic-ulcerative dermatitis on the heels of heifers in a dairy herd infected with Corynebacterium pseudotuberculosis. Vet Rec. 2003;152:598–600.
21. Almeida S, Sousa C, Abreu V, Diniz C, Dorneles EMS, Lage AP, et al. Exploration of nitrate Reductase metabolic pathway in *Corynebacterium pseudotuberculosis*. Int J Genomics. 2017;2017:1–12.
22. Gonçalves JL, Tomazi T, Barreiro JR, Braga PA, Ferreira CR, Araújo Junior JP, et al. Identification of Corynebacterium spp. isolated from bovine intramammary infections by matrix-assisted laser desorption ionization-time of flight mass spectrometry. Vet Microbiol. 2014;173:147–151.
23. Raoult D, Fournier PE, Drancourt M. What does the future hold for clinical microbiology? Nat. Rev. Microbiol. 2004;2:151–9.
24. Langoni H, Camargo da Silva CP, Troncarelli MZ, Tata A, Belaz KRA, Eberlin MN, et al. Short communication: identification of Corynebacterium Bovis by matrix-assisted laser desorption/ionization mass spectrometry. J Dairy Sci. [Internet]. 2017 [cited 2017 Apr 1]; Available from: http://linkinghub.elsevier.com/retrieve/pii/S0022030217302539
25. Ade Guimarães S, EMS D, Andrade GI, Lage AP, Miyoshi A, Azevedo V, et al. Molecular characterization of Corynebacterium pseudotuberculosis isolates using ERIC-PCR. Vet Microbiol. 2011;153:299–306.
26. Dorneles EMS, Santana JA, Ribeiro D, Dorella FA, Guimarães AS, Moawad MS, et al. Evaluation of ERIC-PCR as genotyping method for Corynebacterium pseudotuberculosis isolates. PLoS One. 2014;9:e98758.
27. Dorneles EMS, Santana JA, Andrade GI, Santos ELS, Guimarães AS, Mota RA, et al. Molecular characterization of Corynebacterium pseudotuberculosis isolated from goats using ERIC-PCR. Genet Mol Res GMR. 2012;11:2051–9.
28. MacFaddin JF. Biochemical tests for identification of medical bacteria. 3rd ed. Philadelphia: Lippincott Williams & Wilkins; 2000.
29. Coyle MB, Lipsky BA. Coryneform bacteria in infectious diseases: clinical and laboratory aspects. Clin Microbiol Rev. 1990;3:227–46.
30. Pitcher DG, Saunders NA, Owen RJ. Rapid extraction of bacterial genomic DNA with guanidium thiocyanate. Lett Appl Microbiol. 1989;8:151–6.
31. Cetinkaya B, Karahan M, Atil E, Kalin R, De Baere T, Vaneechoutte M. Identification of Corynebacterium pseudotuberculosis isolates from sheep and goats by PCR. Vet Microbiol. 2002;88:75–83.
32. Khamis A, Raoult D, La Scola B. rpoB gene sequencing for identification of Corynebacterium species. J Clin Microbiol. 2004;42:3925–31.
33. Revelle, W. psych: Procedures for Psychological, Psychometric, and Personality Research [Internet]. Northwestern University, Evanston, Illinois, USA.; 2015. Available from: https://cran.r-project.org/web/packages/psych/index.html
34. Rotondi, M. A. epibasix: Elementary Epidemiological Functions for Epidemiology and Biostatistics [Internet]. 2012. Available from: https://cran.r-project.org/web/packages/epibasix/index.html.
35. R Development Core Team. R: A Language and Environment for Statistical Computing. Vienna, Austria : the R Foundation for Statistical Computing; 2011.
36. Clegg S, Yu F, Griffiths L, Cole JA. The roles of the polytopic membrane proteins NarK, NarU and NirC in Escherichia Coli K-12: two nitrate and three nitrite transporters. Mol Microbiol. 2002;44:143–55.
37. Cohen J. A coefficient of agreement for nominal scales. Educ Psychol Meas. 1960;20:37–46.
38. Asfour HAE, Darwish SF. Evaluation of phenotypic methods versus molecular methods for differentiation of Coagulase positive staphylococci causing bovine mastitis with a special reference to atypical Staphylococcus Aureus. Int J Curr Microbiol Appl Sci. 2014;3(5):543–58.
39. Campbell EA, Pavlova O, Zenkin N, Leon F, Irschik H, Jansen R, et al. Structural, functional, and genetic analysis of sorangicin inhibition of bacterial RNA polymerase. EMBO J. 2005;24:674–82.
40. Gagneux S, Long CD, Small PM, Van T, Schoolnik GK, Bohannan BJM. The competitive cost of antibiotic resistance in mycobacterium tuberculosis. Science. 2006;312:1944–6.
41. Ocheretina O, Escuyer VE, Mabou M-M, Royal-Mardi G, Collins S, Vilbrun SC, et al. Correlation between Genotypic and Phenotypic Testing for Resistance to Rifampin in Mycobacterium tuberculosis Clinical Isolates in Haiti: Investigation of Cases with Discrepant Susceptibility Results. Mokrousov I, editor. PLoS ONE. 2014;9:e90569.
42. Yang B. Relationship between antimycobacterial activities of rifampicin, rifabutin and KRM-1648 and rpoB mutations of mycobacterium tuberculosis. J Antimicrob Chemother. 1998;42:621–8.
43. Boehme CC, Nicol MP, Nabeta P, Michael JS, Gotuzzo E, Tahirli R, et al. Feasibility, diagnostic accuracy, and effectiveness of decentralised use of the Xpert MTB/RIF test for diagnosis of tuberculosis and multidrug resistance: a multicentre implementation study. Lancet. 2011;377:1495–505.
44. Yang H, Qin L, Wang Y, Zhang B, Liu Z, Ma H, et al. Detection of mycobacterium tuberculosis based on H37Rv binding peptides using surface functionalized magnetic microspheres coupled with quantum dots - a nano detection method for mycobacterium tuberculosis. Int J Nanomedicine. 2015;10:77–88.
45. Songer JG, Beckenbach K, Marshall MM, Olson GB, Kelley L. Biochemical and genetic characterization of Corynebacterium pseudotuberculosis. Am J Vet Res. 1988;49:223–6.

46. Sutherland SS, Hart RA, Buller NB. Genetic differences between nitrate-negative and nitrate-positive C. Pseudotuberculosis strains using restriction fragment length polymorphisms. Vet. Microbiol. 1996;49:1–9.
47. Tan MP, Sequeira P, Lin WW, Phong WY, Cliff P, Ng SH, et al. Nitrate Respiration Protects Hypoxic Mycobacterium tuberculosis Against Acid- and Reactive Nitrogen Species Stresses. Neyrolles O, editor. PLoS ONE. 2010;5:e13356.
48. Fournier P-E, Drancourt M, Colson P, Rolain J-M, Scola BL, Raoult D. Modern clinical microbiology: new challenges and solutions. Nat Rev Microbiol. 2013;11:574–85.
49. Oliveira A, Teixeira P, Azevedo M, Jamal SB, Tiwari S, Almeida S, et al. Corynebacterium pseudotuberculosis may be under anagenesis and biovar Equi forms biovar Ovis: a phylogenic inference from sequence and structural analysis. BMC Microbiol. 2016;16:100.
50. Soares SC, Trost E, Ramos RTJ, Carneiro AR, Santos AR, Pinto AC, et al. Genome sequence of Corynebacterium pseudotuberculosis biovar equi strain 258 and prediction of antigenic targets to improve biotechnological vaccine production. J Biotechnol. 2013;167:135–41.
51. Faino L, Seidl MF, Datema E, van den Berg GCM, Janssen A, AHJ W, et al. Single-molecule real-time sequencing combined with optical mapping yields completely finished fungal genome. MBio. 2015;6:e00936–15.

7

Comparison of the fecal bacterial microbiota of healthy and diarrheic foals at two and four weeks of life

A. Schoster[1,2*], H.R. Staempfli[3], L.G. Guardabassi[2,4], M. Jalali[5] and J.S. Weese[5]

Abstract

Background: Diarrhea in foals affects up to 60% of foals during the first six months of life. The effect of diarrhea on the fecal bacterial microbiota in foals has not been investigated. Little is known on the fecal bacterial microbial richness and diversity of foals at a young age. The objective was to compare the fecal bacterial microbiota of healthy foals to foals with diarrhea at two and four weeks of life.

Methods: Fecal samples were collected from foals (n = 20) at 1–14 (T1) and 15–28 (T2) days of age and analyzed using high throughput sequencing. Differences in relative abundance of bacterial taxa, alpha diversity and beta diversity indices were assessed between age-matched foals with diarrhea (n = 9) and healthy foals (n = 11), and between time points.

Results: Differences in microbial community composition based on time point and health status were observed on all taxonomic levels. Of 117 enriched species in healthy foals at T2, 50 (48%) were Lachnospiraceae or Ruminococcaceae. The Chao richness index was increased in healthy foals at T2 compared to T1 (p = 0.02). Foals with diarrhea had a significantly lower richness index than non-diarrheic foals at T2 (p = 0.04). Diarrhea had an inconsistent effect, while time point had a consistent effect on microbial community structure.

Conclusions: Preventative and therapeutic measures for diarrhea should focus on maintaining bacterial microbiota richness. Lachnospiraceae and Ruminococcaceae were underrepresented in foals with diarrhea. These should be evaluated further as potential therapeutic options.

Keywords: Gastrointestinal microbiota, Metagenomic sequencing, Horse, Lachnospiraceae, Ruminococcaceae, Clostridiales

Background

The bacterial microbiota plays a key role in human and animal health. Recent studies indicate that imbalances in the microbial communities and their function (dysbiosis) can be associated with diseases in the gastrointestinal tract and beyond [1]. Dysbiosis in horses has been associated with colitis [2], laminitis [3, 4], equine grass sickness [5], colic [6], and transient diarrhea in foals, known as foal heat diarrhea [7].

* Correspondence: aschoster@vetclinics.uzh.ch
[1]Equine Department, University of Zurich, Vetsuisse Faculty, Winterthurerstrasse 260, 8057 Zurich, Zurich, Switzerland
[2]Department of Veterinary Disease Biology, University of Copenhagen, Faculty of Health and Medical Science, Stigbojlen 4, 1870, Copenhagen, Denmark
Full list of author information is available at the end of the article

Age affects the composition of the gastrointestinal microbiota in humans and animals [8, 9]. The meconium of human infants already contains a distinct microbiota, and gastrointestinal colonization further develops upon contact with the maternal microbiota and environmental bacteria [10]. There have been limited studies in horses using techniques that can adequately evaluate the complex structure of gut microbial communities [11, 12]. A recent next generation sequencing based study reported that the fecal bacterial microbiota of foals is highly variable early in life, but reaches a relatively stable population by approximately 60 days of age [9]. However, the bacterial microbiota continues to develop throughout adolescence. Differences in community structure, evidenced by how many and which species are present as well as their relative abundance, are still present in foals after 60 days of age compared to adult horse [9].

Foal diarrhea is common and important, reportedly affecting 60% of foals during their first six months of life [13]. A single causative agent is often not identified [14]. Acute diarrhea is associated with significant changes in the fecal bacterial microbiota of adult horses. Marked differences in composition of the fecal bacterial microbiota over all taxonomic levels and decreases in bacterial diversity, evenness and richness have been described [2, 15]. Despite the high prevalence of foal diarrhea, there is currently little knowledge about the fecal bacterial microbiota of foals affected by diarrhea. A culture-based study showed that changes in the fecal bacterial microbiota over time did not differ between foals with diarrhea and healthy foals [7]; however, culture-based methods have limited ability to appreciate the complexity of the bacterial microbiota [16].

The objectives of this study were to describe differences between foals with and without diarrhea at two and four weeks of life.

Methods

The University of Guelph Animal Care Committee (AUP 1455) approved this study.

Animals and study protocol

Foals born on one Standardbred and seven Thoroughbred farms in southern Ontario, Canada, were studied. Mares and foals were turned out on pasture during the day and stabled overnight if weather permitted. Mares were fed coastal hay ad libitum and were allowed to graze on pasture. Type and amount of supplemental feed (grain, minerals etc.) differed between farms. Probiotics were not administered to mares or foals. Fecal swabs and medical records were collected from foals as part of a separate study [14]. Experienced farm personnel recorded fecal consistency daily for 28 days on a standardized medical record sheet, which was provided. Foals were included in this study if they were born by natural delivery, were clinically normal at the time of enrollment (24 h after birth), had two fecal samples collected sequentially and had a complete medical record sheet. Exclusion criteria were presence of severe gastrointestinal disease or illness by 24 h of life as well as administration of antimicrobials, anti-inflammatories, probiotics or Biosponge[1] at any point during the study period. Sampling days were dependent on farm management, which resulted in samples being taken during two time periods 1–14 (T1) and 15–28 (T2) days of age. It was determined based on the medical record whether a foal had diarrhea at the time of sampling. Fecal samples from foals with diarrhea were collected within two days after diarrhea occurrence. Foals included in the healthy group did not have diarrhea on any day throughout the study period. The samples were stored at 4 °C for a maximum of two weeks before being transported to the laboratory where all were frozen at −80 °C until DNA extraction.

DNA extraction, 16S rRNA gene amplification, purification and sequencing

Fecal swabs were reconstituted in 1 mL of phosphate buffered saline. The suspension was centrifuged at 9800 g for 4 min and DNA was extracted from the pellet using a commercial kit (E.Z.N.A. Stool DNA Kit[2]) according to manufacturer's recommendations. Adequate DNA quality and quantity were assessed by spectrophotometry (NanoDrop[3]).

Amplification of the V4 region of the 16S rRNA gene, purification and sequencing were performed as previously described [17]. Briefly, primers targeting the V4 region of the 16S rRNA gene were designed with overhanging adapters for annealing to the Illumina index primers in the second PCR step. PCR products were purified and Illumina index primers were attached during the second PCR step. PCR products were purified and evaluated by gel-electrophoresis in 1.5% agarose gel. The samples were sequenced at the University of Guelph's Advanced Analysis Centre using an Illumina MiSeq (Illumina RTA v1.17.28; MCS v2.2).

Bioinformatics and statistics

Distribution of sex, breed and farm was compared between foals with and without diarrhea using Fisher's exact test. The age at the time of sampling between foal with and without diarrhea at a given time point was compared using the Mann-Whitney U test as data was not normally distributed.

The open-source software package, MOTHUR (v1.33.0) was used to process the sequences [18]. Paired end reads were aligned and then sequences were aligned with the SILVA 16S rRNA gene reference database (www.arb-silva.de) [19]. Sequences with ambiguous base calls, inappropriate length (>244 base pairs (bp) or <239 bp), runs of homopolymers of >8 bp, and sequences corresponding to chloroplasts, mitochondria, Archaea and Eukaryotes were removed. Chimeras were identified using uchime [20] and removed. The remaining sequences were classified using the ribosomal database project (RDP) classifier (http://rdp.cme.msu.edu/index.jsp). Subsampling was performed to normalize sequence numbers for further comparison. This consisted of random selection of a number of sequences from each sample that corresponded to the lowest sequence abundance of all samples. Completeness of sampling effort was assessed visually using rarefaction curves.

Alpha diversity was described using the Chao richness, Shannon's evenness and inverse Simpson's index. The two main factors to quantify biological diversity are richness and evenness. Richness (represented here by the Chao richness index) describes the number of species per sample. Evenness (represented by the Shannon evenness index) describes the relative abundance of the different species making up the richness. A community dominated by one or two species is considered less diverse than a community in which several species have a similar abundance. Simpsons diversity index is a measure of diversity which takes into account both richness and evenness.

Only bacterial taxa accounting for more than 1 % of the total were used for statistical analysis. Data were determined to be non-parametric based on examination of quantile plots and Shapiro-Wilk testing. Relative abundances and alpha diversity indices were compared between healthy and diarrheic foals and between age groups in healthy foals using the Wilcoxon test. Observed species richness was compared between healthy foals and foals with diarrhea and between age groups in healthy foals using the Wilcoxon matched pairs signed rank test. False discovery rate (FDR) adjustments using the Benjamin Hochberg procedure were performed for comparisons of relative abundance of taxa between age groups and between foals with and without diarrhea.

Dendograms based on community overlap (classical Jaccard index) and structure (Yue&Clayton index of dissimilarity) were created and visualized by FigTree v1.4.0 (http://tree.bio.ed.ac.uk/). Community overlap and structure were compared between groups by parsimony test, analysis of molecular variance (AMOVA), and analysis of similarities (ANOSIM) applied to the Jaccard and Yue&Clayton data, respectively. The Jaccard index is a measure of the number of species shared between two samples (richness), while the Yue&Clayton index takes into account relative abundance of each species. Dissimilarity was also visualized using principal coordinate analysis (PCoA). Linear discriminant analysis effect size (LEfSe) was performed to identify differentially abundant operational taxonomic units (OTUs) with 97% sequence similarity between groups. [21] A p-value of <0.05 was considered significant for all comparisons. A commercial program was used for all statistical analyses (JMP Statistical discoveries, Version 11).

Results

Demographic data of animals

Twenty foals, 2/20 (10%) Standardbreds and 18/20 Thoroughbreds (90%) were included. Thirteen foals (65%) were male and 7 (35%) were female. Nine of 20 (45%) foals developed diarrhea at some point during the study period (Table 1). Significantly more females developed diarrhea compared to males (p = 0.02). Breed and farm were not significantly different between foals with and without diarrhea (p = 0.19 and p = 0.23, respectively.)

Table 1 Population data on foals studied

Foal	Breed	Sex	Farm	Diarrhea	Age at T1 (days)	Age at T2 (days)	Diarrhea at T1	Diarrhea at T2
1	TB	M	1	No	8	23		
2	TB	M	2	No	4	22		
3	TB	M	1	No	14	26		
4	TB	F	2	Yes	7	17	No	Yes
5	TB	F	1	Yes	7	14	Yes	Yes
6	TB	F	3	Yes	1	15	Yes	No
7	TB	M	4	No	9	25		
8	TB	M	5	No	8	22		
9	TB	F	2	Yes	11	18	Yes	No
10	TB	M	6	No	5	25		
11	TB	M	2	No	10	28		
12	TB	M	7	Yes	7	21	No	Yes
13	TB	M	1	No	5	15		
14	TB	M	1	No	14	28		
15	SB	F	8	Yes	5	19	Yes	No
16	TB	F	6	No	9	20		
17	TB	M	7	No	10	25		
18	TB	M	7	Yes	8	22	No	Yes
19	SB	F	8	Yes	12	26	No	Yes
20	TB	M	2	Yes	5	15	No	Yes

SB Standardbred, *TB* Thoroughbred, *F* Female, *M* Male, T1: 1–14 days of age, T2: 15–28 days of age

Sequencing quality data

The DNA concentration after extraction ranged from 5 to 50 ng/μL. Final concentration of PCR products before sequencing averaged approximately 30 ng/μL. A total of 4,914,371 V4 16S RNA gene sequences passed all quality control filters. Subsampling was performed based on 29,980 sequences per sample. Sequencing depth was deemed adequate based on rarefaction curves (Additional file 1).

Microbial community composition

Twenty-nine different phyla, 71 classes, 129 orders were identified. Seven phyla, 14 classes, and 16 orders had a mean relative abundance of more than 1% (Fig. 1). Of 250 families identified, 19 had a mean relative abundance of >1%. The most abundant family was Ruminococcaceae (13.1%), followed by Lachnospiraceae (12.7%), Verrucomicrobiaceae (8.4%), Moraxellaceae (5.2%), Carnobacteriaceae (4.3%), Pseudomonaceae (3.9%), Enterobacteriaceae (3.8%), Veillonellaceae (3.6%), Lactobacillaceae (3.1%), Erysipelotrichaeceae (2.4%), Fusobacteriaceae (2.3%), Clostridiaceae I (1.9%), Bacillaceae (1.7%), Bacteroidaceae (1.5%), unclassified Subdivsion 5 (1.2%), unclassified Clostridales XI (1.1%), Caulobacteriaceae (1.3%), Enterococcaceae (1.3%) and Planococcaceae (1.2%).

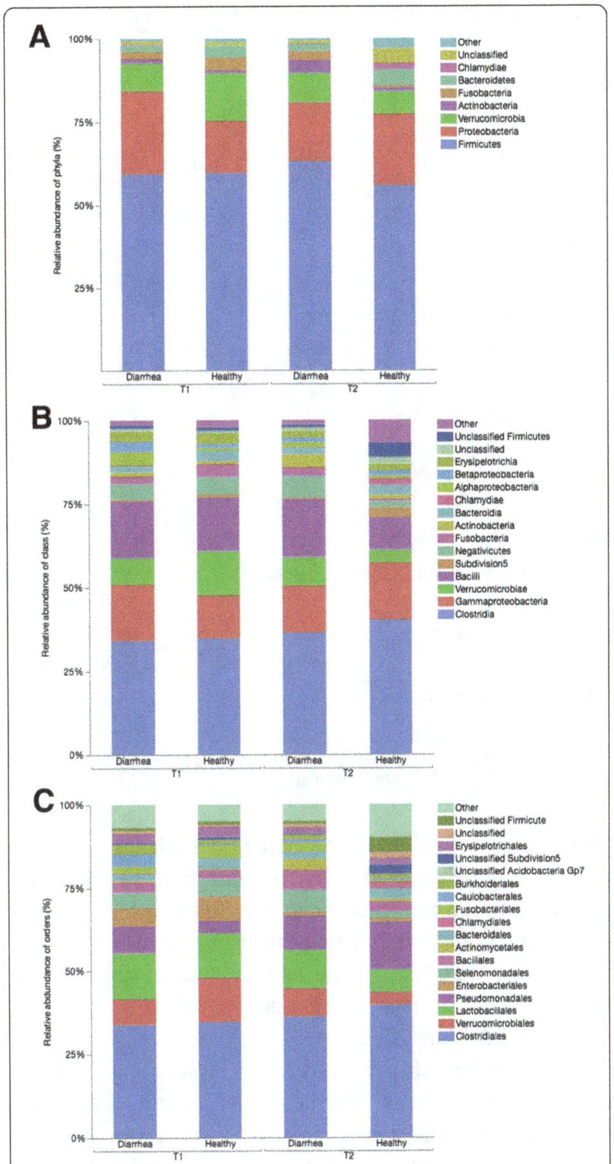

Fig. 1 Relative abundance of predominant phyla (**a**), classes (**b**), and orders (**c**), in healthy foals ($n = 11$) and foals with diarrhea ($n = 4$ at T1, $n = 3$ at T2). Other: Bacterial taxa with ≤1% abundance, Unclassified: Sequences which could not be calssified, T1: 1–14 days of age, T2: 15–28 days of age

Fecal microbial composition of healthy foals at two and four weeks of age

For comparisons between the two time points, only samples from healthy foals ($n = 11$) that did not develop diarrhea throughout the study were analyzed. There were significant differences at all taxonomic levels (Table 2). The number of observed species was significantly lower in foals at T1 compared to T2 ($p < 0.001$, Fig. 2). The estimated richness (Chao index) significantly increased over time ($p = 0.02$). The other alpha diversity indices (Simpson diversity index Shannon evenness index) were not significantly different between T1 and T2 ($p = 0.09$ and $p = 0.08$, respectively, Fig. 3).

Two distinct clusters (T1 and T2) were evident visually with PCOA based on the Jaccard and Yue&Clayton indices (Fig. 4). Samples from foals in the same age group tended to cluster together. Significant differences between T1 and T2 were identified by parsimony test for both indices (Yue&Clayton $p = 0.04$, Jaccard $p = 0.006$). Significant differences were also observed with AMOVA (Jaccard $p = 0.003$, Yue&Clayton $p = 0.001$) and ANOSIM (Jaccard $p = 0.002$, Yue&Clayton $p = 0.001$).

Fecal microbial composition between healthy and diarrheic foals

To assess the influence of diarrhea on microbial community diversity, foals with diarrhea at the time of fecal sample collection were compared to age matched healthy foals ($n = 11$). A total of nine foals developed diarrhea throughout the study period. At T1 four foals had diarrhea, at T2 six foals had diarrhea. There was no statistically significant age difference between foals with and without diarrhea at T1 or T2 ($p = 0.29$ and $p = 0.07$, respectively).

Relative abundance was not significantly different after FDR adjustment on all taxonomic levels at either time point (Table 3). At T1, eight taxa were identified as enriched using LEfSe in the healthy group (*Actinobacillus, Pseudoflavonifractor*, unclassified Lachnospiraceae, *Lactobacillus*, unclassified Clostridiales, *Subdoligranulum,*

Table 2 Relative abundance of significantly different taxa over time in the fecal bacterial microbiota of healthy foals ($n = 11$)

	Median relative abundance % (CI %)		*p*-value	FDR adjusted *p*-value
	T1	T2		
Phyla				
Chlamydiae	0.001 (0–0.004)	0.2 (0.007–0.9)	0.005	0.04
Classes				
Chlamydiae	0.001 (0–0.004)	0.2 (0.007–0.9)	0.005	0.04
Verrucomicrobia Subdivision 5	0.2 (0.01–0.6)	3.2 (1.4–4.1)	0.005	0.04
Orders				
Chlamydiales	0.001 (0–0.004)	0.2 (0.007–0.9)	0.005	0.046
Unclassified Verrucomicrobia Subdivision 5	0.2 (0.01–0.6)	3.2 (1.4–4.1)	0.005	0.046
Families				
Unclassified Verrucomicrobia Subdivision 5	0.2 (0.01–0.6)	3.2 (1.4–4.1)	0.005	0.12
Clostridiaceae XI	0.01 (0.003–0.04)	0.2 (0.05–0.9)	0.02	0.44
Unclassified Clostridiales	1.9 (0.5–4.7)	9.2 (3.3–16.9)	0.02	0.14

FDR: False discovery rate adjusted (Benjamin Hochberg procedure)
T1: 1–14 days of age, T2: 15–28 days of age

Streptococcus, unclassified Verrucomicrobiaceae). Three taxa were enriched in the diarrhea group at T1 (*Aerococcus,* unclassified Erysipelotrichaceae, *Blautia*). At T2, 117 taxa were enriched in the healthy group, 50 (48%) of which were members of the families Lachnospiraceae or Ruminococcaceae (full list, *P*-values and LDA values are shown in Additional file 2).

The number of observed species was significantly lower in foals with diarrhea at T1 and T2 (both $p < 0.001$, Fig. 2). There was also a significant decrease in estimated richness (Chao index) in foals with diarrhea compared to healthy foals at T2 ($p = 0.04$, Fig. 3); however, not at T1 ($p = 0.15$). No other differences in alpha diversity were identified (all $p > 0.61$).

Distinct clusters (healthy foals vs. foals with diarrhea) were not visually evident on Jaccard and Yue&Clayton PcOA (Fig. 5) and a statistical difference in community structure was not consistent across statistical tests (Table 4).

Discussion

The bacterial microbiota of foals is assumed to play an important role in diarrhea, and early colonization and

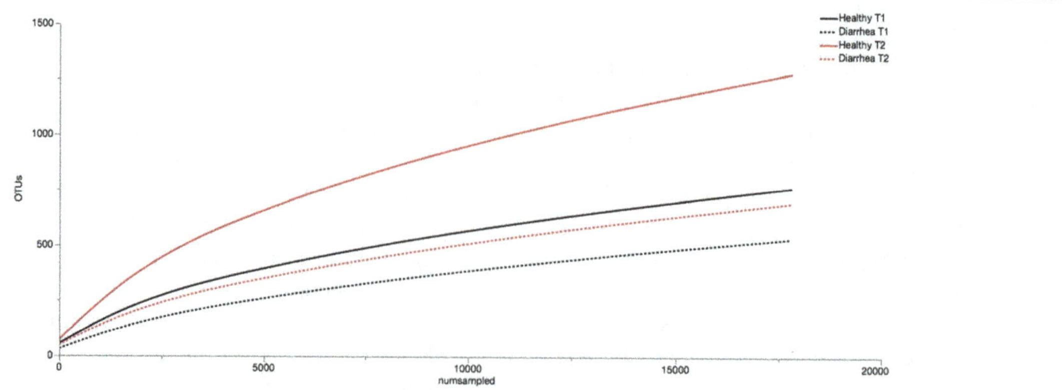

Fig. 2 Rarefication analysis (number of observed species) of the 16S rRNA gene sequences obtained from foal fecal samples, T1: 1–14 days of age, T2: 15–28 days of age. Each line represents the average of a group: healthy foals ($n = 11$) and foals with diarrhea ($n = 4$ at T1 and $n = 3$ each at T2). The analysis was performed on a selected subset of 17,800 sequences (lowest sequence number of all samples)

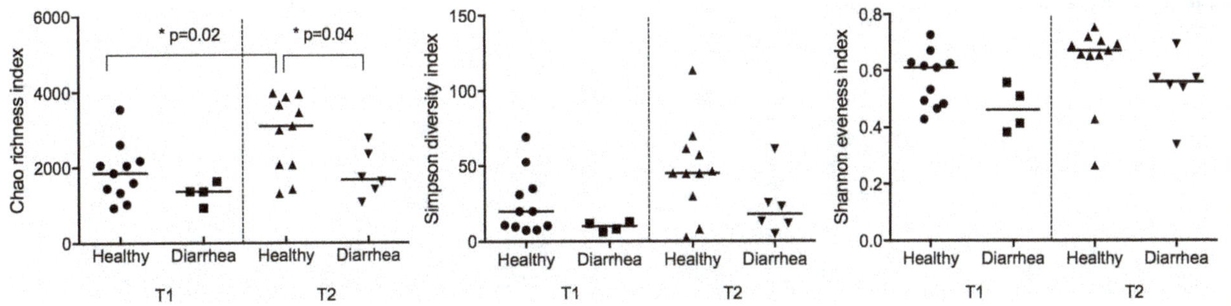

Fig. 3 Median alpha diversity indices of the fecal bacterial microbiota of healthy foals (n = 11) and foals with diarrhea (n = 4 at T1 and n = 6 at T2). T1: 1–14 days of age, T2: 15–28 days of age. Horizontal line represents the median

development is a dynamic process. In this study, significant impacts of both age and diarrhea were noted, with the most evident influential factor being age.

Knowledge of the bacterial microbiota in foals is still in its infancy. Initial culture-based studies tended to focus on a narrow spectrum of the fecal bacterial microbiota, such as lactobacilli, enterococci and clostridia [22]. Subsequent culture-independent studies have provided much more insight into the rapid development of the bacterial microbiota. Foals develop a rich and diverse bacterial microbiota early in life, and it has been previously reported that the foal's fecal bacterial microbiota resembles that of adult horses by 60 days of age. [9]. Here, changes over time in microbial composition were less evident than reported in the above study, something that is unsurprising because of the short study period. Regardless, there were many significant differences in the fecal bacterial microbiota even over this relatively short timeframe, highlighting the dynamic nature of the microbiota. Similar to the only comparable study of the fecal bacterial microbiota of foals, the most abundant bacterial phyla here were Firmicutes, Verrucomicrobia and Proteobacteria [9]. The most abundant families were members of the Clostridia class, Ruminococcaceae and Lachnospiraceae which is also in agreement with a prior study [9].

The field nature of the study and farm management factors made it impossible to collect fecal samples on specified days in this study. This resulted in a wide age range (up to 14 days) in each group. Further, the period between the two samples was not consistent between foals. This complicates interpretation and analysis of the data, particularly trying to determine the effect of age on the microbiota. Nevertheless, further data was added to the growing knowledge on the development of the bacterial microbiota, and the age factor has to be considered when designing and interpreting microbial studies.

In a study in adult horses with colitis changes on all taxonomic levels were identified [2]. Changes in members of higher taxonomic levels, such as phylum, order and class, presumably indicate a more profound change of the bacterial microbiota and are more likely to result in functional differences compared to changes in lower taxonomic levels. In our study none of the changes was

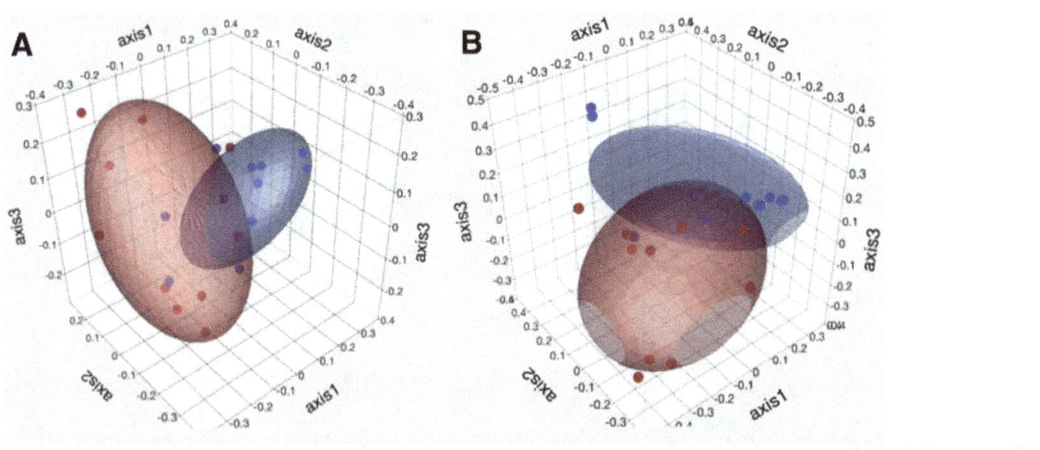

Fig. 4 Principal coordinate analysis of the fecal bacterial microbiota of healthy foals (n = 11) at different time points. Principal coordinate analysis based on the Jaccard (**a**) and Yue&Clayton (**b**) index. Red: T1: 1–14 days of age, Blue: T2: 15–28 days of age. Ellipsoid coverage: 50%

Table 3 Relative abundance of significantly different taxa in the fecal bacterial microbiota of foals with (n = 4 at T1, n = 6 at T2) and without (n = 11) diarrhea

	Age group	Median relative abundance % (CI %)		p-value	FDR adjusted p-value
		Healthy	Diarrhea		
Phylum					
Chlamydiae	T2	0.2 (0.01–0.9)	<0.001(0- < 0.001)	0.02	0.08
Class					
Chlamydiae	T2	0.2 (0.01–0.9)	<0.001(0- < 0.001)	0.02	0.11
Verrucomicrobia Subdivision 5	T2	3.2 (1.4–4.1)	0.05 (<0.011–0.3)	0.004	0.06
Order					
Chlamydiales	T2	0.2 (0.01–0.9)	<0.001(0- < 0.001)	0.02	0.14
Unclassified Verrucomicrobial Subdivison 5	T2	3.2 (1.4–4.1)	0.05 (<0.011–0.3)	0.004	0.08
Family					
Ruminococcaceae	T1	18.2 (0.6–8.5)	1.8 (4.5–23.3)	0.04	1
Clostridiaceae	T2	0.7 (0.3–3)	0.2 0.1–0.4)	0.04	0.35

FDR: False discovery rate adjusted (Benjamin Hochberg procedure)
T1: 1–14 days of age, T2: 15–28 days of age

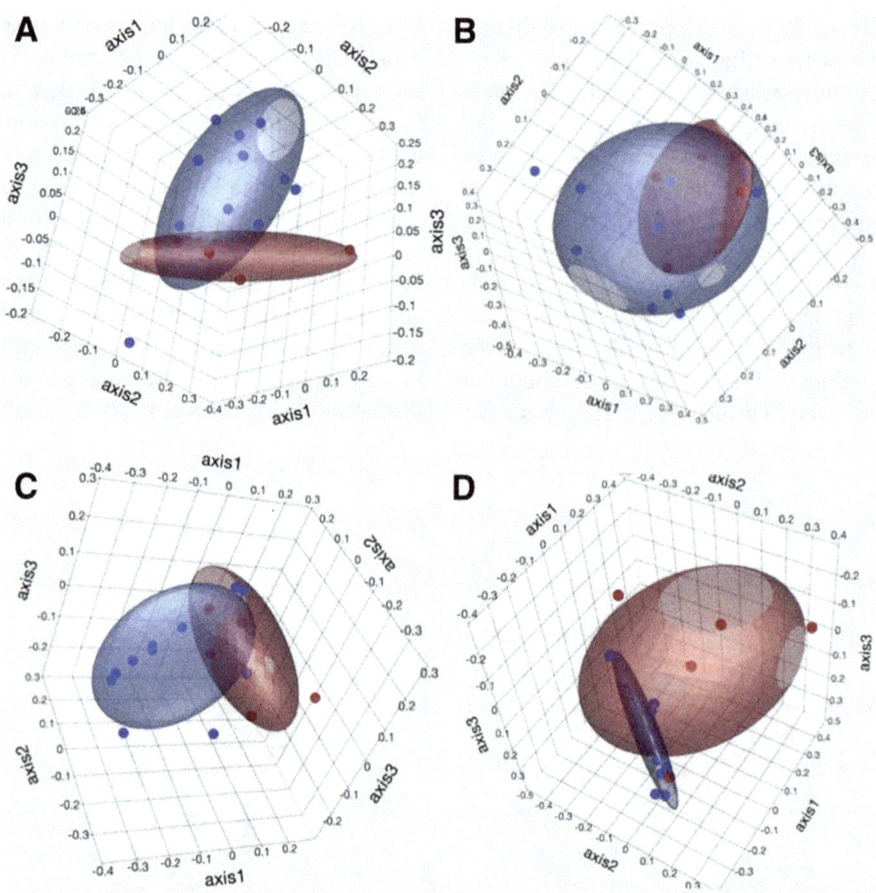

Fig. 5 Principal coordinate analysis of the fecal bacterial microbiota of healthy foals and foals with diarrhea. Principal coordinate analysis based on the Jaccard index (panel **a** for T1 and panel **c** for T2) and the Yue&Clayton index (panel **b** for T1 and panel **d** for T2). T1: 1–14 days of age, T2: 15–28 days of age. Blue: healthy foals (n = 11), red: foals with diarrhea (n = 4 at T1 and n = 6 at T2, red). Ellipsoid coverage: 50%

Table 4 Difference in bacterial microbial composition (Jaccard index) and structure (Yue&Clayton index) of the fecal bacterial microbiota of foals with (n = 4 at T1, n = 6 at T2) and without (n = 11) diarrhea

	T1		T2	
	Jaccard index p-value	Yue&Clayton index p-value	Jaccard index p-value	Yue&Clayton index p-value
Parsimony	0.1	1	0.61	0.07
AMOVA	0.42	0.17	0.01	0.17
ANOSIM	0.21	0.04	0.009	0.009

T1: 1–14 days of age, T2: 15–28 days of age

significant after FDR adjustment. However, some differences in fecal bacterial microbiota composition and structure were evident.

An apparent underrepresentation of Lachnospiraceae and Ruminococcaceae, the two most abundant families, were seen in foals with diarrhea in this study. Lachnospiraceae and Ruminococcaceae, members of the Clostridia class, have been implicated as having important roles in gastrointestinal health in numerous animal species. In humans and animals with gastrointestinal disease these species were consistently under represented, independent of the cause of gastrointestinal disease [23–27]. Clostridia are major producers of short chain fatty acids (SCFA), which are important for intestinal and general health [28, 29]. *Faecalibacterium*, a member of the Ruminococcaceae, has also been shown to produce anti-inflammatory peptides in-vitro [30] and has been shown to decrease diarrhea incidence and mortality in calves [31]. A decrease of these bacterial families in horses with colitis and colic as well as horses exposed to stress factors such as fasting, transport and anesthesia has also been shown [2, 6, 32] and a decrease in some of these members has been identified prior to the onset of colic in post-partum mares [6]. The underrepresentation of members of these families, such as *Blautia*, *Faecalibacterium* and *Ruminococcus* among others, in foals with diarrhea further supports the potential importance of these bacterial families.

Richness was lower in foals with diarrhea compared to healthy foals. Gut bacteria are involved in many homeostatic processes through metabolite production and communication with the host's immune system. While optimal levels of richness are not known, a diverse bacterial microbiota is thought to be of use as it may be more adept at fulfilling a wide range of necessary functions and be more resilient in the face of changes (e.g. nutritional change, stress). Loss of bacterial diversity and richness has been demonstrated in acute and chronic gastrointestinal enteropathies in humans and animals, including wide-ranging disorders such as Crohn's disease [33], inflammatory bowel disease [30] and acute enteric infections [25] in humans, acute diarrhea [27] and inflammatory bowel disease [34] in dogs and acute colitis in adult horses [15].

The complexity of the fecal bacterial microbiota, and the finding that bacterial alpha diversity is decreased in foals with diarrhea raises questions about common approaches to prevention or treatment of diarrhea. Metronidazole is commonly used to treat diarrhea in horses and sometimes foals [35]. Many members of the Clostridia class are susceptible to this drug [36]. Therefore, treatment could potentially inhibit the beneficial components of the fecal bacterial microbiota. Probiotics are also commonly used, although to date several studies have not shown any clear benefit for treatment or prevention of diarrhea in foals [12, 14, 37, 38]. One potential reason could be that the organisms found in most commercial probiotics (e.g. enterococci, lactobacilli) are not those found to be important members of the healthy bacterial microbiota in several studies including our study [2, 39]. This raises questions about the potential efficacy of conventional probiotic organisms for the treatment or prevention of diarrhea, especially when they have to compete in such as rich and abundant existing bacterial microbiota.

Antimicrobial treated foals were excluded as it has been shown that antimicrobial administration causes profound and sustained changes in the equine fecal bacterial microbiota [40]. Foals were included in the study irrespective of the cause of diarrhea. It is unlikely that this influenced the results, as it has been shown in humans that intestinal microbial communities become affected in a similar way, irrespective of the pathogen type and age [25]. Severity, duration and frequency of diarrhea were not taken into account during analysis of these data. Given the small number of foals and large variation in diarrhea duration, this was no feasible.

Factors other than age can impact the fecal bacterial microbiota and could not be accounted for. Foals from seven farms over a period of two breeding seasons were enrolled to acquire a sufficient number of foals [14], creating some potential for farm- and year-based variation. High starch diets and feed changes have been shown to have a significant impact on the microbial communities [41]. Foals less than four weeks of age are not commonly fed large amounts of high starch feed; therefore, significant bias based on farm is unlikely. There are no studies evaluating the effect of other management practices, it is therefore difficult to assess how, and to what extent the factor farm could have influenced these results. Exact feeding and management practices were not available for each farm but should be collected or unified in future studies to better assess the effect of diarrhea with confounding factors.

More females than males were affected by diarrhea. Females could have inherent differences in fecal bacterial microbiota composition compared to males, which could influence results of the effect of diarrhea. This has not been studied in horses, however has been investigated in human medicine, and differences in microbial composition between man and women are present [42]. It cannot be predicted to what extent and in which way this would have influenced our results.

Given that age has an effect on microbial composition, alpha- and beta diversity, we tried to control for this factor when sampling the foals; however, foals with diarrhea had fecal samples taken at an earlier age than healthy foals at time point two. This could have also influenced the results and makes it difficult to interpret the exact effect of diarrhea versus a lingering effect of age in these foals.

Another limitation of this study was the differences in storage conditions for some of the samples. Some samples were stored at 4 °C for up to 2 weeks before being frozen at −80 °C. There is no data on how different storage conditions affect the equine fecal bacterial microbiota; however, it has been shown in dogs and cats that storage at 4 °C for up to 14 days has limited effects on the fecal bacterial microbiota composition. Changes in limited groups occurred but there were no differences in richness, diversity, evenness or community structure [43]. It is likely that this is similar for the equine fecal bacterial microbiota. Storage conditions should not have significantly affected the results of our study, particularly in regards to richness and diversity on the species level.

Conclusions

Bacterial richness is decreased in foals with diarrhea, suggesting that potential preventative and therapeutic measures should focus on providing and maintaining a diverse and rich bacterial microbiota in addition to defining and modifying the key bacterial species involved in gastrointestinal health, such as members of the Lachnospiraceae and Ruminococcaceae.

Endnotes

[1]Bio-Sponge, Platinum Peformance, Buellton, CA.

[2]E.Z.N.A. Stool DNA Kit, Omega Bio-Tek Inc, GA, USA

[3]NanoDrop, Roche, ON, Canada

Additional files

Additional file 1: Rarefecation curve. Rarefaction curves of V4 16S rRNA gene sequences from fecal samples from neonatal foals (n = 20) sampled at 1–14 and 15–28 of age.

Additional file 2: LEfSe Results. Title of date: Analysis from LEfSe analysis. Species significantly enriched in the fecal microbiota of healthy foals (n = 11) and foals with diarrhea (n = 4 at T1 and n = 6 at T2) sampled over time determined by linear discriminant analysis effect size. (LEfSe)

Abbreviations

AMOVA: Analysis of molecular variance; ANOSIM: Analysis of similarities; bp: Base pairs; FDR: False discovery rate; LEfSe: Linear discriminant analysis effect size; OUT: Operational taxonomic unit; PcOA: Principal coordinate analysis; RDP: Ribosomal database project

Acknowledgements

Not applicable.

Funding

This study was supported by a fellowship of the Danish Centre of Antimicrobial Research and Development (DanCARD) funded by the Danish Council for Strategic Research and an operating grant by Equine Guelph. The funding agencies did not have any involvement in study design, collection, analysis and interpretation of data; in the writing of the manuscript; and in the decision to submit the manuscript for publication.

Authors' contributions

AS was involved in study design, carried out sample collection, data analysis and drafted the manuscript. MJ was performed the laboratory work, assisted in data analysis and manuscript drafting. JSW took part in the study design and assisted in data analysis. LG took part in study design and interpretation of data. HS participated in study design and interpretation of data as well as revision of the manuscript. All authors read and approved the final manuscript.

Competing interests

The authors have no conflict of interest to declare.

Consent for publication

Not applicable.

Author details

[1]Equine Department, University of Zurich, Vetsuisse Faculty, Winterthurerstrasse 260, 8057 Zurich, Zurich, Switzerland. [2]Department of Veterinary Disease Biology, University of Copenhagen, Faculty of Health and Medical Science, Stigbojlen 4, 1870, Copenhagen, Denmark. [3]Department of Clinical Studies, University of Guelph, Ontario Veterinary College, Guelph N1G2W1, Canada. [4]Department of Biomedical Sciences, Ross University School of Veterinary Medicine, Basseterre, St Kitts and Nevis. [5]Department of Pathobiology, University of Guelph, Ontario Veterinary College, Guelph N1G2W1, Canada.

References

1. Costa MC, Weese JS. The equine intestinal microbiome. In: Animal health research reviews / conference of research Workers in Animal Diseases; 2012. p. 1–8.
2. Costa MC, Arroyo LG, Allen-Vercoe E, Stampfli HR, Kim PT, Sturgeon A, et al. Comparison of the fecal Microbiota of healthy horses and horses with colitis

by high throughput sequencing of the V3-V5 region of the 16S rRNA Gene. PLoS One. 2012;7(7):e41484.
3. Milinovich GJ, Trott DJ, Burrell PC, Croser EL, Al Jassim RAM, Morton JM, et al. Fluorescence in situ hybridization analysis of hindgut bacteria associated with the development of equine laminitis. Environ Microbiol. 2007;9(8): 2090–100.
4. Steelman SM, Chowdhary BP, Dowd S, Suchodolski J, Janecka JE. Pyrosequencing of 16S rRNA genes in fecal samples reveals high diversity of hindgut microflora in horses and potential links to chronic laminitis. BMC Vet Res. 2012;8:231.
5. Garrett LA, Brown R, Poxton IR. A comparative study of the intestinal microbiota of healthy horses and those suffering from equine grass sickness. Vet Microbiol. 2002;87(1):81–8.
6. Holcombe SJ, Embertson RM, Kurtz KA, Roessner HA, Jalali M, Wismer SE. Equine Vet J. 2015;47(6):641-9.
7. Kuhl J, Winterhoff N, Wulf M, Schweigert FJ, Schwendenwein I, Bruckmaier RM, et al. Changes in faecal bacteria and metabolic parameters in foals during the first six weeks of life. Vet Microbiol. 2011;151(3–4):321–8.
8. Palmer C, Bik EM, DiGiulio DB, Relman DA, Brown PO. Development of the human infant intestinal microbiota. PLoS Biol. 2007;5(7):e177.
9. Costa MC, Stämpfli HR, Allen-Vercoe E, Weese JS. Equine Vet J. 2016;48(6):681-88.
10. Chu DM, Ma J, Prince AL, Antony KM, Seferovic MD, Aagaard KM. Nat Med. 2017;23(3):314-26.
11. Faubladier C, Sadet-Bourgeteau S, Philippeau C, Jacotot E, Julliand V. Molecular monitoring of the bacterial community structure in foal feces pre- and post-weaning. Anaerobe. 2014;25:61–6.
12. Yuyama T. Evaluation of a host-specific Lactobacillus probiotic in neonatal foals. In. Edited by Yusa S. J Appl Res Vet Med. 2004;2:26–32.
13. Frederick J, Giguere S, Sanchez LC. Infectious agents detected in the feces of diarrheic foals: a retrospective study of 233 cases (2003-2008). J Vet Intern Med. 2009;23(6):1254–60.
14. Schoster A, Staempfli HR, Abrahams M, Jalali M, Weese JS, Guardabassi L. J Vet Intern Med. 2015;29(3):925-31.
15. Rodriguez C, Taminiau B, Brevers B, Avesani V, Van Broeck J, Leroux A, et al. Faecal microbiota characterisation of horses using 16 rdna barcoded pyrosequencing, and carriage rate of clostridium difficile at hospital admission. BMC Microbiol. 2015;15(1):181.
16. Eckburg PB, Bik EM, Bernstein CN, Purdom E, Dethlefsen L, Sargent M, et al. Diversity of the human intestinal microbial flora. Science. 2005;308(5728):1635–8.
17. Schoster A, Guardabassi L, Staempfli HR, Abrahams M, Jalali M, Weese JS. Equine Vet J. 2016;48(6):689-96.
18. Schloss PD, Westcott SL, Ryabin T, Hall JR, Hartmann M, Hollister EB, et al. Introducing mothur: open-source, platform-independent, community-supported software for describing and comparing microbial communities. Appl Environ Microbiol. 2009;75(23):7537–41.
19. Quast C, Pruesse E, Yilmaz P, Gerken J, Schweer T, Yarza P, et al. The SILVA ribosomal RNA gene database project: improved data processing and web-based tools. Nucleic Acids Res. 2013;41(Database issue):D590–6.
20. Edgar RC, Haas BJ, Clemente JC, Quince C, Knight R. UCHIME improves sensitivity and speed of chimera detection. Bioinformatics. 2011;27(16):2194–200.
21. Segata N, Izard J, Waldron L, Gevers D, Miropolsky L, Garrett WS, et al. Metagenomic biomarker discovery and explanation. Genome Biol. 2011;12(6):R60.
22. JVdVAVLR Y. Preliminary studies on the bacterial flora of faeces taken from foals, from birth to twelve weeks. Effect of the oral administration of a commercial colostrum replacer. Pferdeheilkunde. 1996;12(3):4.
23. Suchodolski JS, Markel ME, Garcia-Mazcorro JF, Unterer S, Heilmann RM, Dowd SE, et al. The fecal microbiome in dogs with acute diarrhea and idiopathic inflammatory bowel disease. PLoS One. 2012;7(12):e51907.
24. Honneffer JB, Minamoto Y, Suchodolski JS. Microbiota alterations in acute and chronic gastrointestinal inflammation of cats and dogs. World J Gastroenterol. 2014;20(44):16489–97.
25. Singh P, Teal TK, Marsh TL, Tiedje JM, Mosci R, Jernigan K, et al. Intestinal microbial communities associated with acute enteric infections and disease recovery. Microbiome. 2015;3:45.
26. Minamoto Y, Otoni CC, Steelman SM, Buyukleblebici O, Steiner JM, Jergens AE, et al. Alteration of the fecal microbiota and serum metabolite profiles in dogs with idiopathic inflammatory bowel disease. Gut Microbes. 2015;6(1):33–47.
27. Guard BC, Barr JW, Reddivari L, Klemashevich C, Jayaraman A, Steiner JM, et al. Characterization of microbial dysbiosis and metabolomic changes in dogs with acute diarrhea. PLoS One. 2015;10(5):e0127259.
28. Pryde SE, Duncan SH, Hold GL, Stewart CS, Flint HJ. The microbiology of butyrate formation in the human colon. FEMS Microbiol Lett. 2002;217(2):133–9.
29. Antharam VC, Li EC, Ishmael A, Sharma A, Mai V, Rand KH, et al. Intestinal dysbiosis and depletion of butyrogenic bacteria in Clostridium Difficile infection and nosocomial diarrhea. J Clin Microbiol. 2013;51(9):2884–92.
30. Sokol H, Pigneur B, Watterlot L, Lakhdari O, Bermudez-Humaran LG, Gratadoux JJ, et al. Faecalibacterium prausnitzii is an anti-inflammatory commensal bacterium identified by gut microbiota analysis of Crohn disease patients. Proc Natl Acad Sci U S A. 2008;105(43):16731–6.
31. Foditsch C, Pereira RV, Ganda EK, Gomez MS, Marques EC, Santin T, et al. Oral Administration of Faecalibacterium prausnitzii decreased the incidence of severe diarrhea and related mortality rate and increased weight gain in Preweaned dairy heifers. PLoS One. 2015;10(12):e0145485.
32. Schoster A, Mosing M, Jalali M, Staempfli HR, Weese JS. Equine Vet J. 2016;48(5):595-602.
33. Dicksved J, Halfvarson J, Rosenquist M, Jarnerot G, Tysk C, Apajalahti J, et al. Molecular analysis of the gut microbiota of identical twins with Crohn's disease. The ISME journal. 2008;2(7):716–27.
34. Xenoulis PG, Palculict B, Allenspach K, Steiner JM, Van House AM, Suchodolski JS. Molecular-phylogenetic characterization of microbial communities imbalances in the small intestine of dogs with inflammatory bowel disease. FEMS Microbiol Ecol. 2008;66(3):579–89.
35. Feary DJ, Hassel DM. Enteritis and colitis in horses. Vet Clin N Am Equine Pract. 2006;22(2):437–79. ix
36. Brook I, Wexler HM, Goldstein EJ. Antianaerobic antimicrobials: spectrum and susceptibility testing. Clin Microbiol Rev. 2013;26(3):526–46.
37. Weese JS, Rousseau J. Evaluation of Lactobacillus pentosus WE7 for prevention of diarrhea in neonatal foals. J Am Vet Med Assoc. 2005;226(12):2031–4.
38. Desrochers AM, Dolente BA, Roy MF, Boston R, Carlisle S. Efficacy of Saccharomyces boulardii for treatment of horses with acute enterocolitis. J Am Vet Med Assoc. 2005;227(6):954–9.
39. Rodriguez C, Taminiau B, Brevers B, Avesani V, Van Broeck J, Leroux AA, et al. Carriage and acquisition rates of Clostridium Difficile in hospitalized horses, including molecular characterization, multilocus sequence typing and antimicrobial susceptibility of bacterial isolates. Vet Microbiol. 2014; 172(1–2):309–17.
40. Costa MC, Stampfli HR, Arroyo LG, Allen-Vercoe E, Gomes RG, Weese J. Changes in the equine fecal microbiota associated with the use of systemic antimicrobial drugs. BMC Vet Res. 2015;11(1):19.
41. Fernandes KA, Kittelmann S, Rogers CW, Gee EK, Bolwell CF, Bermingham EN, et al. Faecal Microbiota of forage-fed horses in New Zealand and the population dynamics of microbial communities following dietary change. PLoS One. 2014;9(11):e112846.
42. Haro C, Rangel-Zuniga OA, Alcala-Diaz JF, Gomez-Delgado F, Perez-Martinez P, Delgado-Lista J, et al. Intestinal Microbiota is influenced by gender and body mass index. PLoS One. 2016;11(5):e0154090.
43. Weese JS, Jalali M. Evaluation of the impact of refrigeration on next generation sequencing-based assessment of the canine and feline fecal microbiota. BMC Vet Res. 2014;10(1):230.

8

Case definition terminology for paratuberculosis (Johne's disease)

R. J. Whittington*, D. J. Begg, K. de Silva, A. C. Purdie, N. K. Dhand and K. M. Plain

Abstract: Paratuberculosis (Johne's disease) is an economically significant condition caused by *Mycobacterium avium* subsp. *paratuberculosis*. However, difficulties in diagnosis and classification of individual animals with the condition have hampered research and impeded efforts to halt its progressive spread in the global livestock industry. Descriptive terms applied to individual animals and herds such as exposed, infected, diseased, clinical, sub-clinical, infectious and resistant need to be defined so that they can be incorporated consistently into well-understood and reproducible case definitions. These allow for consistent classification of individuals in a population for the purposes of analysis based on accurate counts. The outputs might include the incidence of cases, frequency distributions of the number of cases by age class or more sophisticated analyses involving statistical comparisons of immune responses in vaccine development studies, or gene frequencies or expression data from cases and controls in genomic investigations. It is necessary to have agreed definitions in order to be able to make valid comparisons and meta-analyses of experiments conducted over time by a given researcher, in different laboratories, by different researchers, and in different countries. In this paper, terms are applied systematically in an hierarchical flow chart to enable classification of individual animals. We propose descriptive terms for different stages in the pathogenesis of paratuberculosis to enable their use in different types of studies and to enable an independent assessment of the extent to which accepted definitions for stages of disease have been applied consistently in any given study. This will assist in the general interpretation of data between studies, and will facilitate future meta-analyses.

Background

Paratuberculosis (Johne's disease) is caused by *Mycobacterium avium* subsp. *paratuberculosis (MAP)*. The organism commonly infects ruminants where it resides in macrophages in the small intestinal lamina propria and associated lymph nodes, triggering granulomatous inflammation and an enteropathy that is eventually fatal in many cases. The organism is not host specific, and infections have been reported from species as diverse as rabbits, cats and humans [1–3]. The economic losses in farmed livestock are due to lost milk production, weight loss and mortality [4–8]. In addition there are significant animal welfare considerations associated with this chronic wasting disease [9]. For these reasons, and also whether stated overtly or not the potential for *MAP* to appear in the human food chain, has stimulated the development of disease control programs for paratuberculosis in farmed livestock. In the face of limited resources and many unequivocal public health threats, these control programs satisfy public health agencies who recognize a link but not a causative relationship between *MAP* and Crohn's disease [10], while topic specialists encourage the livestock industry to acknowledge the potential public health issue [11]. The requirement to reduce the prevalence of paratuberculosis has triggered studies to improve laboratory tests, vaccines and to explore the potential for breeding programs for disease resistance in livestock. However, difficulties in diagnosis and in the classification of the disease in individual animals have hampered research and efforts to overcome the progressive spread of paratuberculosis in the global livestock industry.

In one of the largest studies to date, involving detailed examination of more than 1000 cows using a battery of tests, Vazquez et al. (2014) [12] confirmed that most *MAP* infections are subclinical, and that the microbiological and pathological features of paratuberculosis leading to disease transmission are not dissimilar to tuberculosis in humans. In both humans and livestock, infected individuals carry pathogenic mycobacteria silently

* Correspondence: richard.whittington@sydney.edu.au
Sydney School of Veterinary Science and School of Life and Environmental Sciences, Faculty of Science, The University of Sydney, 425 Werombi Road, Camden, NSW 2570, Australia

into new geographic areas [13–15]. It is a feature of chronic mycobacterial diseases in both humans and livestock that our ability to accurately classify individual cases and controls enables meaningful experimental design and analyses in many types of studies; generally these are aimed at better disease diagnosis, control, treatment and prevention (for example see [16, 17]). Descriptive terms that are applied to individual animals and herds such as exposed, infected, diseased, clinical, sub-clinical, infectious, resilient and resistant need to be described objectively and unambiguously so that they can be incorporated consistently into well-understood and reproducible case definitions. Herd-level case definitions can be developed from those applied to individual animals but are not dealt with in this paper.

Case definitions allow for classification of individuals in a population for the purposes of analysis based on accurate counts. The outputs might include the incidence of cases (number of new cases per unit time and population at risk), frequency distributions of the number of cases by age class or more sophisticated analyses involving statistical comparisons of immune responses in vaccine development studies, or of gene frequencies or expression data from cases and controls in genomic investigations. Advances in technology and the availability of new testing platforms enable studies on immune, proteomic, genomic and metabolic disease signatures combined with sophisticated analytical methods, and these can be applied to animal models of paratuberculosis (for example [18]). These approaches aim to provide a greater understanding of disease pathogenesis and host susceptibility, however they ultimately depend on the classification of the status of individual animals. Hence there is a need to use consistent terminology and case definitions in order to establish the foundations for analysis. It is necessary to have agreed definitions in order to be able to make valid comparisons and meta-analyses of experiments conducted over time by a given researcher, in different laboratories, by different researchers, and in different countries. Indeed the lack of standard case definitions is recognized in tuberculosis research to hamper comparison of research findings, prevent best use of existing data and limit the management of disease [19]. This has led to promotion and comparison of standardized clinical case definitions in recent years, but it is already clear that case definitions conceived for one purpose, for example diagnosis of childhood tuberculous meningitis, may not be suitable for another, for example contact tracing, analogous to veterinary trace forward investigation (the problem here was lack of clinical signs in the latter being the first layer of classification in the former) [20, 21]. In this context the case definitions were intended to be used as standardized diagnostic criteria with a view to clinical intervention, and therefore the case definitions had properties of diagnostic tests (accuracy: sensitivity and specificity) [17]. For non-tuberculous mycobacterial infections in humans, adherence to American Thoracic Society diagnostic criteria to distinguish these from airway colonization was poorly associated with any difference in prognosis [22]. The issue is the use of consistent terms for analysis of diagnostic tests and then layering these to reach conclusions to enable classification of individuals. The same problem is evident in paratuberculosis, where animals are classified based on test outcomes; the tests can be used in series or in parallel, and so there will be variable accuracy of classification of the true infection or disease status. For example Zare et al. [23] classified animals as "test-positive" or "test-negative" based on ELISA alone or ELISA and faecal culture in parallel (parallel interpretation, individual is positive if either test is positive). The alternative would have been to require both tests to be positive (series interpretation, individual is positive if both tests are positive). Similarly Gonda et al. [24] used ELISA and faecal culture in parallel to classify animals in a herd as "infected" or non-infected for a genetic study. Collins et al. [25] used faecal culture results in parallel from tests repeated at up to three laboratories to classify animals as "a confirmed case of infection" to evaluate ELISA tests. Socket et al. defined subclinical infection to be isolation of *MAP* from faeces or organs of cows without clinical signs such as diarrhoea or weight loss [26]. Each of these definitions can result in a different pattern of grouping of individuals as cases or controls. Osterstock et al. (2010) [27] simulated faecal culture and ELISA results using reported sensitivity and specificity metrics, and demonstrated that the power to detect a genetic association using case definitions based on these tests was low. Conceptually, the evidence used to define a "case" can range from overwhelming to very limited when the accuracy of the aggregated testing procedure is considered (Fig. 1).

Paratuberculosis presents as a range of sub-clinical and clinical forms during the 1 to 14 year incubation period, and this chronicity of pathogenesis contributes to difficulties with disease characterization at each stage of progression [28]. The variation in disease presentation, the challenges of diagnostic test accuracy, when combined with the lack of consistency in application of terminology and case definitions has led to lack of agreement between studies, be they focused on validation of diagnostic tests, vaccine development or genome wide associations (for example see [29, 30]).

Scope

In this paper, a brief discussion of the specific requirements for individual animal case definitions in studies related to diagnostic tests, genetics/genomics and

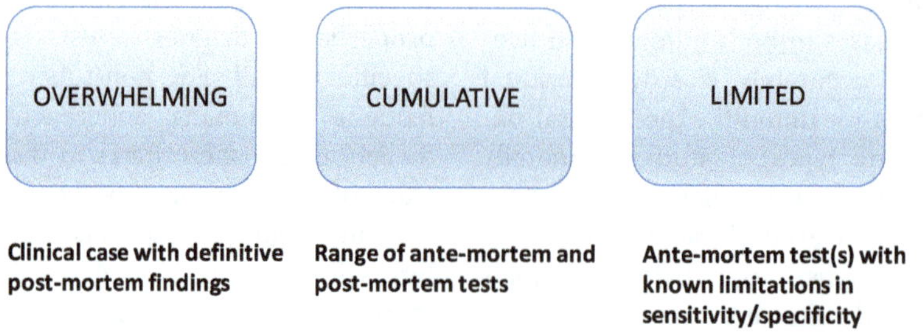

Fig. 1 Conceptual ranking of evidence used to define a "case" in the paratuberculosis literature. Overwhelming evidence: indisputable diagnostic confirmation of clinical paratuberculosis. Cumulative evidence: range of ante-mortem and post-mortem tests applied and/or repeat testing at separate time points, combined with herd history, leading to greater certainty regarding true infection status. Limited evidence: use of ante-mortem tests such as the milk or serum ELISA and faecal culture, either alone or in combination; parallel interpretation of two or more tests (positive in any of the tests applied); uncertain diagnostic implications of combining information from more than one test

vaccines is presented. Diagnostic tests for paratuberculosis, and their attributes are briefly introduced. This is followed by an explanation of terms that are commonly used in the context of paratuberculosis. These terms are then applied systematically in an hierarchical flow chart to enable classification of individual animals using available information such as herd history and objective diagnostic tests. Areas of uncertainty remain with certain animal classifications, and these are highlighted. We propose descriptive terms for different stages in the pathogenesis of paratuberculosis to enable their use in case definitions for different types of studies (diagnostic test evaluations, prevalence estimation, certification of disease freedom, vaccine efficacy and genomic studies). Case definitions can be precisely defined, should be linked to an understanding of pathogenesis, and should be consistent between studies. However, the stringency with which a case definition can be met will differ between studies according to resources and other practical considerations, and the accuracy of animal classification (i.e. the sensitivity and specificity) will also vary. For this reason it is important that guidance be provided to enable self-assessment or indeed an independent assessment of the extent to which case definitions are met in any given study.

Contexts for application of specific terms and case definitions

Diagnostic test evaluation

One of the most important applications of case definition is in diagnostic test evaluation. The World Organisation for Animal Health (OIE) recommends that diagnostic tests be evaluated after explicitly stating the purpose of the test (to ensure that a test is fit for purpose, for example "to detect animals that can transmit the disease") and more generally "to accurately predict the infection or exposure status of the animal or population of animals" [31]. In 2008 Nielsen and Toft reviewed the accuracies of diagnostic tests for paratuberculosis and made distinctions between non-mutually exclusive categories of infected, infectious and affected animals, which they termed "target conditions" [30]. Their epidemiological approach, which recognized the long latent phase of the infection (pathogenesis), enabled test accuracy to be summarized based on stratification of the stages of the disease. This approach is well-recognized, for example in an assessment of direct faecal PCR test accuracy based on stratification of animals in the population according to the severity of their histopathological lesions [32]. Nielsen and Toft (2008) [30] recommended that diagnostic test evaluations be more stringent in future, including consistent classification of subjects and avoidance of variable case definitions. In their conceptualization, the target condition is linked to the purpose of a diagnostic test and to pathogenesis, while the case definition is "a practical description of the target condition" [33]. In other words, the case definition is chosen to suit the needs of the individual study, often involving pragmatic compromise. However, the case definition should be constrained by rules to reflect the target condition [33]. The problem with this approach is that case definition is flexible, and studies conducted for different purposes are not easily comparable because there is lack of consistency in the use of terms that underpin the various possible case definitions. An alternative view is that the target condition is a general statement related to the purpose of a diagnostic test; note that there is little difference between purpose and target condition, as shown in Figure 2 in the article by Nielsen et al. 2011 [33], while case definition is a more precise statement, or an algorithm for diagnostic test inclusion and interpretation. This is also how case definitions have usually been applied in the tuberculosis literature (for example [17]).

Genetics/genomics/genome wide association studies

The purpose of a genome wide association study (GWAS) is to find a relationship between defined genes/alleles and disease characteristics (i.e. a phenotype) at population level, with a view to understanding the relationship between genotype and phenotype at individual animal level. If there is a strong relationship, it may be possible to select genetically resistant individuals for breeding, or alternatively cull susceptible animals to exclude them from the breeding population. Clearly in this context an accurate classification of phenotype is important, and this can be enabled by appropriate and consistent use of case definitions. The lack of consistency of phenotypic classification of animals is one important reason for lack of agreement in the results of different GWAS studies for paratuberculosis [29, 34, 35]. Mostly the discrepancies are due to application of different diagnostic tests with different sensitivities and specificities, at different times in the pathogenesis of the disease, resulting in potential misclassification bias of both cases and controls [34]. Approaches to avoid misclassification bias, given that the genome sequence of an individual is fixed, include repeated testing over time to cover changing disease state in the animals [36], application of multiple ante-mortem diagnostic tests and interpretation of test results in parallel [37, 38] and post-mortem examination which enables culture of tissues and histopathological examination [36, 39]. These steps would increase diagnostic sensitivity, which is often lacking in paratuberculosis studies. However, there may be circumstances where series interpretation of test results is useful to avoid misclassification bias, particularly where specificity of a screening test is suboptimal, for example interferon-γ tests for paratuberculosis in calves [40]. While principles of phenotypic classification are well understood there is as yet no standard upon which to guide genetic studies for paratuberculosis.

Vaccine development and evaluation

Research and development on new vaccines to protect against paratuberculosis will continue [41] until an improved formulation is developed that has better efficacy and safety than those currently available [42–44]. The efficacy of vaccines for paratuberculosis can be measured by reductions in viable *MAP* in tissues, histopathological lesions, faecal shedding of *MAP*, incidence of clinical disease or production of sterile immunity [45, 46]. Researchers should consider using all of these measures as part of a defined animal outcome to determine candidate vaccine efficacy. To avoid misclassification bias of post vaccination outcomes, accurate case definitions using well understood diagnostic measures should be used [30].

The outcome of infection in a vaccinated ruminant could include recovery if vaccination occurs post exposure to *MAP*. Subharat et al. (2012) [47] observed a reduced severity of infection in cattle from 7 to 15 months post vaccination, while Dennis et al. (2011) [48] observed recovery in naturally infected sheep. Description of the spectrum of disease within the unvaccinated control population is also important to accurately measure vaccine efficacy; if the onset of clinical disease in control animals is unnaturally early or prevalent for that species, the protective response of the vaccine may be overwhelmed [49]. Conversely, if none of the animals from the unvaccinated control group develop clinical disease it is hard to establish whether the vaccine is protective against this important outcome, even if histological lesions and *MAP* recovery is recorded. If validated, defined early markers/profiles of infection outcome in the natural host [50] could be used in vaccine efficacy screening instead of conducting screening studies in cell cultures or mice [51].

Disease diagnosis and regulatory action

Paratuberculosis is a notifiable disease in some countries, and accurate diagnosis is important prior to application of control measures which may require stamping out, culling or quarantine measures. Establishing the prevalence of paratuberculosis in a region, or assurance that the infection is absent from a region are also important activities. Trace forward investigations, trace back investigations and confirmation of true infection status following positive results in screening tests are common scenarios. There is some guidance from the OIE on test procedures [52] and also in individual countries (for example Australia [53]) but in general there is no agreed terminology for so-called "target conditions".

Characteristics of diagnostic tests for paratuberculosis

Many of the terms and case definitions for paratuberculosis depend on the results of objective diagnostic tests and historically these have been widely applied to classify animals with paratuberculosis. There are numerous protocols for conducting tests for paratuberculosis (for example see OIE [52]). In general they can be classified as tests for the pathogen (culture or direct PCR of faeces, tissues or milk), or tests for the host's immune response (antibody detection ELISA on serum or milk, various assays for cell mediated immunity such as delayed type hypersensitivity tests) or tissue inflammatory response (gross pathology and histopathology). Test accuracy can be described in terms of sensitivity (the proportion of sick animals that are detected) and specificity (the proportion of healthy animals that test negative), but all are imperfect, i.e. false positive and false negative test outcomes occur [30]. An indication of the accuracy of various tests is provided in Table 1. The lack of perfect tests creates problems in diagnostic test evaluations as newer tests such qPCR are often compared to less sensitive/specific established tests, resulting in apparent lower sensitivity and specificity estimates for newer tests. This has led to an increase in the use of Bayesian latent class models for diagnostic test evaluations, and recommended standards for these [54, 55].

Table 1 Temporal applicability and accuracy of diagnostic tests for paratuberculosis in sheep and cattle

Test	Stage of disease when positive	Potential sensitivity[a]	Potential specificity[b]
Serum ELISA	Mid, late	Low to high[d]	Moderate to high
Delated type hypersensitivity	Early, mid	Moderate to high	Moderate
Interferon gamma assay	Early, mid	Unknown	Unknown
Faecal smear	Mid, late	Low[e]	Low to moderate
Faecal culture	Early[c], mid, late	Low to high[d]	High
Faecal qPCR	Early[c], mid, late	Moderate to high[f]	High
Tissue culture	Early, mid, late	High	High
Gross pathology	Late	Low to moderate	Low to moderate
Histopathology	Mid, late	Moderate to high	High
Clinical signs	Late	Low to moderate	Low to moderate

Adapted from Whittington and Sergeant (2001) [28] and Nielsen and Toft (2008) [30]. The terms low, moderate and high indicate ranges for sensitivity of <40%, 40–70% and >70%, respectively; corresponding values for specificity are <80%, 80–95% and >95%, respectively

[a]Proportion of truly infected/diseased animals that test positive

[b]Proportion of truly non-infected/healthy animals that test negative

[c]Transient, for a few months commencing a few months after infection

[d]High sensitivity possible in late stage of disease

[e]Due to low analytical sensitivity

[f]Based on sensitivity similar to culture in liquid medium

Mismatches between the results of different tests for paratuberculosis are common: tissue culture results may not agree with histopathology; faecal culture may not agree with antibody ELISA. For example, *MAP* was cultured from the tissues of about 30% of sheep and 7% of cattle that did not have histopathological lesions [12, 56]. More recently, in a series of trials conducted at the University of Sydney between 2006 and 2012 involving over 400 sheep that were intensively monitored and received a full necropsy, 13% of the sheep positive for *MAP* by tissue culture had no detectable histopathological lesions across six different regions of the gut and associated lymph nodes (unpublished data).These discrepancies can be readily understood in terms of stage of pathogenesis, site of sample selection and amount of sample examined, and biological/physical properties of the tests (for discussion see [28]). These factors mean that for accurate classification of animals it is often necessary to apply a range of tests, and to do this at more than one time point so as to capitalize on stages of pathogenesis that favour one type of test over another. At any particular time, the stage of pathogenesis in any given individual may be unknown.

Culture of MAP

This test is usually considered to have 100% specificity [30, 57] assuming the appropriate confirmatory tests are used. However, the sensitivity is imperfect because of stage of disease, sample selection and sample decontamination [28, 58]. Sensitivity estimates for culture of faeces range from 16 to 74% across species and stages of disease [30]. Culture of intestinal tissues is the most sensitive way to confirm infection at individual animal level. In addition, culture results can be quantitative [59, 60] and culture performed in liquid medium is more sensitive than culture on solid media (reviewed in [57]). Due to intermittent shedding of *MAP* in faeces, the more frequently samples are collected and tested the greater the number of shedding individuals that can be detected [61].

Direct faecal PCR tests

Direct faecal PCR tests have been developed in recent years [32, 62–65]. If results are normalized against a DNA standard curve, such tests provide quantitative results which correlate with stage of disease [65]. High *MAP* DNA quantities are more likely to represent true infection rather than passive (pass through) shedding of the bacterium [66]. There are few validation studies of test accuracy for direct faecal PCR tests, but sensitivity and specificity of some tests may be similar to faecal culture [65].

Anti-MAP antibody ELISA

A positive result in antibody ELISA is defined by the test kit manufacturer, or the user in terms of sample-to-positive (S/P) or another normalized value. The results of many studies have shown that the specificity of the assay is usually high [30] except in certain geographical locations where specificity may be low due to exposure to environmental mycobacteria [67]. Antibody ELISA on serum samples or milk samples has relatively low sensitivity [30, 68] except in late stages of the disease. Positive results can indicate exposure to *MAP* [69].

Interferon-gamma (IFN-γ)

A positive result is defined in terms of S/P or another normalized value. There have been few validation studies [30] and the specificity of the assay may vary depending on the species, age of the cohort tested and the experimental protocol used. Positive results have been associated with exposure to *MAP* but not necessarily with infection [50, 70]. The assay offers the potential to detect exposure to *MAP* early in the life of an animal, however the sensitivity of the IFN- γ assay is unknown [71].

Lymphocyte proliferation assay

This is a research tool. A positive result is defined by the laboratory; there have been no validation studies but positive results have been associated with exposure to *MAP* [16, 72–74].

Necropsy

This enables a thorough examination of relevant tissues (particularly those of the ileum and associated lymph nodes) and their collection for *MAP* culture as well as histopathological examination. The greater the number of sites in the intestine examined the more likely it is that infection and or disease will be detected [75].

Gross pathology

The gross pathology associated with *MAP* infection, which includes enlargement of mesenteric and ileocaecal lymph nodes and thickening of the intestinal mucosa is not specific to paratuberculosis, and gross changes do not occur in all affected animals [76–80]. Cording of lymphatic vessels in the serosa, mesentery and associated lymph nodes is due to advanced granulomatous inflammation, usually in late stages of pathogenesis.

Histopathology

Objective lesion scoring criteria have been published and are widely used in research applications [12, 48, 81–84]. These systems have multiple categories to describe the extent, severity and nature of the granulomatous lesions that characterize paratuberculosis. The Perez classification [81], like others is categorical and not necessarily ordinal. However, it is likely that there is an order of progression of lesions from mild to severe, and from paucibacillary to multibacillary, based on the results of sequential biopsies [48]. Using the system of Perez et al. (1996) [81] this is from 1 (mild focal) to 2 (focal) to 3a (multifocal), and then to either 3b (multifocal to diffuse, multibacillary) or 3c (multifocal to diffuse, paucibacillary). It is important that relevant tissues are examined. In general, the terminal ileum and ileocaceal valve region and nearby lymph nodes are considered to be predilection sites, but lesions extend more widely along the intestine as the disease progresses [82, 85, 86]; examination of a wider range of intestinal sites and associated lymph nodes is recommended to be more confident that lesions are not present.

Definitions of terms

The following terms are based on the systematic collection of objective historical evidence, clinical signs and laboratory test results that can be organized hierarchically into a logical framework for conceptualization of case definitions. The hierarchy is presented in Fig. 2.

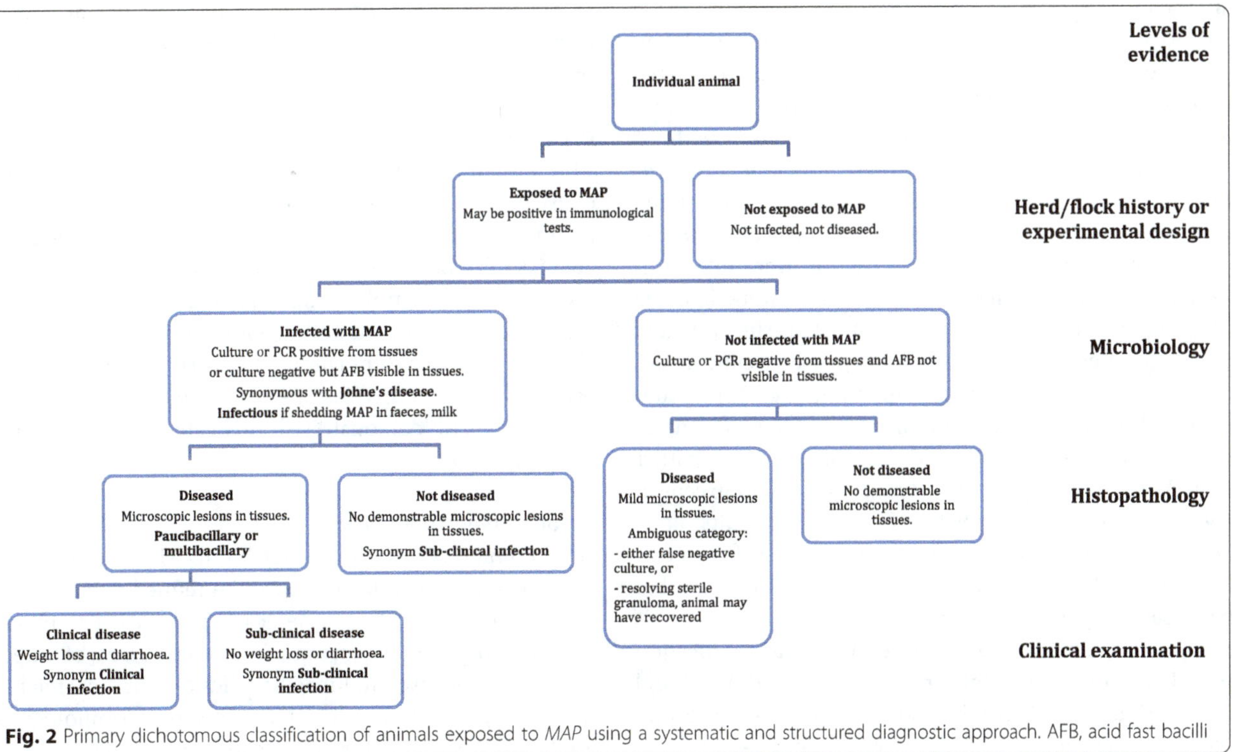

Fig. 2 Primary dichotomous classification of animals exposed to *MAP* using a systematic and structured diagnostic approach. AFB, acid fast bacilli

Paratuberculosis or Johne's disease

This is a comprehensive term to describe all forms of infection with and disease caused by *MAP*. It does not necessarily imply that the animal has outward signs of disease.

Exposed

The animal has been exposed to *MAP*, either through direct or indirect contact with known-infected animals, pasture or bedding or milk, or through an experimental infection. This classification is based on history, a field epidemiological assessment, or direct knowledge of the experimental design. It might be possible to determine whether there was exposure to a potentially infectious dose, or alternatively whether the exposure was unlikely to be sufficient to lead to infection.

Infected

The animal is infected with *MAP* based on a microbiological assessment. Infection is defined by culturing *MAP* from the tissues of the animal, or by demonstrating *MAP* in the tissues by PCR. This is a definitive test process that is conducted post mortem or through biopsy. Culture of faeces can provide indirect evidence of infection. The presence of *MAP* in faeces can be due to pass through (passive shedding) when the animal is ingesting *MAP* from the environment, and although this provides very strong evidence of exposure, it is not confirmation of infection. Pass through occurs for 7–10 days after a single oral exposure in small ruminants and cattle [40, 87–93]. Detection of *MAP* in faeces on more than one occasion (i.e. from independent samples collected on different days) provides more information and is suggestive of infection. In one study, 80% of cows with ≥1 faecal sample positive in culture also had a positive culture test result from their intestinal tissues, confirming true infection [94]. In a 2.5 year trial, 80% of *MAP* exposed sheep grazing together on pasture were infectious (≥ 1 positive fecal culture) but only 45% were infected [95]. Faecal shedding in the uninfected sheep halted 6 months after exposure. Except in special circumstances (see below), microscopic examination alone of tissues collected at post mortem or biopsy is not sufficient to define infection because acid fast bacilli (AFB) other than *MAP* may be present in tissues [80]. Also except in special circumstances, positive ELISA test results alone are not sufficient to define infection because false positive immunological reactions are possible in animals that have been exposed to environmental mycobacteria; this can occur sporadically or because of geographic location [67]. Due to the potential for pass through of *MAP*, and for spurious ELISA results, positive faecal culture and blood or milk antibody ELISA test outcomes on more than one sampling occasion increase the confidence about infection of the animal, but are not definitive.

Clinically infected

The animal is infected and has clinical signs (see Clinical Disease below).

Subclinically infected

The animal is infected but does not have clinical signs (see Subclinical Disease below).

Infectious

The animal is shedding viable *MAP* in its faeces or milk. This classification is based on a microbiological assessment and is defined by positive results in faecal or milk culture. The analytical sensitivity of faecal culture is ≥100 bacilli per gram of faeces [57]. As the infectious dose is not accurately known [49, 96], any detection of *MAP* in faeces by culture indicates that the animal is potentially infectious. The amount of shedding and therefore the relative degree of infectiousness can be determined by culture, and animals can be graded into light, medium or heavy shedders or super-shedders [97, 98]. In the case of pass through shedding, the animal may be considered to be infectious at the time it was shedding. In special circumstances (see below) such as experimental inoculation trials where live bacteria have been administered orally and infection is likely, or where prior faecal culture tests were positive, shedding may be defined by faecal PCR or faecal smear stained with Ziehl Neelsen (ZN), acknowledging that these tests do not distinguish between live and dead bacteria. Quantitative faecal PCR can provide information on the level of shedding [65].

Diseased

The animal has demonstrable histopathological lesions consistent with *MAP* infection. It may also have gross pathological lesions in the intestinal tissues and associated lymph nodes. Most but not all diseased animals will also have demonstrable infection (Fig. 2). Gross lesions are not specific for paratuberculosis and may be absent [76]. There is an ambiguous category where exposure occurred, microscopic lesions are present but the organisms cannot be demonstrated; this category includes recovered cases.

Histopathology positive

Granulomatous lesions attributable to *MAP* are present. The morphological diagnosis can be refined using one of the lesion classification schemes [12, 48, 81–84] to assess the stage of disease and infer the degree of infectiousness, because multibacillary lesions are correlated with heavy faecal shedding [50]. Specific terminology is used in Australia for diagnostic purposes [53]: "a diagnosis of 'lesions consistent with *MAP* infection' is indicated if in any one section, one or more single giant cells and/or one or more accumulations of epithelioid macrophages are observed in the intestinal lamina propria and/or lymph node cortex with the presence of at least one acid fast organism (AFO) morphologically consistent with *MAP*"; a finding 'suggestive of *MAP* infection' is indicated if AFO are not observed. Arguably, microscopic evidence is incomplete unless AFB in the lesions are confirmed to be *MAP*, for example by PCR, or are cultured from the tissues, because other species of mycobacteria can induce similar lesions. Lesion progression is not well described and the distinct categories defined below represent a continuum; for example early lesions in the category of 3a [81] may be paucibacillary or multibacillary precursors.

Paucibacillary lesion

These histopathological lesions do not contain large numbers of AFB [81, 82]. In the classification of Perez et al. (1996) [81] these are typically score 3c lesions, which are quite widespread, but the more focal lesion grades of 1, 2, and 3a usually contain no or few detectable AFB.

Multibacillary lesion

These histopathological lesions are typically widespread or diffuse and contain large numbers of AFB [81, 82]. In the system of Perez et al. (1996) [81] these are termed 3b lesions, but some of the earlier lesions in the 3a category can also contain large numbers of AFB.

Clinical disease

The animal has disease and associated clinical signs, specifically demonstrable weight loss, measured as ≥10% body weight loss over one month [99], and/or is in low body condition score relative to the majority of animals in the flock/herd. Objective visual body condition scoring systems are used internationally [100]. Cattle may have diarrhoea; usually this is profuse and watery. Small ruminants usually do not have watery diarrhoea, and often have normal faecal pellets.

Sub-clinical disease

The animal is diseased but does not have clinical signs attributable to paratuberculosis.

The clinical signs of paratuberculosis are not specific. Weight loss and diarrhoea may occur for a variety of reasons, therefore clinical signs alone cannot be used to define paratuberculosis. Where clinical signs are observed, they can be ascribed to paratuberculosis only when microscopic pathology in the intestine is observed that is consistent with paratuberculosis, with or without gross pathology. Except in special circumstances, culture of *MAP* from tissues or faeces cannot be used as the only test to confirm that clinical signs are due to *MAP* because clinical signs are not due to infection per se; this is clear because animals with paucibacillary or multibacillary lesions can succumb to clinical disease; these are cases with widespread severe lesions rather than mild lesions [85].

Resistant/resilient

It may be possible to classify animals with resistant phenotypes in some circumstances (Fig. 3). Conceptually, resistant/resilient animals are known to have received an infectious dose of *MAP* at an age when they were susceptible but the infection does not establish, does not progress, or remains in a dormant state so that when the animal is examined at necropsy, the infection cannot be detected by culture of tissues and there is no evidence of disease in the histopathological examination.

Recovered from paratuberculosis

The concept of recovery from paratuberculosis depends on strong evidence in order to be accepted. It is a subset of resistant/resilient (Fig. 3). Recovery from paratuberculosis has seldom been demonstrated; it means the elimination of a demonstrable infection [48]. Proof of recovery requires detailed examinations at more than one time point: the animal is shown to be infected and may be diseased at the first time point and is not infected at a subsequent time point. Recovered animals may have residual histopathological lesions from which *MAP* cannot be cultured (sterile granuloma), i.e. have evidence of disease, but the lesions should be mild or of a lower grade than those observed at an earlier time point.

To show resistant/resilient and recovered, exposure to a known infectious dose of *MAP* can be inferred in two

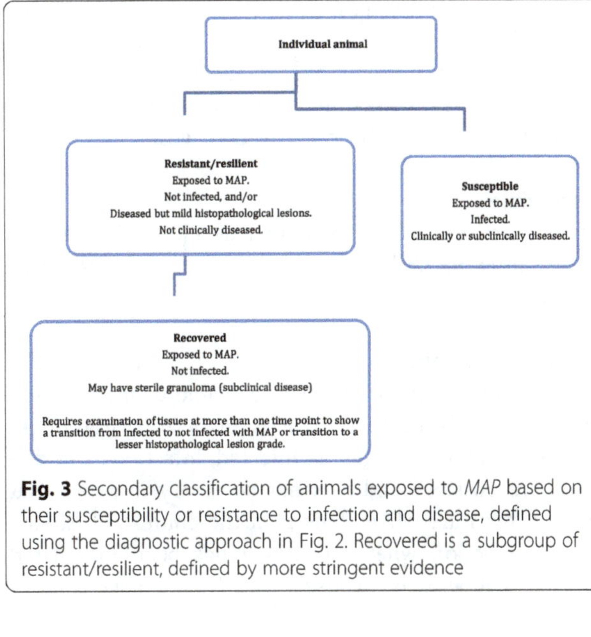

Fig. 3 Secondary classification of animals exposed to *MAP* based on their susceptibility or resistance to infection and disease, defined using the diagnostic approach in Fig. 2. Recovered is a subgroup of resistant/resilient, defined by more stringent evidence

ways. Firstly, using a recognized experimental infection model in which the animal was exposed to *MAP* at a susceptible age by direct inoculation on more than one occasion [49, 99, 101]. Susceptibility of cattle and sheep to MAP infection is greatest before about 6 months of age [102, 103]. A second way is in natural settings where paratuberculosis has been observed. In both contexts, a spectrum of disease is subsequently observed in the cohort of animals, showing that the exposure led to infection and that the host/environmental conditions were conducive to disease expression. Laboratory tests can be used to confirm exposure of individuals, for example a positive result in the IFN-γ test, lymphocyte proliferation assay, anti-*MAP* antibody ELISA and/or faecal culture [30, 50, 69, 70, 72, 99, 104–106] can indicate exposure. *MAP* DNA quantities in faeces assessed by direct quantitative faecal PCR test must be low, that is, there is no evidence of heavy shedding of *MAP* [32, 65]. It is well known that young animals shed *MAP* for a short time commencing several months post exposure; then, after a potentially long latent period, active shedding may recommence as the disease progresses [95, 107, 108]. Therefore, to confirm resistance it is necessary to show that if faecal shedding occurred in a young animal, it ceased, and then there was a lengthy period during which the animal did not shed *MAP*; consequently this assessment can be made only in adult animals after several years. Following necropsy, *MAP* cultures on tissues collected from multiple sites in the gut including the ileocaecal valve and associated lymph nodes must be negative and histopathological lesions if detected must be mild (for example Perez score < 2 [81]). Necropsy examination must be conducted after the animal has had enough time to develop identifiable histopathological lesions, i.e. in adults preferably after several years. Further research is required to properly define these intervals for verification, but the scale is likely to be measured in years.

Susceptible

Susceptible animals are those that develop infection and disease after natural or experimental exposure to *MAP* (Fig. 3).

Special circumstances

Where objective information is available to increase the level of confidence that *MAP* is involved, variation in the criteria above that define infected, infectious and diseased are possible, and it is not necessary to prove that mycobacteria are *MAP*. This is in the context of experimental infection when an animal has been inoculated with or deliberately exposed to *MAP*, a spectrum of disease has been demonstrated after exposure in the cohort, and mycobacterial agents such as *M. bovis* are not present in the population. Natural exposure to *MAP* may be certain, specifically when herd history and expert opinion exists to determine that an animal has been exposed, for example in a herd or flock pasture grazing scenario where there is a high prevalence of infection, or where dairy calves have been exposed to known-infected dams and other mycobacterial diseases are believed not to be present in the population. In these circumstances, AFB observed in tissues or faeces are assumed to be *MAP*; characteristic histopathological lesions without AFB are assumed to be due to *MAP*; anti-*MAP* antibody ELISA positive tests on more than one sampling occasion are assumed to be due to *MAP* exposure; an animal is assumed to be infectious where a prior faecal culture test was positive and later there are positive faecal smear or PCR results (acknowledging that faecal smear and PCR do not distinguish between live and dead bacteria).

Incorporation of terms in case definitions

To be useful, case definitions should be written using terms that are well understood; the descriptions provided above are designed to this end. In addition, where the results of diagnostic tests are used to assign individuals to categories, these tests must be described, and their accuracy documented. This enables an assessment of the extent to which particular case definitions are based on sound data, are consistent and are likely to be "correct". For example if the only evidence of paratuberculosis is an ELISA test result, the level of confidence that an animal is infectious is very low, and if the ELISA test result is negative, it should not be assumed that the animal is not infected.

Conclusions

In this paper, we have proposed descriptive terms for inclusion in case definitions for different stages in the pathogenesis of paratuberculosis. This evolved while planning large scale trials and from our perception that there was a need more broadly for discussion leading to consensus regarding the inclusion of information and reporting of case definitions. Our aim is to propose a framework for animal classification and promote further research. The terminology provided here will be useful in diagnostic test evaluations, prevalence studies, certification of disease freedom, studies of vaccine efficacy, genome wide association studies and also in routine diagnosis of paratuberculosis. Considerations such as time, budget and practicality often determine study designs, however, it should be possible to make an independent assessment of the rigor and extent to which case definitions are met in any given study by determining whether definitions for stages of disease have been applied consistently. This will assist in the general interpretation of data between studies, and will facilitate future meta-analyses.

Abbreviations

AFB: Acid fast bacilli; AFO: Acid fast organism; DNA: Deoxyribonucleic acid; ELISA: Enzyme-linked immunosorbent assay; GWAS: Genome wide association study; IFN-γ: Interferon-gamma; MAP: *Mycobacterium avium* subsp. *paratuberculosis*; OIE: Office International des Epizooties, World Organisation for Animal Health; PCR: Polymerase chain reaction; qPCR: Quantitative real time PCR; ZN: Ziehl Neelsen

Acknowledgements

The authors are grateful to many field veterinarians, animal health officers, and laboratory technical staff at the University of Sydney who contributed to underlying research projects over many years, ideas from which led to this study.

Funding

This work was supported by The University of Sydney, Meat and Livestock Australia and by the Cattle Council of Australia, Sheepmeat Council of Australia and WoolProducers Australia through Animal Health Australia. None of the funding bodies contributed in any way to the design of the study or the collection, analysis, interpretation of data or writing of the manuscript.

Authors' contributions

RW conceived and wrote the manuscript. RW, DB, KDS, AP, ND and KP contributed to and refined the contents during a 10 year research project on paratuberculosis. RW, DB, KDS, AP, ND and KP read, edited and approved the final manuscript.

Consent for publication

Not applicable. This paper does not contain any individual person's data in any form (including and individual details, images or videos) and so does not require consent to publish.

Competing interests

The authors declare that they have no competing interests.

References

1. Daniels MJ, Henderson D, Greig A, Stevenson K, Sharp JM, Hutchings MR. The potential role of wild rabbits *Oryctolagus cuniculus* in the epidemiology of paratuberculosis in domestic ruminants. Epidemiol Infect. 2003;130(3): 553–9.
2. Nugent G, Whitford EJ, Hunnam JC, Wilson PR, Cross M, de Lisle GW. *Mycobacterium avium* subsp. *paratuberculosis* infection in wildlife on three deer farms with a history of Johne's disease. N Z Vet J. 2011; 59(6):293–8.
3. Kirkwood CD, Wagner J, Boniface K, Vaughan J, Michalski WP, Catto-Smith AG, Cameron DJ, Bishop RF. *Mycobacterium avium* subspecies *paratuberculosis* in children with early-onset Crohn's disease. Inflamm Bowel Dis. 2009;15(11):1643–55.
4. McGregor H, Abbott KA, Whittington RJ. Effects of *Mycobacterium avium* subsp *paratuberculosis* infection on serum biochemistry, body weight and wool growth in merino sheep: a longitudinal study. Small Rumin Res. 2015; 125:146–53.
5. Bush RD, Windsor PA, Toribio JA, Webster SR. Financial modelling of the potential cost of ovine Johne's disease and the benefit of vaccinating sheep flocks in southern new South Wales. Aust Vet J. 2008;86(10):398–403.
6. Bush RD, Windsor PA, Toribio JA. Losses of adult sheep due to ovine Johne's disease in 12 infected flocks over a 3-year period. Aust Vet J. 2006; 84(7):246–53.
7. Ott SL, Wells SJ, Wagner BA. Herd-level economic losses associated with Johne's disease on US dairy operations. Preventive Veterinary Medicine. 1999;40(3–4):179–92.
8. Benedictus G, Dijkhuizen AA, Stelwagen J. Economic losses due to paratuberculosis in dairy cattle. Vet Rec. 1987;121(7):142–6.
9. Caspersen O. Wasted cows. Emaciated dairy cattle with poor welfare status are a growing problem. [Danish]. Dansk Veterinaertidsskrift. 2003;86:12–4.
10. Waddell LA, Rajic A, Stärk KDC, McEwen SA. The zoonotic potential of *Mycobacterium avium* ssp. *paratuberculosis*: a systematic review and meta-analyses of the evidence. Epidemiol Infect. 2015;143(15):3135–57.
11. Waddell LA, Rajić A, Stärk KDC, McEwen SA. The potential public health impact of *Mycobacterium avium* ssp. *paratuberculosis*: global opinion survey of topic specialists. Zoonoses Public Health. 2016;63(3):212–22.
12. Vazquez P, Garrido JM, Molina E, Geijo MV, Gomez N, Perez V, Sevilla IA, Alonso-Hearn M, Cortes A, Juste RA. Latent infections are the most frequent form of paratuberculosis in slaughtered Friesian cattle. Span J Agric Res. 2014;12(4):1049.
13. Whittington RJ, Begg DJ, de Silva K, Plain KM, Purdie AC. Comparative immunological and microbiological aspects of paratuberculosis as a model mycobacterial infection. Vet Immunol Immunopathol. 2012;148(1–2):29–47.
14. Gurjav U, Jelfs P, Hill-Cawthorne GA, Marais BJ, Sintchenko V. Genotype heterogeneity of *Mycobacterium tuberculosis* within geospatial hotspots suggests foci of imported infection in Sydney, Australia. Infection Genetics and Evolution. 2016;40:346–51.
15. Gurjav U, Burneebaatar B, Narmandakh E, Tumenbayar O, Ochirbat B, Hill-Cawthorne GA, Marais BJ, Sintchenko V. Spatiotemporal evidence for cross-border spread of MDR-TB along the trans-Siberian railway line. International Journal of Tuberculosis and Lung Disease. 2015;19(11):1376–82.
16. Begg DJ, O'Brien R, Mackintosh CG, Griffin JF. Experimental infection model for Johne's disease in sheep. Infect Immun. 2005;73(9):5603–11.
17. Solomons RS, Visser DH, Marais BJ, Schoeman JF, van Furth AM. Diagnostic accuracy of a uniform research case definition for TBM in children: a prospective study. International Journal of Tuberculosis and Lung Disease. 2016;20(7):903–8.
18. De Buck J, Shaykhutdinov R, Barkema HW, Vogel HJ. Metabolomic profiling in cattle experimentally infected with *Mycobacterium avium* subsp. *paratuberculosis*. PLoS One. 2014;9(11):e111872.
19. Stein CM. Genetic epidemiology of tuberculosis susceptibility: impact of study design. PLoS Pathog. 2011;7(1):e1001189.
20. Wiseman CA, Mandalakas AM, Kirchner HL, Gie RP, Schaaf HS, Walters E, Hesseling AC. Novel application of NIH case definitions in a paediatric tuberculosis contact investigation study. International Journal of Tuberculosis and Lung Disease. 2015;19(4):446–53.
21. Marais S, Thwaites G, Schoeman J, Esteee Torok M, Misra U, Prasad K, Donald P, Wilkinson R, Marais B. Tuberculous meningitis: a uniform case definition for use in clinical research. Lancet Infect Dis. 2010;10:803–12.
22. Kotilainen H, Valtonen V, Tukiainen P, Poussa T, Eskola J, Jarvinen A. Prognostic value of American Thoracic Society criteria for non-tuberculous mycobacterial disease: a retrospective analysis of 120 cases with four years of follow-up. Scand J Infect Dis. 2013;45(3):194–202.
23. Zare Y, Shook GE, Collins MT, Kirkpatrick BW. Evidence of birth seasonality and clustering of *Mycobacterium avium* subspecies *paratuberculosis* infection in US dairy herds. Preventive Veterinary Medicine. 2013;112(3–4):276–84.
24. Gonda MG, Kirkpatrick BW, Shook GE, Collins MT. Identification of a QTL on BTA20 affecting susceptibility to *Mycobacterium avium* ssp. *paratuberculosis* infection in US Holsteins. Anim Genet. 2007;38(4):389–96.
25. Collins MT, Wells SJ, Petrini KR, Collins JE, Schultz RD, Whitlock RH. Evaluation of five antibody detection tests for diagnosis of bovine paratuberculosis. Clin Diagn Lab Immunol. 2005;12(6):685–92.
26. Sockett DC, Conrad TA, Thomas CB, Collins MT. Evaluation of 4 serological tests for bovine paratuberculosis. J Clin Microbiol. 1992;30(5):1134–9.

27. Osterstock JB, Sinha S, Seabury CM, Cohen ND. Effect of classifying disease states in genetic association studies for paratuberculosis. Preventive Veterinary Medicine. 2010;95(1–2):41–9.
28. Whittington RJ, Sergeant ES. Progress towards understanding the spread, detection and control of *Mycobacterium avium* subsp. *paratuberculosis* in animal populations. Aust Vet J. 2001;79(4):267–78.
29. Kupper J, Brandt H, Donat K, Erhardt G. Phenotype definition is a main point in genome-wide association studies for bovine *Mycobacterium avium* ssp. *paratuberculosis* infection status. Animal. 2014;8(10):1586–93.
30. Nielsen SS, Toft N. Ante mortem diagnosis of paratuberculosis: a review of accuracies of ELISA, interferon-gamma assay and faecal culture techniques. Vet Microbiol. 2008;129(3–4):217–35.
31. OIE. Principles and methods of validation of diagnostic assays for infectious diseases. In: *Manual of Diagnstic Tests and Vaccines for Terrestrial Animals. Volume 1*, edn. Paris: OIE; 2012. p. 34–51.
32. Kawaji S, Begg DJ, Plain KM, Whittington RJ. A longitudinal study to evaluate the diagnostic potential of a direct faecal quantitative PCR test for Johne's disease in sheep. Vet Microbiol. 2011;148(1):35–44.
33. Nielsen SS, Toft N, Gardner IA: Structured approach to design of diagnostic test evaluation studies for chronic progressive infections in animals. *Veterinary Microbiology* 2011(1873–2542 (Electronic)).
34. Purdie AC, Plain KM, Begg DJ, de Silva K, Whittington RJ: Candidate gene and genome-wide association studies of *Mycobacterium avium* subsp *paratuberculosis* infection in cattle and sheep: a review. Comp Immunol Microb 2011, 34(3):197–208.
35. Kirkpatrick BW, Shi X, Shook GE, Collins MT: Whole-Genome association analysis of susceptibility to paratuberculosis in holstein cattle. Anim Genet 2010, AGE2097 [pii] [doi] https://doi.org/10.1111/j.1365-2052.2010.02097.x.
36. Koets A, Santema W, Mertens H, Oostenrijk D, Keestra M, Overdijk M, Labouriau R, Franken P, Frijters A, Nielen M, et al. Susceptibility to paratuberculosis infection in cattle is associated with single nucleotide polymorphisms in toll-like receptor 2 which modulate immune responses against *Mycobacterium avium* subspecies *paratuberculosis*. Preventive Veterinary Medicine. 2010;93(4):305–15.
37. Pinedo PJ, Buergelt CD, Donovan GA, Melendez P, Morel L, Wu R, Langaee TY, Rae DO. Association between CARD15/NOD2 gene polymorphisms and paratuberculosis infection in cattle. Vet Microbiol. 2009;134(3–4):346–52.
38. Reddacliff LA, Beh K, McGregor H, Whittington RJ. A preliminary study of possible genetic influences on the susceptibility of sheep to Johne's disease. Aust Vet J. 2005;83(7):435–41.
39. Settles M, Zanella R, McKay S, Schnabel R, Taylor J, Whitlock R, Schukken Y, Van Kessel J, Smith J, Neibergs H. A whole genome association analysis identifies loci associated with *Mycobacterium avium* subsp. *paratuberculosis* infection status in US Holstein cattle. Anim Genet. 2009;40(5):655–62.
40. McDonald WL, Ridge SE, Hope AF, Condron RJ. Evaluation of diagnostic tests for Johne's disease in young cattle. Aust Vet J. 1999;77:113–9.
41. Bannantine JP, Talaat AM. Controlling Johne's disease: vaccination is the way forward. Front Cell Infect Microbiol. 2015;5:2.
42. Windsor PABR, Links I, Eppleston J. Injury caused by self-inoculation with a vaccine of a Freund's complete adjuvant nature (Gudair™) used for control of ovine paratuberculcosis. Aust Vet J. 2005;83(4):216–20.
43. Reddacliff L, Eppleston J, Windsor P, Whittington R, Jones S. Efficacy of a killed vaccine for the control of paratuberculosis in Australian sheep flocks. Vet Microbiol. 2006;115(1–3):77–90.
44. Dhand NK, Johnson WO, Eppleston J, Whittington RJ, Windsor PA. Comparison of pre- and post-vaccination ovine Johne's disease prevalence using a Bayesian approach. Prev Vet Med. 2013;111(1–2):81–91.
45. Singh SV, Singh PK, Kumar N, Gupta S, Chaubey KK, Singh B, Srivastav A, Yadav S, Dhama K. Evaluation of goat based 'indigenous vaccine' against bovine Johne's disease in endemically infected native cattle herds. Indian J Exp Biol. 2015;53(1):16–24.
46. Bull TJ, Vrettou C, Linedale R, McGuinnes C, Strain S, McNair J, Gilbert SC, Hope JC. Immunity, safety and protection of an adenovirus 5 prime-modified vaccinia virus Ankara boost subunit vaccine against *Mycobacterium avium* subspecies *paratuberculosis* infection in calves. Vet Res. 2014;45:112.
47. Subharat S, Shu D, Wedlock DN, Price-Carter M, de Lisle GW, Luo D, Collins DM, Buddle BM. Immune responses associated with progression and control of infection in calves experimentally challenged with *Mycobacterium avium* subsp. *paratuberculosis*. Vet Immunol Immunopathol. 2012;149(3–4):225–36.
48. Dennis MM, Reddacliff LA, Whittington RJ. Longitudinal study of clinicopathological features of Johne's disease in sheep naturally exposed to *Mycobacterium avium* subspecies *paratuberculosis*. Vet Pathol. 2011;48:565–75.
49. Begg DJ, Whittington RJ. Experimental animal infection models for Johne's disease, an infectious enteropathy caused by *Mycobacterium avium* subsp. *paratuberculosis*. Vet J. 2008;176(2):129–45.
50. de Silva K, Begg DJ, Plain KM, Purdie AC, Kawaji S, Dhand NK, Whittington RJ. Can early host responses to mycobacterial infection predict eventual disease outcomes. Preventive Veterinary Medicine. 2013;112(3–4):203–12.
51. Bannantine JP, Hines ME, Bermudez LE, Talaat AM, Sreevatsan S, Stabel JR, Chang YF, Coussens PM, Barletta RG, Davis WC *et al*: Rational framework for evaluating the next generation of vaccines against *Mycobacterium avium* subspecies *paratuberculosis*. *Front Cell Infect Microbiol* 2014, 4(SEP).
52. OIE. Chapter 2.1.11 Paratuberculosis. In: *Manual of Diagnostic Tests and Vaccines for Terrestrial Animals*. Edn. Paris: OIE. p. 2014.
53. Eamens G, Marsh I, Plain K, Whittington R. Australian and New Zealand standard diagnostic test protocols. Paratuberculosis (Johne's disease). Subcommittee on Animal Health Laboratory Standards: Canberra; 2016.
54. Alinovi CA, Ward MP, Lin TL, Moore GE, CC W. Real-time PCR, compared to liquid and solid culture media and ELISA, for the detection of *Mycobacterium avium* ssp. *paratuberculosis*. Vet Microbiol. 2009;136(1–2): 177–9.
55. Kostoulas P, Nielsen S, Branscumc A, Johnson W, Dendukurie N, Dhand N, Toft N, Gardner I. STARD-BLCM: standards for the reporting of diagnostic accuracy studies that use bayesian latent class models. Preventive Veterinary Medicine. 2017;138:37–47.
56. Whittington RJ, Marsh I, McAllister S, Turner MJ, Marshall DJ, Fraser CA. Evaluation of modified BACTEC 12B radiometric medium and solid media for culture of *Mycobacterium avium* subsp. *paratuberculosis* from sheep. J Clin Microbiol. 1999;37(4):1077–83.
57. Whittington RJ. Cultivation of *Mycobacterium avium* subsp. *paratuberculosis*. In: *Paratuberculosis Organism, Disease, Control*. Edn. Edited by Behr MA, Collins DM. Wallingford: CABI; 2010. p. 244–66.
58. Reddacliff LA, Vadali A, Whittington RJ. The effect of decontamination protocols on the numbers of sheep strain *Mycobacterium avium* subsp. *paratuberculosis* isolated from tissues and faeces. Vet Microbiol. 2003; 95(4):271–82.
59. Reddacliff LA, Nicholls PJ, Vadali A, Whittington RJ. Use of growth indices from radiometric culture for quantification of sheep strains of *Mycobacterium avium* subsp. *paratuberculosis*. Appl Environ Microbiol. 2003; 69(6):3510–6.
60. Shin SJ, Han JH, Manning EJ, Collins MT. Rapid and reliable method for quantification of *Mycobacterium paratuberculosis* by use of the BACTEC MGIT 960 system. J Clin Microbiol. 2007;45(6):1941–8.
61. Whitlock RH, Hutchinson LT, Sweeney RW, Spencer PA, Rosenberger AE, Van Buskirk MA. Pattern of detection of *M. paratuberculosis* infected cattle in ten dairy herds cultured every six months for four years. In: *Proceedings of the Fourth International Colloquium on Paratuberculosis*. Edn. Edited by Chiodini RJ, Collins MT, Bassey EOE. Madison: International Association for Paratuberculosis; 1994. p. 47–53.
62. Khare S, Ficht TA, Santos RL, Romano J, Ficht AR, Zhang SP, Grant IR, Libal M, Hunter D, Adams LG. Rapid and sensitive detection of *Mycobacterium avium* subsp. *paratuberculosis* in bovine milk and feces by a combination of immunomagnetic bead separation-conventional PCR and real-time PCR. J Clin Microbiol. 2004;42(3):1075–81.
63. Irenge LM, Walravens K, Govaerts M, Godfroid J, Rosseels V, Huygen K, Gala J-L. Development and validation of a triplex real-time PCR for rapid detection and specific identification of *M. avium* sub sp. *paratuberculosis* in faecal samples. Vet Microbiol. 2009;136(1–2):166–72.
64. Zhang MZ, Zhang S. An efficient DNA extraction method for polymerase chain reaction-based detection of *Mycobacterium avium* subspecies *paratuberculosis* in bovine fecal samples. J Vet Diagn Investig. 2011;23(1):41–8.
65. Plain KM, Marsh IB, Waldron AM, Galea F, Whittington A-M, Saunders VF, Begg DJ, de Silva K, Purdie AC, Whittington RJ. High-throughput direct fecal PCR assay for detection of *Mycobacterium avium* subsp *paratuberculosis* in sheep and cattle. J Clin Microbiol. 2014;52(3):745–57.
66. Sweeney RW, Collins MT, Koets AP, McGuirk SM, Roussel AJ. Paratuberculosis (Johne's disease) in cattle and other susceptible species. J Vet Intern Med. 2012;26(6):1239–50.

67. Pitt DJ, Pinch DS, Janmaat A, Condron RJ. An estimate of specificity for a Johne's disease absorbed ELISA in northern Australian cattle. Aust Vet J. 2002;80(1–2):57–60.
68. Jubb TF, Sergeant ESG, Callinan APL, Galvin JW. Estimate of the sensitivity of an ELISA used to detect Johne's disease in Victorian dairy cattle herds. Aust Vet J. 2004;82(9):569–73.
69. Begg DJ, de Silva K, Carter N, Plain KM, Purdie A, Whittington RJ. Does a Th1 over Th2 dominancy really exist in the early stages of *Mycobacterium avium* subspecies *paratuberculosis* infections. Immunobiology. 2011;216(7):840–6.
70. Jungersen G, Mikkelsen H, Grell SN. Use of the johnin PPD interferon-gamma assay in control of bovine paratuberculosis. Vet Immunol Immunopathol. 2012;148(1–2):48–54.
71. Vazquez P, Garrido JM, Juste RA. Specific antibody and interferon-gamma responses associated with immunopathological forms of bovine paratuberculosis in slaughtered Friesian cattle. PLoS One. 2013;8(5)
72. de Silva K, Begg D, Carter N, Taylor D, Di Fiore L, Whittington R. The early lymphocyte proliferation response in sheep exposed to *Mycobacterium avium* subsp. *paratuberculosis* compared to infection status. Immunobiology. 2010;215(1):12–25.
73. Koo HC, Park YH, Hamilton MJ, Barrington GM, Davies CJ, Kim JB, Dahl JL, Waters WR, Davis WC. Analysis of the immune response to *Mycobacterium avium* subsp. *paratuberculosis* in experimentally infected calves. Infect Immun. 2004;72(12):6870–83.
74. Kurade NP, Tripathi BN, Rajukumar K, Parihar NS. Sequential development of histologic lesions and their relationship with bacterial isolation, fecal shedding, and immune responses during progressive stages of experimental infection of lambs with *Mycobacterium avium* subsp. *paratuberculosis*. Vet Pathol. 2004;41(4):378–87.
75. Whitlock R, Rosenberger A, Sweeney R. In: Chiodini R, Hines M, Collins M, editors. Al e: distribution of *M paratuberculosis* in tissues of cattle form herds infected with Johne's disease. In: *Proceedings of the 5th International Colloquium on Paratuberculosis, Maddison, USA 29 September - 4 October 1996.* Edn. Rehoboth: International Association for Paratuberculosis; 1996. p. 168–74.
76. Abbott KA, Whittington RJ. Monte Carlo simulation of flock-level sensitivity of abattoir surveillance for ovine paratuberculosis. Preventive Veterinary Medicine. 2003;61(4):309–32.
77. Fodstad FH, Gunnarsson E. Post-mortem examination in the diagnosis of Johne's disease in goats. Acta Vet Scand. 1979;20(2):157–67.
78. Tafti AK, Rashidi K. The pathology of goat paratuberculosis: gross and histopathological lesions in the intestines and mesenteric lymph nodes. Zentralblatt Fur Veterinarmedizin - Reihe B. 2000;47:487–95.
79. Hope AF, Kluver PF, Jones SL, Condron RJ. Sensitivity and specificity of two serological tests for the detection of ovine paratuberculosis. Aust Vet J. 2000;78:850–6.
80. Cleland PC, Lehmann DR, Phillips PH, Cousins DV, Reddacliff LA, Whittington RJ. A survey to detect the presence of *Mycobacterium avium* subspecies *paratuberculosis* in Kangaroo Island macropods. Vet Microbiol. 2010;145(3–4): 339–46.
81. Perez V, Garcia Marin JF, Badiola JJ. Description and classification of different types of lesion associated with natural paratuberculosis infection in sheep. J Comp Pathol. 1996;114(2):107–22.
82. Gonzalez J, Geijo MV, Garcia-Pariente C, Verna A, Corpa JM, Reyes LE, Ferreras MC, Juste RA, Garcia Marin JF, Perez V. Histopathological classification of lesions associated with natural paratuberculosis infection in cattle. J Comp Pathol. 2005;133(2–3):184–96.
83. Dennis MM, Antognoli MC, Garry F, Hirst H, Lombard JE, Gould DH, Salman MD. Association of severity of enteric granulomatous inflammation with disseminated *Mycobacterium avium* subspecies *paratuberculosis* infection and antemortem test results for paratuberculosis in dairy cows. Vet Microbiol. 2008;131:154–63.
84. Clark RG, Griffin JF, Mackintosh CG. Johne's disease caused by *Mycobacterium avium* subsp. *paratuberculosis* infection in red deer (Cervus Elaphus): an histopathological grading system, and comparison of paucibacillary and multibacillary disease. N Z Vet J. 2010;58(2):90–7.
85. Clarke CJ, Little D. The pathology of ovine paratuberculosis: gross and histological changes in the intestine and other tissues. J Comp Pathol. 1996; 114(4):419–37.
86. Marshall D, Fraser C, Seaman J, Moloney B, Bailey G. Importance of sample site in histological diagnosis of Johne's disease in sheep. In: Manning E, Collins M, editors. *Proceedings of the 6th International Colloquium on Paratuberculosis.* Edn. Madison: International Association for Paratuberculosis; 1999. p. 511.
87. Larsen AB, Merkal RS, Cutlip RC. Age of cattle as related to resistance to infection with *Mycobacterium paratuberculosis*. Am J Vet Res. 1975; 36(3):255–7.
88. Sweeney RW, Whitlock RH, Rosenberger AE. *Mycobacterium paratuberculosis* cultured from milk and supramammary lymph nodes of infected asymptomatic cows. J Clin Microbiol. 1992;30:166–71.
89. Lyle PAS, Merkal RS. Comparison of ELISA and gel diffusion precipitin tests for paratuberculosis in cattle, sheep and goats. In: *Proceedings of the International Colloquium on Research in Paratuberculosis*, June 16–18. Merkal RS. Ames, Iowa: National Animal Disease Centre; 1983. p. 109–12.
90. Juste RA, Garcia Martin JF, de Ocariz CS, Badiola JJ. Experimental infection of vaccinated and non-vaccinated lambs with *Mycobacterium paratuberculosis*. J Comp Pathol. 1994;110:185–94.
91. Riemann H, Zaman MR, Ruppanner R, Aalund O, Jorgensen JB, Worsaae H, Behymer D. Paratuberculosis in cattle and free-living exotic deer. J Am Vet Med Assoc. 1979;174:841–3.
92. Whittington RJ, Reddacliff LA, Marsh I, McAllister S, Saunders V. Temporal patterns and quantification of excretion of *Mycobacterium avium* subsp *paratuberculosis* in sheep with Johne's disease. Aust Vet J. 2000;78(1):34–7.
93. Whittington RJ, Marsh I, Turner MJ, McAllister S, Choy E, Eamens GJ, Marshall DJ, Ottaway S. Rapid detection of *Mycobacterium paratuberculosis* in clinical samples from ruminants and in spiked environmental samples by modified BACTEC 12B radiometric culture and direct confirmation by IS900 PCR. J Clin Microbiol. 1998;36:701–7.
94. Pradhan AK, Mitchell RM, Kramer AJ, Zurakowski MJ, Fyock TL, Whitlock RH, Smith JM, Hovingh E, Van Kessel JA, Karns JS, et al. Molecular epidemiology of *Mycobacterium avium* subsp. *paratuberculosis* in a longitudinal study of three dairy herds. J Clin Microbiol. 2011;49(3):893–901.
95. Begg DJ, de Silva K, Plain KM, Purdie AC, Dhand N, Whittington RJ. Specific faecal antibody responses in sheep infected with *Mycobacterium avium* subspecies *paratuberculosis*. Vet Immunol Immunopathol. 2015;166(3–4): 125–31.
96. Reddacliff LA, Whittington RJ. Experimental infection of weaner sheep with S strain *Mycobacterium avium* subsp. *paratuberculosis*. Vet Microbiol. 2003; 96(3):247–58.
97. Whitlock RH, Wells SJ, Sweeney RW, Van Tiem J. ELISA and fecal culture for paratuberculosis (Johne's disease): sensitivity and specificity of each method. Vet Microbiol. 2000;77:387–98.
98. Whitlock R, Sweeney R, Fyock T, Smith J. MAP super-shedders: another factor in the control of Johne's disease. In: Manning E, Nielsen S, editors. *Proceedings of the 8th International Colloquium on paratuberculosis.* Edn. Madison: International Association for Paratuberculosis; 2005. p. 164.
99. Begg DJ, de Silva K, Di Fiore L, Taylor DL, Bower K, Zhong L, Kawaji S, Emery D, Whittington RJ. Experimental infection model for Johne's disease using a lyophilised, pure culture, seedstock of *Mycobacterium avium* subspecies *paratuberculosis*. Vet Microbiol. 2010;141:301–11.
100. Roche JR, Dillon PG, Stockdale CR, Baumgard LH, VanBaale MJ. Relationships among international body condition scoring systems. J Dairy Sci. 2004;87(9): 3076–9.
101. Hines ME, 2nd, Stabel JR, Sweeney RW, Griffin F, Talaat AM, Bakker D, Benedictus G, Davis WC, de Lisle GW, Gardner IA *et al*: Experimental challenge models for Johne's disease: a review and proposed international guidelines. Vet Microbiol 2007, 122(3–4):197–222.
102. Windsor PA, Whittington RJ. Evidence for age susceptibility of cattle to Johne's disease. Vet J. 2010;184(1):37–44.
103. McGregor H, Dhand NK, Dhungyel OP, Whittington RJ. Transmission of *Mycobacterium avium* subsp. *paratuberculosis*: dose-response and age-based susceptibility in a sheep model. Preventive Veterinary Medicine. 2012;107(1–2):76–84.
104. de Silva K, Begg D, Whittington R. The interleukin 10 response in ovine Johne's disease. Vet Immunol Immunopathol. 2011;139:10–6.
105. Mortier RA, Barkema HW, Negron ME, Orsel K, Wolf R, De Buck J. Antibody response early after experimental infection with *Mycobacterium avium* subspecies *paratuberculosis* in dairy calves. J Dairy Sci. 2014;97(9):5558–65.
106. Mortier RA, Barkema HW, Wilson TA, Sajobi TT, Wolf R, De Buck J. Dose-dependent interferon-gamma release in dairy calves experimentally infected with *Mycobacterium avium* subspecies *paratuberculosis*. Vet Immunol Immunopathol. 2014;161(3–4):205–10.

107. van Roermund HJ, Bakker D, Willemsen PT, de Jong MC. Horizontal transmission of *Mycobacterium avium* subsp. *paratuberculosis* in cattle in an experimental setting: calves can transmit the infection to other calves. Vet Microbiol. 2007;122(3–4):270–9.
108. Mortier RAR, Barkema HW, Orsel K, Wolf R, De Buck J. Shedding patterns of dairy calves experimentally infected with *Mycobacterium avium* subspecies *paratuberculosis*. Vet Res. 2014;45(1).

9

Comparison of competitive exclusion with classical cleaning and disinfection on bacterial load in pig nursery units

K. Luyckx[1], S. Millet[2], S. Van Weyenberg[1], L. Herman[1], M. Heyndrickx[1,3], J. Dewulf[4] and K. De Reu[1*]

Abstract

Background: Colonisation of the environment of nursery units by pathogenic micro-organisms is an important factor in the persistence and spread of endemic diseases in pigs and zoonotic pathogens. These pathogens are generally controlled by the use of antibiotics and disinfectants. Since an increasing resistance against these measures has been reported in recent years, methods such as competitive exclusion (CE) are promoted as promising alternatives.

Results: This study showed that the infection pressure in CE units after microbial cleaning was not reduced to the same degree as in control units. Despite sufficient administration of probiotic-type spores, the analysed bacteria did not decrease in number after 3 production rounds in CE units, indicating no competitive exclusion. In addition, no differences in feed conversion were found between piglets raised in CE and control units in our study. Also, no differences in faecal consistency (indicator for enteric diseases) was noticed.

Conclusion: These results indicate that the CE protocol is not a valuable alternative for classical C&D.

Keywords: Competitive exclusion, Cleaning and disinfection, Bacterial load, Pig nursery units

Abbreviations: AC, After cleaning; AD, After disinfection; BC, Before cleaning; BPW, Buffered peptone water; C&D, Cleaning and disinfection; CE, Competitive exclusion; CFU, Colony forming units; CS (%), Proportion of countable samples given in percentage; D (%), Proportion of positive samples after detection given in percentage; *E. coli*, *Escherichia coli*; ILVO, Institute for agricultural and fisheries research; MBC, Minimum bactericidal concentration; MIC, Minimum inhibitory concentration; MRSA ST398, Methicillin resistant *Staphylococcus aureus* sequence type 398; MRSM, chromID® MRSA-SMART medium; PIP AHC, Probiotics in process animal house cleaner; PIP AHS, Probiotics in process animal house stabilizer; Q1, First quartile; Q2, Median; Q3, Third quartile; QAC, Quaternary ammonium compounds; TD100, Treatment days per 100 days at risk; W1, After one week of production; W5, After five weeks of production

Background

Colonisation of the environment in nursery units by pathogenic micro-organisms is an important factor in the persistence and spread of endemic diseases in pigs and of zoonotic pathogens. These infections are often controlled by the use of antibiotics and disinfectants [1]. However, an increasing level of resistance against these substances has been observed in recent years [2–5]. Since 2005, methicillin resistant *Staphylococcus aureus* sequence type 398 (MRSA ST398) has been found on farms and farm animals, especially pigs [6–8]. MRSA ST398 has a multiresistant phenotype [9], a zoonotic character [10] and can also pick up new resistance genes [11]. Wong et al. [12] described the presence of disinfectant resistance genes in porcine MRSA. The minimum inhibitory and bactericidal concentrations (MIC and MBC) of these MRSA strains were lower than the recommended concentrations of disinfectants. However, there is concern that an impairment of the used disinfectant, resulting in exposure to lower active levels of these agents (e.g., due to presence

* Correspondence: koen.dereu@ilvo.vlaanderen.be
[1]Institute for Agricultural and Fisheries Research (ILVO), Technology and Food Science Unit, Melle, Belgium
Full list of author information is available at the end of the article

of organic material), resistant MRSA strains harbouring these disinfectant resistance genes may be selected [12]. Slifierz et al. [13] showed that the use of quaternary ammonium compound-based (QAC) disinfectants is a risk for selecting (antibiotic resistant) MRSA in commercial swine herds. Antibiotic multiresistant *Salmonella* strains on pig farms have been described in several countries [14–16]. Randall et al. [17] suggested that the use of biocides alone or combined with antibiotic treatment may also increase selective pressure towards antibiotic resistance of *Salmonella enterica*. Beier et al. [18] showed that β-haemolytic enterotoxigenic *Escherichia coli* (*E. coli*) strains isolated from neonatal pigs, were resistant to chlorhexidine and QAC. Some of these resistant strains had also multiple antibiotic resistance.

Because of the ongoing concern about excessive use of biocides and potential resistance development and cross-resistance to clinically important antibiotics, the use of bacterial biocontrol agents has often been suggested as an alternative method to antagonise the growth of these pathogens. The working mechanism of these biocontrol agents is based on the concept of micro-organisms that should compete with pathogens in the environment by competitive exclusion, influencing quorum sensing, producing antimicrobial compounds (e.g., bacteriocins) and/or competition for attachment sites [19]. However, only very few reports describing the use and the effectiveness of microbial biocontrol agents on farms are available in literature. The aim of this study was to compare the effectiveness of a commercial competitive exclusion (CE) protocol with a classical cleaning and disinfection (C&D) protocol in decreasing *Salmonella*; (haemolytic) *E. coli*, faecal coliforms, *Enterococcus* spp. and MRSA contamination of nursery units during 3 successive rounds.

Methods

Management in control and CE units

This study was carried out in 6 identical nursery units at the experimental pig farm of the Institute for Agricultural and Fisheries Research (ILVO) during 3 successive production rounds. Piglets were moved to these units immediately after weaning (4 weeks of age) and stayed there for 6 weeks. Three units were assigned to the control group (classical C&D protocol) and 3 to the treatment group (CE protocol). Each compartment consists of eight identical pens of 1.8 m^2. Piglets were raised per six in one pen. After 6 weeks, piglets were transported to fattening units and pens were cleaned (and disinfected) according to the tested protocols.

Classical C&D protocol was carried out after pigs were removed. Manure was removed by cleaning with cold water. Twenty-four hours later, pens were soaked with 2 % MS Topfoam (sodium hydroxide) (Schippers, Bladel, The Netherlands) for 30 min. The cleaning product and any remaining dirt was removed under high pressure with cold water (150 bar) and pens were disinfected with 1 % (v/v) MS Megades (glutaraldehyde and quaternary ammonium compounds) (Schippers). Finally, the pens were kept empty during two weeks of down-time.

The CE units pens were first hosed down with cold water to remove manure; 24 h later they were soaked with 1.5 % (v/v) PIP AHC (Probiotics In Process Animal House Cleaner, Chrisal, Lommel, Belgium) at 40 °C for 10 min and rinsed with warm water (40 °C). PIP AHC consists of cleaning compounds, *Bacillus* spp. spores and enzymes. In CE units, no disinfection was carried out. In addition, during the 2-week down-time period as well as during production, CE units were sprayed 2–3 times per week with pure PIP AHS (Animal Housing Stabilizer, Chrisal) to bring and retain biocontrol agents into the stall environment. In the first week of production during the third round, CE units were sprayed every day of the week with PIP AHS. The AHC and AHS PIP products contained *Bacillus* spp. spores of five different species in a concentration of 8.5 and 7.5 log colony forming units (CFU)/mL, respectively.

Both protocols were carried out according to the manufacturers guidelines. For each protocol an individual and identical high pressure jet (Kärcher, HDS 6/14-4CX, Temse, Belgium) was used.

Sampling scheme

Sampling was performed at different time points ("sampling moments"): (1) immediately after pig loading (before cleaning, BC); (2) 24 h after cleaning (CE units) (AC) or 24 h after disinfection (control units) (AD); (3) after 1 week (W1) and (4) after 5 weeks of production (W5) (piglets present). Three pens per compartment were sampled at each sampling moment. Premoistened sponge swab samples with 10 mL Buffered Peptone Water (BPW) (3 M, SSL10BPW, St-Paul, USA) were taken at five locations per pen: synthetic grid floor, concrete wall, synthetic wall, drinking nipples and feeding trough. Samples were taken in triplicate per type of location resulting in 15 swab samples per nursery unit at each sampling moment. After disinfection, 10 mL Dey Engley neutralising broth (Sigma Aldrich, Fluka, D3435, St-Louis, USA) was used to premoisten the sponge swab samples (SSL100, 3 M) used. A surface of 625 cm^2 (A4 paper format) was sampled. Because the surface of the drinking nipples was smaller than 625 cm^2, 2 drinking nipples per pen were sampled and pooled as one sample.

Sample processing

Samples were transported to the lab under refrigeration and stored at 3 ± 2 °C for 18 h before further processing. Samples were first diluted with 30 ml of BPW (Oxoid,

CM0509, Basingstroke, Hampshire, England) and then homogenized by placing them in a Masticator (IUL instruments, S.A., Barcelona, Spain). Prior to plating, swab samples were further serial diluted (1:10) in peptone physiological salt water (Bio Trading, K110B009AA, Mijdrecht, The Netherlands) to produce countable results on the selected agar media: Slanetz-and-Bartley (Oxoid, CM0377) for *Enterococcus* spp., Rapid *E. coli* (Biorad, 356–4024, Marnes-la-Coquettes, France) for *E. coli* and faecal coliforms and chromID® MRSA-SMART (MRSM, bioMérieux, 413050,Marcy l'Etoile, France) for MRSA enumerations. Slanetz and Bartley, Rapid *E. coli* and MRSA-SMART agar plates were incubated at 37 °C during 48 h, 44 °C during 24 h and at 37 °C during 24–48 h, respectively. A 3 ml BPW-fraction of the sample was heated for 10 min at 80 °C, diluted in peptone water and plated on Plate Count Agar (Oxoid, CM0325) for spore enumerations in order to determine the CFU count in both PIP products and to test if *Bacillus* spp. spores were well distributed and sufficiently present in pens. Plate Count Agar plates were incubated for 72 h at 30 °C. Also, a 10 ml BPW-fraction of the sample was mixed with 10 ml double concentrated Mueller Hinton Broth (Oxoid, CM0405) and 13 % (w/v) sodium chloride (Merck, 1.06404.500, Darmstadt, Germany). After overnight incubation at 37 °C, 100 µl was plated on MRSM for detection of MRSA. In addition, the original sample diluted in BPW (i.e., the remaining BPW fraction) was overnight incubated at 37 °C for detection methods. Detection of *E. coli* and faecal coliforms was carried out by plating 10 µl of the enriched BPW fraction on Rapid *E. coli* medium. *Salmonella* detection on the broth was carried out according to ISO 6579:2002 Annex D protocol [20].

Confirmation of, MRSA, *Salmonella* and haemolytic *E. coli*

Five positive MRSA colonies (if present) were subcultured on Tryptone Soy Agar (Oxoid, CM0131) and DNA was extracted according to the method of Stranden et al. [21]. A multiplex PCR, as described by Maes et al. [22], was performed for MRSA and a CC398 specific PCR, as described by Stegger et al. [23], for MRSA ST398 confirmation.

Positive *Salmonella* colonies on Xylose Lysine Deoxycholate agar medium (Oxoid, CM0469) were subcultured on Nutrient Agar (Oxoid, CM0003). After incubation, PCR confirmation on cel lysates was performed as described by Aabo et al. [24].

From the third down-time and production round, five positive *E. coli* colonies (when possible) were subcultured on Columbia base Blood Agar (Oxoid, CM0331) with 5 % sheep blood and incubated for 24 h at 37 °C for analysis of haemolytic *E. coli*. If a plate was negative after 24 h, it was incubated for a further 24 h. To calculate the enumerations of haemolytic *E. coli*, the ratio of the number of positive haemolytic *E. coli* colonies on the 5 selected colonies was multiplied by the mean *E. coli* enumeration of that sample.

Other analyses

Piglets were weighed individually at the age of 4, 6 and 9 weeks. Also feed intake was monitored per pen on the same moments allowing to calculate feed conversion ratio of every pen.

In addition, faecal consistency was evaluated according to [25]: a score from 1 (no diarrhea) to 4 (serious diarrhea) was assigned per pen.

Finally, clinical manifestations and treatment with antibiotics were registered. Treatments days per 100 days at risk (TD100) was calculated per pen for each protocol. This was done by calculating the ratio of treatments days (number of days that piglets received antibiotics) and the number of days at risk (time that pigs could be exposed to antibiotics), taking the number of dead piglets into account. This ratio was then multiplied by 100.

Statistical analysis

The distribution of the dependent variables was characterised with a histogram and Q-Q plot. Log transformed enumerations of spores and *Enterococcus* spp. and results of average daily gain, daily feed intake, feed conversion ratio and TD100 ratio followed a normal distribution. Log transformed enumerations of *E. coli*, haemolytic *E. coli*, faecal coliforms and MRSA did not follow this distribution.

The 4 point scale faecal consistency score was reduced to a binary scale: 0 = pens with score 1 and 1 = pens with score > 1.

The effect of the predictor variables on the normal distributed data (dependent variables) was assessed using multivariate linear regression. The effect of predictor variables on the non normally distributed outcome variables describing the enumeration and detection of the different bacteria (absence or below the detection limit =0, presence =1) was tested by means of multivariate logistic regression analysis.

A backward stepwise elimination was performed to determine the final statistical model for each bacteriological parameter, starting with the global model (predictor variables: protocol used, sampling moment, production round and location) and subsequently removing all non-significant terms. Only biologically relevant interaction effects were considered. In each model, the variables compartment and pen were included as a random effect to correct for measurements within one pen and compartment. The predictor variable sampling moment was included as a repeated measure. Post-hoc comparison was performed with a Tukey-Kramer test. Throughout the analyses, P-values ≤ 0.05 were considered as significant.

All statistical analyses were carried out with Statistical Analysis System software (SAS®, version 9.4, SAS Institute Inc.).

Results

In total 1074 swab samples were taken during 3 successive rounds. At each sampling moment approximately 90 samples were taken: i.e., 45 in CE units ($n = 3$) and 45 in control units ($n = 3$).

Spore enumerations

At every sampling moment and in each production round, higher spore enumerations were found for CE units compared to control units ($P < 0.01$) (Fig. 1a and b), with a minimal difference of 0.70 log (BC) and 1.15 log (first round) CFU (colony forming units)/sampling area. Further, spore enumerations increased after every round in CE units ($P < 0.01$) (Fig. 1b). Mean spore enumerations ranged from 2.88 log CFU/sampling area AC to 4.89 log CFU/sampling area at W5 during production piglets present and from 1.25 log CFU/sampling area AD to 2.61 log CFU/sampling area at W5 for CE and control units, respectively.

Enterococcus spp. enumerations

When considering the overall contamination level in both units, higher *Enterococcus* spp. enumerations, with a mean difference of 0.80 log CFU/sampling area, were found in CE units ($P < 0.01$). After disinfection of control units, lower *Enterococcus* spp. enumerations were observed compared to cleaned CE units ($P < 0.01$) (Fig. 2a). The mean difference was 2.88 log CFU/sampling area. Cleaning of CE units caused a reduction of 0.42 log CFU/sampling area, while in disinfected control units a reduction of 3.54 log CFU/sampling area was noticed. Before cleaning and after 1 week of production, no differences in *Enterococcus* spp. enumerations were found between units. However, at W5, higher *Enterococcus* spp. enumerations were found in CE units ($P = 0.05$). In addition, *Enterococcus* spp. enumerations were higher in every production round for CE units ($P < 0.01$) (Fig. 2b).

E. coli enumerations

More *E. coli* countable samples were found for CE units after cleaning compared to control units after disinfection ($P < 0.01$) (Fig. 3a). Proportion of countable samples was reduced by 9 % AC of CE units, while a reduction of 41 % was obtained after disinfecting control units. During production and before cleaning, no differences were found in amount of countable *E. coli* samples between both types of units.

In control units, lower amounts of countable samples were found AD compared to amounts found BC and W1 ($P < 0.01$) while this was not seen AC of CE units (Fig. 3a).

Descriptive values of *E. coli* enumeration at each sampling moment are given in Table 1.

Haemolytic *E. coli* enumerations

Of all samples taken in CE units ($n = 180$) and control units ($n = 180$) during the 3rd round, 24 % and 23 % were positive for haemolytic *E. coli*, respectively. Of these positive samples, 16 % were obtained AC (CE

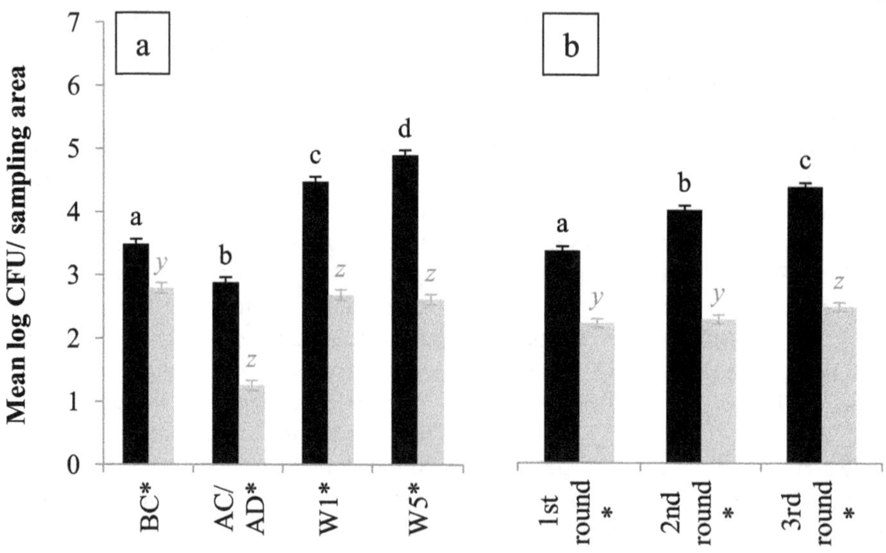

Fig. 1 Mean spore enumerations in log colony forming units/sampling area for CE (*dark grey bars*) and control units (*light grey bars*). At each sampling moment (**a**) and per round (**b**), 135 and 180 samples were taken per unit type, respectively. Significant differences between sampling moments or rounds within one type of unit are indicated by different letters above bars. Significant differences between protocols within one sampling moment or round are indicated by a star (*) on the horizontal axis. Vertical bars denote standard errors. BC, before cleaning; AC/AD, after cleaning (CE unit) or after disinfection (control unit); W1, after 1 week of production; W5: after 5 weeks of production

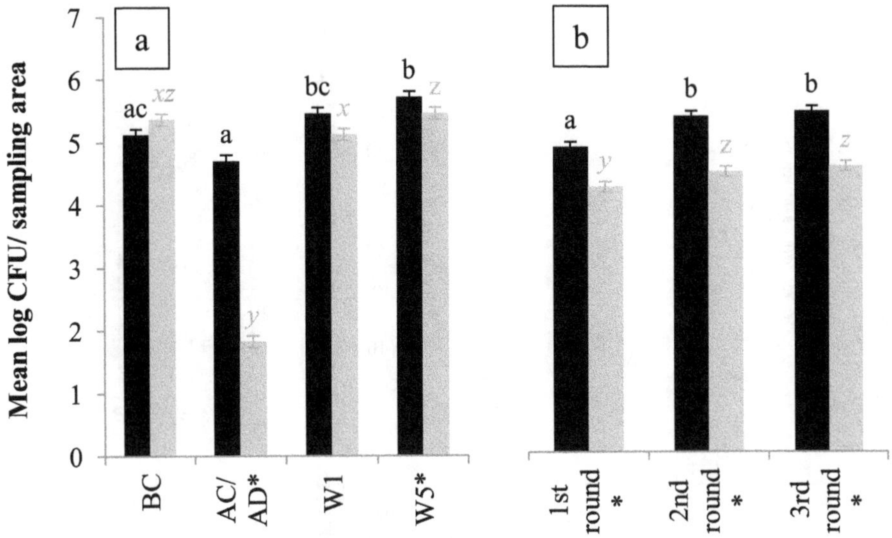

Fig. 2 Mean *Enterococcus* spp. enumerations in log colony forming units/sampling area for CE (*dark grey bars*) and control units (*light grey bars*). At each sampling moment (**a**) and per round (**b**), 135 and 180 samples were taken per unit type, respectively. Significant differences between sampling moments or rounds within one type of unit are indicated by different letters above bars. Significant differences between protocols within one sampling moment or round are indicated by a star (*) on the horizontal axis. Vertical bars denote standard errors. BC; before cleaning, AC/AD, after cleaning (CE unit) or after disinfection (control unit); W1, after 1 week of production and W5: after 5 weeks of production

units) and 0 % were obtained AD (control units), respectively. Mean enumerations were 3.0 log CFU/sampling area for both types of units. No significant differences were noticed between units.

Faecal coliform enumerations

When comparing CE and control units, results of faecal coliform enumeration confirmed the observations obtained with *E. coli* analyses (Fig. 3c). A reduction of 26 and 51 % of faecal coliform countable samples was obtained AC and AD of CE and control units, respectively.

After cleaning as well as AD, a significant reduction of faecal coliform countable samples was obtained ($P < 0.01$).

Faecal coliform enumerations at each sampling moment for both types of units are given in Table 1.

E. coli and faecal coliform detection

Detection results of *E. coli* (Fig. 3b) and faecal coliforms (Fig. 3d) confirmed the enumeration results of both parameters.

MRSA enumerations

After cleaning, countable samples were reduced 61 % for CE units, 20 % less than the observed reduction in disinfected control units ($P < 0.01$) (Fig. 3e). When pens were soiled (BC, W1 and W5), no differences in MRSA contamination were found between both types of units.

Mean and median enumerations for MRSA are given for each sampling moment in Table 1.

MRSA detection

Detection results showed that the number of MRSA positive samples was the highest (90 %) for CE units compared to the control units (81 %) ($P < 0.01$) (Fig. 3f).

Salmonella detection

No *Salmonella* was found in this study.

Sampling locations

Mean enumerations (with standard deviation) and median enumerations (with first and third quartile) of *Enterococcus* spp., *E. coli*, faecal coliforms and MRSA after cleaning (CE units) and disinfection (control units) are given per type of sampling location in Table 2. In addition, the percentage of countable swab samples (enumerations) and positive samples after enrichment (detection) is shown for both types of units. Also, mean spore and *Enterococcus* spp. counts on all samples taken in CE and control units are given for each type of location in Figs. 4 and 5, respectively.

After cleaning of CE units, enumerations of *Enterococcus* spp. were the highest for floors, concrete walls and drinking nipples. In addition, highest percentage of countable *E. coli* samples and median enumerations were found for floors and concrete walls. Moreover, after enrichment also drinking nipples were still often contaminated with *E. coli*. Results of faecal coliforms and MRSA confirmed these observations.

In control units, high numbers of *Enterococcus* spp. were found on floors and drinking nipples. Most *E.*

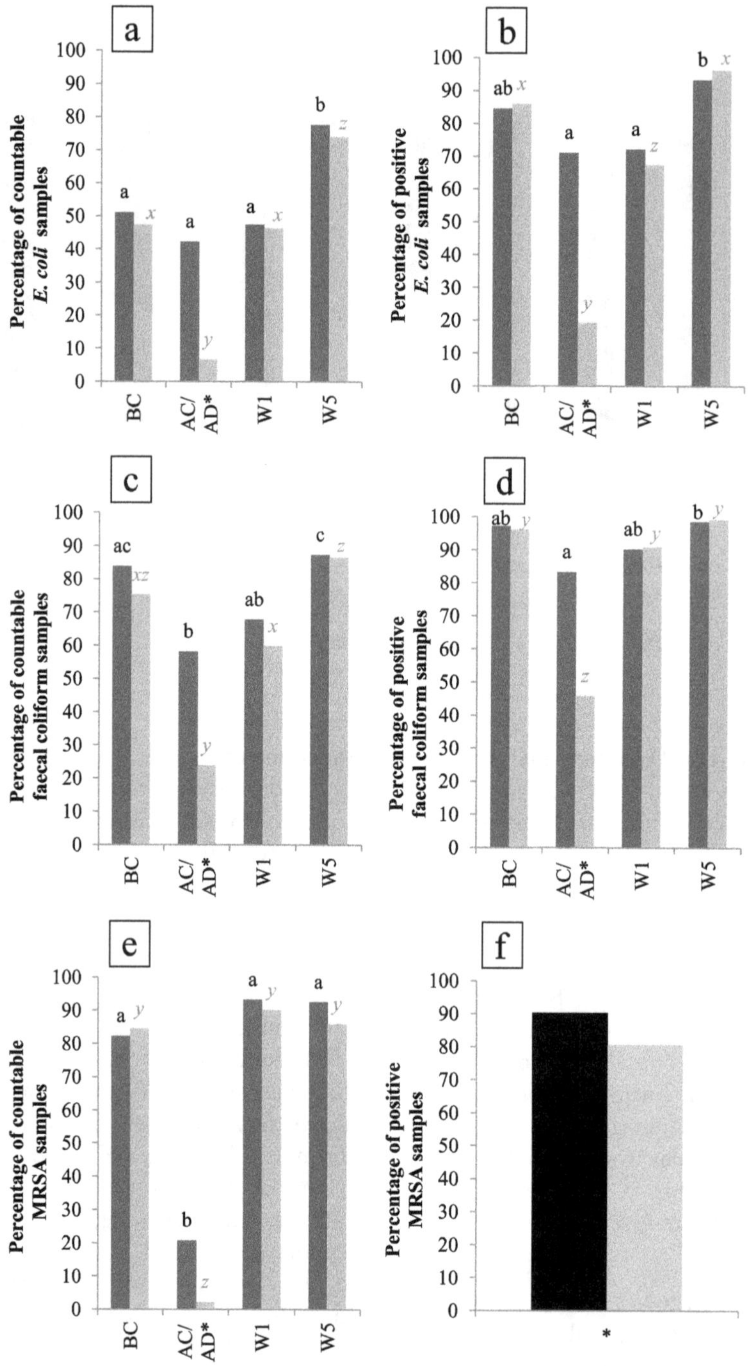

Fig. 3 Percentage of positive samples before (enumerations) and after enrichment (detection) for *E. coli* (**a**-**b**), faecal coliforms (**c**-**d**) and MRSA (**e**-**f**) given for CE (*dark grey bars*) and control units (*light grey bars*). At each sampling moment and in total 135 and 540 samples were taken per unit type, respectively. Significant differences between sampling moments within one type of unit are indicated by letters above bars. Significant differences between protocols within one sampling moment are indicated by a star (*) on the horizontal axis. BC, before cleaning; AC/AD, after cleaning or after disinfection; W1, after 1 week of production and W5: after 5 weeks of production

coli positive samples after enrichment were found for floors, drinking nipples and feeding troughs. In addition, highest enumerations for faecal coliforms were also found at these locations. Finally, for MRSA, drinking nipples were the most contaminated after disinfection.

Table 1 Descriptive values for *Escherichia coli* (*E. coli*), faecal coliforms and methicillin resistant *Staphylococcus aureus* (MRSA) enumerations (log colony forming units/sampling area) given for each sampling moment for CE units and control units

Sampling moment	*E. coli*	Faecal coliforms	MRSA
CE units			
BC[a]	0.0–**1.6**–2.8	2.7 ± 1.5	2.9 ± 1.4
AC/AD[b]	0.0–**0.0**–2.8	0.0–**1.9**–3.8	0.0–**0.0**–0.0
W1[c]	0.0–**0.0**–2.8	0.0–**2.7**–3.8	3.3 ± 1.1
W5[d]	2.5 ± 1.6	3.1 ± 1.5	3.2 ± 1.1
Control units			
BC	0.0–**0.0**–3.0	2.6 ± 1.7	2.9 ± 1.4
AC/AD	0.0–**0.0**–0.0	0.0–**0.0**–0.0	0.0–**0.0**–0.0
W1	0.0–**0.0**–3.0	0.0–**2.0**–3.6	3.2 ± 1.3
W5	2.5 ± 1.8	3.1 ± 1.6	2.9 ± 1.3

Mean and standard deviation are given for enumerations that are normally distributed. First quartile (Q1), median (Q2, bold characters) and third quartile (Q3) are given for enumerations that did not follow this distribution
[a]BC, before cleaning
[b]AC/AD, after cleaning/after disinfection
[c]W1, after 1 week of production
[d]W5, after 5 weeks of production

More spore enumerations were found at every location for CE units (Fig. 4), with a minimal difference of 1.2 log CFU/sampling area.

In addition, when considering the overall *Enterococcus* spp. contamination level, higher levels were found for each location in CE units (Fig. 5).

Performance results

Mean starting weight of piglets in CE and control pens was 7.4 ± 1.5 and 7.1 ± 1.5 kg, respectively. A mean feed intake of 0.539 ± 0.078 and 0.521 ± 0.065 kg/day was observed for CE and control units, respectively. No significant differences were found between feed intake of piglets raised in CE and control pens. When considering results of daily gain, no significant differences were found. Average daily gain was 0.407 ± 0.056 and 0.395 ± 0.053 kg for piglets in CE and control pens, respectively. In addition, no significant differences in mean feed conversion were found: 1.327 ± 0.072 and 1.324 ± 0.085 for pigs in CE and control units, respectively.

Faecal consistency

No significant differences in scores of faecal consistency between protocols were noticed (data not shown).

Table 2 Descriptive values for *Escherichia coli* (*E. coli*), faecal coliforms and methicillin resistant *Staphylococcus aureus* (MRSA) enumerations (log colony forming units/sampling area) and detection after cleaning (CE units) and disinfection (control units) for each type of sampling location. Detection method was carried out after an overnight enrichment of samples

Location	*Enterococcus* spp.		*E.coli*			Faecal coliforms			MRSA		
	CS (%)[f]	Enumerations	CS (%)	Enumerations	D (%)[g]	CS (%)	Enumerations	D (%)	CS (%)	Enumerations	D (%)
CE units											
1[a]	100	5.0 ± 0.8	59	0.0–**1.6**–3.0	85	67	0.0–**3.2**–3.7	96	44	0.0–**0.0**–1.9	81
2[b]	100	4.8 ± 1.0	67	0.0–**1.6**–4.1	78	90	2.6–**3.9**–4.9	92	22	0.0–**0.0**–0.0	74
3[c]	100	4.4 ± 0.9	4	0.0–**0.0**–0.0	48	19	0.0–**0.0**–0.0	50	11	0.0–**0.0**–0.0	56
4[d]	100	4.9 ± 0.4	41	0.0–**0.0**–3.0	85	52	0.0–**2.5**–3.7	96	19	0.0–**0.0**–0.0	63
5[e]	96	4.4 ± 1.3	41	0.0–**0.0**–2.2	59	62	0.0–**2.5**–3.6	83	7	0.0–**0.0**–0.0	44
Control units											
1	70	2.1 ± 1.6	11	0.0–**0.0**–0.0	26	33	0.0–**0.0**–2.5	58	0	0.0–**0.0**–0.0	26
2	48	0.0–**0.0**–3.0	0	0.0–**0.0**–0.0	4	10	0.0–**0.0**–0.0	46	0	0.0–**0.0**–0.0	19
3	33	0.0–**0.0**–1.7	0	0.0–**0.0**–0.0	7	5	0.0–**0.0**–0.0	17	4	0.0–**0.0**–0.0	19
4	89	3.3 ± 1.5	19	0.0–**0.0**–0.0	30	43	0.0–**0.0**–3.2	67	4	0.0–**0.0**–0.0	37
5	48	0.0–**0.0**–2.9	4	0.0–**0.0**–0.0	30	29	0.0–**0.0**–2.8	42	4	0.0–**0.0**–0.0	15

Mean and standard deviation are given for enumerations that are normally distributed. First quartile (Q1), median (Q2, bold characters) and third quartile (Q3) are given for enumerations that did not follow this distribution
[a]1, floors
[b]2, concrete walls
[c]3, synthetic walls
[d]4, drinking nipples
[e]5, feeding trough
[f]CS (%), proportion of countable samples given in percentage
[g]D (%), proportion of positive samples after detection given in percentage

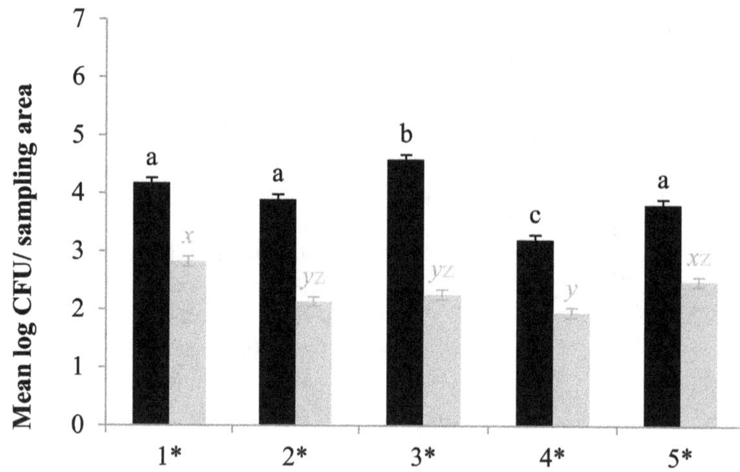

Fig. 4 Mean spore enumerations in log colony forming units/sampling area for CE (*dark grey bars*) and control units (*light grey bars*) for each location. At each location, 108 samples were taken per type of unit. Significant differences between sampling moments within one type of unit are indicated by different letters above bars. Significant differences between protocols within one sampling moment are indicated by a star (*) on the horizontal axis. Vertical bars denote standard errors. 1, grid floor; 2, concrete wall; 3, synthetic wall; 4, drinking nipples; 5, feeding trough

Antibiotic treatment

The mean TD100 for CE and control units was 27.9 ± 0.9 and 28.3 ± 2.1 %, respectively. No significant differences were found between protocols.

Discussion

The emergence of multiresistant (pathogenic) bacteria is of great concern for animal and human health. Excessive use of antibiotics [26, 27] and disinfectants [28–30] in for example the animal primary production, could possibly contribute to this phenomenon. Therefore, alternative methods such as competitive exclusion (CE) are promoted as promising. In this study a commercial CE protocol (by probiotic-type bacteria) was compared with a classical C&D protocol in nursery units.

According to the manufacturer of the PIP products, a reduction of pathogenic bacteria and improvement in hygiene after CE during 3 successive production rounds should be obtained. The first statement could not be confirmed by this study: *E. coli* (*Salmonella*-indicator), haemolytic *E. coli* and MRSA analyses showed that the infection pressure after CE cleaning was not reduced to the same extent as implementing a disinfection step. Furthermore, during production no differences were noticed. Also no improvement in hygiene was seen: during the 5th week of production higher *Enterococcus* spp. enumerations (hygiene indicator) and no differences in

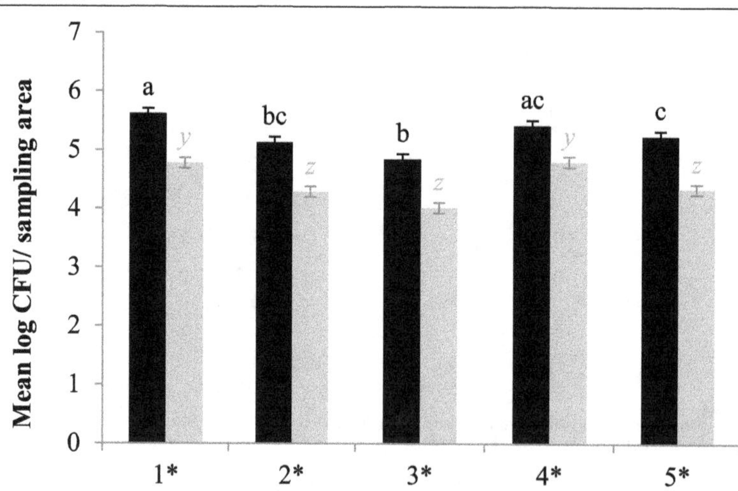

Fig. 5 Mean *Enterococcus* spp. enumerations in log colony forming units/sampling area for CE (*dark grey bars*) and control units (*light grey bars*) for each location. At each location, 108 samples were taken per type of unit. Significant differences between sampling moments within one type of unit are indicated by different letters above bars. Significant differences between protocols within one sampling moment are indicated by a star (*) on the horizontal axis. Vertical bars denote standard errors. 1, grid floor; 2, concrete wall; 3, synthetic wall; 4, drinking nipples; 5, feeding trough

faecal coliforms (faecal indicator) contamination between the two types of units were found. Because, higher contamination levels of MRSA and pathogen-indicator organisms (*E. coli*) were found in CE units after cleaning, there may be a greater chance of infecting young piglets arriving in those nurseries.

Several hypotheses have been proposed to explain the mechanisms of CE cultures. One is that CE bacteria should compete with other bacteria for adhesion sites, nutrients and energy, which results in preventing growth and proliferation of pathogenic bacteria in the environment (Cummings and Macfarlane, [31]). Another hypothesis is that these bacteria influence the quorum sensing communication and therefore inhibit expression of virulence and colonisation genes of pathogens (Vilà et al. [32]; Deep et al. [33]). Besides CE bacteria, also enzymes were administered during cleaning, with the aim of helping to eliminate biofilms. In this study, no reduction of the analysed bacteria after 3 production rounds in CE units was seen. Several explanations were found to clarify this observation: (i) adhesion sites are abundantly present in animal houses, hence there is no need for competition; (ii) removal of organic debris is only carried out when piglets are removed from pens, therefore CE-, pathogenic and other bacteria have an abundance of nutrients during production, eliminating the need for competition between bacteria; (iii) however, in order to compete for nutrients, spores need to germinate, which may not be the case for all spores.

Moreover, Luyckx, et al. [34] (i.e., chapter III) showed that a cleaning step in broiler houses caused a reduction of total aerobic bacteria with 2 log CFU/sampling surface and that a disinfection step caused a further reduction of 1.5 log CFU. Although, cleaning caused a greater reduction of total aerobic bacteria, both the above study and this one showed that a disinfection step is still an important step for further reducing the bacterial infection pressure in barns with naturally high levels of environmental bacteria.

Improvement of feed conversion efficiency by probiotic-type bacteria could be obtained by a shift in intestinal flora, stimulating growth of nonpathogenic facultative anaerobic bacteria, inhibiting growth of pathogens, and enhancing digestion and utilisation of nutrients [35]. However, no differences were found between piglets raised in CE and control units in our study. Also, no differences in faecal consistency was noticed. A possible explanation could be that not enough CE bacteria could be administered directly to the animals through the environmental spray application.

Finally, the contamination levels of the different sampling locations were analysed after cleaning of CE units and disinfection of control units. In CE units, grid floors, concrete walls and drinking nipples were still mostly contaminated by *Enterococcus* spp., *E. coli*, faecal coliforms and MRSA after cleaning. Although spore counts showed that high numbers of CE bacteria were present at these locations, the contamination level of different bacteria was still much higher compared to the microbial load after disinfection of control units. In addition, the overall *Enterococcus* spp. contamination of all locations during the experiment was higher in CE units. In control units, grid floors and drinking nipples seemed critical locations after disinfection. Luyckx, et al. [36] also showed that drinking cups are critical locations for C&D in broiler houses.

A limitation of our study was that the CE protocol was only carried out in pig nursery units, and not in farrowing units. Therefore, the piglets gut microbiota was already formed, which could contain pathogens and contaminate pig nursery units on arrival. Conversely, this is also a drawback of the CE protocol. A future perspective could be to determine the efficacy of a CE protocol applied on the whole farm, however this approach would substantially increase the work load and associated costs for the farmer.

Conclusions

Very few studies about the impact of microbial cleaning and administration during production on the environment in animal houses are available. Our results showed that competitive exclusion by probiotic-type bacteria could not meet the claims provided by the manufacturer. Moreover, this study showed that a good C&D protocol during down-time is still very important for reducing infection pressure in nursery units. However, more research should be carried out for a valuable alternative, because disinfectant resistance might be an upcoming problem.

Acknowledgments

Many thanks go to Kristof Dierkens and Eline Dumoleijn for their practical support. We also thank Miriam Levenson for the English language editing of this manuscript.

Funding

This research is funded by the Belgian Federal Public Service for Health, Food Chain Safety and Environment (RT 11/8 Cleandesopt).

Authors' contributions

KL was involved in the sample collection, laboratory analyses, statistical analyses, interpretation of the data and drafting the manuscript. JD, SM and KD coordinated the study. SVW and JD evaluated the statistical analyses. KL, SM, SVW, LH, MH, JD and KD contributed to development and writing of the paper. All authors read and approved the final manuscript.

Competing interests

The authors declare that they have no competing interests.

Consent for publication

Not applicable.

Author details
[1]Institute for Agricultural and Fisheries Research (ILVO), Technology and Food Science Unit, Melle, Belgium. [2]Institute for Agricultural and Fisheries Research (ILVO), Animal Sciences Unit, Melle, Belgium. [3]Department of Pathology, Bacteriology and Poultry Diseases, Ghent University, Faculty of Veterinary Medicine, Merelbeke, Belgium. [4]Veterinary Epidemiology Unit, Department of Reproduction, Obstetrics and Herd Health, Faculty of Veterinary Medicine, Ghent University, Merelbeke, Belgium.

References

1. SCENIHR. Assessment of the antibiotic resistance effects of biocides. 2009.
2. Russell AD. Mechanisms of bacterial resistance to antibiotics and biocides. Prog Med Chem. 1998;35:133–97.
3. Mateu E, Martin M. Why is anti-microbial resistance a veterinary problem as well? J Vet Med B Infect Dis Vet Public Heal. 2001;48:569–81.
4. Soumet C, Fourreau E, Legrandois P, Maris P. Resistance to phenicol compounds following adaptation to quaternary ammonium compounds in *Escherichia coli*. Vet Microbiol. 2012;14:147–52.
5. Callens BF, Haesebrouck F, Maes D, Butaye P, Dewulf J, Boyen F. Clinical resistance and decreased susceptibility in *Streptococcus suis* isolates from clinically healthy fattening pigs. Microb Drug Resist. 2013;19:146–51.
6. Vanderhaeghen W, Hermans K, Haesebrouck F, Butaye P. Methicillin-resistant *Staphylococcus aureus* (MRSA) in food production animals. Epidemiol Infect. 2010;138:606–25.
7. Weese JS. Methicillin-resistant *Staphylococcus aureus* in animals. Ilar J. 2010; 51:233–44.
8. Smith TC, Pearson N. The emergence of *Staphylococcus aureus* ST398. Vector Borne Zoonotic Dis. 2011;11:327–39.
9. Kehrenberg C, Cuny C, Strommenger B, Schwarz S, Witte W. Methicillin-resistant and -susceptible *Staphylococcus aureus* strains of clonal lineages ST398 and ST9 from swine carry the multidrug resistance gene *cfr*. Antimicrob Agents Chemother. 2009;53:779–81.
10. Catry B, Van Duijkeren E, Pomba MC, Greko C, Moreno MA, Pyorala S, Ruzauskas M, Sanders P, Threlfall EJ, Ungemach F, Torneke K, Munoz-Madero C, Torren-Edo J. Reflection paper on MRSA in food-producing and companion animals: epidemiology and control options for human and animal health. Epidemiol Infect. 2010;138:626–44.
11. Pletinckx LJ, Verhegghe M, Crombé F, Dewulf J, De Bleecker Y, Rasschaert G, Butaye P, Goddeeris BM, De Man I. Evidence of possible methicillin-resistant *Staphylococcus aureus* ST398 spread between pigs and other animals and people residing on the same farm. Prev Vet Med. 2013;109:293–303.
12. Wong TZ, Zhang M, O'Donoghue M, Boost M. Presence of antiseptic resistance genes in porcine methicillin-resistant *Staphylococcus aureus*. Vet Microbiol. 2013;162:977–9.
13. Slifierz MJ, Friendship RM, Weese JS. Methicillin-resistant *Staphylococcus aureus* in commercial swine herds is associated with disinfectant and zinc usage. Appl Environ Microbiol. 2015;81:2690–5.
14. Rajic A, McFall ME, Deckert AE, Reid-Smith R, Manninen K, Poppe C, Dewey CE, McEwen SA. Antimicrobial resistance of *Salmonella* isolated from finishing swine and the environment of 60 Alberta swine farms. Vet Microbiol. 2004;104:189–96.
15. Sisak F, Havlickova H, Hradecka H, Rychlik I, Kolackova I, Karpiskova R. Antibiotic resistance of *Salmonella* spp. isolates from pigs in the Czech Republic. Vet Med. 2008;5:327–39.
16. Chuanchuen R, Padungtod P. Antimicrobial resistance genes in *Salmonella enterica* isolates from poultry and swine in Thailand. J Vet Med Sci. 2009;71: 1349–55.
17. Randall LP, Cooles SW, Piddock LJ, Woodward MJ. Effect of triclosan or a phenolic farm disinfectant on the selection of antibiotic-resistant *Salmonella enterica*. J Antimicrob Chemother. 2004;54:621–7.
18. Beier RC, Bischoff KM, Poole TL. Disinfectants (Biocides) used in animal production: antimicrobial resistance considerations. In: Beier RC, Pillai SD, Phillips TD, editors. Preharvest and postharvest food safety: contemporary issues and future directions. Hoboken: John Wiley & Sons; 2008. p. 480.
19. Patterson JA, Burkholder KM. Application of prebiotics and probiotics in poultry production. Poult Sci. 2003;82:627–31.
20. Anonymous. Microbiology of food and animal feeding stuffs - Horizontal method for the detection of Salmonella spp. In: Int Stand 6579 Annex D Detect Salmonella spp Anim faeces samples from Prim Prod stage Int Organ Stand Geneva, Switzerland. 2002.
21. Stranden A, Frei R, Widmer AF. Molecular typing of methicillin-resistant *Staphylococcus aureus*: can PCR replace pulsed-field gel electrophoresis? J Clin Microbiol. 2003;41:3181–6.
22. Maes N, Magdalena J, Rottiers S, De Gheldre Y, Struelens MJ. Evaluation of a triplex PCR assay to discriminate *Staphylococcus aureus* from coagulase-negative Staphylococci and determine methicillin resistance from blood cultures. J Clin Microbiol. 2002;40:1514–7.
23. Stegger M, Lindsay JA, Moodley A, Skov R, Broens EM, Guardabassi L. Rapid PCR detection of *Staphylococcus aureus* clonal complex 398 by targeting the restriction-modification system carrying sau1-hsdS1. J Clin Microbiol. 2011;49:732–4.
24. Aabo S, Rasmussen OF, Rossen L, Sørensen PD, Olsen JE. *Salmonella* identification by the polymerase chain reaction. Mol Cell Probes. 1993;7:171–8.
25. Pedersen K, Toft N. Intra- and inter-observer agreement when using a descriptive classification scale for clinical assessment of faecal consistency in growing pigs. Prev Vet Med. 2011;98:288–91.
26. Nikaido H. Multidrug resistance in bacteria. Annu Rev Biochem. 2009;78:119–46.
27. Gullberg E, Albrecht LM, Karlsson C, Sandegren L, Andersson DI. Selection of a multidrug resistance plasmid by sublethal levels of antibiotics and heavy metals. MBio. 2014;5:e01918–14.
28. Whitehead RN, Overton TW, Kemp CL, Webber MA. Exposure of *Salmonella enterica* serovar Typhimurium to high level biocide challenge can select multidrug resistant mutants in a single step. PLoS One. 2011;6:e22833.
29. Randall LP, Clouting CS, Gradel KO, Clifton-Hadley FA, Davies RD, Woodward MJ. Farm disinfectants select for cyclohexane resistance, a marker of multiple antibiotic resistance, in *Escherichia coli*. J Appl Microbiol. 2005;98:556–63.
30. Karatzas KAG, Webber MA, Jorgensen F, Woodward MJ, Piddock LJV, Humphrey TJ. Prolonged treatment of *Salmonella* enterica serovar Typhimurium with commercial disinfectants selects for multiple antibiotic resistance, increased efflux and reduced invasiveness. J Antimicrob Chemother. 2007;60:947–55.
31. Cummings JH, Macfarlane GT. Role of intestinal bacteria in nutrient metabolism. JPEN J Parenter Enter Nutr. 1997;21:357–65.
32. Vilà B, Esteve-Garcia E, Brufau J. Probiotic micro-organisms: 100 years of innovation and efficacy; modes of action. Worlds Poult Sci J. 2010;66:369–80.
33. Deep A, Chaudhary U, Gupta V. Quorum sensing and bacterial pathogenicity: from molecules to disease. J Lab Physicians. 2011;3:4–11.
34. Luyckx K, Dewulf J, Van Weyenberg S, Herman L, Zoons J, Vervaet E, Heyndrickx M, De Reu K. Comparison of sampling procedures and microbiological and non-microbiological parameters to evaluate cleaning and disinfection in broiler houses. Poult Sci. 2015;94:740–9.
35. Lutful Kabir SM. The role of probiotics in the poultry industry. Int J Mol Sci. 2009;10:3531–46.
36. Luyckx K, VanWeyenberg S, Dewulf J, Herman L, Zoons J, Vervaet E, Heyndrickx M, De Reu K. On-farm comparisons of different cleaning protocols in broiler houses. Poult Sci. 2015;94:1986–93.

10

Prevalence, antimicrobial susceptibility and risk factors associated with non-typhoidal *Salmonella* on Ugandan layer hen farms

Terence Odoch[1,2*], Yngvild Wasteson[2], Trine L'Abée-Lund[2], Adrian Muwonge[3], Clovice Kankya[1], Luke Nyakarahuka[1,2], Sarah Tegule[1] and Eystein Skjerve[2]

Abstract

Background: Non-typhoidal *Salmonella* (NTS) are among the leading global foodborne pathogens and a significant public health threat. Their occurrence in animal reservoirs and their susceptibilities to commonly used antimicrobials are poorly understood in developing countries. The aim of this study was to estimate the prevalence, determine antimicrobial susceptibility and identify risk factors associated with NTS presence in laying hen farms in Uganda through a cross-sectional study.

Results: Pooled faecal samples were collected from 237 laying hen farms and these were analysed for NTS following standard laboratory procedures. In total, 49 farms (20.7%; 95% Confidence interval (CI): 15.6–25.6%) were positive for NTS presence. Altogether, ten *Salmonella* serotypes were identified among the confirmed 78 isolates, and the predominant serotypes were *Salmonella* Newport (30.8%), *S.* Hadar (14.1%), *S.* Aberdeen (12.8%), *S.* Heidelberg (12.8%), and *S.* Bolton (12.8%). Phenotypic antimicrobial resistance was detected in 45(57.7%) of the isolates and the highest resistance was against ciprofloxacin (50.0%) followed by sulphonamides (26.9%) and sulphamethoxazole/trimethoprim (7.7%). Resistance was significantly associated with sampled districts ($p = 0.034$). Resistance to three or more drugs, multi-drug resistance (MDR) was detected in 12 (15.4%) of the isolates, 9 (75%) of these were from Wakiso district. A multivariable logistic model identified large farm size (OR = 7.0; 95% CI: 2.5–19.8) and the presence of other animal species on the farm (OR = 5.9; 95% CI: 2.1–16.1) as risk factors for NTS prevalence on farms. Having a separate house for birds newly brought to the farms was found to be protective (OR = 0,4; 95% CI: 0.2–0.8).

Conclusion: This study has highlighted a high prevalence and diversity of NTS species in laying hen farms in Uganda and identified associated risk factors. In addition, it has demonstrated high levels of antimicrobial resistance in isolates of NTS. This could be because of overuse or misuse of antimicrobials in poultry production. Also importantly, the insights provided in this study justifies a strong case for strengthening One Health practices and this will contribute to the development of NTS control strategies at local, national and international levels.

Keywords: Non-typhoidal *Salmonella*, Antimicrobial susceptibility, Risk factor, Layer hens, Prevalence

Background

Non-typhoid *Salmonella* (NTS) is one of the leading bacterial causes of food-borne illnesses, posing huge challenges to public health systems around the world [1–3]. A recent estimate of the global burden of NTS morbidity and mortality showed that enteric NTS cause 93.8 million illnesses with 155,000 deaths annually, while invasive NTS were estimated to cause 3.4 million cases with 681,316 deaths annually [4–6]. African countries have a relatively low level of reported NTS gastroenteritis, but a much higher level of invasive non-enteric NTS infections, estimated at 227 cases per 100,000 persons per year compared to the global average of 49 cases per 100,000 persons per year [4]. This distribution of

* Correspondence: odoch@covab.mak.ac.ug; odochterence@gmail.com
[1]Department of Bio-security, Ecosystems and Veterinary Public Health, College of Veterinary Medicine, Animal Resources and Biosecurity (COVAB), Makerere University, Kampala, Uganda
[2]Department of Food Safety and Infection Biology, Faculty of Veterinary Medicine, Norwegian University of Life Sciences (NMBU), Oslo, Norway
Full list of author information is available at the end of the article

salmonellosis makes Africa the leading continent with invasive non-enteric NTS cases accounting for more than half of the global cases [4]. In humans, many of the gastroenteric infections caused by NTS are self-limiting, and thus, many sporadic cases go unnoticed and/or unreported. However, a serious aspect of this situation is that some of the gastroenteric infections may develop into bacteraemia, which is an emerging opportunistic infection in individuals infected with HIV, the elderly and in children [7, 8].

The reservoirs of food-borne NTS are often located in the primary food animal production. Many of these zoonotic NTS are able to colonize the intestinal tract of a variety of animal species, and in most of these cases, the animals are healthy and asymptomatic. Faecally contaminated foodstuffs like meat, eggs, dairy products and sometimes vegetables are the main sources of salmonellosis in humans [2, 3, 9, 10]. The dissemination of NTS is also a growing concern due to increasing cases of drug resistant isolates and their frequent carriage of transmissible antimicrobial resistance genes. Even more worrying is the rising occurrence of multidrug-resistant NTS, including cases reported in some African countries [5, 11]. Because of multidrug-resistance, treatment with first line drugs is often no longer an alternative, and this puts pressure on the use of second or third line drugs. Some limited studies in Africa on antimicrobial resistance in NTS isolates from animal sources have been undertaken, but with varying results [11–13].

Many prevalence and risk factor studies of NTS in layer and broiler populations have been conducted in the USA and Europe [14–17]. A systematic review of risk factors associated with laying hen farms identified multiple risk factors related to biosecurity measures, management factors and the environment [18]. In addition, developed countries have put in place monitoring and surveillance systems for antimicrobial resistance targeting important zoonotic pathogens like NTS. Unfortunately, such systematic surveillance neither exist for NTS nor other food-borne pathogens in most developing countries, including Uganda [19]. Consequently, the role of poultry as a reservoir and source of NTS in developing countries is poorly understood. Furthermore, the development of antibiotic resistance of NTS to commonly used antibiotics in agricultural production needs prompt investigation, commencing with susceptibility testing. The significant data gaps in developing countries hinder development of effective control systems and risk-mitigation strategies at multiple levels.

Since most human NTS infections originate from animal sources, prevention and control at pre-harvest level in the primary production units is an effective way to minimize NTS dissemination and transmission to humans through the food chains [20–22]. The aim of this study was to estimate the prevalence, test antimicrobial susceptibility and identify risk factors of NTS using production and management information from a sample of commercial laying chicken farms.

Methods

Study area and recruitment of farms

The study was carried out between June 2015 and August 2016 in the districts of Wakiso, Masaka and Lira in Uganda. Wakiso district (00°24′N, 32° 29′E) and Masaka district (00° 30′S, 31° 45′E) are located in the central region of Uganda, while Lira district is located in northern region of Uganda (02°20′N, 33°06′E). These districts were purposively selected because of their high commercial poultry households that make them the hub of poultry industry in Uganda. The sampling frame was generated from a list of farmers participating in National Agricultural Advisory Services (NAADS) program in the three selected districts of Uganda. In Uganda, the majority of poultry farmers are smallholders, and therefore the inclusion criterion was that for a farm to participate, it should have a minimum number of 50 chicken. A sample size calculator, FreeCalc sample size calculation for imperfect tests (www.epitools.ausvet.com.au, accessed on 3rd, June, 2015) was used. The required sample size for demonstrating disease freedom was calculated as previously described [23, 24]. The calculator had the following input; population size (Masaka = 147, Lira = 145, Wakiso = 77), sensitivity (60%), specificity (100%), design prevalence (5%), and the desired type 1 and type 2 errors were all assumed at 0.05. Because of small populations, the modified hypergeometric option was used. A total sample size of 237 (Masaka = 85, Lira = 84, Wakiso = 68) was calculated for individual districts. Computer-generated random numbers were used to select farms. After selection, farmers (respondents) were asked for their cooperation and willingness to participate, and after that a verbal consent was obtained. Those who were not willing to participate were replaced by random selection of others from the same list. Questionnaires were administered to all participating farms and faecal samples were taken for bacteriological analysis.

Sample collection

Flocks and poultry house sizes varied a lot in the study areas; and because of this, the sampling scheme was standardized. In cases where a farm had more than one poultry house, but with the same age group of birds in each house, one house was randomly selected and sampled. On the other hand, if a farm had more than one house but with different age groups, all the houses were sampled. Each house was divided into sectors of about 5 m by 5 m (25 m^2), an approach adapted from previous studies [25, 26]. One sample was collected from each sector using sterile gloves and boot swabs. The samples from each house were pooled together, transferred to a properly labelled sterile container and put in a cool box with ice packs. The samples were transported to the laboratory within less than 8 h and processing began immediately. All flocks were sampled once.

Bacterial diagnostics and identification of *Salmonella* serotypes

Culture and isolation of *Salmonella* spp. followed standard procedures according to *ISO 6579:2002/Amd 1:2007 Annex D: Detection of Salmonella spp. in animal faeces and in environmental samples from the primary production* [27]. Briefly, pooled samples were homogenized, 25 g weighed and added to 225 ml of Buffered Peptone Water (BPW) for pre-enrichment and incubated for 20 h at 37 °C. The culture obtained was subjected to selective Modified Semisolid Rappaport Vassiliadis (MSRV) agar plates and incubated at 41.5 °C for 24–48 h. One colony from each culture indicative of NTS was further plated on selective Xylose Lysine Deoxycholate (XLD) agar and incubated at 37 °C for 24 h. Presumptive NTS colonies were stored at −20 °C in Mueller-Hinton agar. The samples were later transported to Norway where they were sub-cultured on blood agar plates and stored at 4 °C. Biochemical confirmatory tests were done by using the API-20E (BioMerieux, Marcy l'Etoile, France) identification system. All isolates were serotyped according to the Kauffman–White–Le–Minor technique [28] at the Norwegian Veterinary Institute.

Antibiotic susceptibility testing

Antibiotic susceptibility testing of all identified isolates was performed on 13 antibiotics (NEO-SENSITABS™, Rosco, Denmark) using the standard Kirby-Bauer disk diffusion methods on Muller-Hinton agar. Interpretation of sensitive (S), intermediate (I) or resistant (R) was done according to Clinical and Laboratory Standards Institute [29], except for ciprofloxacin (CIPR1μg) which was interpreted using CLSI [30]. The 13 antibiotics were selected based on the common antibiotics used in Uganda and those recommended by World Health Organization (WHO) for routine integrated antimicrobial resistance monitoring [31]. These were gentamycin (GEN10μg), sulfonamide (SULFA240μg), trimethoprim-sulfamethoxazole (SxT 25 μg), ciprofloxacin (CIPR1μg), cefotaxime (CTX 30 μg), meropenem (MPR 10 μg), chloramphenicol (CLR30μg), ceftazidime (CAZ30 μg), ampicillin (AMP10μg), amoxycillin clavulanic acid (AMC30μg), trimethoprim (TRIM5μg), tetracycline (TET 30μg), and enrofloxacin (ENROF10μg). *Escherichia coli* ATCC 25922 was used as quality control. NTS isolates showing resistance to three or more antibiotics were classified as multidrug-resistant.

Questionnaire administration

All questionnaires were directly administered onsite after pre-testing. Pre-testing of the questionnaire was done by three trained research assistants in neighbouring districts of Kampala and Mukono in central Uganda and Kole in northern Uganda. These districts have similar production and management systems to the study districts. After pre-testing, the research team reviewed the questionnaires before final administration. The final questionnaire had 80% close-ended questions and was used to collect variables to determine risk factors. The questionnaires collected information on general farm management practices and characteristics, disease prevention, control and management as well as demographic data of the farmers and managers. The questionnaire was written in English, but the research assistants would determine whether the respondent was competent in English or not. Where the respondent was not competent in English, the research assistant would translate in the local language of Luganda (in the case of Wakiso and Masaka districts) and Lwo (in the case of Lira district). The selected households were identified with the help of the local veterinary personnel and chairpersons of local council one. Local council one is the smallest administrative unit in Uganda. Data entry was done by a trained assistant at the College of Veterinary Medicine, Animal Resources and Biosecurity, Makerere University, Kampala, Uganda.

Data management and analysis

After establishing the database, data were exported to the Statistical Package for Social Scientists (SPSS, version 20) computer program for further data analyses. A farm was considered positive if one of the pooled faecal samples taken tested positive for NTS. An initial descriptive statistics using tables and chi-square testing was performed to assess the association of each variable independently. This was followed by a multivariable logistic model built based upon variables with p-values < 0.20 in the initial analyses. All candidate variables were tested for collinearity with other variables using tabulation, and if collinearity was found, the most biologically relevant variable was chosen. The model was built utilizing a backward selection among the candidate variables ($p < 0.20$ from initial analyses) strategy using the Likelihood Ratio test with for comparing models [32]. The final model was assessed for fit using the Hosmer-Lemeshow test [33].

Results

Number of samples, NTS prevalence and serotypes

A total of 237 farms participated in the study (Wakiso, $n = 68$; Lira, $n = 84$; Masaka, $n = 85$). Sampling according to the standardized sampling scheme resulted in 366 pooled samples from the 237 farms. Of the 237 farms, 49 (20.7%; 95% CI = 15.6,-25.6%) were positive for NTS. Salmonella isolates were recovered from 78 of the 366 samples (21.3%).

Ten *Salmonella* serotypes were identified from the 78 isolates recovered (Table 1). Of the 49 NTS-positive farms, five farms were contaminated with two different serotypes. All these farms had three or more poultry houses and the serotypes were from different houses. The farms were from the two districts of Wakiso and Masaka representing the central part of Uganda.

Antimicrobial susceptibility of NTS

Forty five, 57.7% (95% CI: 47.4–67.9%) of the 78 isolates were resistant to at least one antibiotic in the disc diffusion test. Resistance varied significantly by district ($p = 0.034$); highest in Wakiso with 75.9% of the isolates from the district resistant to at least one of the tested antibiotics; this was followed by Lira with 52.0% and Masaka with 41.7% of the isolates resistant. The highest resistance was against ciprofloxacin (50.0% of the isolates) followed by sulphonamide (26.9%), sulfamethoxazole/trimethoprim (7.7%), trimethoprim (7.7%), and tetracycline (5.1%), then ampicillin (5.1%), chloramphenicol (5.1%), and enrofloxacin (5.1%). All the isolates were susceptible to meropenem, gentamycin, amoxicillin-clavulanic acid, ceftazidime, and cefotaxime. Multidrug-resistance was seen in 12 (15.4%) of the isolates and five multidrug-resistant phenotypes were identified (Table 2).

Factors associated with NTS

Some key demographic factors, farm management, disease prevention and control practices showing significant association with the prevalence of NTS on farms are presented in Table 3. These were included as candidate variables for the multivariable logistic model (insert Table 3).

Table 1 Distribution of NTS serotypes in layer hen farms in Uganda

Serotype	Number of farms	Percentage (%) of positive farms	Percentage (%) of farms investigated
S. Newport	13	26.5	5.5
S. Hadar	7	3.0	3.0
S. Aberdeen	10	20.4	4.2
S. Heidelberg	7	3.0	3.0
S. Bolton	6	6.0	2.5
S. Enteritidis	4	8.2	1.7
S. Mbandaka	3	6.1	1.3
S. Kampala	2	4.1	0.8
S. Typhimurium	1	2.0	0.4
S. Uganda	1	2.0	0.4

A final multivariable logistic model identified some risk factors for presence of *Salmonella* spp. (Table 4). Due to collinearity between some variables, type of poultry house and number of houses were dropped (collinear with farm size). Having a written biosecurity plan, and having a separate house for sick birds were also dropped (collinear with having a separate house for new chicken). The final multivariate logistic model found that larger farms had significantly more NTS. Similarly, presence of other livestock species like cattle, goats, sheep, pigs were significantly associated with presence of NTS (Table 4). Another variable that came out to be associated with presence of NTS was keeping of records. On the other hand, the use of separate houses for birds newly brought into the farms reduced the probability for presence of NTS. The model fit was, however, limited, as shown by the Hosmer Lemeshow test ($p < 0.05$).

Discussion

This study represents, to our knowledge, the first estimate of the prevalence of NTS in laying hen farms in Uganda. NTS prevalence was estimated at 21% of the farms with ten different serotypes identified. High phenotypic resistance to antimicrobials was found among the isolates with almost 58% of the isolates found resistant. In this study, the logistic regression model identified large farm size, presence of other poultry, and keeping of records as factors associated with occurrence of NTS in Uganda.

NTS prevalence of 21% is not surprisingly high considering how the poultry industry operates in the country, where disease control efforts are poor and deficient. In Uganda, chickens are not vaccinated against NTS. The available vaccines is for fowl typhoid targeting *Salmonella* Gallinarum and the protocol used is not ideal for identification of *S.* Gallinarum. Vaccinations of poultry in Uganda are not mandatory. Most commercial layer hen farms include fowl typhoid vaccinations in their routine vaccination schedules. A similar study in Senegal reported detection of NTS in faecal samples in 35.1% of farms [34] and in Nigeria, a related study reported isolation of NTS in

Table 2 Multidrug resistant profiles of NTS isolates from Wakiso, Lira and Masaka districts, Uganda 2017

Serotype	Resistance profile	No of isolates	District where isolates were recovered
S. Bolton	CIPR, SULFA, TET	1	Lira
S. Mbandaka	CIPR, CLR, AMP	4	Masaka (2), Wakiso (2)
S. Hadar	SULFA, TRIM, SxT	4	Wakiso
S. Hadar	CIPR, SUL, TRIM, SxT	2	Wakiso
S. Newport	CIPR, SULFA, TET, ENROF	1	Wakiso

AMP Ampicillin, *CIPR* Ciprofloxacin, *CLR* Chloramphenicol, *ENROF* Enrofloxacin, *SULFA* Sulphonamides, *SxT* Sulfamethoxazole-trimethoprim, *TET* Tetracycline, *TRIM* Trimethoprim

Table 3 Key demographic factors, disease management practices and farm characteristics associated with the prevalence of *Salmonella*, with *p*-values from simple chi-square analyses

Variable	Category	*Salmonella* positive farms (%)	*p*-value
Sex of farmer	Male ($n = 108$)	31 (28.7)	0.004
	Female ($n = 129$)	18 (14.0)	
Sex of manager	Male ($n = 85$)	27 (31.89)	< 0.001
	Female ($n = 115$)	12 (10.4)	
	Not applicable ($n = 37$)		
Age of the manager	< 20 years ($n = 5$)	4 (80.0)	0.001
	20–35 years ($n = 103$)	18 (17.5)	
	36–50 years ($n = 85$)	23 (27.1)	
	> 50 years ($n = 35$)	3 (8.6)	
	Missing ($n = 9$)		
Education level of the farmer	Primary ($n = 44$)	5 (11.4)	0.012
	Secondary ($n = 76$)	12 (15.8)	
	Tertiary ($n = 102$)	31 (30.4)	
	Missing ($n = 15$)		
Farm size (no. of birds)	Small (50–500) ($n = 162$)	19 (11.7)	< 0.001
	Medium (501–1000) ($n = 33$)	14 (42.4)	
	Large (> 1000) ($n = 38$)	14 (36.8)	
	Missing ($n = 4$)		
Number of poultry houses	One house ($n = 135$)	12 (8.9)	< 0.001
	Two houses ($n = 45$)	8 (17.8)	
	Three houses ($n = 32$)	21 (65.6)	
	> 3 houses ($n = 25$)	8 (32.0)	
Management system	Free range ($n = 47$)	2 (4.3)	< 0.001
	Semi intensive ($n = 90$)	11 (12.2)	
	Intensive ($n = 98$)	35 (35.7)	
	Others ($n = 2$)		
Use of protective clothing	Yes ($n = 136$)	35 (25.7)	0.031
	No ($n = 99$)	14 (14.1)	
	Missing ($n = 2$)		
Who does vaccination	Private ($n = 88$)	19 (21.6)	0.029
	Self/family ($n = 136$)	25 (18.4)	
	Employee ($n = 9$)	5 (55.6)	
	Missing ($n = 4$)		
Reuse of egg trays	Yes ($n = 105$)	29 (27.6)	0.034
	No ($n = 119$)	19 (16.0)	
	Missing ($n = 13$)		
Who treats the birds	Self ($n = 155$)	22 (14.2)	< 0.001
	Government/Animal Health Worker ($n = 11$)	0 (0.0)	
	Private/Animal Health worker ($n = 52$)	24 (46.2)	
	Missing ($n = 19$)		
Presence of other livestock	Present ($n = 101$)	26 (25.7)	0.097
	Not present ($n = 136$)	23 (16.9)	

Table 3 Key demographic factors, disease management practices and farm characteristics associated with the prevalence of *Salmonella*, with *p*-values from simple chi-square analyses *(Continued)*

Variable	Category	*Salmonella* positive farms (%)	*p*-value
Having a separate house for new birds	Yes ($n = 136$)	24 (17.6)	0.134
	No ($n = 97$)	25 (25.8)	
	Missing ($n = 4$)		
Disposal of dead birds	Burying ($n = 109$)	21 (19.3)	< 0.001
	Burning ($n = 17$)	12 (70.6)	
	Throw away ($n = 45$)	9 (20.0)	
	Giving to animals (dogs and pigs) ($n = 32$)	4 (12.5)	
	Drop in a pit ($n = 24$)	3 (12.5)	
	Missing ($n = 10$)		
Keeping of pets	Yes ($n = 137$)	35 (25.5)	0.025
	No ($n = 99$)	14 (14.1)	
	Missing ($n = 1$)		
If yes, species of pets	Dogs ($n = 62$)	20 (32.3)	0.006
	Cats ($n = 24$)	0 (0.0)	
	Both dogs and cats ($n = 51$)	15 (29.4)	
Keeping of records	Yes ($n = 153$)	43 (28.1)	< 0.001
	No ($n = 80$)	5 (6.2)	

12.5% of poultry droppings [35]. A more recent study in Nigeria by Fagbamilla et al. [36] estimated NTS prevalence of 43.6% in commercial poultry farms. In Algeria, a study in laying hen flocks by Bouzidi et al. [37] found that eight out 18 flocks were contaminated with NTS.

The identification of ten different serotypes can be regarded as a manifestation of the heterogeneous reservoirs and sources of NTS contamination. *S.* Newport was the most prevalent serotype, compared to the more commonly reported *S.* Enteritidis and *S.* Typhimurium in poultry isolates [37–40]. All the NTS serotypes identified in this study are zoonotic, and are known to have caused human disease outbreaks elsewhere. Consequently, this high prevalence of zoonotic NTS in the poultry reservoir constitutes a public health threat. *S.* Typhimurium, *S.* Newport, *S.* Hadar and *S.* Heidelberg have also been reported by Centers for Disease Control and Prevention (CDC) as the most threatening serotypes to public health because of their association with multidrug-resistance [41]. *S.* Mbandaka has been reported in many poultry products across the world [41–45]. A recent publication by Afema et al. [40] reported detection of mainly *S.* Kentucky, *S.* Heidelberg, *S.* Enteritidis, *S.* Typhimurium, and *S.* Virchow from poultry faeces. Also another study by Ikwap et al. [46] reported most of the serotypes of this study in isolates from piggeries in Uganda.

Studies of antibacterial susceptibility in NTS from African countries show highly variable results. An occurrence of almost 58% of isolates resistant to at least one antibiotic, is higher than what was reported in a similar study in Chad, that found overall resistance to 16 antibiotics tested at 33% [13]. However, it is lower compared to a study in Sudan that reported antibiotic resistance in NTS isolates at 98% [47] and similar to a more recent one in Ghana that reported resistance at 60.6% [48]. In Ethiopia, a study on NTS isolates from dairy cattle by Eguale et al. [49] found resistance at 30%. This high level of resistance could be associated with overuse and misuse of antibiotics in poultry farming. The significantly higher resistance level of NTS from Wakiso, which is

Table 4 Results from multivariable logistic regression showing identified factors associated with *Salmonella* spp. prevalence, with odds ratios with 95% Confidence Interval (CI) and corresponding p-values for the variables

Variable	Level	Odds Ratio	95% CI	*p*-value
Farm size (no. of birds)	Medium vs small	7.0	2.5–19.8	< 0.001
	Large vs small	5.9	2.1–16.1	0.001
Presence of other animal species	Present vs absent	5.0	2.1–16.1	< 0.001
Houses for new birds	Present vs absent	0.4	0.2–0.8	0.014
Records	Present vs absent	6.7	2.2–20.2	0.001

the immediate district surrounding the capital Kampala should be of concern. Kampala is the biggest hub of trade and movements of people, animals and animal products in the country, and resistant bacteria can potentially spread from here to all regions in the country.

Multidrug-resistance was seen in *S.* Bolton, *S.* Mbandaka, *S.* Hadar, and *S.* Newport isolates. High levels of multidrug-resistance have been reported elsewhere in Africa [11, 12, 48, 50]. The bacteria expressing resistance towards antimicrobials of which some are commonly used in humans and animals exposes a daunting challenge. Increasing development of antimicrobial resistance against commonly used drugs like ciprofloxacin, tetracyclines, sulphonamides sulfamethoxazole_trimethoprim (co-trimoxazole) in Uganda poises a great threat to public health and economy. Tetracyclines and sulphonamides are among the most widely used drugs for treatment and prophylaxis in food animals [51]. Increasing resistance toward these antimicrobials will render them less available leaving farmers with no cheaper options. In Uganda, ciprofloxacin is not licensed for use in poultry production, but is widely used for treatment of many human infections, including salmonellosis. The mechanisms behind the observed high resistance to ciprofloxacin in this study needs to be investigated.

Resistance to sulfamethoxazole-trimethoprim (co-trimoxazole) was also seen in this study. Co-trimoxazole is a drug that is used in Uganda for controlling opportunistic infections in persons living with HIV/AIDS [52, 53]. This causes concern as many of these patients will succumb to opportunistic infections [52–54] and also considering that most patients cannot afford other options of antimicrobials. All isolates were susceptible to the extended-spectrum beta-lactams (meropenem, cefotaxime, ceftazidime) that were tested. Efforts should be put in place to maintain this status. Strategies to reduce antimicrobial resistance in Ugandan farm settings should focus on improving management, biosecurity, and sensitization of key stakeholders such as farmers, farm workers, policy makers, drug dealers, animal health workers and veterinarians.

At univariate analysis, a number of demographic farm management and production variables were associated with occurrence of NTS on farms. The final logistic regression model built identified large farm size, presence of other poultry species, and keeping of records as factors associated with NTS in Uganda. The final model was also tested for the random effect of village to assess the degree of independence. While initial analyses indicated that village had some effect, the final model revealed no such effect – indicating that the factors found were stable across the study districts. A large farm was one of the risk factors associated with NTS determined by the model. This is in concordance with the fact that farm size has been significantly associated with presence of NTS in studies conducted in Britain [26], Trinidad and Tobago, Grenada, and St. Lucia [55], France [15, 56] and Belgium [57]. A previous study of presence of NTS in layer and broiler flocks in the Kampala region in Uganda by Nasinyama et al. [58] identified bird type, flock size and downtime as significant risk factors. In the Ugandan setting, bigger farms tend to attract many activities; visitors and the obtaining of feeds, feed ingredients, chickens and other supplies from multiple sources, many of which informal and unregulated. Under these situations with low biosecurity practices, keeping adequate hygiene standards can be difficult. In addition, most routine operations like mixing of feeds, feeding of birds, watering and vaccinations are manual requiring many workers, some of them coming from outside the farms. Some farms have a limited workforce and are therefore less effective in keeping high standards of routine hygienic practices. All these factors can be further complicated by farms experiencing erratic outage of power and water supplies. As a range of management factors are related to farm size, we may not have identified the most biologically important causal factors.

The current study identified presence of other animal species as another risk factor for NTS. When present on farms, other animal species will most likely share water feeds and space with the chicken and thereby increasing the opportunities for the spread of the bacteria due to direct or indirect contacts. The other animal species may be reservoirs of NTS and thus, contribute to the maintenance of high prevalence of NTS at a farm.

Surprisingly, keeping records emerged as a factor increasing the risk of infection. This could be because in Uganda record keeping is poor among smallholder farmers, and this study found a significant association of NTS with large farms. Keeping records is therefore probably correlating with large farms. It remains open if this variable should be in the model, but leaving out this variable did not affect the estimates for the other variable much. The variable is therefore not considered to be a confounder, but it may perhaps represent other factors.

Having separate housing for birds newly introduced in the farm was associated with lower levels of NTS. The lower level of NTS in farms using separate houses for new chicken is as expected and may represent other factors related to general hygiene, potentially reducing the risk of introduction and maintenance of NTS at farms. Normally housing new birds separately provides an opportunity to observe and provide timely treatment before they are released to mix with other birds on the farms.

The prevalence estimate in the current study is associated with several uncertainties. The study was a cross-sectional study including only one sampling occasion per farm. Depending on the infection levels, it is possible that in some farms a small proportion of birds shed NTS in faeces and this is normally intermittent [59].

Consequently, the prevalence and number of NTS in faecal droppings may therefore change over time and analysis of this requires a longitudinal monitoring scheme. The sampling of faecal droppings only, in order to determine the presence or absence of NTS, may be a limiting factor as NTS in farm settings can be carried in litter, feeds and water as well. However, pooled faecal and environmental sampling of poultry houses is still better than sampling individual birds for detection of NTS on farms as reported in previous studies [60, 61]. In addition, this study targeted commercial egg laying farms who are registered, and yet a lot of farmers are not registered with NAADS. However, these results provide an important insight into the occurrence of NTS in Ugandan poultry, particularly in the absence of previous similar studies. In this study, data on the sources of day old chicks were not captured and this could be included in future studies of NTS in Uganda as sources of day old chicks are potential risk factors for *Salmonella.* In addition, the sampling strategies limited identification of more than one serotype in small farms with only one house as only one sample was taken and one colony was picked for serotyping.

Conclusions

A high prevalence and high levels of antimicrobial resistant NTS in commercial laying chicken farms in Uganda was revealed in this study. Large farms and presence of other animal species at the farm were identified as risk factors for NTS. Both these risk factors are associated with biosecurity challenges. Although limited, this study should pave way for informing the establishment of proper NTS control systems based on empirical scientific evidence.

Further characterization of NTS from the poultry reservoir that is documented through the present work will be necessary in order to elucidate the transmission dynamics and dissemination of these important zoonotic bacteria. Particular emphasis needs to be given to the determination of antimicrobial resistance genes and their mobility in future studies.

Abbreviations

CDC: Centre for Disease Control and Prevention; CI: Confidence interval; MDR: Multi-drug resistance; MSRV: Modified Semi solid Rappaport Vassiliadis (MSRV); NAADS: National Agricultural Advisory Services; NTS: Non-typhoidal *Salmonella*; UNCST: Uganda National Council of Science and Technology; WHO: World Health Organization; XLD: Xylose Lysine Deoxycholate

Acknowledgements

The authors thank all farmers, farm managers, district authorities and research assistants for their various contributions including their valuable time and knowledge. We are equally very grateful for the support from the researchers and technicians at the Department of Food Safety and Infection Biology at NMBU, particularly Toril Lindbäck and Kristin O' Sullivan. We would like to acknowledge Nasinyama George of Kampala International University for the advice and guidance at the conception of this study. Our thanks to Bergsjo Bjarne of Norwegian Veterinary Institute for serotyping the isolates.

Funding

This work was supported by the Norwegian Programme for Capacity Development in Higher Education and Research for Development (NORHED project No.UGA-13/0031) based at Makerere University, Kampala Uganda and Norwegian University of Life Sciences, Oslo.

Authors' contributions

TO was the principal investigator, contributed to conception, design, data collection, analysis and drafting of the manuscript. YW contributed to conception design, supervision, editing and approval. TML supervised the lab analysis, participated in drafting and reviewing of the manuscript. AM contributed to the design and review of the manuscript. CK helped with the acquisition of funding, supervision, editing and reviewing the manuscript. LN helped with field data collection and writing. ST participated in field data collection, isolation and writing. ES contributed to acquisition of funding, design, data analysis, writing and editing. All authors read and approved the final manuscript.

Consent for publication

Not applicable.

Competing interests

The authors declare that they have no competing interests.

Author details

[1]Department of Bio-security, Ecosystems and Veterinary Public Health, College of Veterinary Medicine, Animal Resources and Biosecurity (COVAB), Makerere University, Kampala, Uganda. [2]Department of Food Safety and Infection Biology, Faculty of Veterinary Medicine, Norwegian University of Life Sciences (NMBU), Oslo, Norway. [3]Divisions of Genetics and Genomics, Roslin Institute, The Royal (Dick) Vet School of Veterinary Studies, University of Edinburgh, Edinburgh, UK.

References

1. Routh JA, Pringle J, Mohr M, Bidol S, Arends K, Adams-Cameron M, Hancock WT, Kissler B, Rickert R, Folster J, et al. Nationwide outbreak of multidrug-resistant *Salmonella* Heidelberg infections associated with ground turkey: United States, 2011. Epidemiol Infect. 2015;143:3227–34.
2. Painter JA, Hoekstra RM, Ayers T, Tauxe RV, Braden CR, Angulo FJ, Griffin PM. Attribution of foodborne illnesses, hospitalizations, and deaths to food commodities by using outbreak data, United States, 1998-2008. Emerg Infect Dis. 2013;19:407–15.
3. Scallan E, Hoekstra RM, Angulo FJ, Tauxe RV, Widdowson MA, Roy SL, Jones JL, Griffin PM. Foodborne illness acquired in the United States-major pathogens. Emerg Infect Dis. 2011;17:7–15.
4. Ao TT, Feasey NA, Gordon MA, Keddy KH, Angulo FJ, Crump JA. Global burden of invasive nontyphoidal *Salmonella* disease, 2010(1). Emerg Infect Dis. 2015;21:941–9.
5. Feasey NA, Dougan G, Kingsley RA, Heyderman RS, Gordon MA. Invasive non-typhoidal *Salmonella* disease: an emerging and neglected tropical disease in Africa. Lancet. 2012;379(9835):2489–99.
6. Majowicz SE, Musto J, Scallan E, Angulo FJ, Kirk M, O'Brien SJ, Jones TF, Fazil A, Hoekstra RM. International collaboration on enteric disease 'Burden of illness S: the global burden of nontyphoidal Salmonella gastroenteritis. Clin Infect Dis. 2010;50:882–9.
7. Graham SM, Molyneux EM, Walsh AL, Cheesbrough JS, Molyneux ME, Hart CA. Nontyphoidal *Salmonella* infections of children in tropical Africa. Pediatr Infect Dis J. 2000;19:1189–96.
8. Gordon MA, Graham SM, Walsh AL, Wilson L, Phiri A, Molyneux E, Zijlstra EE, Heyderman RS, Hart CA, Molyneux ME. Epidemics of invasive *Salmonella enterica* serovar enteritidis and *S-enterica* serovar typhimurium infection associated with multidrug resistance among adults and children in Malawi. Clin Infect Dis. 2008;46:963–9.

9. Dechet AM, Herman KM, Chen Parker C, Taormina P, Johanson J, Tauxe RV, Mahon BE. Outbreaks caused by sprouts, United States, 1998-2010: lessons learned and solutions needed. Foodborne Pathog Dis. 2014;11:635–44.
10. Callejon RM, Rodriguez-Naranjo MI, Ubeda C, Hornedo-Ortega R, Garcia-Parrilla MC, Troncoso AM. Reported foodborne outbreaks due to fresh produce in the United States and European Union: trends and causes. Foodborne Pathog Dis. 2015;12:32–8.
11. Abdel-Maksoud M, Abdel-Khalek R, El-Gendy A, Gamal RF, Abdelhady HM, House BL. Genetic characterisation of multidrug-resistant Salmonella enterica serotypes isolated from poultry in Cairo, Egypt. Afr J Lab Med. 2015;4(1):1–7.
12. Ahmed AM, Shimamoto T, Shimamoto T. Characterization of integrons and resistance genes in multidrug-resistant *Salmonella* enterica isolated from meat and dairy products in Egypt. Int J Food Microbiol. 2014;189:39–44.
13. Tabo DA, Diguimbaye CD, Granier SA, Moury F, Brisabois A, Elgroud R, Millemann Y. Prevalence and antimicrobial resistance of non-typhoidal *Salmonella* serotypes isolated from laying hens and broiler chicken farms in N'Djamena. Chad Vet Microbiol. 2013;166:293–8.
14. Henzler DJ, Kradel DC, Sischo WM. Management and environmental risk factors for *Salmonella* enteritidis contamination of eggs. Am J Vet Res. 1998;59:824–9.
15. Adeline HS, Marianne C, Sophie L, Francoise L, Isabelle P, Sandra R, Virginie M, Philippe F, Nicolas R. Risk factors for *Salmonella* enterica subsp enterica contamination in 519 French laying hen flocks at the end of the laying period. Prev Vet Med. 2009;89:51–8.
16. Mollenhorst H, van Woudenbergh CJ, Bokkers EGM, de Boer IJM. Risk factors for *Salmonella* enteritidis infections in laying hens. Poult Sci. 2005;84:1308–13.
17. Schulz J, Van Hoorebeke S, Hald B, Hartung J, Van Immerseel F, Radtke I, Kabell S, Dewulf J. The dynamics of *Salmonella* occurrence in commercial laying hen flocks throughout a laying period. Avian Pathol. 2011;40:243–8.
18. Denagamage T, Jayarao B, Patterson P, Wallner-Pendleton E, Kariyawasam S. Risk factors associated with *Salmonella* in laying hen farms: systematic review of observational studies. Avian Dis. 2015;59:291–302.
19. Kirk MD, Pires SM, Black RE, Caipo M, Crump JA, Devleesschauwer B, Dopfer D, Fazil A, Fischer-Walker CL, Hald T, et al. World Health Organization estimates of the global and regional disease burden of 22 foodborne bacterial, protozoal, and viral diseases, 2010: a data synthesis. PLoS Med. 2015;12(12):e1001921.
20. Bouchrif B, Le Hello S, Pardos M, Karraouan B, Perrier-Gros-Claude JD, Ennaji MM, Timinouni M, Weill FX. Ceftazidime-resistant *Salmonella* enterica. Morocco Emerg Infect Dis. 2009;15(10):1693–5.
21. De Knegt LV, Pires SM, Hald T. Attributing foodborne salmonellosis in humans to animal reservoirs in the European Union using a multi-country stochastic model. Epidemiol Infect. 2015;143(6):1175–86.
22. Moffatt CRM, Musto J, Pingault N, Miller M, Stafford R, Gregory J, Polkinghorne BG, Kirk MD. *Salmonella* Typhimurium and outbreaks of egg-associated disease in Australia, 2001 to 2011. Foodborne Pathog Dis. 2016;13(7):379–85.
23. Cameron A. Survey toolbox for livestock diseases : a practical manual and software package for active surveillance in developing countries. 1st ed. Australian Centre for International Agricultural Research: Canberra; 1999.
24. Cameron AR, Baldock FC. A new probability formula for surveys to substantiate freedom from disease. Prev Vet Med. 1998;34(1):1–17.
25. Van Hoorebeke S, Van Immerseel F, De Vylder J, Ducatelle R, Haesebrouck F, Pasmans F, de Kruif A, Dewulf J. Faecal sampling underestimates the actual prevalence of *Salmonella* in laying hen flocks. Zoonoses Public Health. 2009;56:471–6.
26. Snow LC, Davies RH, Christiansen KH, Carrique-Mas JJ, Cook AJC, Evans SJ. Investigation of risk factors for *Salmonella* on commercial egg-laying farms in Great Britain, 2004-2005. Vet Rec. 2010;166:579–86.
27. International Organization for Standardization. ISO 6579:2002/Amd 1:2007: detection of *Salmonella* spp. in animal faeces and in environmental samples from the primary production stage, amendment 1, annex D. In: Microbiology of food and animal feeding stuffs. Horizontal method for the detection of *Salmonella spp*. Geneva, Switzerland: International Organization for Standardization; 2007.
28. Grimont PAD, Weill F-X. Antigenic formulae of the *Salmonella* serovars, World Health Organization Collaborating Centre for Reference and Research on Salmonella 2007. 9th ed. Paris: Institut Pasteur; 2007. p. 167.
29. CLSI. Performance standards for antimicrobial susceptibility testing: twenty-fifth informational supplement. Wayne: Clinical Laboratory Standards Institute; 2015.
30. CLSI. Interpretation of the Antibiogramme with Neo-Sensitabs MIC break-points according to CLSI (M31-A4/M31-S2 2013) Inoculum according to Kirby-Bauer / confluent colonies. Wayne: Clinical and Laboratory Standards Institute; 2013.
31. WHO. Integrated surveillance of antimicrobial resistance: guidance from a WHO Advisory Group. Geneva: WHO; 2013. http://www.who.int/foodsafety/publications/agisar_guidance/en/. Accessed on 31 May 2017
32. Dohoo I, Martin W, Stryhn H. Veterinary epidemiologic research. 2nd ed. Charlottetown: VER inc.; 2009.
33. Hosmer DW, Lemeshow S. Applied logistic regression. 2nd ed. Hoboken: Wiley; 2000.
34. Dione MM, Ieven M, Garin B, Marcotty T, Geerts S. Prevalence and antimicrobial resistance of *Salmonella* isolated from broiler farms, chicken carcasses, and street-vended restaurants in Casamance, Senegal. J Food Prot. 2009;72:2423–7.
35. Orji MU, Onuigbo HC, Mbata TI. Isolation of *Salmonella* from poultry droppings and other environmental sources in Awka, Nigeria. Int J Infect Dis. 2005;9:86–9.
36. Fagbamila IO, Barco L, Mancin M, Kwaga J, Ngulukun SS, Zavagnin P, Lettini AA, Lorenzetto M, Abdu PA, Kabir J, et al. *Salmonella* serovars and their distribution in Nigerian commercial chicken layer farms. PLoS One. 2017; 12(3):e0173097. https://doi.org/10.1371/journal.
37. Bouzidi N, Aoun L, Zeghdoudi M, Bensouilah M, Elgroud R, Oucief I, Granier SA, Brisabois A, Desquilbet L, Millemann Y. *Salmonella* contamination of laying-hen flocks in two regions of Algeria. Food Res Int. 2012;45:897–904.
38. Alvarez-Fernandez E, Alonso-Calleja C, Garcia-Fernandez C, Capita R. Prevalence and antimicrobial resistance of *Salmonella* serotypes isolated from poultry in Spain: comparison between 1993 and 2006. Int J Food Microbiol. 2012;153:281–7.
39. Garber L, Smeltzer M, Fedorka-Cray P, Ladely S, Ferris K. Salmonella enterica serotype enteritidis in table egg layer house environments and in mice in US layer houses and associated risk factors. Avian Dis. 2003;47:134–42.
40. Afema JA, Byarugaba DK, Shah DH, Atukwase E, Nambi M, Sischo WM. Potential sources and transmission of salmonella and antimicrobial resistance in Kampala, Uganda. PLoS One. 2016;11(3):e0152130.
41. Olobatoke RY, Mulugeta SD. Incidence of non-typhoidal *Salmonella* in poultry products in the North West Province, South Africa. S Afr J Sci. 2015;111:70–6.
42. Im MC, Jeong SJ, Kwon Y-K, Jeong O-M, Kang M-S, Lee YJ. Prevalence and characteristics of *Salmonella spp*. isolated from commercial layer farms in Korea. Poult Sci. 2015;94:1691–8.
43. Iwabuchi E, Maruyama N, Hara A, Nishimura M, Murakami M, Ochiai T, Hirai K. Nationwide survey of *Salmonella* prevalence in environmental dust from layer Frams in Japan. J Food Prot. 2010;73:1993–2000.
44. Kramarenko T, Nurmoja I, Kärssin A, Meremäe K, Hörman A, Roasto M. The prevalence and serovar diversity of *Salmonella* in various food products in Estonia. Food Control. 2014;42:43–7.
45. Zhang J, Yang X, Kuang D, Shi X, Xiao W, Zhang JY, Zheng G, Xu X, Meng JH. Prevalence of antimicrobial resistance of non-typhoidal *Salmonella* serovars in retail aquaculture products. Int J Food Microbiol. 2015;210:47–52.
46. Ikwap K, Erume J, Owiny DO, Nasinyama GW, Melin L, Bengtsson B, Lundeheim N, Fellstrom C, Jacobson M. Salmonella species in piglets and weaners from Uganda: prevalence, antimicrobial resistance and herd-level risk factors. Prev Vet Med. 2014;115(1–2):39–47.
47. Elmadiena M, El Hussein AA, Muckle CA, Cole L, Wilkie E, Mistry K, Perets A. Antimicrobial susceptibility and multi-drug resistance of *Salmonella enterica subspecies enterica* serovars in Sudan. Trop Anim Health Prod. 2013;45(5):1113–8.
48. Andoh LA, Dalsgaard A, Obiri-Danso K, Newman MJ, Barco L, Olsen JE. Prevalence and antimicrobial resistance of Salmonella serovars isolated from poultry in Ghana. Epidemiol Infect. 2016;144(15):3288–99.
49. Eguale T, Engidawork E, Gebreyes WA, Asrat D, Alemayehu H, Medhin G, Johnson RP, Gunn JS. Fecal prevalence, serotype distribution and antimicrobial resistance of *Salmonellae* in dairy cattle in central Ethiopia. BMC Microbiol. 2016;16:11.
50. Fashae K, Ogunsola F, Aarestrup FM, Hendriksen RS. Antimicrobial susceptibility and serovars of salmonella from chickens and humans in Ibadan, Nigeria. J Infect Dev Ctries. 2010;4(8):484–94.

51. OIE. Annual report on the use of antimicrobial agents in animals - better understanding of the global situation. Paris: OIE; 2016.
52. Kasirye R, Baisley K, Munderi P, Grosskurth H. Effect of cotrimoxazole prophylaxis on malaria occurrence in HIV-infected patients on antiretroviral therapy in sub-Saharan Africa. Tropical Med Int Health. 2015;20(5):569–80.
53. Kasirye RP, Baisley K, Munderi P, Levin J, Anywaine Z, Nunn A, Kamali A, Grosskurth H. Incidence of malaria by cotrimoxazole use in HIV-infected Ugandan adults on antiretroviral therapy: a randomised, placebo-controlled study. AIDS. 2016;30(4):635–43.
54. Campbell JD, Moore D, Degerman R, Kaharuza F, Were W, Muramuzi E, Odongo G, Wetaka M, Mermin J, Tappero JW. HIV-infected Ugandan adults taking antiretroviral therapy with CD4 counts > 200 cells/mu L who discontinue Cotrimoxazole prophylaxis have increased risk of malaria and diarrhea. Clin Infect Dis. 2012;54(8):1204–11.
55. Adesiyun A, Webb L, Musai L, Louison B, Joseph G, Stewart-Johnson A, Samlal S, Rodrigo S. Survey of *Salmonella* contamination in chicken layer farms in three Caribbean countries. J Food Prot. 2014;77:1471–80.
56. Chemaly M, Huneau-Salauen A, Labbe A, Houdayer C, Petetin I, Fravalo P. Isolation of salmonella enterica in laying-hen flocks and assessment of eggshell contamination in France. J Food Prot. 2009;72:2071–7.
57. Namata H, Meroc E, Aerts M, Faes C, Abrahantes JC, Imberechts H, Mintiens K. *Salmonella* in Belgian laying hens: an identification of risk factors. Prev Vet Med. 2008;83:323–36.
58. Nasinyama GW, McEwen SA, Waltner-Toews D, Gyles CL, Wilson J, Opuda-Asibo J, Poppe C. Factors associated with occurrence of Salmonella in broiler and layer flocks of chickens in Kampala district, Uganda. Epidemiol Sante Anim. 1997;4:31–2.
59. Carrique-Mas JJ, Davies RH. Sampling and bacterial detection *Salmonella* in poultry and poultry premises. Rev Sci Tech. 2008;27:665–77.
60. Arnold ME, Carrique-Mas JJ, Davies RH. Sensitivity of environmental sampling methods for detecting *Salmonella* Enteritidis in commercial laying flocks relative to the within-flock prevalence. Epidemiol Infect. 2010;138(3):330–9.
61. Arnold ME, Carrique-Mas JJ, McLaren I, Davies RH. A comparison of pooled and individual bird sampling for detection of *Salmonella* in commercial egg laying flocks. Prev Vet Med. 2011;99(2):176–84.

11

A robust PCR for the differentiation of potential virulent strains of *Haemophilus parasuis*

N. Galofré-Milà[1], F. Correa-Fiz[1], S. Lacouture[2], M. Gottschalk[2], K. Strutzberg-Minder[3], A. Bensaid[1], S. Pina-Pedrero[1] and V. Aragon[1*]

Abstract

Background: *Haemophilus parasuis* is the etiological agent of Glässer's disease in swine. *H. parasuis* comprises strains with heterogeneous virulence capacity, from non-virulent to highly virulent. Determination of the pathogenic potential of the strains is important for diagnosis and disease control. The virulence-associated trimeric autotransporters (*vtaA*) genes have been used to predict *H. parasuis* virulence by PCR amplification of their translocator domains. Here, we report a new and improved PCR designed to detect a different domain of the *vtaA* genes, the leader sequence (LS) as a diagnostic tool to predict virulence.

Methods: A collection of 360 *H. parasuis* strains was tested by PCR with LS specific primers. Results of the PCR were compared with the clinical origin of the strains and, for a subset of strains, with their phagocytosis and serum resistance using a Chi-square test.

Results: LS-PCR was specific to *H. parasuis*, and allowed the differential detection of the leader sequences found in clinical and non-clinical isolates. Significant correlation was observed between the results of the LS-PCR and the clinical origin (organ of isolation) of the strains, as well as with their phagocytosis and serum susceptibility, indicating that this PCR is a good predictor of the virulence of the strains. In addition, this new PCR showed a full correlation with the previously validated PCR based on the translocator domain. LS-PCR could be performed in a wide range of annealing temperatures without losing specificity.

Conclusion: This newly described PCR based on the leader sequence of the *vtaA* genes, LS-PCR, is a robust test for the prediction of the virulence potential of *H. parasuis* strains.

Keywords: *Haemophilus parasuis*, PCR diagnosis, Bacterial virulence, Glässer's disease diagnosis

Background

Haemophilus parasuis comprises strains of different virulence, from non-virulent to highly virulent. This bacterial species can be found colonizing the upper respiratory tract of clinically healthy piglets, although some strains can cause invasive systemic disease. Systemic bacterial spreading induces a strong inflammation, which leads to the characteristic lesions of fibrinous polyserositis. The systemic disease caused by *H. parasuis* is known as Glässer's disease. While *H. parasuis* can be found in basically all farms, disease is developed in a small percentage of them. Several factors are important in disease development, including the presence of other pathogens in the farm and the virulence of the *H. parasuis* strains [1].

Piglets can be colonized by several strains of *H. parasuis*, and therefore, several strains of the bacterium are found in a single farm [2]. This epidemiological situation makes crucial the correct determination of the strain causing the disease outbreak for disease control.

Many studies have been performed in an effort to find virulence markers for *H. parasuis* [3–5]. Some specific genomic sequences were identified by microarray studies to be differentially present in *H. parasuis* strains depending on their clinical origin. Those genes were identified and named virulence associated trimeric autotransporters (*vtaA*) and were classified in three groups based on the

* Correspondence: virginia.aragon@irta.es
[1]IRTA, Centre de Recerca en Sanitat Animal (CReSA, IRTA-UAB), Campus de la Universitat Autònoma de Barcelona, 08193 Bellaterra, Spain
Full list of author information is available at the end of the article

yadA-like translocator domain sequence [6]. *VtaAs* from groups 1 and 2 were associated to clinical strains [6]. Moreover, two VtaAs from group 1 were demonstrated to play a role in phagocytosis resistance, a virulence mechanism of *H. parasuis* [7, 8]. PCR tests were designed for *H. parasuis* identification and virulence prediction using the *yadA*-like translocator domain of group 1 and 3 *vtaA* [9]. Detection of group 3-translocator was *H. parasuis* species-specific, while detection of group 1-translocator was associated to *H. parasuis* virulent strains [9]. However, the conditions for the proper execution of that PCR were very stringent and complex regarding temperatures and bacterial DNA concentrations, with the risk of losing specificity if not strictly respecting the previously described conditions. Therefore, it was difficult to implement for routine diagnosis. Recently, a genomic comparison of 212 strains confirmed previous reports on the use of *H. parasuis vtaA* for virulence prediction [5]. Two different leader sequences were detected in these genes, and each type was over-represented either in clinical (associated with disease) or non-clinical isolates [5]. Here, we present a new and more robust PCR, based on the leader sequences of the *vtaA* genes.

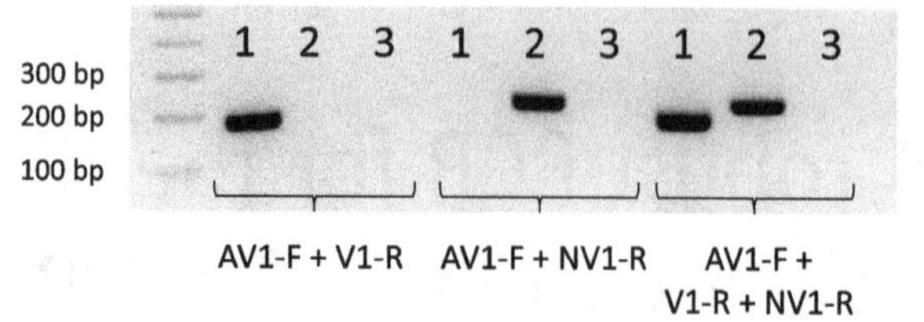

Fig. 1 PCR results with the virulent strain Nagasaki (1) and the non-virulent strain F9 (2). Lanes 3 are negative controls. The combination of primers used in each reaction are indicated in the figure

Methods

PCR conditions

Leader sequences of the *vtaA* genes were aligned and compared for primer design, taking into account the clinical origin of the strains (strains isolated from either lesions or nasal cavities of healthy piglets). As forward primer, a common sequence within the leader sequence of *vtaAs* was identified (AAATATTTAGAGTTATTGGAGTC) and named AV1-F. For specific amplification, two reverse primers were chosen; V1-R (AATATACCTAGTAATACTA GACTTAAAAG), for *vtaA* found in clinical (putative virulent) strains, and NV1-R (CAGAATAAGCAAAATCAGC), for non-clinical nasal (putative non-virulent) strains. Conditions for the PCR reactions were, 1.5 mM $MgCl_2$, 0.4 mM each deoxynucleotide triphosphate (dNTP), 400 nM each primer, 1 U GoTaq polymerase (Promega) and 0.3–500 ng of genomic DNA in a final volume of 25 μL in GoTaq buffer (Promega). Cycling conditions were 5 min at 94 °C, followed by 30 cycles of 45 s at 94 °C, 45 s at 52 °C and 1 min at 72 °C, then a final incubation at 72 °C for 7 min.

Bacterial strains

The PCRs based on the leader sequence of the *vtaA* genes were tested with *H. parasuis* strains previously described [9], together with *H. parasuis* clinical isolates from the diagnostic laboratory services of the Faculty of Veterinary Medicine of the University of Montreal (Canada), the Innovative Veterinary Diagnostics (IVD) Laboratory in Seelze-Letter (Germany) and the laboratory Exopol in Zaragoza (Spain). Nasal isolates were obtained from the nasal cavities of healthy piglets, while the rest of strains were obtained from clinical cases of disease, including systemic, pulmonary and clinical isolates of unknown origin. Association between the PCR results and the clinical origin of the strains was assessed using Pearson's Chi-square test for categorical data.

Specificity of the leader sequence PCR was confirmed with strains of *Actinobacillus pleuropneumoniae*, *Actinobacillus porcinus*, *Actinobacillus indolicus*, *Actinobacillus minor*, *Actinobacillus suis*, *Pasteurella multocida*, *Streptococcus suis* and *Escherichia coli* isolated from swine.

Virulence assays

The putative virulence of the strains was inferred by the clinical origin of the isolates. For a set of strains phagocytosis and serum resistance assays were performed following previously described protocols [8, 10]. Association between the virulence assays and the PCR results was evaluated using two tailed Fisher exact probability test.

Results and discussion

Preliminary assays demonstrated that the reverse primers V1-R (for detection of clinical, putative virulent, strains) and NV1-R (for detection of non-clinical, putative non-virulent, strains) could be used either in pairs with the forward primer AV1-F or in a combination of the three together (Fig. 1), maintaining specificity. The latter multiplex PCR will be referred as LS-PCR for clarity throughout the rest of text.

LS-PCR sensitivity limit was estimated to 0.3 ng of genomic DNA, both for the virulent Nagasaki strain and the non-virulent SW114 strain. Importantly, annealing temperature was modified between 47.5 and 57 °C without losing sensitivity.

Table 1 Summary of the results of the leader PCR in a collection of 360 strains from different clinical origin

	Number of strains				
PCR results	Total	Isolation site			
		Systemic	Pulmonary	Nasal	Unknown[a]
V	262	75	120	43	24
NV	98	5	14	77	2

[a]clinical isolates, from cases of disease
V virulent, *NV* non-virulent

Table 2 Association of the PCR results with the serum and phagocytosis susceptibility of selected strains (Fisher, $p < 0.04$ and $p < 0.0005$, respectively); (S: sensible; R: resistant). NV: non-virulent and V: virulent, as determined by the *vtaA* leader sequence PCR

		Serum susceptibility		Phagocytosis susceptibility	
		S	R	S	R
PCR	V	14	16	9	19
	NV	10	2	12	1
		24	18	21	20

A summary of the results obtained with the LS-PCR and the collection of strains is presented in Table 1. To evaluate the association between this new PCR and the potential virulence of *H. parasuis*, results of the LS-PCR and the clinical origin of the strains (nasal versus clinical isolates) were compared using a Chi-Square test. The correlation between the LS-PCR results and the clinical origin (organ of isolation) of the strains was highly significant (Pearson, $p < 0.0001$), indicating that this PCR is a good predictor of the putative virulence of the strains. If the results of the LS-PCR are compared only between the nasal and systemic isolates, the correlation was also highly significant (Pearson, $p < 0.0001$), with 77 out of 120 nasal strains yielding amplification with primer NV1-R and 75 out of 80 systemic strains showing amplification with V1-R.

In addition, when the strains previously analyzed using the described PCR for the *yadA* translocator domain of *vtaAs* [9] were tested with the new LS-PCR, a full correlation between both tests was observed. All the strains yielding the amplicon of non-virulent (NV) strains in the LS-PCR were negative in the group 1-*vtaA* PCR, and all the strains that produced the amplicon of clinical virulent (V) strains in the LS-PCR were positive in the group 1-*vtaA* PCR.

To support the results of the LS-PCR, phagocytosis and serum resistance for some strains were contrasted with the PCR results. The association of the LS-PCR results with virulence mechanisms was also significant, although statistically weaker than those found with the clinical origin of the strains, probably due to the lower number of strains used. Table 2 shows the association of the LS-PCR results with serum susceptibility of the strains (Fisher, $p = 0.04$) and with phagocytosis susceptibility (Fisher, $p = 0.0005$). Worth mentioning, two reference strains, serovar 7 strain 174 and serovar 11 strain H465, classified as non-virulent serovars, were identified as virulent by the PCR. In phagocytosis assays, strain 174 was sensitive and strain H465 was resistant to phagocytosis by porcine alveolar macrophages (PAMs). Thus, the results of the LS-PCR and the phagocytosis test were discordant for strain 174. One of the strains that was classified as virulent by this new LS-PCR, strain SL3–2, was sensitive to both phagocytosis and serum. Interestingly, the genome sequence of this strain is available [5] and genome analysis showed the presence of *vtaA5* and absence of *vtaA* 1, 4, 6, 7, 8 and 9 (from virulent group 1 *vtaAs*) in the genome regions found in other strains. Therefore, strain SL3–2 may be lacking some VtaAs involved in the in vitro virulence assays used in this study, phagocytosis and serum susceptibility, and it may represent a strain with an intermediate phenotype due to reduction in the number of *vtaAs*. On the other hand, five strains isolated from systemic sites (pericardium, brain and abdomen) yielded NV amplification in the LS-PCR. Two of these 5 strains, isolated from

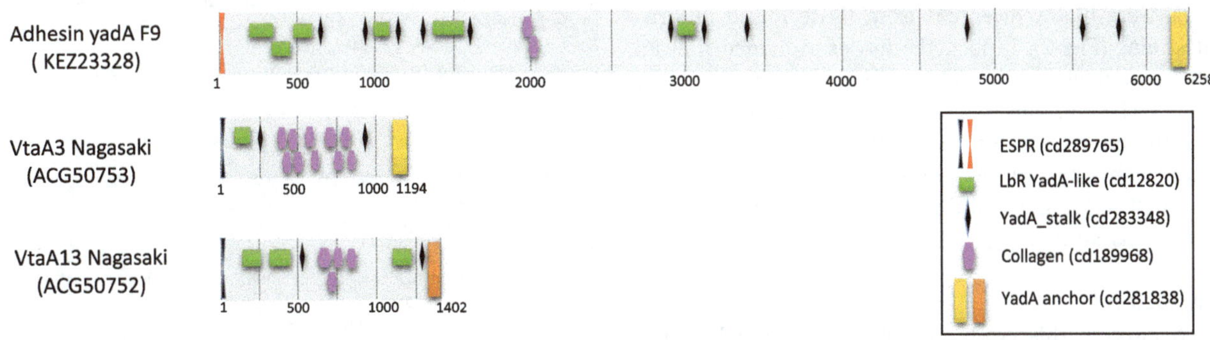

Fig. 2 Schematic representation of three *H. parasuis* autotransporters. Each panel shows the domains predicted using CD-search algorithm from NCBI in each protein. At the top, the protein found in non-virulent F9 strain (adhesin YadA) with leader sequence from VtaAs overrepresented in non-clinical isolates (in *red*) and translocator domain from group 1 VtaAs (in *yellow*) is shown. Below, representative proteins from group 1 (VtaA3, ACG50753; group 1 translocator domain indicated in *yellow*) and group 3 (VtaA13, ACG50752; group 3 translocator domain indicated in orange) from Nagasaki strain are shown. The depicted domains are: ESPR (Extended Signal Peptide of Type V secretion system, cd289765), LbR YadA-like (YadA-like, left-handed beta-roll cd12820), YadA stalk (Coiled stalk of trimeric autotransporter adhesion, cd 283,348), Collagen (Collagen triple helix repeat 20 copies, cd189968) and YadA anchor or translocator domain (YadA-like C-terminal region, cd281838). Accession numbers for proteins and domains are shown between brackets. Domains are represented with the same shapes between proteins. Mismatching colors within the same shapes denote low homology between domains from different proteins. Numbers below each protein representation correspond to amino acids

brain and pericardium, were studied by serum and phagocytosis susceptibility assays, and were found to be sensitive in both tests (with reduction of bacteria of more than 5 logs after 1 h of incubation with fresh serum, and with more than 50% of PAM with associated bacteria in phagocytosis assays), showing a good correlation between the in vitro tests and the PCR results. It is known that some predisposing factors, such as co-infections [11–13], can facilitate systemic spread of low virulent strains, due to the immune suppression induced by the concomitant pathogens, and this could explain how these serum and phagocytosis sensitive strains were found in systemic organs. In these cases, the main probable cause of disease was not *H. parasuis*, which in fact, was probably acting as a secondary agent. As any other test, this PCR needs to be complemented with clinical, pathological and epidemiological data to reach a meaningful diagnosis of the disease in the farm.

Analysis of the genome of four non-virulent strains (serovar 3 reference strain SW114, serovar 8 reference strain C5, and nasal strains MU21–2 and F9) detected the expected presence of one gene encoding a large trimeric autotransporter with the typical translocator domain of group 3 *vtaA*s, but also a very large trimeric autotransporter of more than 6000 amino acids, with the translocator sequence characteristic of group 1-*vtaA* associated with virulent strains. This latter gene was transcribed under laboratory and biofilm conditions in the F9 strain, indicating that it is a functional gene (GEO:GSE56428). This very large group 1-*vtaA* autotransporter can explain the positive results with the previously described PCR in group 1-*vtaA* for some non-virulent strains, when the conditions of this test were not exactly as described by Olvera et al. [9]. The other domains of this gene, passenger and leader domains, were highly divergent from those found in virulent strains (Fig. 2). In fact, the leader sequence showed high homology to the *vtaAs* found in non-virulent strains. This finding explains the necessity of the stringent conditions for the PCR based on the translocator domain of *vtaAs*, while supporting the use of the LS-PCR for determining the putative virulence of *H. parasuis* strains.

Conclusion

As conclusion, this newly described PCR based on the leader sequence of the *vtaA* genes, LS-PCR, is a robust test for the prediction of the virulence potential of *H. parasuis* strains.

Highlights

- Leader sequences of *vtaA* differ depending on the clinical origin of the *H. parasuis* strain
- A robust PCR based on the *vtaA* leader sequence predicts the virulence of *H. parasuis* strains
- This PCR is species-specific and works efficiently at a wide range of annealing temperature

Abbreviations

dNTP: Deoxynucleotide triphosphate; LS: Leader sequence; NV: Non-virulent; PAM: Porcine alveolar macrophage; V: Virulent; VtaA: Virulence-associated trimeric autotransporters

Acknowledgments

This work was supported by grant AGL2013-45662 from the Ministerio de Economía y Competitividad (Mineco) of Spain awarded to VA and the Diagnostic Service of the University of the Montreal. The authors are also grateful to Exopol laboratory from Zaragoza (Spain) and to CERCA Programme/Generalitat de Catalunya.

Funding

This work was supported by grant AGL2013-45662 from the Ministerio de Economía y Competitividad (Mineco) of Spain awarded to VA and the Diagnostic Service of the University of the Montreal.

Authors' contributions

NGM, FCF, SL and SPP performed the experiments and participated in the analysis of data; MG, KSM and AB contributed materials and participated in the analysis and writing of the paper; VA conceived the experiments and analyzed the data; NGM, FCF and VA wrote the paper. All authors revised and approved the final version of the manuscript.

Competing interests

The authors declare that they have no competing interests.

Consent for publication

Not applicable.

Author details

[1]IRTA, Centre de Recerca en Sanitat Animal (CReSA, IRTA-UAB), Campus de la Universitat Autònoma de Barcelona, 08193 Bellaterra, Spain. [2]Faculté de médecine vétérinaire, Université de Montréal, 3200, rue Sicotte, Saint-Hyacinthe, Québec J2S 2M2, Canada. [3]IVD Innovative Veterinary Diagnostics (IVD GmbH), Albert-Einstein-Str. 5, 30926 Seelze, Germany.

References

1. Aragon V, Segales J, Oliveira S. Glässer's disease. In: Zimmerman JJ, Karriker LA, Ramirez A, Schwartz KJ, Stevenson GW, editors. Diseases of swine. 10th ed. Ames: Wiley-Blackwell; 2012. p. 760–9.
2. Cerdà-Cuéllar M, Naranjo JF, Verge A, Nofrarias M, Cortey M, Olvera A, Segales J, Aragon V. Sow vaccination modulates the colonization of piglets by *Haemophilus parasuis*. Vet Microbiol. 2010;145:315–20.
3. Sack M, Baltes N. Identification of novel potential virulence-associated factors in *Haemophilus parasuis*. Vet Microbiol. 2009;136:382–6.
4. Zhou H, Yang B, Xu F, Chen X, Wang J, Blackall PJ, et al. Identification of putative virulence-associated genes of *Haemophilus parasuis* through suppression subtractive hybridization. Vet Microbiol. 2010;144:377–83.
5. Howell KJ, Weinert LA, Chaudhuri RR, Luan SL, Peters SE, Corander J, Harris D, Angen Ø, Aragon V, Bensaid A, et al. The use of genome wide association methods to investigate pathogenicity, population structure and serovar in *Haemophilus parasuis*. BMC Genomics. 2014;15:1179.
6. Pina S, Olvera A, Barcelo A, Bensaid A. Trimeric autotransporters of *Haemophilus parasuis*: generation of an extensive passenger domain repertoire specific for pathogenic strains. J Bacteriol. 2009;191:576–87.

7. Costa-Hurtado M, Ballester M, Galofre-Mila N, Darji A, Aragon V. VtaA8 and VtaA9 from *Haemophilus parasuis* delay phagocytosis by alveolar macrophages. Vet Res. 2012;43:57.
8. Olvera A, Ballester M, Nofrarias M, Sibila M, Aragon V. Differences in phagocytosis susceptibility in *Haemophilus parasuis* strains. Vet Res. 2009;40:24.
9. Olvera A, Pina S, Macedo N, Oliveira S, Aragon V, Bensaid A. Identification of potentially virulent strains of *Haemophilus parasuis* using a multiplex PCR for virulence-associated autotransporters (*vtaA*). Vet J. 2012;191:213–8.
10. Cerdà-Cuéllar M, Aragon V. Serum-resistance in *Haemophilus parasuis* is associated with systemic disease in swine. Vet J. 2008;175:384–9.
11. Yu J, Wu J, Zhang Y, Guo L, Cong X, Du Y, Li J, Sun W, Shi J, Peng J, et al. Concurrent highly pathogenic porcine reproductive and respiratory syndrome virus infection accelerates *Haemophilus parasuis* infection in conventional pigs. Vet Microbiol. 2012;158:316–21.
12. Palzer A, Haedke K, Heinritzi K, Zoels S, Ladinig A, Ritzmann M. Associations among *Haemophilus parasuis*, *Mycoplasma hyorhinis*, and porcine reproductive and respiratory syndrome virus infections in pigs with polyserositis. Can Vet J. 2015;56:285–7.
13. Friendship CRC, Armstrong G, Friendship RM. Management of an outbreak of porcine reproductive and respiratory syndrome (PRRS) in a nursery facility. In: AASV annual meeting; 2011. p. 303–4.

12

European multicenter study on antimicrobial resistance in bacteria isolated from companion animal urinary tract infections

Cátia Marques[1], Luís Telo Gama[1], Adriana Belas[1], Karin Bergström[2], Stéphanie Beurlet[3], Alexandra Briend-Marchal[3], Els M. Broens[4], Marta Costa[5], Delphine Criel[6], Peter Damborg[7], Marloes A. M. van Dijk[4], Astrid M. van Dongen[8], Roswitha Dorsch[9], Carmen Martin Espada[10], Bernhard Gerber[11], Maria Kritsepi-Konstantinou[12], Igor Loncaric[13], Domenico Mion[14], Dusan Misic[15], Rebeca Movilla[16], Gudrun Overesch[17], Vincent Perreten[17], Xavier Roura[16], Joachim Steenbergen[6], Dorina Timofte[18,19,20], Georg Wolf[21], Renato Giulio Zanoni[14], Sarah Schmitt[22], Luca Guardabassi[7,23] and Constança Pomba[1*]

Abstract

Background: There is a growing concern regarding the increase of antimicrobial resistant bacteria in companion animals. Yet, there are no studies comparing the resistance levels of these organisms in European countries. The aim of this study was to investigate geographical and temporal trends of antimicrobial resistant bacteria causing urinary tract infection (UTI) in companion animals in Europe. The antimicrobial susceptibility of 22 256 bacteria isolated from dogs and cats with UTI was determined. Samples were collected between 2008 and 2013 from 16 laboratories of 14 European countries. The prevalence of antimicrobial resistance of the most common bacteria was determined for each country individually in the years 2012–2013 and temporal trends of bacteria resistance were established by logistic regression.

Results: The aetiology of uropathogenic bacteria differed between dogs and cats. For all bacterial species, Southern countries generally presented higher levels of antimicrobial resistance compared to Northern countries. Multidrug-resistant *Escherichia coli* were found to be more prevalent in Southern countries. During the study period, the level of fluoroquinolone-resistant *E. coli* isolated in Belgium, Denmark, France and the Netherlands decreased significantly. A temporal increase in resistance to amoxicillin-clavulanate and gentamicin was observed among *E. coli* isolates from the Netherlands and Switzerland, respectively. Other country-specific temporal increases were observed for fluoroquinolone-resistant *Proteus* spp. isolated from companion animals from Belgium.

Conclusions: This work brings new insights into the current status of antimicrobial resistance in bacteria isolated from companion animals with UTI in Europe and reinforces the need for strategies aiming to reduce resistance.

Keywords: Antimicrobial resistance, Temporal trends, MRSA, MRSP, Dog, Cat

* Correspondence: cpomba@fmv.ulisboa.pt
[1]Faculdade de Medicina Veterinária, Centro de Investigação Interdisciplinar em Sanidade Animal (CIISA), Lisboa, Portugal
Full list of author information is available at the end of the article

Background

Bacterial urinary tract infections (UTI) are frequently diagnosed in dogs and are considered rare in cats [1, 2]. Lately, increased frequencies of UTI in cats have been reported in some European countries [3–5] in particularly when concurrent diseases are present [6].

Escherichia coli is the most frequent isolated bacteria causing UTI in dogs and cats. Several studies show frequencies greater than 30 % [7–9]. Other commonly isolated bacteria genera include *Staphylococcus* spp., *Enterococcus* spp., *Proteus* spp. and *Klebsiella* spp. [7–10].

Previous studies in the United Kingdom and in Missouri-Columbia (USA) analysing the temporal trends of antimicrobial resistance in small collections of bacterial isolates from companion animal infections point to a significant increase in antimicrobial resistance [11, 12]. Furthermore, the emergence of multidrug-resistant bacteria (isolates resistant to three or more antimicrobial categories) in companion animals is an increasing concern [11, 13–15]. This creates new therapeutic challenges in veterinary medicine and is also a public health issue, since these pathogens may be zoonotic [16] and companion animals may play a role in the spread of resistant bacteria due to their close contact to humans [14, 17].

Antimicrobial resistance may vary according to the geographic location [9, 18]. Data on antimicrobial resistance in bacteria isolated from companion animals with UTI in Europe are not easily comparable due to differences in study design, such as variations in host species, inclusion criteria and/or time period. Thus, it is difficult to get a European overview of antimicrobial resistance as seen in human medicine surveillance programmes such as the European Antimicrobial Resistance Surveillance Network [18].

Antimicrobial therapy in UTI should ideally rely on susceptibility testing of the isolated bacteria [19]. Yet, antimicrobials are frequently administered empirically based on the presence of compatible clinical signs, urine cytological findings and in the absence of urine culture and are required to alleviate UTI symptoms while waiting for antimicrobial susceptibility testing results [19]. Besides the pharmacokinetic-pharmacodynamic properties, the empiric antimicrobial selection should consider the most likely causative agent as well as its regional susceptibility patterns [8]. Moreover, according to the World Organisation for Animal Health [20], veterinarians should adopt strategies aimed at the reduction of antimicrobial resistance. Therefore, current information on the aetiology and antimicrobial resistance focused on UTI is of crucial importance.

Under the umbrella of the European Society of Veterinary Nephrology and Urology, a multicenter retrospective study was launched in November 2013 with the goal of getting antimicrobial resistance data on bacteria isolated from companion animal with UTI across Europe. A Urinary Tract Infection Resistance – Veterinary Network (UTIR-VNet) was constituted with this purpose in mind. Partial results were presented at the annual Society meeting included in the 25th congress of the European College of Veterinary Internal Medicine, 4–6 September 2014, Mainz, Germany. The aim of this study was to determine the frequency of uropathogens in dogs and cats with urinary tract infection in Europe and to characterise the frequency and temporal trends of antimicrobial resistance over a period of six years. We hereby present a complete report and discussion of this study.

Methods

Participating countries

Between January and September 2014, 16 veterinary microbiology laboratories from 14 European countries (Austria, Belgium, Denmark, France, Germany, Greece, Italy, the Netherlands, Portugal, Serbia, Spain, Sweden, Switzerland, United Kingdom), were invited to participate in this study (Fig. 1). Laboratories were requested to send available retrospective data on animal species, age and gender, bacterial identification and antimicrobial susceptibility testing conducted in bacteria obtained from dogs and cats with UTI between 2008 and 2013. Samples were obtained with owners consent as part of the routine care of canine and feline UTI.

Bacterial Isolates

The bacteria identification varied between laboratories. Most laboratories used standard phenotypic tests, including API, while others used techniques such as PCR and MALDI-TOF. This discrepancy was particularly evident for staphylococci, which were classified to either the species or genus level depending on the laboratory.

Susceptibility testing

The following antimicrobials were included: amoxicillin-clavulanate (AMC), ampicillin (AMP), cefotaxime (CTX), cefovecin (CVN), cefoxitin (FOX), ceftazidime (CAZ), cefpodoxime (CPD), ceftiofur (EFT), ciprofloxacin (CIP), enrofloxacin (ENR), gentamicin (CN), marbofloxacin (MAR), oxacillin (OX), penicillin (P) and trimethoprim/sulfamethoxazole (SXT).

The retrospective nature of the study forced us to include two in vitro antimicrobial susceptibility testing methods. Laboratories from Austria, France, Germany, Greece, Italy, the Netherlands, Portugal, Serbia, Spain, United Kingdom, used standard disc diffusion method according to Clinical Laboratory Standards Institute (CLSI) guidelines [21], whereas Sweden (VetMIC, SVA, Uppsala, Sweeden), Denmark and United Kingdom (COMPAN1F Sensititre panels, Thermo Fisher), Switzerland and

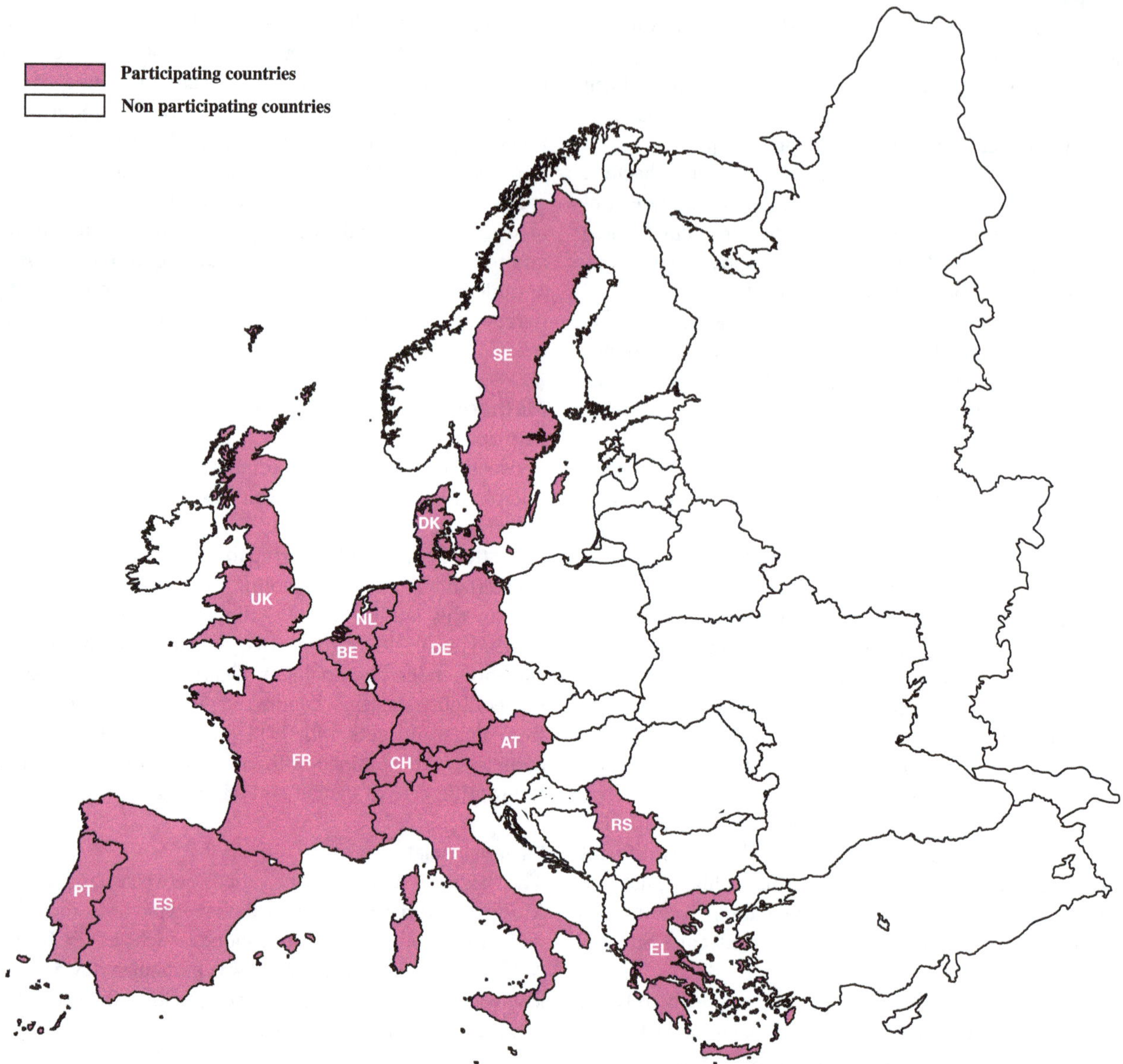

Fig. 1 Participating countries in the Urinary tract infection antimicrobial resistance veterinary network – UTIR-VNet. Countries: AT- Austria; BE- Belgium; DK- Denmark; FR- France; DE- Germany; EL- Greece; IT- Italy; NL- the Netherlands; PT- Portugal; RS- Serbia; ES- Spain; SE- Sweden; CH- Switzerland; UK- United Kingdom

Belgium (VITEK 2, BioMérieux) used broth microdilution method.

Human CLSI breakpoints [22] were used for interpretation of minimal inhibitory concentration and disk diffusion results for CAZ (30 μg), CTX (30 μg), and CIP (5 μg), whereas veterinary CLSI breakpoints [23] were used for AMC (30 μg), AMP (30 μg), CN (10 μg), CPD (10 μg), ENR (5 μg), FOX (30 μg), MAR (5 μg), OX (1 μg), P (10U), and SXT (25 μg). Clinical breakpoints from the Societé Française de Microbiology [24] were used for EFT (30 μg). Results for CVN (30 μg) were interpreted according to the manufacturer guidelines. As seen in the human European Antimicrobial Resistance Surveillance Network (EARS-Net) report [18], when data on minimal inhibitory concentrations or inhibition zone diameter were not available, the laboratories' own interpretations (susceptible, intermediate and resistant) were accepted. This was the case for Spain, Serbia, and Germany that used contemporary CLSI guidelines, for the United Kingdom that used the breakpoints from the British Society of Antimicrobial Chemotherapy [25] and for the Netherlands and Switzerland (2008–2010) that used breakpoints recommended by the Dutch Committee on Guidelines for Susceptibility testing [26].

Data analysis and statistical methods

Statistical analysis was performed using the SAS statistical software package for Windows, version 9.3, (SAS Institute Inc, Cary, North Carolina, USA).

The Fisher exact test was used to compare pathogen frequencies by species or gender of the host, by simple/multiple infection and by country. An alpha value of 0.05 was used.

Isolates were considered fully resistant when found to be resistant according to the clinical breakpoint applied. An isolate was considered susceptible when found to be susceptible or intermediate according to the clinical breakpoint applied. The antimicrobials included in this study are known to be highly concentrated in the urine so their report as susceptible may be appropriated for isolates categorized as intermediate [19].

Regarding third generation cephalosporins (3GC), laboratories tested different 3GC resistance surrogates. Therefore, to evaluate the antimicrobial resistance to 3GC, an isolate was considered as 3GC resistant when it was resistant to at least one of the five 3GC tested (CTX, CAZ, CVN, EFT or CPD). The same rational was applied to evaluate resistance to fluoroquinolones (FLU), namely using ENR, CIP or MAR as a marker of resistance. Methicillin-resistance in staphylococci was determined according to CLSI guidelines [23] using cefoxitin or oxacillin to evaluate resistance depending on the bacterial species considered. Yet, Germany and Spain did not send data on methicillin-resistance. France did not test staphylococci against oxacillin and thus did not report methicillin-resistance regarding *Staphylococcus pseudintermedius* (MRSP). The Netherlands did not have data on staphylococci susceptibility to OX or FOX but instead reported data on the detection of the *mec*A gene by PCR. The frequency of methicillin-resistance did not include staphylococci only identified to the genus level.

Enterobacteriaceae were considered multidrug-resistant (MDR) when fully resistant to three or more categories of antimicrobials, namely AMC, 3GC, SXT, CN and/or FLU. Unlike the MDR definition proposed by other authors [27], intermediate isolates from this study were considered as susceptible. This difference was applied because we are considering drugs that can be highly concentrated in urine. Furthermore, this approach will reduce any overestimation of MDR frequency due to the use of different breakpoint guidelines. Full-susceptibility (FullS) was defined as an isolate being susceptible for all the above-mentioned categories of antimicrobials. Since Belgium had no data available on 3GC and the Netherlands had little data on CN, MDR and FullS percentages do not include resistance to 3GC for Belgium and resistance to CN for the Netherlands.

As a rule, statistical analysis was only done when at least ten isolates for a specific organism-antimicrobial agent combination were reported for a given country. All frequencies are presented with a confidence interval of 95 % (95 % CI).

Maps of European resistance distribution were drawn considering the percentage of fully resistant isolates to the considered antimicrobial agent, over the years 2012–2013. A scale of colours was applied composed of six resistance intervals after the example of EARS-Net surveillance program reports [18].

Statistical analysis of temporal trends of antimicrobial resistance for a specific organism-antimicrobial agent combination were determined within each country. Temporal trends were only determined for countries reporting data on at least three consecutive years and ten isolates per year. A SAS LOGISTIC regression, with the year as a continuous variable and an alpha value of 0.05 was conducted. Temporal trends of resistance were mainly determined for *E. coli* since this was the most represented bacterial species. Yet, temporal trends of AMC, FLU and SXT in *Proteus* spp. were also determined for Belgium, France, the Netherlands and Sweden.

Results

Overall, data on 22,256 uropathogenic bacteria were obtained from 15,097 dog and 5963 cat positive urine cultures. Table 1 summarises the numbers of bacterial isolates obtained by year and country.

Considering the records containing information about the age, dogs ($n = 4425$) and cats ($n = 1514$) had similar

Table 1 Total number of isolated bacteria by year and country

Country[a]	Year						
	2008	2009	2010	2011	2012	2013	Total
AT	-	-	-	-	144	185	329
BE	-	-	547	578	623	739	2487
DK	29	30	53	116	153	205	587
FR	-	-	620	733	780	995	3128
DE	-	64	93	140	161	146	604
EL	24	29	13	11	32	43	152
IT	-	36	29	36	77	65	243
NL	480	867	958	1132	1195	1307	5939
PT	77	54	57	34	32	45	299
RS	17	19	10	2	3	3	54
ES	14	23	27	40	47	79	230
SE	730	924	1071	1202	1355	1647	6929
CH	109	120	112	125	114	174	754
UK	31	44	81	117	126	122	521
Total	1511	2210	3671	4267	4842	5755	22256

[a]AT, Austria; BE, Belgium; DK, Denmark; FR, France; DE, Germany; EL, Greece; IT, Italy; NL, the Netherlands; PT, Portugal; RS, Serbia; ES, Spain; SE, Sweden; CH, Switzerland; UK, United Kingdom

mean ages, namely 8.77 years (SD ± 4.04, 9.00 median, 6.00 IQR, range 0.1–20) and 8.82 years (SD ± 5.03, 8.50 median, 8.1 IQR, range 0.2–22) respectively. Gender was only specified in 3885 records where 61.41 % (95 % CI 59.69–63.12 %, $n = 1900/3094$) of dogs and 48.29 % (95 % CI 44.81–51.78 %, $n = 382/791$) of cats were females.

Among all urine cultures, 94.64 % (95 % CI 94.33–94.94 %, $n = 19932/21060$) resulted in the growth of bacterial pure cultures, with no significant difference between cats and dogs ($P = 0.1856$). Both in dogs and cats, *E. coli* was the most frequently identified bacteria and accounted for 59.45 % (95 % CI 58.80–60.09 %, $n = 13231/22256$) of all isolates. The frequency of the remaining bacterial species differed significantly between dogs and cats (Table 2). *Enterococcus* spp. and *Staphylococcus* spp. frequencies were higher in cats, whereas *Proteus* spp. and *Klebsiella* spp. were more prevalent in dogs.

Considering the years 2012–2013, the major differences in *E. coli* (Table 3, Fig. 2) and *Proteus* spp. (Table 4, Fig. 3) antimicrobial resistance frequencies were seen between Northern (Denmark and Sweden) and Southern (Italy, Greece, Portugal and Spain) countries.

The lowest frequencies of AMC resistance in *E. coli* were detected in isolates from Denmark (2.88 %) and Belgium (4.29 %). *E. coli* from Portugal (48.15 %) had a significantly higher AMC resistance frequency ($P < 0.05$) when compared with all countries except for Spain, Italy and Greece (Table 3). Less than 15 % of *Proteus* spp. were resistant to AMC in all countries with exception of Portugal (50 %) and Spain (26.67 %) (Table 4).

E. coli resistance to 3GC had a similar distribution to what was seen for AMC (Fig. 2). The highest 3GC resistance frequencies were found in Southern countries, namely Portugal (31.25 %), Italy (24.64 %) and Spain (21.15 %) (Table 3). *Proteus* spp. 3GC resistance was lower than 5 % in Austria, Denmark, Sweden, Switzerland, United Kingdom and the Netherlands, whereas Portugal (33.33 %) and Spain (15.38 %) were the countries with the highest resistance levels (Table 4).

SXT resistance in Southern countries was higher than 25 and 45 % for *E. coli* and *Proteus* spp., respectively (Tables 3 and 4; Figs. 2 and 3). Sweden and Denmark had the lowest SXT resistance values (lower than 9 %). The remaining included countries had frequencies ranging between 10.21-21.13 % and 20–37.93 % in *E. coli* and *Proteus* spp., respectively (Tables 3 and 4).

E. coli FLU resistance was higher in the Southern countries and ranged from 29.03 % in Portugal to 31.88 % in Italy (Table 3). Concerning *Proteus* spp., Spain and Germany had around 50 % FLU resistance, followed by Italy and Portugal with around 40 % (Table 4). Sweden, Denmark, Belgium and the Netherlands had less than 10 % FLU resistant *E. coli*. Denmark, Sweden, United Kingdom and the Netherlands had less than 10 % FLU resistant *Proteus* spp. (Figs. 2 and 3).

Table 2 Uropathogenic bacteria aetiology, single versus mixed infections and cat versus dog as host species

Organism	Overall		Single organism		Mixed infections			Dogs		Cats		
	n	% (95 % CI)[a]	*n*	% (95 % CI)[a]	*n*	% (95 % CI)[a]	*P*	*n*	% (95 % CI)[a]	*n*	% (95 % CI)[a]	*P*
Enterobacter spp.	308	1.38 (1.23–1.54)	244	1.22 (1.07–1.38)	64	2.75 (2.09–3.42)	**<0.0001**	194	1.21 (1.04–1.38)	114	1.81 (1.48–2.14)	**0.0008**
Enterococcus spp.	1506	6.77 (6.44–7.10)	1129	5.66 (5.34–5.99)	377	16.22 (14.72–17.72)	**<0.0001**	745	4.66 (4.34–4.99)	761	12.11 (11.31–12.92)	**<0.0001**
Escherichia coli	13231	59.45 (58.80–60.09)	12417	62.30 (61.62–62.97)	814	35.03 (33.09-36-97)	**<0.0001**	9506	59.51 (58.75–60.27)	3725	59.30 (58.08–60.51)	0.7832
Klebsiella spp.	478	2.15 (1.96–2.34)	400	2.01 (1.81–2.20)	78	3.36 (2.62–4.09)	**<0.0001**	385	2.41 (2.17–2.65)	93	1.48 (1.18–1.78)	**<0.0001**
Proteus spp.	1992	8.95 (8.58–9.33)	1770	8.88 (8.49–9.28)	222	9.55 (8.36–10.75)	0.2824	1869	11.70 (1.20–1.22)	123	1.96 (1.62–2.30)	**<0.0001**
Pseudomonas spp.	389	1.75 (1.58–1.92)	315	1.58 (1.41–1.75)	74	3.18 (2.47–3.90)	**<0.0001**	293	1.83 (1.63–2.04)	96	1.53 (1.22–1.83)	0.1249
Staphylococcus spp.	2893	13.00 (12.56–13.44)	2519	12.64 (12.18–13.10)	374	16.09 (14.60–17.59)	**<0.0001**	1836	11.49 (11.00–11.99)	1057	16.83 (15.90–17.75)	**<0.0001**
Streptococcus spp.	802	3.60 (3.36–3.85)	586	2.94 (2.71–3.17)	216	9.29 (8.11–10.47)	**<0.0001**	675	4.23 (3.91–4.54)	127	2.02 (1.67–2.37)	**<0.0001**
Other	657	2.95 (2.73–3.17)	552	2.77 (2.54–3.00)	105	4.52 (3.67–5.36)	-	471	2.95 (2.69–3.21)	186	2.96 (2.54–3.38)	-

[a]95 % CI, 95 % Confidence interval
n - Total number of isolates
P- P value obtained by Fisher exact test when comparing single versus mixed infections and cat versus dog as host. Statistically significant values are highlighted in bold

Table 3 Percentage of resistance in *Escherichia coli* by antimicrobial and country in 2012–2013

Country[a]	AMC		3GC		FLU		CN		SXT		Combined resistance		
	n	% R (95 % CI)[b] [Stat. Dif.][c]	*n*	% R (95 % CI)[b] [Stat. Dif.][c]	*n*	% R (95 % CI)[b] [Stat. Dif.][c]	*n*	% R (95 % CI)[b] [Stat. Dif.][c]	*n*	% R (95 % CI)[b] [Stat. Dif.][c]	*n*	% MDR (95 % CI)[b] [Stat. Dif.][c]	% FullS (95 % CI)[b] [Stat. Dif.][c]
AT	142	14.08 (8.36–19.81) [a,b]	142	5.63 (1.84–9.43) [a, b]	142	11.97 (6.63–17.31) [a]	142	5.63 (1.84–9.43) [a, b]	142	14.08 (8.36–19.81) [a, b]	142	8.45 (3.88–13.03) [a]	78.87 (72.16–85.59) [a]
BE	840	4.29 (2.92–5.66) [c]	0	- -	769	6.63 (4.87–8.39) [b]	840	1.67 (0.80–2.53) [c]	839	10.37 (8.31–12.43) [a]	769[d]	1.43[d] (0.59–2.27) -	85.05[d] (82.52–87.57) -
DK	206	2.88 (0.61–5.16) [c]	208	4.33 (1.41–7.09) [a, c]	208	2.88 (0.61–5.16) [c]	208	1.92 (0.06–3.79) [a, c]	208	8.17 (4.45–11.90) [a, c]	208	2.88 (0.61–5.16) [b]	88.94 (84.68–93.20) [b, c]
FR	954	12.79 (10.67–15.91) [a, d]	933	10.83 (8.83–12.82) [b]	948	12.76 (10.64–14.89) [a]	951	3.36 (2.22–4.51) [a, d]	959	16.27 (13.93–18.60) [b, d]	909	11.00 (8.97–13.04) [a, c]	77.23 (74.50–79.95) [a]
DE	153	11.76 (6.66–16.87) [a, d]	152	11.84 (6.71–16.98) [b, d]	153	16.34 (10.48–22.20) [a, d]	153	1.96 (0.00–4.16) [a, c, d]	153	17.65 (11.61–23.69) [b, d, e]	152	8.55 (4.11–13.00) [a]	67.76 (60.33–75.19) [d]
EL	31	25.81 (10.40–41.21) [b, d, e, f]	9	7R/2S -	30	30.00 (13.60–46.40) [d, e]	0	- -	26	34.62 (16.33–52.90) [e, f]	0	- -	- -
IT	69	26.09 (15.73–36.45) [e, f]	69	24.64 (14.47–34.80) [e]	69	31.88 (20.89–42.88) [e]	69	14.49 (6.19–22.80) [e]	69	28.99 (18.28–39.69) [e, f]	69	28.99 (18.28–39.69) [d]	63.77 (52.43–75.11) [d, e, f]
NL	1461	10.81 (9.22–12.41) [a]	1380	3.77 (2.76–4.77) [a, c]	1457	4.94 (3.83–6.05) [b, c]	81	3.70 (0.00–7.82) [a, c, f]	1459	10.21 (8.66–11.77) [a]	1380[d]	2.25[d] (1.46–3.03) -	81.30[d] (79.25-83.36) -
PT	27	48.15 (29.30-66.99) [e]	32	31.25 (15.19-47.31) [e]	31	29.03 (13.05-45.01) [d, e]	30	10.00 (0.00-20.74) [b, d, e, f]	31	32.26 (15.80-48.71) [e, f]	25	24.00 (7.26-40.74) [c, d, e]	32.00 (13.71–50.29) [g, h]
RS	3	2R/1S -	2	1R/1S -	3	0R/3S -	3	0R/3S -	3	1R/2S -	2	1MDR -	1Full-S -
ES	60	31.67 (19.90–43.44) [e, f]	52	21.15 (10.05–32.25) [d, e]	61	29.51 (18.06–40.95) [e]	46	15.22 (4.84–25.60) [b, e]	60	26.67 (15.48–37.86) [e, f]	37	29.73 (15.00–44.46) [d, e]	43.24 (27.28–59.21) [e, g]
SE	2091	6.98 (5.89–8.07) [g]	2082	0 [f]	2091	1.05 (0.61–1.49) [f]	2091	0.19 (0.00–0.38) [g]	2091	4.97 (4.04–5.91) [c]	2082	0.24 (0.03–0.45) [f]	90.2 (88.92–91.48) [b, h]
CH	133	10.53 (5.31–15.74) [a, g]	133	8.27 (3.59–12.95) [b, c]	132	13.64 (7.78–19.49) [a, d]	132	6.82 (2.52–11.12) [b, d, e, f]	131	13.74 (7.85–19.64) [a, d, g]	130	10.00 (4.84–15.16) [a, e]	83.08 (76.63–89.52) [a, c]
UK	143	21.68 (14.92–28.43) [b, f]	143	20.98 (14.31–27.65) [d, e]	143	11.89 (6.58–17.19) [a]	92	6.52 (1.48–11.57) [a, e, f]	142	21.13 (14.41–27.84) [b, f, g]	89	15.56 (8.07–23.04) [a, e]	67.78 (58.12–77.43) [a, d, f]

AMC amoxicillin clavulanate, *3GC* third generation cephalosporins, *FLU* fluoroquinolones, *CN* gentamicin, *SXT* trimethoprim/sulfamethoxazole, *MDR* multidrug-resistant, *Full-S* fully-susceptible

[a]Countries: AT, Austria; BE, Belgium; DK, Denmark; FR, France; DE, Germany; EL, Greece; IT, Italy; NL, the Netherlands; PT, Portugal; RS, Serbia; ES, Spain; SE, Sweden; CH, Switzerland; UK, United Kingdom.

[b]95 % CI, 95 % Confidence interval

[c]Stat. Dif., Statistical significant differences. Countries with no statistical difference are marked with the same letter. Countries were compared by Fisher exact test with an alpha value of 0.05. Countries with less than ten tested isolates were not compared. Regarding MDR and FullS, only countries tested for all the considered antimicrobials were compared

n, Total number of *Escherichia coli* tested for the considered antimicrobial category

[d]MDR and FullS percentages do not include resistance to 3GC for Belgium and resistance to CN for the Netherlands

Overall, *E. coli* CN resistance was lower than 16 % (Table 3). Regarding resistance to CN in *Proteus* spp. the same resistance frequency occurred with the exception of Portugal where a higher resistance frequency was recorded (33.33 %) (Table 4).

E. coli from Portugal, Spain and Italy, and *Proteus* spp. from Portugal showed the highest frequencies of MDR (Tables 3 and 4). As expected, Portugal was one of the countries with lowest FullS, both in *E. coli* (32.00 %) and *Proteus* spp. (35.71 %). Italy had even lower FullS in

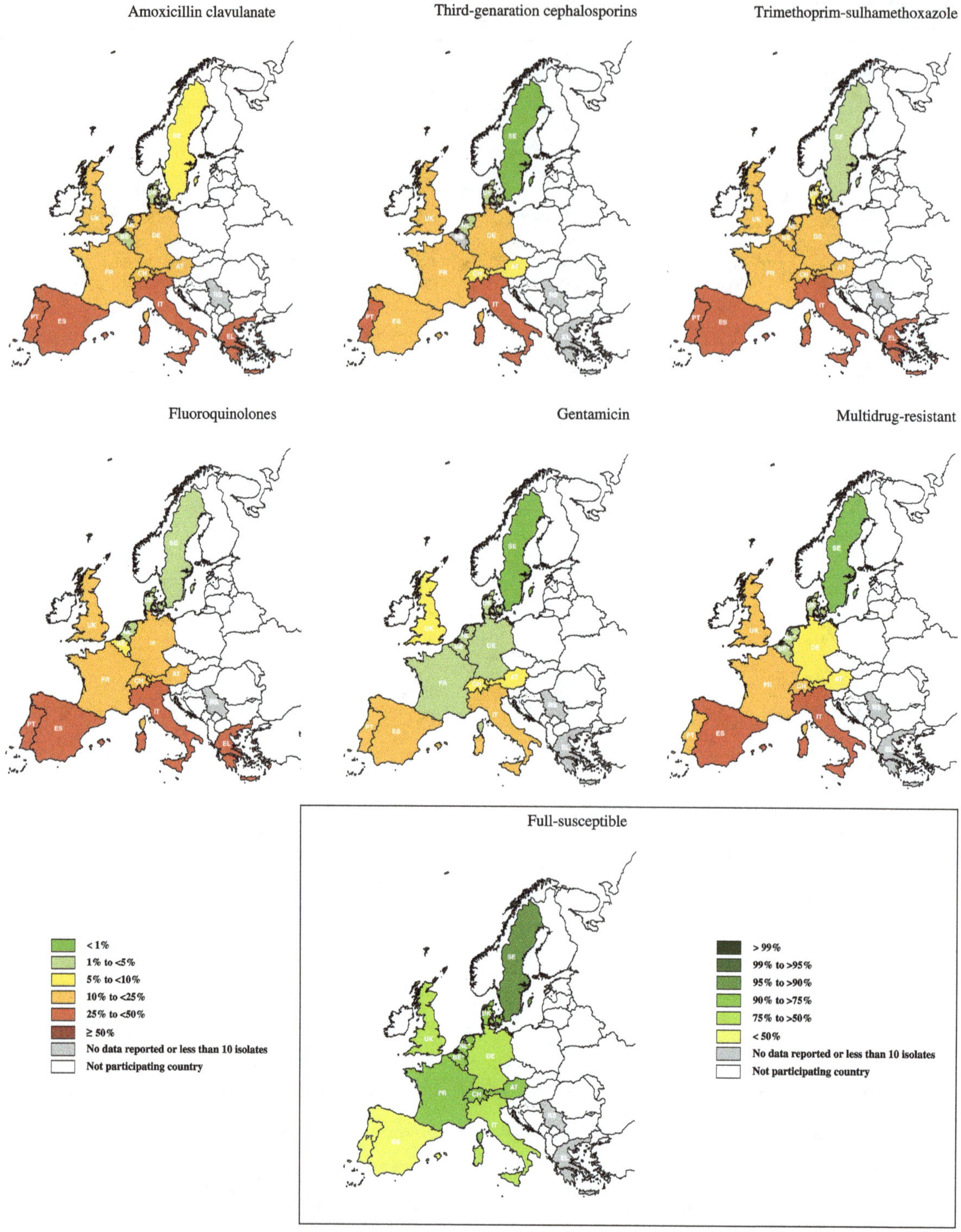

Fig. 2 Percentage (%) of *Escherichia coli* antimicrobial resistance by antimicrobial and country in the years 2012–2013. Countries: AT- Austria; BE- Belgium; DK- Denmark; FR- France; DE- Germany; EL- Greece; IT- Italy; NL- the Netherlands; PT- Portugal; RS- Serbia; ES- Spain; SE- Sweden; CH- Switzerland; UK- United Kingdom. Multidrug-resistance considering combined resistance to three or more of the following antimicrobial categories: AMC, 3GC, FLU, CN and SXT. Full-susceptibility (FullS) was defined as an isolate being susceptible for all the above-mentioned categories of antimicrobials. Regarding multidrug-resistance and full-susceptibility frequencies, countries marked by asterisk: 3GC was not included for Belgium and CN for the Netherlands. Thus, these frequencies may be underestimated when compared with the remaining countries

Table 4 Percentage of resistance in *Proteus* spp. by antimicrobial and country in 2012-2013

Country[a]	AMC		3GC		FLU		CN		SXT		Combined resistance		
	n	% R (95 % CI)[b] [Stat. Dif.][c]	*n*	% R (95 % CI)[b] [Stat. Dif.][c]	*n*	% R (95 % CI)[b] [Stat. Dif.][c]	*n*	% R (95 % CI)[b] [Stat. Dif.][c]	*n*	% R (95 % CI)[b] [Stat. Dif.][c]	*n*	% MDR (95 % CI)[b] [Stat. Dif.][c]	% FullS (95 % CI)[b] [Stat. Dif.][c]
AT	29	10.34 (0.00–21.43) [a, b, c]	29	0 [a, b]	29	17.24 (3.49–30.99) [a, b, c]	29	6.90 (0.00–16.12) [a, b]	29	37.93 (20.27–55.59) [a, b]	29	6.90 (0.00–16.12) [a]	55.17 (37.07–73.27) [a, b]
BE	143	2.10 (0.00–4.45) [a, g]	0	- -	135	28.15 (20.56–35.73) [a, d]	155	9.68 (5.02–14.33) [a]	154	35.06 (27.53–42.60) [a, b]	125[d]	4.80[d] (1.05-8.55) -	57.60[d] (48.94–66.26) -
DK	31	0 [a, d]	31	0 [a, b]	31	0 [e, f]	31	0 [a, b]	31	6.45 (0.00–15.10) [c]	31	0 [a, b]	93.55 (44.41–84.90) [c]
FR	215	7.44 (3.93–10.95) [b, d]	211	6.64 (3.28-9.99) [a]	212	17,92 (12.76-23.09) [b, g]	214	9.81 (5.83-13.80) [a]	216	27.78 (21.80-33.75) [a]	204	10.29 (6.12-14.46) [a]	66.67 (60.20-73.14) [a]
DE	10	0 [a, b, f]	10	10.00 (0.00–28.59) [a, b, c]	10	50.00 (19.01–80.99) [a, d]	10	0 [a, b, c]	10	20.00 (0.00–44.79) [a, c, d]	10	0 [a, b]	50.00 (19.01–80.99) [a, d]
EL	8	1R/7S -	0	- -	8	4R/4S -	0	- -	7	4R/3R -	0	- -	- -
IT	12	0 [a, b, c]	12	8.33 (0.00–23.97) [a, b, c]	12	41.67 (13.77–69.56) [a, d, g]	12	8.33 (0.00–23.97) [a, b, c]	12	66.67 (39.99–93.34) [b, e]	12	8.33 (0.00–23.97) [a, b, c]	16.67 (0.00–37.75) [d]
NL	261	6.13 (3.22–9.04) [a, b, e]	244	2.87 (0.77–4.96) [a]	260	8.85 (5.39–12.30) [c, e, h]	17	11.76 (0.00–27.08) [a, c]	260	27.31 (21.89–32.72) [a]	243[d]	3.29[d] (1.05–5.54) -	69.96[d] (64.19–75.72) -
PT	14	50.00 (23.81–76.19) [e]	15	33.33 (9.48–57.19) [c, d]	15	40.00 (15.21–64.79) [a, g, i]	15	33.33 (9.48–57.19) [c]	15	46.67 (21.42–71.91) [a, e]	14	42.86 (16.93–68.78) [c]	35.71 (10.61–60.81) [b, d, e]
RS	1	0R/1S -	1	1R/0S -	1	0R/1S -	1	0R/1S -	0	- -	0	- -	- -
ES	15	26.67 (4.29–49.05) [c, e, f]	13	15.38 (0.00–35.00) [a, d]	15	53.33 (28.09–78.58) [d, i]	9	2R/7S -	15	53.33 (28.09–78.58) [b, d, e]	7	2MDR -	4Full-S -
SE	170	2.35 (0.07–4.63) [a, f, g]	169	0 [b, e]	170	0.59 (0.00–1.74) [f]	170	0.59 (0.00–1.74) [b]	170	7.06 (3.21–10.91) [c]	169	0 [b]	91.12 (86.84–95.41) [c]
CH	17	0 [a, b, f]	17	0 [a, e]	17	23.53 (3.37–43.69) [a, g, h, I, j]	17	5.88 (0.00–17.07) [a, b, c]	17	35.29 (12.58–58.01) [a, e]	17	0 [a, b]	64.71 (41.99–87.42) [a, e]
UK	16	12.50 (0.00–28.70) [a, b, f]	16	0 [a, e]	16	0 [b, e, f, j]	11	0 [a, b, c]	15	33.33 (9.48–57.19) [a, e]	10	0 [a, b]	70.00 (41.60–98.40) [a, c, e]

AMC amoxicillin clavulanate, *3GC* third generation cephalosporins, *FLU* fluoroquinolones, *CN* gentamicin, *SXT* trimethoprim/sulfamethoxazole, *MDR* multidrug-resistant, *FullS* fully-susceptible

[a]Countries: AT, Austria; BE, Belgium; DK, Denmark; FR, France; DE, Germany; EL, Greece; IT, Italy; NL, the Netherlands; PT, Portugal; RS, Serbia; ES, Spain; SE, Sweden; CH, Switzerland; UK, United Kingdom.

[b]95 % CI, 95 % Confidence interval.

[c]Stat. Dif., Statistical significant differences. Countries with no statistical difference are marked with the same letter. Countries were compared by Fisher exact test with an alpha value of 0.05. Countries with less than ten tested isolates were not compared. Regarding MDR and FullS, only countries tested for all the considered antimicrobials were compared

n, Total number of *Proteus* spp. tested for the considered antimicrobial category

[d]MDR and FullS percentages do not include resistance to 3GC for Belgium and resistance to CN for the Netherlands

Proteus spp. (16.67 %). Most of the remaining countries had MDR levels lower than 10 %, with the exception of MDR *E. coli* from United Kingdom (15.56 %) and France (11 %). The highest *E. coli* and *Proteus* spp. FullS frequencies were found in Denmark and Sweden (Tables 3 and 4).

Due to the limited number of *Staphylococcus* spp. isolates available, the percentage of resistance to antimicrobials was determined on fewer countries for this group of bacteria (Tables 5 and 6). In most countries, *Staphylococcus pseudintermedius* was the most frequently

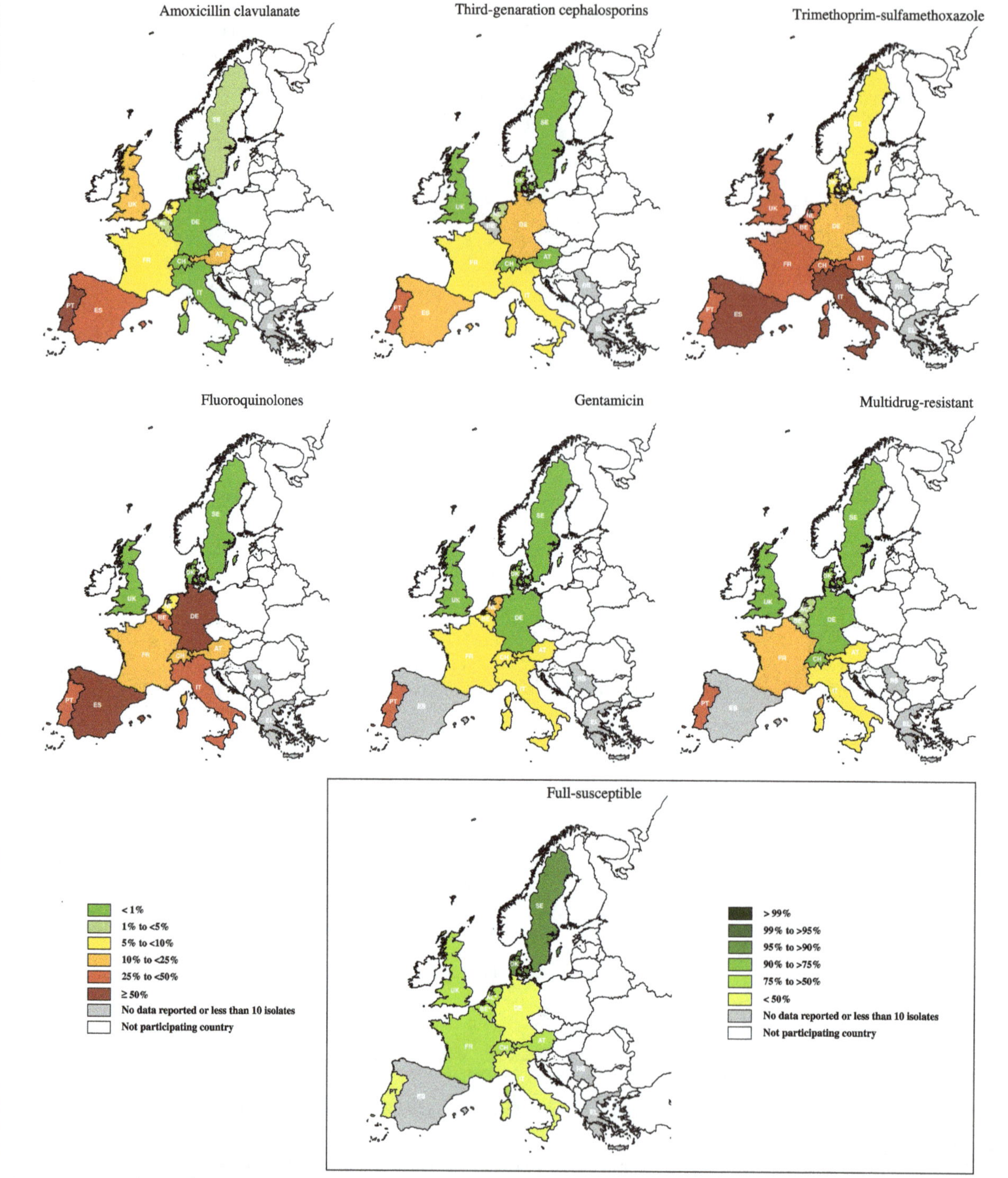

Fig. 3 Percentage (%) of *Proteus* spp. antimicrobial resistance by antimicrobial and country in the years 2012–2013. Countries: AT- Austria; BE- Belgium; DK- Denmark; FR- France; DE- Germany; EL- Greece; IT- Italy; NL- the Netherlands; PT- Portugal; RS- Serbia; ES- Spain; SE- Sweden; CH- Switzerland; UK- United Kingdom. Multidrug resistance considering combined resistance to three or more of the following antimicrobial categories: AMC, 3GC, FLU, CN and SXT. Full-susceptibility was defined as an isolate being susceptible for all the above-mentioned categories of antimicrobials. Regarding multidrug-resistance and full-susceptibility frequencies, countries marked by asterisk: 3GC was not included for Belgium and CN for the Netherlands. Thus, these frequencies may be underestimated when compared with the remaining countries

Table 5 *Staphylococcus* spp. and methicillin-resistance by country in 2012–2013

Country[a]	N	Staphylococci species by country					Methicillin-resistance within each group					
		SA	SP	CoPS	CoNS	SPP	MRSA		MRSP		MRCoNS	
		% (95 % CI)[b]	% (95 % CI)[b]	% (95 % CI)[b]	% (95 % CI)[b]	% (95 % CI)[b]	*n* tested	R % (95 % CI)[b]	*n* tested	R % (95 % CI)[b]	*n* tested	R % (95 % CI)[b]
AT	78	7.69 (1.78–13.61)	19.23 (10.48–27.98)	6.41 (0.97–11.85)	56.41 (45.41–67.41)	10.26 (3.52–16.99)	5	1R/4S -	15	33.33 (9.48–57.19)	43	27.91 (14.50–41.31)
BE	122	14.75 (8.46–21.05)	52.46 (43.60–61.32)	0 -	32.79 (24.46–41.12)	0 -	18	5.56 (0–16.14)	64	12.50 (4.40–20.60)	40	25.0 (11.58–38.42)
DK	52	1.92 (0–5.66)	53.85 (40.30–67.40)	1.92 (0–5.66)	28.85 (16.53–41.16)	13.46 (4.18–22.74)	1	1S -	27	0 -	15	46.67 (21.42–71.91)
FR	242	8.26 (4.80–11.73)	72.73 (67.12–78.34)	0 -	19.01 (14.06–23.95)	0 -	20	40.0 (18.53–61.47)	0	- -	46	17.39 (6.44–28.34)
DE	64	4.69 (0–9.87)	50.0 (37.75–62.25)	0 -	39.06 (27.11–51.02)	6.25 (0.32–12.18)	0	- -	0	- -	0	- -
EL	10	0 -	10.0 (0–28.59)	0 -	0 -	90 (71.41–100)	-	- -	1	1R -	-	- -
IT	19	0 -	94.74 (84.70–100)	0 -	5.26 (0–15.30)	0 -	-	- -	18	50.0 (26.90–73.10)	0	- -
NL	365	4.93 (1.12–2.71)	47.95 (42.82–53.07)	0 -	47.12 (42.0–52.24)	0 -	0	- -	174	10.92 (6.29–15.55)	172	0.58 (0–1.72)
PT	7	1SA -	4SP -	0CoPS -	0CoNS -	2SPP -	1	1R -	4	2R/2S -	0	- -
RS	0	- -	- -	- -	- -	- -	-	- -	-	- -	-	- -
ES	13	0 -	0 -	15.38 (0–35.0)	46.15 (19.05–73.25)	38.46 (12.02–64.91)	-	- -	-	- -	0	- -
SE	325	8.62 (5.56–11.67)	53.54 (48.12–58.96)	2.46 (0.78–4.15)	32.31 (27.22–37.39)	3.08 (1.20–4.95)	28	0 -	174	1.15 (0–2.73)	105	4.76 (0.69–8.84)
CH	46	4.35 (0–10.24)	52.17 (37.74–66.61)	4.35 (0–10.24)	34.78 (21.02–48.55)	4.35 (0–10.24)	2	0R/2S -	20	10.00 (0–23.15)	15	66.67 (42.81–90.52)
UK	32	12.50 (1.04–23.96)	53.13 (35.84–70.41)	6.25 (0–14.64)	18.75 (5.23–32.27)	9.38 (0–19.47)	3	1R/2S -	12	8.33 (0–23.97)	3	1R/2S -

Staphylococci identification varied according to the country. Some countries identified staphylococci to species level, others to genus level and others included data on the coagulase test. Thus, the staphylococci results were grouped as follows: 1. *Staphylococcus aureus* (SA); 2. *Staphylococcus pseudintermedius* (SP); 3. coagulase positive staphylococci (CoPS), 4. coagulase negative staphylococci (CoNS) and 5. other staphylococci (SPP). Group 2 includes staphylococci identified only as CoPS or staphylococci species known to be coagulase positive other than SA and SP. Group 3 includes staphylococci identified only as CoNS or staphylococci species known to be coagulase negative. Group 4 includes staphylococci identified as *Staphylococcus* spp

MRSA methicillin-resistant *Staphylococcus aureus, MRSP* methicillin-resistant *Staphylococcus pseudintermedius, MRCoNS* methicillin-resistant coagulase negative staphylococci

[a]Countries: AT, Austria; BE, Belgium; DK, Denmark; FR, France; DE, Germany; EL, Greece; IT, Italy; NL, the Netherlands; PT, Portugal; RS, Serbia; ES, Spain; SE, Sweden; CH, Switzerland; UK, United Kingdom

[b]95 % CI, 95 % Confidence interval

N, Total number of staphylococci

n tested, number of staphylococci tested for methicillin-resistance within each group

isolated followed by coagulase negative staphylococci (CoNS) (Table 5). In general, the overall antimicrobial resistance levels in Southern countries were higher than in Northern countries (Fig. 4) as seen in Gram-negative bacteria (Figs. 2 and 3).

Besides the limited number of staphylococci, methicillin-resistance results were also limited due to the identification only to genus level or lack of testing the appropriate antimicrobial surrogate. Denmark and Sweden showed the lowest *S. pseudintermedius* methicillin-resistance (MRSP) (0 and 1.15 %, respectively). The remaining countries had MRSP frequencies higher than 8 %, attaining 50 % in Italy. Methicillin-resistance was also high in CoNS (Table 5).

Staphylococci SXT resistance ranged from 2.77 to 63.16 % and showed similar geographical distribution to Gram-negative bacteria (Fig. 4). Among the participating countries, Staphylococci FLU resistance frequencies were higher in Italy (42.11 %) and again lower in Sweden (1.54 %) and Denmark (1.96 %), with the remaining countries varying between 6.59 and 26.92 % (Table 6). Italy, Austria, Germany and Switzerland CN resistant staphylococci frequencies ranged between 26.32 and 9.76 % while the remaining countries had less than 6 % (Table 6).

Regarding resistance temporal trends, most countries had no significant changes in *E. coli* resistance over the

Table 6 Percentage of resistance in *Staphylococcus* spp. by antimicrobial and country in 2012–2013

Country[a]	FLU		CN		SXT	
	n	% R (95 % CI)[b] [Stat. Dif.][c]	*n*	% R (95 % CI)[b] [Stat. Dif.][c]	*n*	% R (95 % CI)[b] [Stat. Dif.][c]
AT	78	26.92 (17.08–36.77) [a, b]	78	19.23 (10.48–27.98) [a]	78	20.51 (11.55–29.47) [a, b]
BE	116	7.76 (2.89–12.63) [c, d]	107	3.74 (0.14–7.33) [b]	122	13.11 (7.12–19.10) [a, b, c]
DK	51	1.96 (0.00–5.77) [c, e, f]	51	3.92 (0.00–9.25) [b]	51	0 - [d]
FR	238	23.53 (18.14–28.92) [a, g]	237	5.06 (2.27–7.85) [b]	242	11.57 (7.54–15.60) [a, c]
DE	55	18.18 (7.99–28.38) [a, d, g]	55	10.91 (2.67–19.15) [a, b]	55	23.64 (12.41–34.86) [b]
EL	10	20.00 (0.00–44.79) [a, d, e,gN h]	0	- - -	9	1R/8S - -
IT	19	42.11 (19.90–64.31) [a]	19	26.32 (6.52–46.12) [a]	19	63.16 (41.47–84.85) [e]
NL	364	6.59 (4.04–9.14) [c, i]	9	1R/8S - -	365	11.51 (8.23–14.78) [c]
PT	6	3R/3S - -	7	2R/5S - -	7	1R/6S - -
RS	0	- - -	0	- - -	0	- - -
ES	13	15.38 (0.00-35.00) [a, d, e, h, i]	8	0R/8S - -	11	18.18 (0.00-40.97) [a, b, c]
SE	325	1.54 (0.20–2.88) [f]	325	0 - [c]	325	2.77 (0.99–4.55) [d]
CH	41	24.39 (11.25–37.54) [a, b]	41	9.76 (0.67–18.84) [a, b]	41	19.51 (7.38–31.64) [a, b, c]
UK	31	12.90 (1.10–24.70) [b, c, e, g]	22	4.55 (0.00–13.25) [a, b, c]	30	16.67 (3.33–30.00) [a, b, c]

FLU fluoroquinolones, *CN* gentamicin, *SXT* trimethoprim/sulfamethoxazole
[a]Countries: AT, Austria; BE, Belgium; DK, Denmark; FR, France; DE, Germany; EL, Greece; IT, Italy; NL, the Netherlands; PT, Portugal; RS, Serbia; ES, Spain; SE, Sweden; CH, Switzerland; UK, United Kingdom
[b]95 % CI, 95 % Confidence interval
[c]Stat. Dif., Statistical significant differences. Countries with no statistical difference are marked with the same letter. Countries were compared by fisher exact test with an alpha value of 0.05. Countries with less than ten tested isolates were not compared
n, Total number of *Staphylococcus* spp. tested for the considered antimicrobial category

time periods considered (Table 7). Belgium showed a significant decrease in *E. coli* resistance to all antimicrobials and an increase in full susceptible isolates. Denmark (AMC, FLU, SXT), France (3GC, FLU), the Netherlands (3GC, FLU, SXT, MDR) and Sweden (CN, MDR) had also significant decreases in *E. coli* resistance over time (Table 7). However, the Netherlands (AMC) and Switzerland (CN) had a significant increase in *E. coli* resistance (Table 7). A rising trend was also detected in *Proteus* spp. FLU resistance from Belgium (Table 8).

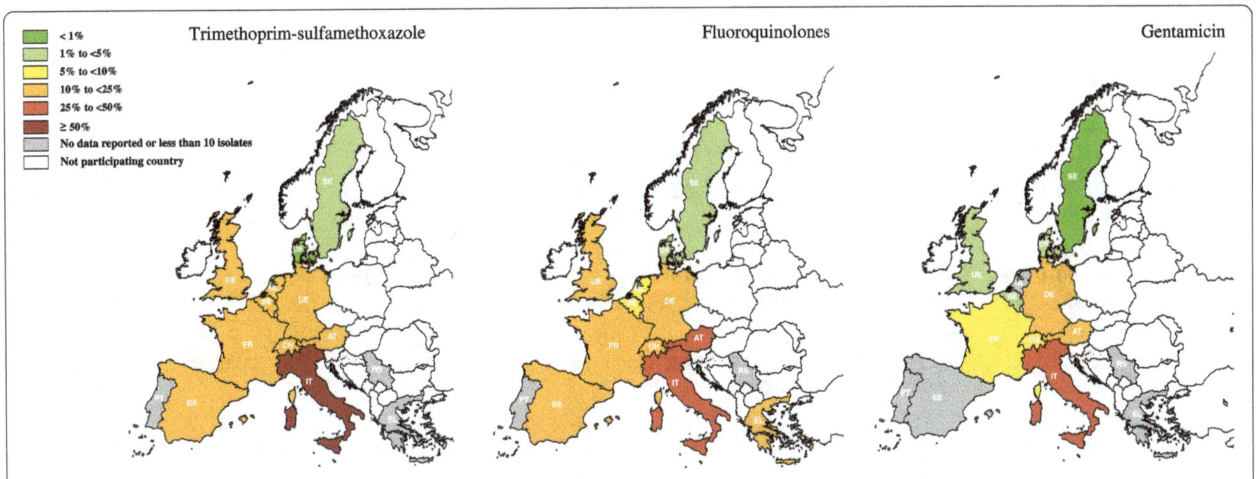

Fig. 4 Percentage (%) of *Staphylococcus* spp. antimicrobial resistance by antimicrobial and country in the years 2012–2013. Countries: AT- Austria; BE- Belgium; DK- Denmark; FR- France; DE- Germany; EL- Greece; IT- Italy; NL- the Netherlands; PT- Portugal; RS- Serbia; ES- Spain; SE- Sweden; CH- Switzerland; UK- United Kingdom

Discussion

Published data on antimicrobial resistance in bacteria isolated from companion animal UTIs over Europe is scarce [19] and the comparison between studies is impaired by the use of different inclusion criteria and different time periods. Moreover, UTI resistance frequencies are usually reported together with susceptibility data from other sites of infection [11, 28], combining different bacteria genera [8, 9] and several countries [29, 30]. These facts impair the establishment of a global epidemiological overview of UTI bacteria resistance in Europe. This is the first large study to analyse antimicrobial susceptibility data of canine and feline isolates from several European countries allowing an epidemiological overview of UTI resistance trends in Europe.

In accordance to previous studies [7–9, 31, 32], *E. coli* was the most frequently isolated bacteria in dogs and cats. *Enterococcus* presented a significantly higher frequency in cats and *Proteus* spp. in dogs. While not compared in previous studies, this difference could be expected based on some published data focused on cats [7, 9] and dogs [32] separately.

One of the most important findings from this study was the overall higher resistance frequencies found in the Southern countries (Italy, Greece, Portugal and Spain) when compared with the Northern countries (Denmark and Sweden). The lower frequency of antimicrobial resistance in Northern countries, such as Sweden, is likely a consequence of the tight regulations and surveillance on antimicrobial prescribing and resistance in companion animals. In light of the present results, such strategies could be useful in aiming the reduction of antimicrobial resistance in the Southern countries.

Resistance to Beta-Lactams

Amoxicillin-clavulanate

Considering that AMC is one of the most used antimicrobials in animals, the levels of resistance detected in this study are worrisome, especially in the Southern countries. Previous published reports showed different frequencies of AMC resistance in *E. coli* and in *Proteus* spp. that are likely due to the fact they report to different time frames and inclusion criteria [10, 32–37]. In the absence of clinical data it is not possible to know if this resistance relates to uncomplicated or complicated UTI [19]. Thus, these results need to be further investigated in order to establish whether AMC is a suitable empiric therapeutic choice for companion animals UTI in Southern Europe.

Third generation cephalosporins

Southern countries had also higher levels of resistance to 3GCs. Although Greece was not included due to limited data, considering that seven out of the nine tested isolates were resistant to 3GCs, one can expect the prevalence of 3GC resistance to be high. Previous studies in Portugal found a considerable lower 3GC resistance value (1.4 %) in *E. coli* from dogs in earlier years [10]. In the present work, the lower Swedish results for 3GC resistance in *E. coli* and *Proteus* spp. are in agreement with early studies [38]. Being of critical importance to humans [39], prudent use of 3GC is of upmost importance.

Methicillin-resistance

The frequency of methicillin-resistant staphylococci, especially *S. pseudintermedius* and CoNS, varied considerably between countries and confirmed previous reports on a low MRSP prevalence in Scandinavia compared to elsewhere in Europe [40]. Resistance to methicillin in

Table 7 Temporal trends of antimicrobial resistance in *Escherichia coli* by country

Country[a] (Years)	AMC OR[b] (95 % CI)[c] *P* value	3GC OR[b] (95 % CI)[c] *P* value	FLU OR[b] (95 % CI)[c] *P* value	CN OR[b] (95 % CI)[c] *P* value	SXT OR[b] (95 % CI)[c] *P* value	MDR OR[b] (95 % CI)[c] *P* value	FullS OR[b] (95 % CI)[c] *P* value
BE (2010–13)	**0.787 (0.646–0.960) 0.0180**	- - -	**0.749 (0.635–0.882) 0.0006**	**0.677 (0.507–0.904) 0.0081**	**0.796 (0.695–0.912) 0.0010**	**0.529[d] (0.393–0.712) <0.0001**	**1.275[d] (1.127–1.442) 0.0001**
DK (2008–13)	**0.698 (0.500–0.976) 0.0357**	0.869 (0.646–1.169) 0.3533	**0.742 (0.565–0.976) 0.0325**	0.926 (0.620–1.384) 0.7086	**0.793 (0.642–0.980) 0.0316**	0.874 (0.615–1.242) 0.4528	**1.396 (1.156–1.684) 0.0005**
FR (2010–13)	0.885 (0.780–1.005) 0.0606	**0.859 (0.749–0.987) 0.0314**	**0.822 (0.727–0.928) 0.0016**	0.938 (0.734–1.200) 0.6121	0.960 (0.853–1.080) 0.4997	0.901 (0.782–1.037) 0.1448	**1.112 (1.002–1.233) 0.0456**
DE (2009–13)	1.029 (0.779–1.358) 0.8424	1.076 (0.805–1.438) 0.6211	1.185 (0.912–1.540) 0.2037	0.856 (0.520–1.409) 0.5397	1.040 (0.831–1.302) 0.7317	1.111 (0.801–1.541) 0.5295	0.941 (0.780–1.136) 0.5281
EL[e] (2009–13)	1.534 (0.851–2.766) 0.1545	1.083 (0.586–2.003) 0.7992	0.924 (0.630–1.355) 0.6855	- - -	0.880 (0.596–1.301) 0.5229	- - -	- - -
IT (2009–2013)	1.175 (0.844–1.637 0.3391)	1.017 (0.749–1.383) 0.9127	0.828 (0.629–1.090) 0.1784	1.007 (0.700–1.449) 0.9686	0.769 (0.582–1.016) 0.0645	1.065 (0.761–1.490) 0.7147	1.248 (0.953–1.634) 0.1076
NL (2008–13)	**1.108 (1.026–1.197) 0.0088**	**0.465 (0.402–0.539) <0.0001**	**0.916 (0.841–0.999) 0.0464**	0.682 (0.327–1.422) 0.3071	**0.917 (0.859–0.978) 0.0083**	**0.380[d] (0.320–0.450) <0.0001**	**1.648[d] (1494.–1.818) <0.0001**
PT (2008–13)	1.139 (0.913–1.419) 0.2482	1.187 (0.945–1.492) 0.1411	1.029 (0.823–1.287) 0.8029	1.222 (0.899–1.660) 0.2010	1.087 (0.867–1.364) 0.4680	1.156 (0.898–1.488) 0.2601	0.797 (0.629–1.010) 0.0608
ES (2010–13)	1.372 (0.855–2.201) 0.1899	1.551 (0.857–2.808) 0.1474	0.801 (0.529–1214) 0.2965	0.859 (0.467–1.578) 0.6238	0.752 (0.489–1.156) 0.1939	1.237 (0.677–2.258) 0.4897	0.944 (0.570–1.564) 0.8234
SE (2008–13)	0.976 (0.915–1.041) 0.4569	- - -	0.980 (0.827–1.147) 0.8018	**0.700 (0.562–0.872) 0.0015**	0.961 (0.892–1.037) 0.3059	**0.697 (0.493–0.985) 0.0407**	1.035 (0.965–1.110) 0.3341
CH (2008–13)	1.143 (0.905–1.445) 0.2621	1.116 (0.861–1.447) 0.4067	1.007 (0.841–1.205) 0.9426	**1.493 (1.009–2.208) 0.0451**	1.080 (0.901–1.294) 0.4050	1.189 (0.920–1.536) 0.1863	1.025 (0.877–1.197) 0.7594
UK (2008–13)	1.075 (0.857–1.357) 0.5194	1.106 (0.873–1.400) 0.4041	0.945 (0.739–1.208) 0.6511	1.306 (0.792–2.155) 0.2952	0.972 (0.797–1.185) 0.7778	1.355 (0.954–1.925) 0.0892	1.154 (0.950–1.401) 0.1492

AMC amoxicillin clavulanate, *3GC* third generation cephalosporins, *FLU* fluoroquinolones, *CN* gentamicin, *SXT* trimethoprim/sulfamethoxazole, *MDR* multidrug-resistant, *FullS* fully-susceptible

[a]BE, Belgium; DK, Denmark; FR, France; DE, Germany; EL, Greece; IT, Italy; NL, the Netherlands; PT, Portugal; ES, Spain; SE, Sweden; CH, Switzerland; UK, United Kingdom

[b]OR, Odds ratio

[c]95 % CI, 95 % Confidence interval

[d]MDR and FullS temporal trends do not include resistance to 3GC for Belgium and CN for the Netherlands

[e]Data regarding the years 2010 and 2012 were excluded from Greece resistance trends analysis since less than ten isolates were tested in those years

Statistically significant trends are highlighted in bold

coagulase-positive *Staphylococcus* (*S. aureus* and *S. pseudintermedius*) was detected in this study and is a great animal and public health concern [41]. Currently, the recommended methods for the detection of methicillin-resistance in *Staphylococci* are manly phenotypic but in some circumstances the molecular detection of the *mecA* gene is clinically and epidemiologically necessary [22, 23, 42]. This should be taken in consideration for the harmonization of veterinary susceptibility testing in Europe.

Resistance to fluoroquinolones

In this study, high resistance frequencies towards the fluoroquinolones were found in *E. coli*, *Proteus* spp *and Staphylococcus* spp. isolates in the southern European countries but also in *Proteus* spp. from Germany, Belgium and Switzerland and *Staphylococcus* spp. from Austria, Switzerland and France. Several authors [32, 34, 43, 44] have reported lower FLU resistance frequencies than the ones found in this study, especially regarding the Southern countries [43, 44]. The results of high

Table 8 Temporal trends of antimicrobial resistance in *Proteus* spp. by country

Country[a] (Years)	AMC OR[b] (95 % CI)[c] *P* value	FLU OR[b] (95 % CI)[c] *P* value	SXT OR[b] (95 % CI)[c] *P* value
BE (2010–13)	0.627 (0.312–1.259) 0.1889	**1.292 (1.006–1.659) 0.0450**	0.891 (0.726–1.092) 0.2649
FR (2010–13)	0.945 (0.625–1.431) 0.7908	1.004 (0.764–1.319) 0.9770	0.954 (0.756–1.205) 0.6944
NL (2008–13)	1.092 (0.860–1.387) 0.4709	0.970 (0.829–1.135) 0.7067	1.010 (0.903–1.129) 0.8660
SE (2008–13)	0.892 (0.657–1.210) 0.4620	0.884 (0.494–1.583) 0.6788	0.941 (0.759–1.165) 0.5756

AMC amoxicillin clavulanate, *FLU* fluoroquinolones, *SXT* trimethoprim/sulfamethoxazole
Statistically significant trends are highlighted in bold
[a]BE, Belgium; DK, Denmark; FR, France; NL, the Netherlands; SE, Sweden; CH, Switzerland
[b]OR, Odds ratio
[c]95 % CI, 95 % Confidence interval

resistance frequencies towards the fluoroquinolones found in this study are concerning because fluoroquinolones are considered a good first choice for pyelonephritis treatment and should otherwise be used as a second line antimicrobial [19].

Resistance to folate inhibitors and to aminoglicosides

In this study, resistance to SXT in Europe was high, especially in *E. coli* and *Proteus* spp.. The higher SXT resistance found in *Proteus* spp., than in *E. coli* from several European countries, is consistent with other reports [34, 36, 45]. Compared with previous studies, these results show a superior SXT resistance in *E. coli* and *Proteus* spp. from Italy and Portugal [10, 43] and *Staphylococcus* spp. from Belgium [36].

Also in agreement to previous studies, gentamicin was the antimicrobial with lower resistance in *E. coli*, *Proteus* spp. and *Staphylococcus* spp. all-over Europe [32, 34, 35, 37, 38, 43, 45]. Nevertheless, the distribution seemed to follow the same pattern, with increased resistance in Southern over Northern countries.

Multidrug-resistance

Finally, MDR bacteria presented the worst scenario once again in *E. coli* from Southern countries and in *Proteus* spp. from Portugal. The emergence of MDR bacteria in companion animals has been previously described [46, 47] and represents a great therapeutic challenge and public health concern. However, MDR/FullS frequencies are seldom reported and published data account for different antimicrobials, thus impairing any comparisons with the present results [10, 32, 35, 38, 45].

Trends in antimicrobial resistance

The surveillance of antimicrobial resistance is an important tool to guide the implementation of antimicrobial stewardship strategies. In this study, most countries had no significant changes in antimicrobial resistance over the time frame considered. Nevertheless, decreasing trends in antimicrobial resistance were found in *E. coli*. These encouraging trends were not detected in AMC and CN resistance in *E. coli* from the Netherlands and Switzerland, respectively, where an increasing trend was observed. Although no changes over time were detected in *E. coli* resistance against AMC and 3CGs in Portugal, the considerably lower resistance frequencies previously reported in earlier years [10], point to a possible increasing trend [33]. The same may be the case for *E. coli* AMC resistance in Germany and Switzerland [34, 35].

Despite reporting clear trends such as the difference in resistance between Northern and Southern countries, data from this study should be interpreted with caution. Due to the retrospective nature of this study, data on clinical history such as the type of UTI and previous antimicrobial treatment were unavailable. Furthermore, the use of laboratory data may represent a bias towards resistance, since urine cultures from complicated cases tend to be requested more often than simple uncomplicated UTI [8, 31]. These limitations are not restricted to certain countries, and are therefore not likely to hamper comparison of data across borders. Given the limitations of retrospective studies, a veterinary European surveillance network gathering data prospectively on antimicrobial resistance, as well as, on clinical data is of the upmost importance to facilitate development of national evidence-based guidelines that take into consideration type of UTI, local regulations and patterns of antimicrobial resistance.

The use of different susceptibility testing methods and different clinical breakpoints is considered a major limitation. The lack of harmonization became evident in this study when trying to compare 3GC and methicillin-resistance. Although it also happens in the well-established

EARS network reports of resistance on bacteria from human invasive infections [18], this limitation weakens the comparison of resistance between countries in the present and future surveillance studies. This harmonization would allow future within and between countries resistance frequencies comparisons over time and would also provide relevant information on the impact of different antimicrobial usage policies. Thus, the authors agree that the harmonization of methods and interpretative criteria in veterinary medicine should be a priority. The role of the new veterinary committee on antimicrobial susceptibility testing VetCAST [48] may be crucial in this harmonization process. Despite these limitations, the results from this study provide relevant and updated information on the current antimicrobial resistance in UTI bacteria from companion animals in Europe. Similar studies should also be conducted regarding other types of infection to improve the awareness on the European distribution of antimicrobial resistance in companion animals. Ideally, monitoring of companion animal antimicrobial resistance should be implemented in Europe, as it is the case for food producing animals. Such surveillance would provide crucial information to promote the appropriate use of antimicrobial and therefore limit the spread of resistance.

Conclusions

This work brings new insights into the current scenario of the European antimicrobial resistance bacteria isolated from companion animals with UTI. An important finding from this study was the higher frequency of resistance in Southern European countries (Italy, Greece, Spain, Portugal) when compared to Northern European countries (Denmark, Sweden). Furthermore, there is an evident need to harmonize methods and interpretative criteria in veterinary medicine. Given the limitations of retrospective studies, an European surveillance network gathering data on antimicrobial resistance is of the upmost importance to facilitate the development of national evidence-based guidelines.

Abbreviations

3GC: Third generation cephalosporins; 95 % CI: 95 % confidence interval; AMC: Amoxicillin-clavulanate; AMP: Ampicillin; AT: Austria; BE: Belgium; CAZ: Ceftazidime; CH: Switzerland; CIP: Ciprofloxacin; CLSI: Clinical and Laboratory Standards Institute; CN: Gentamicin; CN120: Gentamicin high-level; CoNS: Coagulase negative staphylococci; CoPS: Coagulase positive staphylococci; CPD: Cefpodoxime; CTX: Cefotaxime; CVN: Cefovecin; DE: Germany; DK: Denmark; EARS-Net: European Antimicrobial Resistance Surveillance Network; EFT: Ceftiofur; EL: Greece; ENR: Enrofloxacin; ES: Spain; FLU: Fluoroquinolones; FOX: Cefoxitin; FR: France; FullS: Full-susceptibility; IT: Italy; MAR: Marbofloxacin; MDR: Multidrug-resistant; MRCoNS: Methicillin-resistant coagulase negative staphylococci; MRSA: Methicillin-resistant *Staphylococcus aureus*; MRSP: Methicillin-resistant *Staphylococcus pseudintermedius*; NL: the Netherlands; OR: Odds ratio; OX: Oxacillin; P: Penicillin; PT: Portugal; R: Full resistant; RS: Serbia; S: Susceptible; SA: *Staphylococcus aureus*; SE: Sweden; SP: *Staphylococcus pseudintermedius*; Stat. Dif.: Statistical significant differences; SXT: Trimethoprim/sulfamethoxazole; UK: United Kingdom; UTI: Urinary tract infection

Acknowledgements

We thank Professor Miguel Moreno and Dr. Christina Greko for helping to set up links with some collaborating laboratories.

Funding

This study was conducted with the financial support of CIISA and Fundação para a Ciência e a Tecnologia through Project UID/CVT/00276/2013. CM and AB hold Fundação para a Ciência e a Tecnologia PhD grants SFRH/BD/77886/2011 and SFRH/BD/113142/2015, respectively.

Authors' contributions

CP conceived the study and its coordination. CP and CM participated in the design of the study and contacted the collaborating laboratories included. All authors were responsible for data regarding the bacteria identification and susceptibility testing from the respective laboratory. CM and LTG conducted statistical analysis. CM wrote the initial draft and KB, EMB, PD, MAMD, RD, IL, DM, GO, VP, XR, JS, DT, GW, RGZ, SS, LG and CP made critical improvements for the final manuscript. All authors read and approved the final manuscript.

Competing interests

The authors declare that they have no competing interests.

Consent for publication

Not applicable.

Author details

[1]Faculdade de Medicina Veterinária, Centro de Investigação Interdisciplinar em Sanidade Animal (CIISA), Lisboa, Portugal. [2]The National Veterinary Institute (SVA), Uppsala, Sweden. [3]Laboratoire Vebiotel, Arcueil, France. [4]Department of Infectious Diseases and Immunology, Utrecht University, Utrecht, The Netherlands. [5]Department of Clinical Veterinary Sciences, Faculty of Medical and Veterinary Sciences, University of Bristol, Langford, UK. [6]AML-Medvet laboratory, Antwerp, Belgium. [7]Department of Veterinary Disease Biology, Faculty of Health and Medical Sciences, University of Copenhagen, Frederiksberg, Denmark. [8]Department of Clinical Sciences of Companion Animals, University of Utrecht, Utrecht, The Netherlands. [9]Clinic of Small Animal Medicine, LMU Munich, Munich, Germany. [10]Hospital Clínico Veterinario Complutense, Universidad Complutense, Servicio de Microbiologia y Parasitologia, Madrid, Spain. [11]Vetsuisse Faculty, University of Zurich, Clinic for Small Animal Internal Medicine, Zurich, Switzerland. [12]Department of Clinical Studies, Companion Animal Clinic, Faculty of Health Sciences, School of Veterinary Medicine, Aristotle University of Thessaloniki, Thessaloniki, Greece. [13]Institute of Microbiology, University of Veterinary Medicine, Vienna, Austria. [14]Department of Veterinary Medical Science, University of Bologna, Bologna, Italy. [15]Department of microbiology, Faculty of Veterinary Medicine, University of Belgrade, Belgrade, Serbia. [16]Hospital Clínic Veterinari, Universitat Autònoma de Barcelona, Bellaterra, Spain. [17]Institute of Veterinary Bacteriology, Vetsuisse Faculty, University of Bern, Bern, Switzerland. [18]School of Veterinary Science, University of Liverpool, Cheshire, UK. [19]Faculty of Veterinary Medicine, University of Agronomical Sciences Veterinary Medicine, Lasi, Romania. [20]Institute of Infection and Global Health, University of Liverpool, Liverpool, UK. [21]Institute for Infectious Diseases and Zoonoses, LMU Munich, Munich, Germany. [22]Institute of Veterinary Bacteriology, Vetsuisse Faculty, University of Zurich, Zurich, Switzerland. [23]Department of Biomedical Sciences, Ross University School of Veterinary Medicine, Basseterre, St Kitts and Nevis.

References

1. Dowling PM. Antimicrobial therapy of urinary tract infections. Can Vet J. 1996;37:438–41.
2. Thompson MF, Litster AL, Platell JL, Trott DJ. Canine bacterial urinary tract infections: New developments in old pathogens. Vet J. 2011;190:22–7.

3. Gerber B, Boretti FS, Kley S, Laluha P, Müller C, Sieber N, et al. Evaluation of clinical signs and causes of lower urinary tract disease in European cats. J Small Anim Pract. 2005;46:571–7.
4. Eggertsdóttir AV, Lund HS, Krontveit R, Sørum H. Bacteriuria in cats with feline lower urinary tract disease: a clinical study of 134 cases in Norway. J Feline Med Surg. 2007;9:458–65.
5. Saevik BK, Trangerud C, Ottesen N, Sørum H, Eggertsdóttir AV. Causes of lower urinary tract disease in Norwegian cats. J Feline Med Surg. 2011;13:410–7.
6. Mayer-Roenne B, Goldstein RE, Erb HN. Urinary tract infections in cats with hyperthyroidism, diabetes mellitus and chronic kidney disease. J Feline Med Surg. 2007;9:124–32.
7. Litster A, Moss SM, Honnery M, Rees B, Trott DJ. Prevalence of bacterial species in cats with clinical signs of lower urinary tract disease: Recognition of *Staphylococcus felis* as a possible feline urinary tract pathogen. Vet Microbiol. 2007;121:182–8.
8. Hall JL, Holmes MA, Baine SJ. Prevalence and antimicrobial resistance of canine urinary tract pathogens. Vet Rec. 2013;173:549.
9. Dorsch R, von Vopelius-Feldt C, Wolf G, Straubinger RK, Hartmann K. Feline urinary tract pathogens: prevalence of bacterial species and antimicrobial resistance over a 10-year period. Vet Rec. 2015;176:201.
10. Féria C, Correia J, Machado J, Vidal R, Gonçalves J. Urinary tract infection in dogs. Analysis of 419 urocultures carried out in Portugal. Adv Exp Med Biol. 2000;485:301–4.
11. Normand EH, Gibson NR, Reid SWJ, Carmichael S, Taylor DJ. Antimicrobial-resistance trends in bacteria isolates from companion-animal community practice in the UK. Prev Vet Med. 2000;46:267–78.
12. Cohn LA, Gary AT, Fales WH, Madsen RW. Trends in fluoroquinolone resistance of bacteria isolated from canine urinary tracts. J Vet Diagn Invest. 2003;15:338–43.
13. Pellerin JL, Bourdeau P, Sebbag H, Person JM. Epidemiosurveillance of antimicrobial compound resistance of *Staphylococcus intermedius* clinical isolates from canine pyodermas. Comp Immunol Microbiol Infect Dis. 1998;21:115–33.
14. European Medicine Agency. Reflection paper on the risk of antimicrobial resistance transfer from companion animals. http://www.ema.europa.eu/ema/pages/includes/document/open_document.jsp?webContentId=WC500181642. Accessed 15 Sept 2015.
15. Pomba C, Endimiani A, Rossano A, Saial D, Couto N, Perreten V. First report of OXA-23-mediated carbapenem resistance in sequence type 2 multidrug-resistant *Acinetobacter baumannii* associated with urinary tract infection in a cat. Antimicrob Agents Chemother. 2014;58:1267–8.
16. Johnson JR, Clabots C. Sharing of virulent *Escherichia coli* clones among household members of a woman with acute cystitis. Clin Infect Dis. 2006;43:e101–8.
17. Guardabassi L, Schwarz S, Lloyd H. Pet animals as reservoirs of antimicrobial-resistant bacteria. J Antimicrob Chemother. 2004;54:321–32.
18. European Centre for Disease Prevention and Control. Antimicrobial resistance surveillance in Europe 2013. Annual Report of the European Antimicrobial Resistance Surveillance Network (EARS-Net). Stockholm: ECDC; 2014.
19. Weese S, Blondeau JM, Boothe D, Breitschwerdt EB, Guardabassi L, Hillier A, et al. Antimicrobial use guidelines for treatment of urinary tract disease in dogs and cats: antimicrobial guidelines working group of the international society for companion animal infectious disease. Vet Med Int. 2011;2011:263768.
20. World Organization for Animal Health. OIE Terrestrial Animal Health Code Chapter 6.9. Responsible and Prudent Use of Antimicrobial Agents in Veterinary Medicine. http://www.oie.int/index.php?id=169&L=0&htmfile=chapitre_antibio_use.htm. Accessed 15 Sept 2015.
21. Clinical and Laboratory Standards Institute. Performance Standards for Antimicrobial Disk and Dilution Susceptibility Tests for Bacteria Isolated from Animals-Fourth Edition: Approved Standard VET01-A4. Wayne: CLSI; 2013.
22. Clinical and Laboratory Standarts Institute. Performance Standards for Antimicrobial Susceptibility Testing: Twenty-third Informational Supplement M100-S25. Wayne: CLSI; 2015.
23. Clinical and Laboratory Standarts Institute. Performance Standards for Antimicrobial Disk and Dilution Susceptibility Tests for Bacteria Isolated from Animals: Second Information Supplement VET01-S2. Wayne: CLSI; 2013.
24. Societe Française de Microbiology. Antibiogramme veterinaire du comite de l'antibiogramme de la societe francaise de microbiologie. Paris: SFM; 2012.
25. Howe RA, Andrews JM, Party BW. BSAC standardized disc susceptibility testing method (version 11). J Antimicrob Chemother. 2012;67:2783–4.
26. Commissie Richtlijnen Gevoeligheidsbepalingen. Interpretatie van gevoeligheidsonderzoek en gevoeligheidscriteria voor antibacteriële middelen in Nederland. Ned Tijdschr Med Microbiol. 2000;8:79–81.
27. Magiorakos AP, Srinivasan A, Carey RB, Carmeli Y, Falagas ME, Giske CJ, et al. Multidrug-resistant, extensively drug-resistant and pandrug-resistant bacteria: an international expert proposal for interim standard definitions for acquired resistance. Clin Microbiol Infect. 2012;18:268–81.
28. Ruscher C, L bke-Becker A, Wleklinski CG, Soba A, Wieler LH, Walther B. Prevalence of Methicillin-resistant *Staphylococcus pseudintermedius* isolated from clinical samples of companion animals and equidaes. Vet Microbiol. 2008;136:197–201.
29. Meunier D, Acar JF, Martel JL, Kroemer S, Valle M. A seven-year survey of susceptibility to marbofloxacin of pathogenic strains isolated from pets. Int J Antimicrob Agents. 2004;24:592–8.
30. Kroemer S, Garch FE, Galland D, Petit JL, Woehrle F, Boulouis HJ. Antibiotic susceptibility of bacteria isolated from infections in cats and dogs throughout Europe (2002–2009). Comp Immunol Microbiol Infect Dis. 2014;37:97–108.
31. Ball KR, Rubin JE, Chirino-Trejo M, Dowling PM. Antimicrobial resistance and prevalence of canine uropathogens at the Western College of Veterinary Medicine Veterinary Teaching Hospital, 2002–2007. Can Vet J. 2008;49:985–90.
32. Windahl U, Holst BS, Nyman A, Grönlund U, Bengtsson B. Characterisation of bacterial growth and antimicrobial susceptibility patterns in canine urinary tract infections. BMC Vet Res. 2014;10:217.
33. Féria C, Ferreira E, Correia JD, Gonçalves J, Caniça M. Patterns and mechanisms of resistance to β-lactams and β-lactamase inhibitors in uropathogenic *Escherichia coli* isolated from dogs in Portugal. J Antimicrob Chemother. 2002;49:77–85.
34. Grobbel M, Lübke-Becker A, Alešík E, Schwarz S, Wallmann J, Werckenthin C, et al. Antimicrobial susceptibility of *Escherichia coli* from swine, horses, dogs and cats as determined in the BfT-GermVet monitoring program 2004–2006. Berl Munch Tierarztl Wochenschr. 2007;120:391–401.
35. Lanz R, Kuhnert P, Boerlin P. Antimicrobial resistance and resistance gene determinants in clinical *Escherichia coli* from different animal species in Switzerland. Vet Microbiol. 2003;91:73–84.
36. Criel D, Steenbergen J, Stalpaert M. Prevalence and antimicrobial susceptibility of canine uropathogens in Northern Belgium: a retrospective study (2010 to 2012). J Small Anim Pract. 2015;56:73.
37. Pedersen K, Pedersen K, Jensen H, Finster K, Jensen VF, Heuer OE. Occurrence of antimicrobial resistance in bacteria from diagnostic samples from dogs. J Antimicrob Chemother. 2007;60:775–81.
38. Hagman R, Greko C. Antimicrobial resistance in *Escherichia coli* isolated from bitches with pyometra and from urine samples from other dogs. Vet Rec. 2005;157:193–7.
39. World Health Organization. Critically important antimicrobials for human medicine. http://apps.who.int/iris/bitstream/10665/77376/1/9789241504485_eng.pdf. Accessed 15 Sept 2015.
40. Swedres-Svarm. Consumption of antibiotics and occurrence of antibiotic resistance in Sweden. Solna/Uppsala: Public Health Agency of Sweden and National Veterinary Institute; 2014.
41. Guardabassi L, Prescott JF. Antimicrobial stewardship in small animal veterinary practice: From theory to practice. Vet Clin North Am Small Anim Pract. 2015;45:361–76.
42. European Committee on Antimicrobial Susceptibility Testing. EUCAST guidelines for detection of resistance mechanisms and specific resistances of clinical and/or epidemiological importance. Version 1.0. http://www.eucast.org/fileadmin/src/media/PDFs/EUCAST_files/Resistance_mechanisms/EUCAST_detection_of_resistance_mechanisms_v1.0_20131211.pdf. Accessed 15 Sept 2015.
43. Tramuta C, Robino P, Nucera D, Salvarani S, Banche G, Malabaila A, et al. Molecular characterization and antimicrobial resistance of faecal and urinary *Escherichia coli* isolated from dogs and humans in Italy. Vet Ital. 2014;50:23–30.
44. Oliveira M, Dias FR, Pomba C. Biofilm and fluoroquinolone resistance of canine *Escherichia coli* uropathogenic isolates. BMC Res Notes. 2014;7:499.
45. Grobbel M, Lübke-Becker A, Alešík E, Schwarz S, Wallmann J, Werckenthin C, et al. Antimicrobial susceptibility of *Klebsiella* spp. and *Proteus* spp. from various organ systems of horses, dogs and cats as determined in the BfT-GermVet monitoring program 2004–2006. Berl Munch Tierarztl Wochenschr. 2007;120:402–11.

46. Pomba C, Couto N, Moodley A. Treatment of a lower urinary tract infection in a cat caused by a multi-drug methicillin-resistant *Staphylococcus pseudintermedius* and *Enterococcus faecalis*. J Feline Med Surg. 2010;12:802–6.
47. Wagner S, Gally DL, Argyle SA. Multidrug-resistant Escherichia coli from canine urinary tract infections tend to have commensal phylotypes, lower prevalence of virulence determinants and *ampC*-replicons. Vet Microbiol. 2014;169:171–8.
48. Veterinary Committee on Antimicrobial Susceptibility Testing (VetCAST). http://www.eucast.org/ast_of_veterinary_pathogens (2015). Accessed 15 Sept 2015.

OmpA protein sequence-based typing and virulence-associated gene profiles of *Pasteurella multocida* isolates associated with bovine haemorrhagic septicaemia and porcine pneumonic pasteurellosis in Thailand

Teerasak E-kobon[1,2*], Ratiporn Leeanan[1], Saengtian Pannoi[1], Pornchai Anuntasomboon[1], Pacharee Thongkamkoon[3] and Arinthip Thamchaipenet[1]

Abstract

Background: *Pasteurella multocida* is a Gram-negative bacterium that causes economically significant infections of a broad range of animal species. Pneumonic and septicaemic pasteurellosis caused by this bacterium remain important problems in pigs, cattle, and water buffaloes in Thailand. The aim of this study was to characterise the virulence-associated gene profiles and to develop an OmpA molecular typing scheme for classifying 191 bovine and porcine isolates of *P. multocida* collected between 1989 and 2012 in Thailand using polymerase chain reactions (PCRs), nucleotide sequencing, and sequence and structural bioinformatics analyses.

Results: PCR screening successfully characterised the profiles of 25 virulence-associated genes in all isolates. The gene profiles separated these isolates into bovine and porcine clusters based on eight genes (*hgbB*, *hsf1*, *tadD*, *nanH*, *pfhA*, *plpE*, *pmHAS*, and *tbpA*). Phylogenetic analyses of the nucleotide and protein sequences corresponding to the *ompA* gene, which encodes a major outer membrane surface protein, showed two major bovine and porcine clusters. Structural prediction and analysis of the dN/dS ratio revealed four hypervariable extracellular loops of the OmpA transmembrane domains. These four loops were used to develop an OmpA typing scheme. This scheme classified 186 isolates into five major loop sequence types (LST8, LST12, LST15, LST18, and LST19), consistent with the phylogenetic results. The loop regions of the bovine isolates were predicted to be more antigenic than those of the porcine isolates. Thus, molecular evolution of the OmpA proteins could be used to classify *P. multocida* isolates into different capsular types, host types, and, possibly, pathogenicity levels.

Conclusions: Together with the virulence-associated gene profiles, the typing reported in this work provides a better understanding of *P. multocida* virulence. Effective monitoring and potential strain-specific subunit vaccines could be developed based on these loop oligopeptides.

Keywords: *Pasteurella multocida*, *ompA*, Pneumonic pasteurellosis, Haemorrhagic septicaemia, Virulence-associated genes, Molecular evolution, Molecular typing

* Correspondence: fscitse@ku.ac.th
[1]Department of Genetics, Faculty of Science, Kasetsart University, 50, Ngam Wong Wan Rd, Lad Yao, Chatuchak, Bangkok 10900, Thailand
[2]Bioinformatics and Systems Biology Unit, Computational Biomodelling Laboratory for Agricultural Science and Technology (CBLAST), Faculty of Science, Kasetsart University, 50 Ngam Wong Wan Rd, Lat Yao, Chatuchak, Bangkok 10900, Thailand
Full list of author information is available at the end of the article

Background

Pasteurella multocida is a facultative anaerobic Gram-negative bacterium responsible for economically significant infections in a broad range of animal species [1]. *P. multocida* commonly presents as a commensal bacterium in the respiratory tract but can become a primary or secondary pathogen depending on health status, animal species, climatic conditions, and poor husbandry practices [1, 2]. The organism causes a variety of respiratory diseases, including pneumonic pasteurellosis of ruminants and pigs, porcine progressive atrophic rhinitis (PAR), avian cholera, bovine haemorrhagic septicaemia (HS), snuffles in lagomorphs, and human infections via bites or scratches from carnivores [2]. Pneumonic and septicaemic pasteurellosis remain important problems in pigs, cattle, and water buffaloes worldwide. The disease severity varies from acute to subacute to chronic in different animal hosts [3] and depending on the bacterial serotype [4]. Generally, this organism can be classified into five capsular serotypes (A, B, D, E, and F) and 16 lipopolysaccharide (LPS) serotypes (1–16) [3]. Associations of certain serotypes of *P. multocida* with specific disease symptoms or geographical areas have been systematically shown by Davies et al. [5–9]. How these serotypic preferences and host predilections contribute to the virulence of *P. multocida* is not fully understood.

Recently, several comparative genomic studies have revealed different genes and genetic elements between virulent strains of *P. multocida* and avirulent strains [10–12]. The pathogenicity and virulence of *P. multocida* involve multiple genes related to the bacterial capsule, endotoxins (LPS), dermonecrotic exotoxin or *P. multocida* toxin, phages, plasmids, type IV pili, adhesins, extracellular enzymes, and outer membrane proteins (OMPs) [2, 13, 14]. Several genes encoding these features of *P. multocida*, including *exbB*, *exbD*, *fimA*, *fur*, *hgbA*, *hgbB*, *hsf1*, *hsf2*, *nanB*, *nanH*, *oma87*, *ompA*, *ompH*, *pfhA*, *plpB*, *plpE*, *pmHAS*, *psl*, *ptfA*, *sodA*, *sodC*, *tadD*, *tbpA*, *tonB*, and *toxA*, have been used in molecular typing studies to define virulence-associated gene profiles. The products of the *exbB*, *exbD*, *fur*, and *tonB* genes are needed for energy transfer from the inner membrane to the outer membrane iron transporters [15]. The *hgbAB* and *tbpA* genes encode outer membrane haemoglobin and transferrin transporters that are tightly regulated by the product of the *fur* gene [16]. The *fimA*, *hsf1*, *hsf2*, *pfhA*, *ptfA*, and *tadD* genes encode adhesion and colonisation factors that allow *P. multocida* to colonise host mucosal membranes [2, 17–19]. The products of the *nanB*, *nanH*, *ompH*, *plpB*, and *psl* genes are OMPs involved in nutrient acquisition and transport. The sialidase proteins NanB and NanH cleave sialic acids from the host membrane for use as nutrients and in modifying the cell envelope to evade the host immune system [2, 20]. OmpH, a porin, is a general transporter that facilitates the diffusion of various molecules [21]. The superoxide dismutases *sodA* and *sodC* are important in the oxidative stress response and in protection against oxidative stress [22]. The *ompA* and *oma87* genes are required for the biosynthesis and integrity of the outer membrane, the outermost surface of the bacterium that interfaces with the external environment [23]. The highly abundant OmpA protein possesses a C-terminal globular domain that interacts with the peptidoglycan layer of the cell wall, providing stability and integrity to the outer membrane. The OmpA protein is also involved in adherence to host cells through heparin and fibronectin binding [24]. The outer membrane lipoproteins PlpB, PlpE and Psl (P6-like) may stimulate immune protection against the bacterium in animal hosts, but their precise functions remain unclear [25–27]. The *toxA* gene encodes a dermonecrotic toxin (DMT) that blocks chemotaxis-induced migration of dendritic cells to lymph nodes and restricts the progress of the adaptive immune response [2]. Some of these virulence-associated genes appear only in virulent strains of the bacterium and are highly correlated with disease severity. Others may also be present in non-pathogenic strains but are highly expressed only in virulent strains in vivo, as shown by Li et al. [28].

The existing evidence suggests that the virulence-associated genes described above may be required for pathogenic strains of *P. multocida* to survive under host conditions. Several studies have screened these genes in a range of *P. multocida* isolates in attempts to identify their involvement in virulence and host specificity [29–33]. These studies revealed the prevalence of the *toxA* gene in *P. multocida* strains (mainly capsular type D) associated with porcine PAR and frequent observation of the *tbpA* gene in the strains that affect cattle. Many of these genes, particularly the OMP-encoding genes, have been widely studied, and some have been used as the basis for the development of vaccines that can heterologously protect against infections by multiple strains of *P. multocida* [13, 14, 34–39]. This evidence has led to the hypothesis that molecular variations within the same virulence-associated genes may affect host specificity and virulence. Verma et al. found seven classes of *ompA* alleles in 46 isolates of *P. multocida* [40]. Associations of these *ompA* alleles with capsular type and disease status have been proposed. Another recent study identified associations between *ompH* alleles and the capsular types of 83 isolates of *P. multocida* and found variable *ompH* alleles within capsular type A isolates [41]. This information is important for detailed typing of virulence isolates and will be helpful in the monitoring of *P. multocida* infections. However, the prevalence of specific virulence-associated genotypes and OmpA types in pigs, cattle, and water buffaloes in Thailand has not been determined. Therefore, this study aimed to characterise the virulence-associated gene profiles of 191 bovine and porcine *P. multocida* isolates collected in Thailand over a 24-year period and to develop a protein-sequence-based OmpA typing scheme using molecular genetics and bioinformatics techniques. The results of this study provide an alternative molecular typing of *P. multocida* isolates and serve as a basis for the development of OmpA type-specific vaccines.

Results

Clustering of 25 virulence gene profiles of 191 bovine and porcine isolates of *P. multocida* revealed two major clusters: bovine and porcine (Fig. 1). Ninety-nine percent of the isolates had the profiles of 17 virulence genes in common (the presence of *exbB*, *exbD*, *fimA*, *fur*, *hgbA*, *hsf2*, *nanB*, *oma87*, *ompA*, *ompH*, *plpB*, *psl*, *ptfA*, *sodA*, *sodC*, and *tonB* and the nearly complete absence of *toxA*). The dendrogram in Fig. 1 shows that the profiles of eight virulence genes (*hgbB*, *hsf1*, *tadD*, *nanH*, *pfhA*, *plpE*, *pmHAS*, and *tbpA*) could be used to separate the isolates into two major clusters. The bovine cluster (shown in *dark blue* in Fig. 1) included five genes (*hsf1*, *hgbB*, *nanH*, *pfhA*, and *toxA*) that were shared across the seven subgroups. The profiles of the eight virulence genes varied across the four subgroups of the porcine cluster (shown in *green* in Fig. 1). The profiles of the Thai bovine isolates of *P. multocida* were less diverse than those of the porcine isolates.

In this study, the bovine isolates (C cluster) were divided into six subgroups — C1, C2, C3, C4, C5, and C6 — based on the profiles of the genes *hgbB*, *hsf1*, *tadD*, and *pmHAS*. The third subgroup, C3, accounted for 76% of the bovine isolates. There was no clear separation between the isolates obtained from cattle and those obtained from water buffaloes or between samples collected in different years. The subgroups C1, C2, C3, C6, and C0 displayed similar virulence gene profiles lacking *pmHAS*, *plpE*, and *tadD* (Fig. 1). The subgroups C4 and C5 additionally displayed the presence of the *pmHAS* and *tadD* genes, respectively. Unlike the porcine cluster, almost all of the bovine isolates possessed the *hsf1*, *hgbB*, *pfhA*, and *tbpA* genes; thus, these genes could be key to the success of these strains in causing acute HS.

The second cluster of porcine isolates was divided into four subgroups: P1, P2, P3, and P4 (Fig. 1). Subgroup P4 (40%), followed by subgroup P1 (37%), included the highest number of porcine isolates. Most isolates of subgroup P1 had the *nanH*, *pfhA*, *plpE*, *pmHAS*, and *tadD* genes in common and showed complete loss of *tbpA*. The *pfhA* gene was only present in subgroup P1, whereas *hsf1* and *hgbB* were present in some isolates of this subgroup. All members of the P1 subgroup belonged to capsular type A, including two bovine type A isolates: 1C and 12C. Similarly, nearly all members of subgroup P4, with the exception of the 104P strain, also belonged to capsular type A. These strains had the *nanH*, *pmHAS*, *hgbB*, and *tadD* genes in common. Two other subgroups of the porcine cluster, subgroups P2 and P3, were isolates of capsular type D. All isolates of subgroup P2 showed the presence of *hsf1*, *nanH*, *hgbB*, and *tadD* genes together with the lack of *pfhA*, *pmHAS*, and *tbpA* genes. Some isolates in this subgroup had the *plpE* gene. The third subgroup, P3, only shared the *tadD*, *hgbB*, and *nanH* genes; the other five genes were absent. These results demonstrate the presence of variable virulence gene-associated profiles in porcine isolates of *P. multocida* in Thailand.

The *ompA* gene was successfully amplified and sequenced from 186 isolates of *P. multocida* in this study. The obtained nucleotide sequences were trimmed to a length of 940 nucleotides and were confirmed to

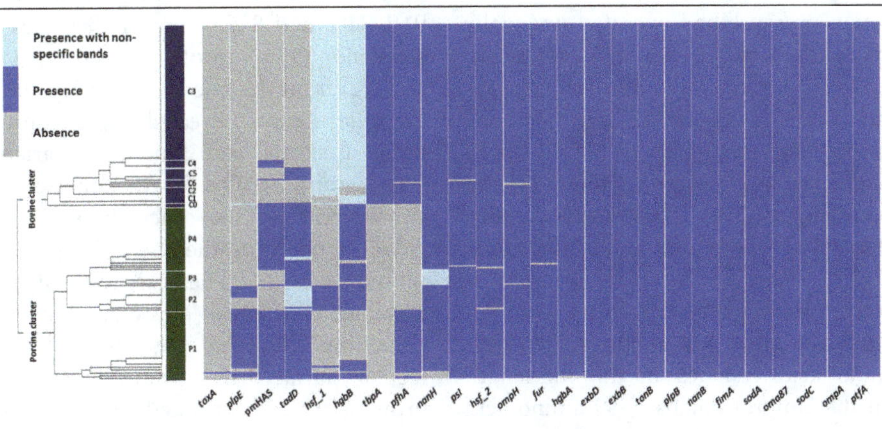

Fig. 1 Hierarchical clustering results of 25 virulence-associated gene profiles. The dendrogram shows the hierarchical clustering results of 25 virulence-associated gene profiles (represented as a three-colour heatmap) obtained from 191 isolates of *P. multocida* associated with diseased pigs, cattle, and water buffaloes in Thailand. The letter C is used to indicate the clusters of cattle and water buffaloes (C1, C2, C3, C4, C5, and C6), which are shown in dark blue; P indicates the pig clusters (P1, P2, P3, and P4), which are shown in green

correspond to the *ompA* gene. The obtained sequences covered nearly the full length of the transmembrane domain of this gene. Forty-one available *ompA* nucleotide sequences were also downloaded from the NCBI nucleotide database and compared with the sequences identified in this study. After multiple sequence alignment and phylogenetic construction of 227 DNA sequences, the phylogenetic tree of the *ompA* gene of *P. multocida* (Fig. 2a and Additional file 1: Table S1) clearly showed two major clusters of the bovine (cluster C) and porcine (cluster P) isolates, consistent with the clustering of the virulence-associated genes shown in Fig. 1. The bovine cluster consisted of a single large group of 97 bovine isolates (79 Thai isolates and 18 database strains) of capsular type B. The second porcine cluster consisted of five subgroups: P1, P2, P3, P4, and P5. Sixty-five of the porcine isolates were almost equally clustered in subgroups P1 and P2. Subgroup P3 members (13 strains) included only the samples in the NCBI database. Thirty isolates of subgroup P4 were further divided into subgroups P4I (9 isolates) and P4II (21 isolates). With the exception of a single capsular type D isolate, 87P (subgroup P2), the isolates in subgroups P1, P2, P4I, and P5 were capsular type A. All isolates in the P4II subgroup were capsular type D. These results demonstrate the presence of molecular differences in the *ompA* genes of the two capsular types of porcine *P. multocida* isolates. Interestingly, two bovine isolates of capsular type A (1C and 12C) also grouped within the porcine cluster (subgroups P5 and P4I).

Analysis of nucleotide substitutions within the *ompA* gene was conducted on 95 unique *ompA* sequences, returning a dN of 1.3667, a dS of 1.0341, and a dN/dS ratio of 0.8751. The dN and dS of each codon position in 227 nucleotide sequences of the *ompA* genes analysed in this study were compared (Fig. 3). The results showed that selection pressure had operated unequally on different regions of the *ompA* genes of *P. multocida*. Codon positions 61–220 accumulated more nonsynonymous than synonymous changes, as did positions 409–457. Codon positions 247–325 displayed more synonymous changes, as did positions 460–508 and 781–820, whereas positions 544–780 showed a counterbalance between synonymous and nonsynonymous substitutions.

The OmpA proteins encoded by the *ompA* gene sequences in this study contained 314 amino acids. Compared to the amino acid residues in the full-length OmpA proteins in the Uniprot database, 39 amino acid residues were not included in this study. Twenty-two amino acids were missing from the N-terminus, whereas the C-terminus was shortened by 16 amino acids. The sequences of the transmembrane domain were obtained, and the equally trimmed 186 sequences of this domain were aligned and summarised in a logo plot (Fig. 4a), which showed three variable regions at amino acid positions 24–42, 80–93, and 132–147. These regions correlated well with the dN/dS results for regions 60–159, 248–296, and 415–455, respectively (Fig. 3).

Approximately 252 amino acids within the transmembrane domain were compared (Fig. 4a); the resulting protein phylogenetic tree is shown in (Fig. 2b and Additional file 1: Table S1). The tree shows two major clusters of OmpA proteins from the Thai bovine and porcine isolates. The first cluster consists of two subgroups (P1 and P2) of the porcine isolates associated with capsular type A. The second cluster contains a very large subgroup C (C1 and C2) of the bovine isolates of capsular type B and a small subgroup of the porcine (P3 and P4) isolates. The members of subgroup P3 are all porcine isolates associated with capsular type D, whereas the members of subgroup P4 are capsular type A isolates, including the bovine isolate 12C. Although this protein tree differs slightly from the nucleotide tree derived for the *ompA* gene, the distinctions between animal hosts and capsular types are clearly shown.

The multiple aligned OmpA sequences were subjected to structural prediction. The consensus OmpA structure of *P. multocida* strains in Thailand was predicted based on the template structures of the OmpA-like domain from *Acinetobacter baumannii* (4g4x_A) and the OmpA transmembrane domain from *Escherichia coli* (1qjp) (Fig. 4b). The predicted OmpA structure of the Thai isolates of *P. multocida* contained two domains: a globular C-terminal peptidoglycan-binding domain and a transmembrane ß-barrel N-terminal domain. The transmembrane domain consisted of eight antiparallel ß-sheets interspersed with four short periplasmic turns and four long extracellular loops, similar to the OmpA proteins of other bacteria. Six OmpA structures (21P, 32P, 42P, 91P, 34C, and 84C) were predicted as representative of six major OmpA protein clusters (P1, P2, P3, P4, C1, and C2) from the tree shown in Fig. 2b. Superposition of these structures revealed eight conserved transmembrane ß-sheets and four hypervariable loop regions (Fig. 5a and b). The fourth loop was more structurally conserved than the other three loops (Fig. 5c). Individual models of these six OmpA proteins are presented in Fig. 6. These representative structures were classified into two clusters, similar to the protein clustering shown in Fig. 2b. By computing the molecular surface, the extracellular loops of these six proteins were determined to be rich in charged amino acid residues (middle and bottom rows in Fig. 6). Taken together, the data show that the observed variations in the nucleotide sequences of the *ompA* genes contribute to the structures of the hypervariable extracellular loop regions of the OmpA proteins.

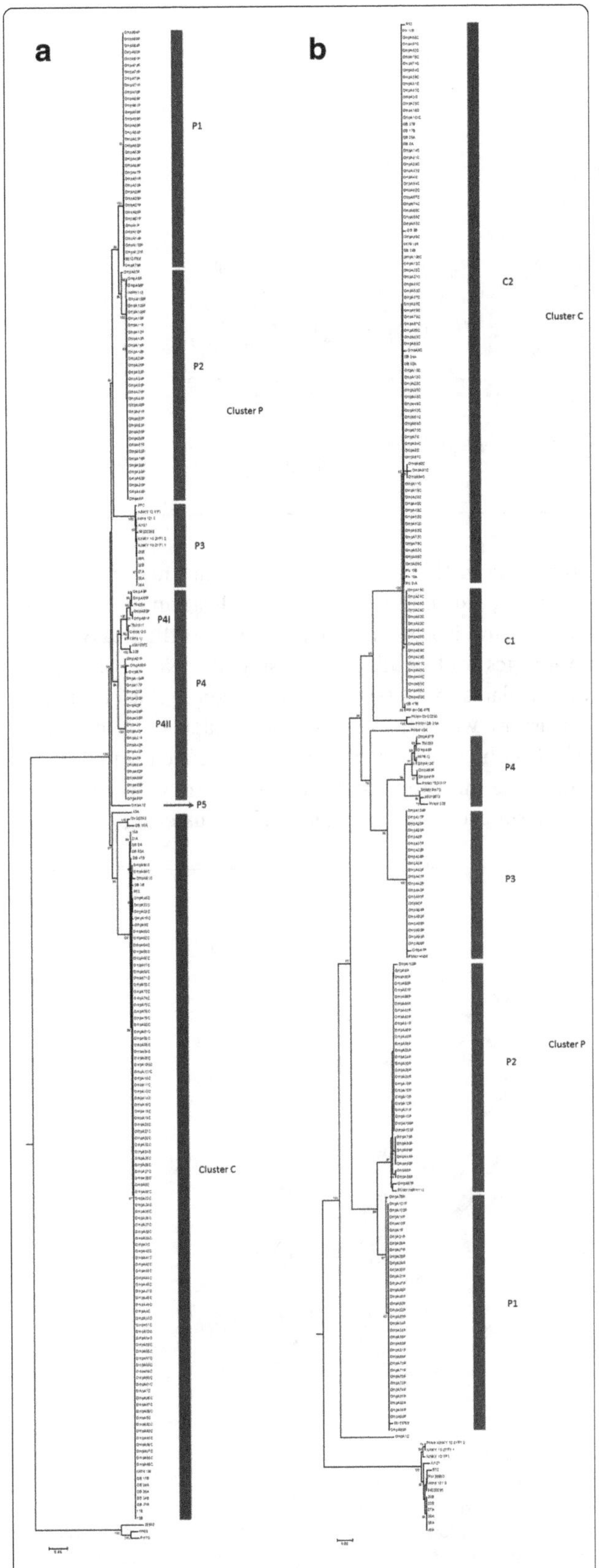

Fig. 2 Phylogenetic trees of partial *ompA* genes and proteins. Molecular evolutionary history of partial *ompA* genes (**a**) and proteins (**b**) obtained from 186 *P. multocida* isolates associated with diseased cattle, water buffaloes, and pigs in Thailand in comparison with 41 available *ompA* genes and proteins from the NCBI database. The phylogenetic relationships were inferred using the neighbour-joining method. Evolutionary analyses were conducted in MEGA 6. The bovine clusters (C1 and C2) are labelled in the dark blue bars, and the porcine clusters (P1, P2, P3, and P4) are labelled in the green bars. The P4 subcluster consists of the P4I and P4II groups. Details regarding each cluster are presented in Additional file 2: Table S2

The amino acid sequences corresponding to the four hypervariable extracellular loops (L1, L2, L3, and L4) were extracted from the alignment and trimmed to the same length. The first loop (L1) was closest to the N-terminus, whereas the last loop (L4) was close to the C-terminal domain. A difference in at least one amino acid position within the same loop was considered to represent a distinct loop sequence type (LST). This study developed the OmpA protein sequence-based typing scheme using the observed LSTs. Each LST consisted of four loop types: loop 1 sequence type (L1ST), loop 2 sequence type (L2ST), loop 3 sequence type (L3ST), and loop 4 sequence type (L4ST), which was formularised as LST = L1ST: L2ST: L3ST: L4ST. The use of LST molecular typing on these isolates revealed 30 LSTs comprising 21 L1STs, 11 L2STs, 14 L3STs, and 10 L4STs. Fourteen LSTs were found in 186 Thai bovine and porcine isolates; the other 16 LSTs were present only in the database strains. Five LSTs (LST8, LST12, LST15, LST18, and LST19) included 80% of the Thai isolates. The bovine OmpA proteins in subgroup C1 (capsular type B) harboured LST19 (11:5:5:3), whereas subgroup C2 (capsular type B) belonged to the LST8 group (6:5:5:3). The porcine subgroups P1, P2, and P3 had LST12 (8:3:3:3), LST15 (9:7:3:3), and LST18 (10:2:2:3), respectively. Clearly, the porcine strains of capsular types A (subgroups P1 and P2) and D (subgroup P3) could be differentiated based on their LSTs.

To understand the importance of these variations, the four hypervariable loop sequences of the six subgroups (C1, C2, P1, P2, P3, and P4) were subjected to antigenicity prediction. The prediction algorithm was based on the physicochemical properties of experimentally determined antigens. No loops of the porcine isolates of subgroups P1, P2, and P3 displayed antigenic epitopes. Subgroup P4, which contained the bovine isolate 12C and other porcine isolates, displayed a possibly antigenic first loop. Intriguingly, the bovine subgroups C1 and C2 each had three possibly antigenic loops (L1, L2, and L3). This antigenic variation could have resulted from high levels of nonsynonymous substitution within the loop regions.

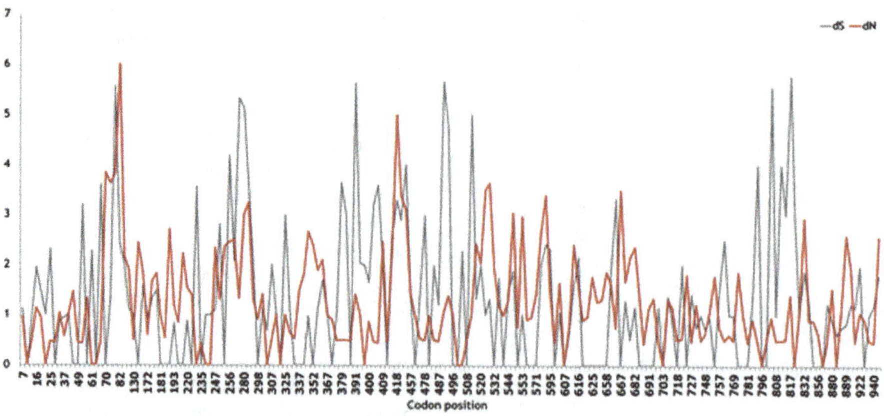

Fig. 3 Codon-based dN/dS ratio of the OmpA protein. Calculation of the dN and dS values of each codon of the *ompA* gene of *P. multocida* as a basis for examining the effects of natural selection at each codon position. The x-axis shows the codon positions; the y-axis shows the dN and dS values. The analysis was conducted using the MEGA 6 program

Discussion

Analysis of 25 virulence-associated gene profiles identified 16 genes that may have important functions in all 191 isolates of *P. multocida*. The absence of these genes is expected to greatly affect the survival and likely the virulence of *P. multocida*. Some of these genes may also appear in non-pathogenic strains but may be highly expressed in virulent strains under in vivo conditions, as shown by Li et al. [28]. However, the near absence of the *toxA* gene in this study (it appeared in only one porcine isolate) could reflect successful eradication of *toxA*-positive porcine isolates in Thailand due to the heavy use of antibiotics and vaccines in past years. None of the bovine isolates possessed the *toxA* gene. This finding is consistent with the results of a similar study of Indian and South Asian cattle strains associated with HS, in which the infectious bacteria did not carry the *toxA* gene but harboured the *tbpA* gene [42]. Clustering of the 191

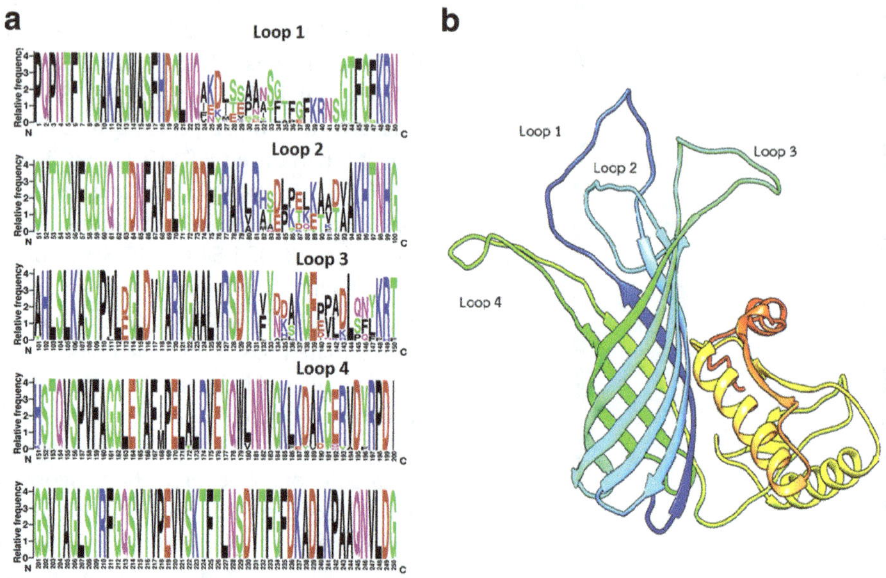

Fig. 4 Alignment of the OmpA proteins in association with the predicted OmpA structure. Logo plot summarising the multiple sequence alignment of the partial OmpA sequences of 186 bovine and porcine isolates of *P. multocida* in Thailand using the WebLogo program (**a**). The height of the stack indicates the sequence conservation level at that position. The symbol height also indicates the relative frequency of amino acids at that position. The alignment was mapped onto the homology-predicted OmpA structure (**b**) using the Chimera program to identify substructures of the OmpA protein. These substructures were mapped back onto the alignments as loop 1, loop 2, loop 3, and loop 4. The ompA structures were predicted based on the templates of the OmpA-like domain from *Acinetobacter baumannii* (4g4x_A) and the OmpA transmembrane domain from *Escherichia coli* (1qjp) using the HHPRED and MODELLER programs. The domain shown in yellow is the partial C-terminal peptidoglycan-binding domain, and the domain shown in green is the transmembrane ß-barrel N-terminal domain. The model was visualised using the Chimera program

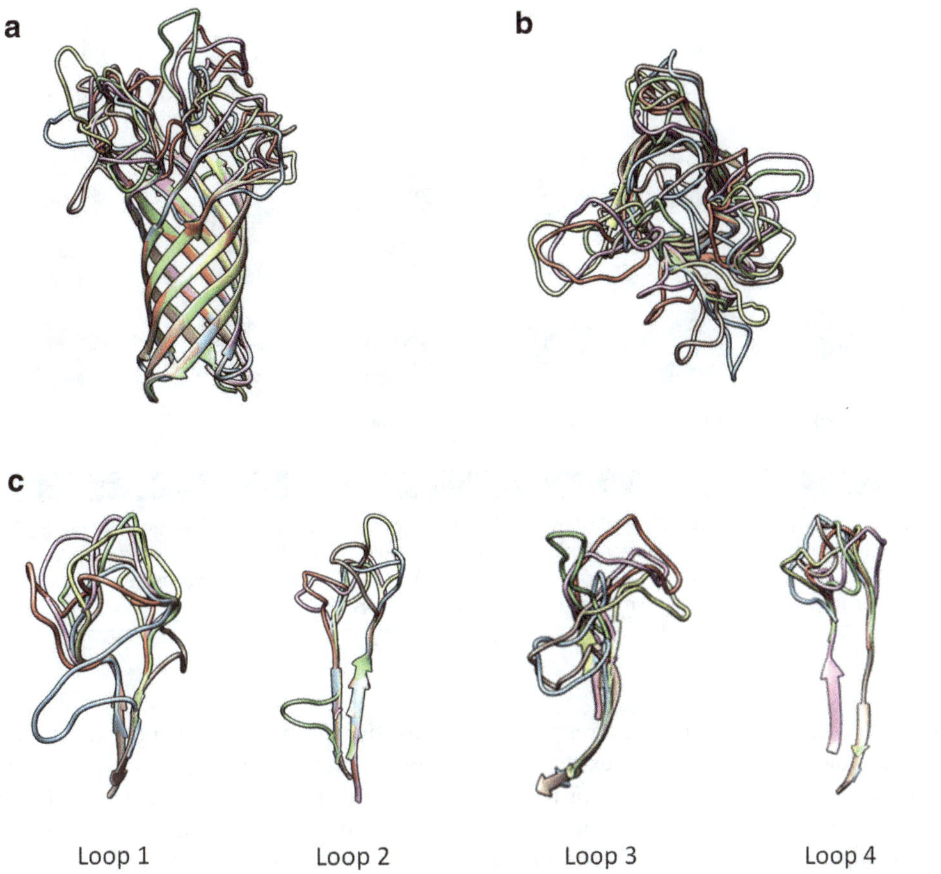

Fig. 5 Comparative structures of the OmpA proteins. Comparative structures of the OmpA proteins from six protein clusters (P1, P2, P3, P4, C1, and C2) according to the protein phylogenetic tree (Fig. 2b) of the OmpA proteins of *P. multocida*. A side view of the conserved transmembrane ß-sheets is shown in **a**, and the four hypervariable loops are shown in the top view (**b**). The individual extracellular loops are compared in **c**. The colours represent different proteins: *orange* indicates isolate 21P, *blue* indicates isolate 32P, *green* indicates isolate 42P, *yellow* indicates isolate 91P, *pink* indicates isolate 34C, and *red* indicates isolate 84C

isolates analysed, which was based mainly on the profiles of eight genes, showed that the profiles of the Thai bovine isolates of *P. multocida* were less diverse than those of the porcine isolates. The results were supported by pulsed-field gel electrophoresis (PFGE) and multilocus sequence typing (MLST) of eight field isolates and one vaccine strain of *P. multocida* associated with HS cases from Thailand [43]. All isolates shared the same MLST sequence type 122 and the same PFGE pattern, whereas the method used in the current study was able to distinguish additional minor groups of the bovine isolates.

The prevalence rates of *tbpA*, *pfhA*, and *hgbB* genes in the bovine isolates are also consistent with the results of a study of Japanese cattle strains that exhibited associations of *tbpA*, *pfhA*, and *hgbB* genes with strains collected from diseased animals rather than healthy ones [32]. The virulence-gene-associated profiles of the porcine isolates were highly diverse and showed clear separation between isolates of capsular types A and D. These isolates were associated with chronic and subchronic pneumonic pasteurellosis that persisted and multiplied for long periods (several generations) within the host's respiratory tract, which could explain why more variations accumulated in these porcine isolates.

PCR amplification of virulence-associated genes *P. multocida* typically uses primers that specifically bind the conserved regions of the virulence-associated genes identified in different isolates of *P. multocida*. This strategy provides a rapid broad scanning of these genes across a large number of isolates, but the results of this method do not provide details on how the genes differ. This study selected the *ompA* gene, which encodes a highly abundant cell-surface-adhesive OMP, for further molecular evolutionary studies. The phylogenetic analyses of the *ompA* gene and its encoded protein conducted in this study confirmed that there is a clear separation between a few clusters of the bovine isolates and more diverse porcine clusters and a distinction between capsular types that is consistent with that

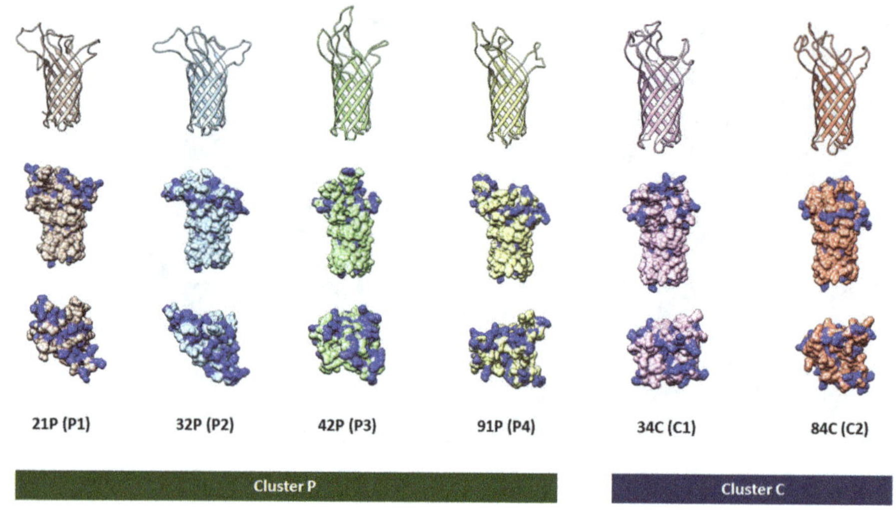

Fig. 6 Surface structures of the predicted OmpA proteins. Predicted structures of the OmpA proteins from six major groups (P1, P2, P3, P4, C1, C2) according to the protein tree (Fig. 2b) of bovine and porcine isolates of *P. multocida* in Thailand. These structures are shown in ribbon (*top*) and surface-view (*middle* and *bottom*) formats. In the surface-view format, the residues highlighted in blue represent charged amino acids. Side and top views of the surface-view format are shown in the middle and bottom rows

previously shown by Verma et al. [40]. The results support the idea that low genetic diversity exists in the clonal population of the bovine isolates of capsular type B in Thailand. This conclusion is consistent with previous studies that compared 16S rRNA genes and found a monophyletic relationship and low genetic diversity of bovine strains of *P. multocida* in the UK [9] and India [44]. Interestingly, two bovine isolates of capsular type A (1C and 12C) collected from water buffaloes and cattle in 1989 and 1995 were grouped within the porcine cluster collected between 2005 and 2009, similar to the gene profiles shown in Fig. 1, suggesting that these bovine isolates were transferred from porcine hosts.

The *ompA* genes displayed a dN/dS ratio of less than one, indicating that these genes are under purifying or stabilising selection that does not allow the genes to change drastically over time, consistent with the calculation by Johnson et al. [11]. The selection pressures on different regions of the *ompA* genes of *P. multocida* were also observed to be unequal based on the fact that the multiple aligned OmpA sequences showed the presence of limited variable regions, a characteristic that could have caused the observed clustering in the protein phylogenetic tree. Mapping the aligned amino acid sequences of the transmembrane domain of the OmpA proteins in this study to the predicted OmpA structures clearly confirmed that the four hypervariable extracellular loops have experienced different selection pressures. Three of these loops were predicted to be more antigenic in the bovine cluster than in the porcine cluster, and these three loops contained more charged residues (positive or negative charges) than other loops, which could determine the specificity of adherence of the bacterium to host cells or to extracellular matrix molecules. These findings suggest that these three extracellular loops are potentially important in host adaptation and that they may play roles in the development of acute HS in cattle and water buffaloes. However, these strong antigenic epitopes might not be necessary for the development of porcine chronic pneumonic pasteurellosis; the adherence function of the loop regions of the OmpA proteins would likely be more important for this prolonged disease. Therefore, the amino acid sequences of these four loops were used to develop the LST scheme through which *P. multocida* strains were directly classified based on the specific sequences of the potential virulence-associated regions of their OmpA proteins.

Evidence for an adherence function of the OmpA protein in *P. multocida* was obtained in this study. OmpA of the bovine strain of *P. multocida* serotype A:3 adheres to heparin, heparin sulphate, type IX collagen, and fibronectin in the extracellular matrix layer of Madin-Darby bovine kidney (MDBK) cells [24, 45]. The OmpA protein preferentially bound to the N-terminal heparin-binding domain of fibronectin [45]. In our study, a heparin-binding site that includes a K/R-X-K/R motif was identified in the second extracellular loop (L2) of the protein (Fig. 4a). This second loop was the most enriched in positively charged amino acids (lysine, arginine, and histidine), accounting for an average of 25% of the loop length. Variations in the amino acid sequence of this loop could indicate certain levels of binding optimisation for specific host cell adherence. Recently, Katoch et al. [46] amplified and sequenced the *ompA* genes of four bovine strains of *P. multocida* (two of capsular type A and two of capsular type B). The authors found two different sequence types of the *ompA* genes that were specific to the strains of capsular types A (allele II) and B (allele I). These differences occurred within the four extracellular loop regions. The authors compared the in vitro and in vivo adhesion and invasion capacities of the two groups of strains and found that the capsular type B group with allele I of the *ompA* gene was more invasive than the other group. Unlike other studies, the current study could also differentiate porcine isolates of capsular types A and D, and bovine isolates of capsular type B based on the protein sequence-based LSTs (not the *ompA* alleles), and the differences in the LSTs could be directly linked to the molecular function of the OmpA protein. These assigned LSTs could potentially be used to determine the virulence of *P. multocida* isolates and further classify other *P. multocida* isolates e.g. bovine and porcine isolates of the same capsular type A. However, in vitro and in vivo assays may be required to confirm these findings.

Conclusions

Molecular variation of the OmpA proteins could be used to classify *P. multocida* isolates into different capsular types, hosts, and, possibly, pathogenicity levels. Taking into account this protein sequence-based typing together with virulence-associated gene profiles will provide a better understanding of *P. multocida* virulence. Effective monitoring and potential strain-specific subunit vaccines could be developed based on these loop oligopeptides.

Methods

Bacterial strains

A total of 191 strains of *Pasteurella multocida* were kindly collected and provided by the National Institute of Animal Health, Department of Livestock, Ministry of Agriculture and Cooperatives, Thailand. These isolates were obtained from clinical cases of pigs, cattle, and water buffaloes in Thailand from 1989 to 2012 (Additional file 2: Table S2). Ninety-two of these isolates were from pneumonic pasteurellosis (70 isolates of capsular type A and 22 isolates of type D) in pigs; the others were HS cases (96 isolates of capsular type B and three isolates of type A) in cattle and water buffaloes. Most of the isolates were collected from lungs (81 samples); some were from hearts (11), livers (9), kidneys (3), lymph nodes (3), tonsils (2), blood (1), and brain (1). However, disease information of 75 isolates was unavailable due to the loss of old data records. All samples were stored at −80 °C. The isolates were plated on blood agar supplemented with 5% inactivated sheep blood and incubated at 37 °C for 24 h.

Genomic DNA extraction from *P. multocida* isolates

Genomic DNA of each sample was prepared by heat treatment. An aliquot of 1 ml of overnight culture in brain-heart infusion broth (BHIB, Oxoid) was centrifuged at 13,000 xg for 5 min and washed in phosphate-buffered saline (PBS). The pellet was resuspended in DNase- and RNase-free distilled water and heated at 100 °C for 5 min. After final centrifugation at the same speed, the supernatant was used for PCR.

Selection of virulence-associated genes of *P. multocida*

Twenty-five virulence-associated genes (*exbB, exbD, fimA, fur, hgbA, hgbB, hsf1, hsf2, nanB, nanH, oma87, ompA, ompH, pfhA, plpB, plpE, pmHAS, psl, ptfA, sodA, sodC, tadD, tbpA, tonB,* and *toxA*) were selected based on previous research [18, 27, 33] and bioinformatics predictions [47]. These genes are involved in nutrient and energy acquisition, cellular transport, adherence, protection from immune attack, biosynthesis of the outer membrane and capsule, and detoxification (Table 1). Primers specific for the candidate genes were selected and modified based on previous work. We confirmed the specificity of the primers using BLASTN searches against an NCBI nucleotide sequence database. Details concerning the selected genes and their corresponding primer pairs are presented in Table 1. The primers were synthesised commercially (Macrogen Co., Ltd., Korea).

PCR amplification of 25 virulence-associated genes

Twenty-five pairs of oligonucleotide primers were used to detect 25 virulence-associated genes from 191 isolates of *P. multocida* associated with disease in pigs, cattle, and water buffaloes in triplicate. One microliter of bacterial genomic DNA was used as a template for each 10-µl PCR mixture containing 1 µl of 10X PCR buffer (Vivantis Technologies Sdn. Bhd., Malaysia), 1 µl of 2 mM dNTPs (Vivantis Technologies Sdn. Bhd., Malaysia), 0.3 µl of 50 mM $MgCl_2$ (Vivantis Technologies Sdn. Bhd., Malaysia), 0.2 µl of 5 U Taq DNA polymerase (Vivantis Technologies Sdn. Bhd., Malaysia), and 0.2 µl of each of 2 µM forward and reverse primers. To hasten the PCR screening process, six virulence-associated genes were detected in two sets of multiplex PCRs: the first set consisted of *omp87, ptfA,* and *sodC,* and the latter set consisted of *fimA, nanB,* and *sodA.* Each multiplex PCR mixture contained 1 µl of genomic DNA, 1 µl of 10X PCR buffer, 1 µl of 2 mM dNTPs, 0.3 µl of 50 mM $MgCl_2$, 0.2 µl (5 U) of Taq DNA polymerase, and 1 µl of each of 2 µM forward and reverse primers in a volume of 10 µl. A negative control for amplification was generated using an equal volume of distilled water instead of the genomic DNA. The PCRs were conducted in the T100™ thermal cycler (Bio-Rad Laboratories, Inc., US). For all PCRs except the PCR for

Table 1 Selected virulence-associated genes and their corresponding primer pairs

No	Gene symbol	Function	Primer name	Primer sequence (5′ → 3′)	Product size (kb)	References
1	*exbB*	Energy transport for iron acquisition	exbB-F exbB-R	TTGGCTTGTGATTGAACGC TGCAGGAATGGCGACTAAA	283	[18]
2	*exbD*	Energy transport for iron acquisition	exbD-F exbD-R	CGTTCTGATTACAGCCTCTT AACGAAATCTTGGAAACTGG	247	[18]
3	*fimA*	Adherence and colonization	fimA-F fimA-R	CCATCGGATCTAAACGACCTA AGTATTAGTTCCTGCGGGTG	806	[18]
4	*fur*	Iron-dependent regulation	fur-F fur-R	GTTTACCGTGTATTAGACCA CATTACTACATTTGCCATAC	244	[18]
5	*hgbA*	Iron acquisition	hgbA-F hgbA-R	TCAACGGCAGATAATCAGGG GCGGGAATGCTGAAGATAAG	268	[18]
6	*hgbB*	Iron acquisition	hgbB-F hgbB-R	ACCGCGTTGGAATTATGATTG CATTGAGTACGGCTTGACAT	768	[33]
7	*hsf1*	Adherence and colonization	hsf1-F hsf1-R	TTGAGTCGGCTGTAGAGTTCG ACTCTTTAGCAGTGGGGACAACCTC	654	[18]
8	*hsf2*	Adherence and colonization	hsf2-F hsf2-R	ACCGCAACCATGCTCTTAC TGACTGACATCGGCGGTAC	430	[18]
9	*nanB*	Nutrition acquisition	nanB-F nanB-R	GTCCTATAAAGTGACGCCGA ACAGCAAAGGAAGACTGTCC	586	[33]
10	*nanH*	Nutrition acquisition	nanH-F nanH-R	GTGGGAACGGGAATTGTGA ACATGCCAAGTTTGCCCTA	287	[18]
11	*oma87*	Outer membrane protein assembly and insertion	oma87-F oma87-R	GGCAGCGAGCAACAGATAACG TGTTCGTCAAATGTCGGGTGA	833	[18]
12	*ompA*	Outer membrane biosynthesis and integrity	ompA-F ompA-R	CGCATAGCACTCAAGTTTCTCC CATAAACAGATTGACCGAAACG	202	[18]
13	*ompH*	Outer membrane general transport	ompH-F ompH-R	CGCGTATGAAGGTTTAGGT TTTAGATTGTGCGTAGTCAAC	452	[18, 33]
14	*pfhA*	Adherence and colonization	pfhA-F pfhA-R	AGCTGATCAAGTGGTGAAC TGGTACATTGGTGAATGCTG	256	[33]
15	*plpB*	Amino acid transport	plpB-F plpB-R	TTTGGTGGTGCGTATGTCTTCT AGTCACTTTAGATTGTGCGTAG	531	[18]
16	*pmHAS*	Capsule biosynthesis	pmHAS-F pmHAS-R	TCAATGTTTGCGATAGTCCGTTAG TGGCGAATGATCGGTGATAGA	430	[18]
17	*psl*	Outer membrane biosynthesis and integrity	psl-F psl-R	TCTGGATCCATGAAAAAACTAACTAAAGTA AAGGATCCTTAGTATGCTAACACAGGACGACG	400	[33]
18	*ptfA*	Adherence and colonization	ptfA-F ptfA-R	TGTGGAATTCAGCATTTTAGTGTGTC TCATGAATTCTTATGCGCAAAATCCT GCTGG	500	[18, 33]
19	*sodA*	Detoxification of radicals	sodA-F soda-R	TACCAGAATTAGGCTACGC GAAACGGGTTGCTGCCGCT	263	[33]
20	*sodC*	Detoxification of radicals	sodC-F sodC-R	AGTTAGTAGCGGGGTTGGCA TGGTGCTGGGTGATCATCATG	237	[33]
21	*tadD*	Adherence and colonization	tadD-F tadD-R	TCTACCCATTCTCAGCAAGGC ATCATTTCGGGCATTCACC	418	[18]
22	*tbpA*	Iron acquisition	tbpA-F tbpA-R	TGCGACAACGGAAATTTCCTC GGACAGTGCATATAACTTGTTTACTA	808	[33]
23	*tonB*	Energy transport for iron acquisition	tonB-F tonB-R	CGACGGTGAAACCTGAGCCA CCGAGCGATAAGCATTGACT	261	[18]
24	*toxA*	Exotoxin	toxA-F toxA-R	CTTAGATGAGCGACAAGGTT GGAATGCCACACCTCTATA	864	[33]
25	*plpE*	Highly immunogenic outer membrane lipoprotein	plpE-F plpE-R	CCATGGGCATGAAACAAATCGTTTTAAA CTCGAGTTGTGCTTGGTGACTTTTTC	1010	[27]

ompH, the following reaction conditions were used: 4 min of initial denaturation at 94 °C; 30 cycles of 30 s denaturation at 94 °C, 30 s annealing at 55 °C, and 1 min extension at 72 °C; and 9 min of final elongation at 72 °C. For the *ompH* PCR, annealing was conducted for 30 s at 57 °C. The amplified products were analysed by electrophoresis on 1.5% agarose gels (Vivantis Technologies Sdn. Bhd., Malaysia), stained with ethidium bromide, and visualised under UV exposure. The appearance of products of the expected sizes was counted as positive identification.

Construction of virulence-associated gene profiles of *P. multocida*

Twenty-five virulence-associated genes were screened in 92 porcine, 89 bovine, and 10 unknown isolates of *P. multocida* in Thailand using gene-specific PCR. The presence/absence of these 25 genes in each isolate was used to define the virulence-associated gene profile. The profiles were constructed by assigning 0 for the absence of the expected band, 1 for the presence of the expected band, and 2 for the presence of the expected band together with other nonspecific bands. The profiles of all isolates were analysed by hierarchical clustering using a complete linkage method with the dist() and hclust() functions in the R program [48]. A dendrogram and a heatmap were constructed using the gplots package to visualise the clustering results. The virulence profiles were analysed in terms of animal host, capsular type, and available disease information.

Nucleotide sequence determination of the *ompA* gene

Primers for amplification of the *ompA* gene were synthesised by Macrogen Co., Ltd., Korea. The gene was amplified using Taq DNA polymerase (PrimeSTAR GXL DNA Polymerase, Takara Bio. Inc., Japan) with the forward (OMPA-F, 5′-AGGATCCATGAAAAAAACAGCAATT GCATTGA-3′) and reverse (OMPA-R, 5′-TCTCGAGT TATTTGTTACCTTTAACAGCGATTTC-3′) primers; the sequences of these primers were modified from Gao et al. [49]. The PCRs contained 5 μl of 50 ng/μl genomic DNA, 10 μl of 5X PCR buffer, 5 μl of 2 mM dNTPs, 1 μl (5 U) of Taq DNA polymerase, and 5 μl of each of 2 μM forward and reverse primers in a total volume of 50 μl. The reaction mixtures were incubated for 30 cycles consisting of initial denaturation at 98 °C for 3 min; denaturation at 98 °C for 10 s, annealing at 55 °C for 15 s, extension at 68 °C for 1 min; and final extension at 68 °C for 3 min. The PCR products were purified using a GF-1 Ambiclean kit (Vivantis Technologies Sdn. Bhd., Malaysia), and the cleaned products were subjected to sequencing with both primers using an Applied Biosystems automatic sequencer (ABI 3730XL) (Macrogen Co., Ltd., Korea). The sequence chromatograms were checked for quality, and the *ompA* sequences were confirmed using the BLASTN program.

Sequence alignment and phylogenetic analysis of the *ompA* gene

The nucleotide sequences of the *ompA* gene were edited, trimmed, and aligned using BioEdit version 7.1.8 [50] and ClustalW in the MEGA 6 program [51]. Noise and low-quality signals were further removed using in-house-written R scripts. Phylogenetic analyses of the edited nucleotide sequences were conducted using the MEGA 6 program. Phylogenetic trees of the *ompA* gene were constructed based on the neighbour-joining model with the p-distance method and a thousand-replicate bootstrap analysis in the MEGA 6 program. The analysis also included the *ompA* nucleotide sequences of *P. multocida* deposited in the NCBI nucleotide database (http://www.ncbi.nlm.nih.gov/genbank/). A phylogenetic tree was constructed, and all isolates were assigned to clusters. The aligned sequences were then analysed using the MEGA 6 and SNAP [52] programs to estimate the numbers of synonymous (dS) and nonsynonymous (dN) substitutions per residue in the gene. The ratio of nonsynonymous to synonymous nucleotide substitutions (dN/dS ratio) is a measure of selection pressure. Maximum likelihood analysis of natural selection was also computed for each codon.

Protein sequence analysis and structural prediction of the OmpA protein

The nucleotide sequences of the *ompA* gene were translated using the ExPASy translation tool (http://web.expasy.org/translate/). The amino acid sequences were trimmed and edited using in-house-written R scripts and then aligned to identify conserved and variable regions using ClustalW. These regions were summarised using the WebLogo program [53]. A protein phylogenetic tree was constructed based on the neighbour-joining model with the Poisson correction method and a thousand-replicate bootstrap using the MEGA 6 program. The proteins were then assigned to clusters. A representative OmpA protein from an individual cluster in the protein phylogenetic tree was subjected to homology modelling using the HHPred and MODELLER programs [54] and was visualised using the Chimera [55] program. The OmpA structure essentially consists of two domains: a globular C-terminal peptidoglycan-binding domain and a transmembrane ß-barrel N-terminal domain. The transmembrane domain was composed of eight antiparallel ß-sheets interspersed with four short periplasmic turns and four long extracellular loops [56]. The predicted OmpA transmembrane domains were extracted for the next step in the analysis.

Development of protein-sequence-based OmpA typing schemes

The conserved and variable regions of the candidate OmpA sequences were mapped onto their corresponding predicted structures by structural superimposition and were compared using the Chimera program. Four extracellular loops and transmembrane ß-sheets of the OmpA transmembrane domain were cleaved at equal lengths across all isolates using R scripts. The amino acid sequences of the variable substructures were multiply aligned using ClustalW, and the unique sequences were assigned subsequence types by the R scripts. The protein sequence-based OmpA typing schemes were a combination of subsequence types (X_1, Y_1, Z_1, ...), where X_1, Y_1, and Z_1 are subsequence type 1 of substructures X, Y, and Z used to represent each isolate of *P. multocida*. Finally, the sequences of these substructures were submitted for prediction of antigenic peptides by comparison with experimentally known peptide epitopes [57].

Additional files

Additional file 1: Table S1. Clustering summary of 186 bovine and porcine isolates of *P. multocida* collected from Thailand and 41 strains from the NCBI database. Three clustering methods were shown including nucleotide and protein phylogenetic analyses, and the OmpA protein sequence-based typing using four extracellular loop sequence types (LSTs) of the transmembrane domain. The LST types in the last column were created by the combination of different types of the four extracellular loops 1, 2, 3, and 4. DNA and protein cluster codes correlated with those in Fig. 2a and b.

Additional file 2: Table S2. Information of 191 *P. multocida* isolates associated with diseased pigs, cattle and water buffaloes in Thailand collected from 1989 to 2012. These isolates were collected and maintained by the National Institute of Animal Health, Department of Livestock, Ministry of Agriculture and Cooperatives. Each isolate was named with two-letter code.

Abbreviations

HS: Haemorrhagic septicaemia; LST: Loop sequence type; OmpA: Outer membrane protein A; PAR: Progressive atrophic rhinitis; PCR: Polymerase chain reaction

Acknowledgements

The authors would like to acknowledge the members of the Laboratory of Bacteriology and Mycology, National Institute of Animal Health, Department of Livestock, Ministry of Agriculture and Cooperatives, Thailand for providing bacterial isolates, a biosafety laboratory, equipment, comments, and other support.

Funding

This research project was supported by the Thailand Research Fund (grant no. MRG5680082) and by the Preproposal Research Fund (PRF) from the Faculty of Science, Kasetsart University, Thailand.

Authors' contributions

TE planned the experiments, analysed the results, and prepared the manuscript. RL and SP conducted the PCR screening of the virulence-associated genes. PA conducted the PCR and nucleotide sequencing of the *ompA* gene. PT and AT participated in the study design, discussed the results, and provided comments. All authors approved the final manuscript.

Consent for publication

Not applicable.

Competing interests

The authors declare that they have no competing interests.

Author details

[1]Department of Genetics, Faculty of Science, Kasetsart University, 50, Ngam Wong Wan Rd, Lad Yao, Chatuchak, Bangkok 10900, Thailand. [2]Bioinformatics and Systems Biology Unit, Computational Biomodelling Laboratory for Agricultural Science and Technology (CBLAST), Faculty of Science, Kasetsart University, 50 Ngam Wong Wan Rd, Lat Yao, Chatuchak, Bangkok 10900, Thailand. [3]Laboratory of Bacteriology and Mycology, National Institute of Animal Health, Department of Livestock, Ministry of Agriculture and Cooperatives, 50/2 Kasetklang, Lad Yao, Chatuchak, Bangkok 10900, Thailand.

References

1. Wilson BA, Ho M. *Pasteurella multocida*: from zoonosis to cellular microbiology. Clin Microbiol Rev. 2013;26(3):631–55.
2. Harper M, Boyce JD, Adler B. *Pasteurella multocida* pathogenesis: 125 years after Pasteur. FEMS Microbiol Lett. 2006;265(1):1–10.
3. Carter GR. Pasteurellosis: *Pasteurella multocida* and *Pasteurella hemolytica*. Adv Vet Sci. 1967;11:321–79.
4. Hunt ML, Adler B, Townsend KM. The molecular biology of *Pasteurella multocida*. Vet Microbiol. 2000;72(1–2):3–25.
5. Davies RL. Genetic diversity among *Pasteurella multocida* strains of avian, bovine, ovine and porcine origin from England and Wales by comparative sequence analysis of the 16S rRNA gene. Microbiology. 2004;150(12):4199–210.
6. Davies RL, Caffrey B, Watson PJ. Comparative analyses of *Pasteurella multocida* strains associated with the ovine respiratory and vaginal tracts. Vet Rec. 2003; 152(1):7–10.
7. Davies RL, MacCorquodale R, Baillie S, Caffrey B. Characterization and comparison of *Pasteurella multocida* strains associated with porcine pneumonia and atrophic rhinitis. J Med Microbiol. 2003;52(1):59–67.
8. Davies RL, MacCorquodale R, Caffrey B. Diversity of avian *Pasteurella multocida* strains based on capsular PCR typing and variation of the OmpA and OmpH outer membrane proteins. Vet Microbiol. 2003;91(2–3):169–82.
9. Davies RL, MacCorquodale R, Reilly S. Characterisation of bovine strains of *Pasteurella multocida* and comparison with isolates of avian, ovine and porcine origin. Vet Microbiol. 2004;99(2):145–58.
10. Du H, Fang R, Pan T, Li T, Li N, He Q, Wu R, Peng Y, Zhou Z. Comparative genomics analysis of two different virulent bovine *Pasteurella multocida* isolates. Int J Genomics. 2016;2016:4512493.
11. Johnson TJ, Abrahante JE, Hunter SS, Hauglund M, Tatum FM, Maheswaran SK, Briggs RE. Comparative genome analysis of an avirulent and two virulent strains of avian *Pasteurella multocida* reveals candidate genes involved in fitness and pathogenicity. BMC Microbiol. 2013;13:106.
12. Yu C, Sizhu S, Luo Q, Xu X, Fu L, Zhang A. Genome sequencing of a virulent avian *Pasteurella multocida* strain GX-pm reveals the candidate genes involved in the pathogenesis. Res Vet Sci. 2016;105:23–7.
13. Adler B, Bulach D, Chung J, Doughty S, Hunt M, Rajakumar K, Serrano M, van Zanden A, Zhang Y, Ruffolo C. Candidate vaccine antigens and genes in *Pasteurella multocida*. J Biotechnol. 1999;73(2–3):83–90.
14. Hatfaludi T, Al-Hasani K, Boyce JD, Adler B. Outer membrane proteins of *Pasteurella multocida*. Vet Microbiol. 2010;144(1–2):1–17.
15. Bosch M, Garrido E, Llagostera M, Pérez de Rozas AM, Badiola I, Barbé J. *Pasteurella multocida exbB*, *exbD* and *tonB* genes are physically linked but independently transcribed. FEMS Microbiol Lett. 2002;210(2): 201–8.
16. Ratledge C, Dover LG. Iron metabolism in pathogenic bacteria. Annu Rev Microbiol. 2000;54(1):881–941.
17. Ruffolo CG, Tennent JM, Michalski WP, Adler B. Identification, purification, and characterization of the type 4 fimbriae of *Pasteurella multocida*. Infect Immun. 1997;65(1):339–43.
18. Tang X, Zhao Z, Hu J, Wu B, Cai X, He Q, Chen H. Isolation, antimicrobial resistance, and virulence genes of *Pasteurella multocida* strains from swine in China. J Clin Microbiol. 2009;47(4):951–8.
19. Tomich M, Planet PJ, Figurski DH. The tad locus: postcards from the widespread colonization island. Nat Rev Microbiol. 2007;5(5):363–75.
20. Mizan S, Henk A, Stallings A, Maier M, Lee MD. Cloning and characterization of sialidases with 2-6′ and 2-3′ sialyl lactose specificity from *Pasteurella multocida*. J Bacteriol. 2000;182(24):6874–83.
21. Luo Y, Glisson JR, Jackwood MW, Hancock RE, Bains M, Cheng IH, Wang C. Cloning and characterization of the major outer membrane protein gene (ompH) of *Pasteurella multocida* X-73. J Bacteriol. 1997;179(24):7856–64.

22. Kroll JS, Langford PR, Wilks KE, Keil AD. Bacterial [Cu,Zn]-superoxide dismutase : phylogenetically distinct from the eukaryotic enzyme, and not so rare after all! Microbiology. 1995;141(9):2271–9.
23. Noinaj N, Kuszak AJ, Gumbart JC, Lukacik P, Chang H, Easley NC, Lithgow T, Buchanan SK. Structural insight into the biogenesis of β-barrel membrane proteins. Nature. 2013;501(7467):385–90.
24. Dabo SM, Confer AW, Quijano-Blas RA. Molecular and immunological characterization of *Pasteurella multocida* serotype a:3 OmpA: evidence of its role in *P. multocida* interaction with extracellular matrix molecules. Microb Pathog. 2003;35(4):147–57.
25. Wei X, Wang Y, Luo R, Qian W, Sizhu S, Zhou H. Identification and characterization of a protective antigen, PlpB of bovine *Pasteurella multocida* strain LZ-PM. Dev Comp Immunol. 2017;71:1–7.
26. Kasten RW, Hansen LM, Hinojoza J, Bieber D, Ruehl WW, Hirsh DC. *Pasteurella multocida* produces a protein with homology to the P6 outer membrane protein of *Haemophilus influenzae*. Infect Immun. 1995;63(3):989–93.
27. Singh AP, Singh S, Ranjan R, Gupta SK, Singh VP, Sharma B. Molecular heterogeneity of plpE gene in Indian isolates of *Pasteurella multocida* and expression of recombinant PlpE in vaccine strain of *P. multocida* serotype B: 2. J Vet Sci. 2010;11(3):227–33.
28. Li N, Long Q, Du H, Zhang J, Pan T, Wu C, Lei G, Peng Y, Hardwidge PR. High and low-virulent bovine *Pasteurella multocida* capsular type a isolates exhibit different virulence gene expression patterns in vitro and in vivo. Vet Microbiol. 2016;196:44–9.
29. Furian TQ, Borges KA, Rocha SLS, Rodrigues EE. Nascimento VPd, Salle CTP, Moraes HLS: detection of virulence-associated genes of *Pasteurella multocida* isolated from cases of fowl cholera by multiplex-PCR. Pesquisa Vet Brasil. 2013;33:177–82.
30. Khamesipour F, Momtaz H, Mamoreh MA. Occurrence of virulence factors and antimicrobial resistance in *Pasteurella multocida* strains isolated from slaughter cattle in Iran. Front Microbiol. 2014;5:536.
31. Ferreira TS, Felizardo MR, Sena de Gobbi DD, Gomes CR, Nogueira Filsner PH, Moreno M, Paixao R, Pereira Jde J, Micke Moreno A. Virulence genes and antimicrobial resistance profiles of *Pasteurella multocida* strains isolated from rabbits in Brazil. ScientificWorldJournal. 2012;2012:685028.
32. Katsuda K, Hoshinoo K, Ueno Y, Kohmoto M, Mikami O. Virulence genes and antimicrobial susceptibility in *Pasteurella multocida* isolates from calves. Vet Microbiol. 2013;167(3–4):737–41.
33. Ewers C, Lübke-Becker A, Bethe A, Kießling S, Filter M, Wieler LH. Virulence genotype of *Pasteurella multocida* strains isolated from different hosts with various disease status. Vet Microbiol. 2006;114(3–4):304–17.
34. Wu JR, Shien JH, Shieh HK, Chen CF, Chang PC. Protective immunity conferred by recombinant *Pasteurella multocida* lipoprotein E (PlpE). Vaccine. 2007;25(21):4140–8.
35. Chomnawang MT, Nabnuengsap J, Kittiworakarn J, Pathanasophon P. Expression and immunoprotective property of a 39-kDa PlpB protein of *Pasteurella multocida*. J Vet Med Sci. 2009;71(11):1479–85.
36. Hatfaludi T, Al-Hasani K, Gong L, Boyce JD, Ford M, Wilkie IW, Quinsey N, Dunstone MA, Hoke DE, Adler B. Screening of 71 *P. multocida* proteins for protective efficacy in a fowl cholera infection model and characterization of the protective antigen PlpE. PLOS ONE. 2012;7(7):e39973.
37. Thanasarasakulpong A, Poolperm P, Tankaew P, Sawada T, Sthitmatee N. Protectivity conferred by immunization with intranasal recombinant outer membrane protein H from *Pasteurella multocida* serovar a:1 in chickens. J Vet Med Sci. 2015;77(3):321–6.
38. Shivachandra SB, Yogisharadhya R, Kumar A, Mohanty NN, Nagaleekar VK. Recombinant transferrin binding protein a (rTbpA) fragments of *Pasteurella multocida* serogroup B:2 provide variable protection following homologous challenge in mouse model. Res Vet Sci. 2015;98:1–6.
39. Kumar A, Yogisharadhya R, Ramakrishnan MA, Viswas KN, Shivachandra SB. Structural analysis and cross-protective efficacy of recombinant 87 kDa outer membrane protein (Omp87) of *Pasteurella multocida* serogroup B:2. Microb Pathog. 2013;65:48–56.
40. Verma S, Salwan R, Katoch S, Verma L, Chahota R, Dhar P, Sharma M. The relationship between capsular type and OmpA of *Pasteurella multocida* is associated with the outcome of disease. Microb Pathog. 2016;101:68–75.
41. Nefedchenko AV, Glotova TI, Glotov AG, Ternovoy VA, Sementsova AO. Prevalence of different OmpH-types among *Pasteurella multocida* isolated from lungs of calves with respiratory problems. Microb Pathog. 2017;104:184–9.
42. Verma S, Sharma M, Katoch S, Verma L, Kumar S, Dogra V, Chahota R, Dhar P, Singh G. Profiling of virulence associated genes of *Pasteurella multocida* isolated from cattle. Vet Res Commun. 2013;37(1):83–9.
43. Moustafa AM, Bennett MD, Edwards J, Azim K, Mesaik MA, Choudhary MI, Pathanasophon P, Worarach A, Ali Q, Abubakar M, et al. Molecular typing of haemorrhagic septicaemia-associated *Pasteurella multocida* isolates from Pakistan and Thailand using multilocus sequence typing and pulsed-field gel electrophoresis. Res Vet Sci. 2013;95(3):986–90.
44. Dey S, Singh VP, Kumar AA, Sharma B, Srivastava SK, Singh N. Comparative sequence analysis of 16S rRNA gene of *Pasteurella multocida* serogroup B isolates from different animal species. Res Vet Sci. 2007;83(1):1–4.
45. Dabo SM, Confer AW, Hartson SD. Adherence of *Pasteurella multocida* to fibronectin. Vet Microbiol. 2005;110(3–4):265–75.
46. Katoch S, Sharma M, Patil RD, Kumar S, Verma S. In vitro and in vivo pathogenicity studies of *Pasteurella multocida* strains harbouring different ompA. Vet Res Commun. 2014;38(3):183–91.
47. E-komon T, Burchmore R, Herzyk P, Davies R. Predicting the outer membrane proteome of *Pasteurella multocida* based on consensus prediction enhanced by results integration and manual confirmation. BMC bioinformatics. 2012;13:63.
48. Team RDC. R: a language and environment for statistical computing. In. Vienna, Austria: R Foundation for Statistical Computing; 2010.
49. Gao M-y, Xyu B, Gong J-s, Wang X, Fan J-h, Liu X-x: cloning and sequence analysis of OmpA gene of 11 avian *Pasteurella multocida* strains. Acta Agr Zhejiangensis 2013, 25(5):0–956.
50. Hall T. BioEdit: an important software for molecular biology. GERF Bull Biosci. 2011;2(1):60–1.
51. Tamura K, Stecher G, Peterson D, Filipski A, Kumar S. MEGA6: molecular evolutionary genetics analysis version 6.0. Mol Biol Evol. 2013;30(12):2725–9.
52. Ota T, Nei M. Variance and covariances of the numbers of synonymous and nonsynonymous substitutions per site. Mol Biol Evol. 1994;11(4):613–9.
53. Crooks GE, Hon G, Chandonia JM, Brenner SE. WebLogo: a sequence logo generator. Genome Res. 2004;14(6):1188–90.
54. Soding J, Biegert A, Lupas AN. The HHpred interactive server for protein homology detection and structure prediction. Nucleic Acids Res. 2005; 33(Web Server issue):W244–8.
55. Pettersen EF, Goddard TD, Huang CC, Couch GS, Greenblatt DM, Meng EC, Ferrin TE. UCSF chimera–a visualization system for exploratory research and analysis. J Comput Chem. 2004;25(13):1605–12.
56. Carpenter T, Khalid S, Sansom MSP. A multidomain outer membrane protein from *Pasteurella multocida*: modelling and simulation studies of PmOmpA. BBA - Biomembranes. 2007;1768(11):2831–40.
57. Kolaskar AS, Tongaonkar PC. A semi-empirical method for prediction of antigenic determinants on protein antigens. FEBS Lett. 1990;276(1–2):172–4.

14

Determination of N-acylhomoserine lactones of *Pseudomonas aeruginosa* in clinical samples from dogs with otitis externa

Darja Kušar*, Karin Šrimpf, Petra Isaković, Lina Kalšek, Javid Hosseini, Irena Zdovc, Tina Kotnik, Modest Vengušt and Gabrijela Tavčar-Kalcher

Abstract

Background: Bacterial intercellular communication, called quorum sensing, takes place via the production and collective response to signal molecules. In Gram-negative bacteria, like *Pseudomonas aeruginosa*, these signaling molecules are N-acylhomoserine lactones (AHLs). *P. aeruginosa* is a common cause of inflammation of the ear canal (otitis externa) in dogs. It employs quorum sensing to coordinate the expression of host tissue-damaging factors, which are largely responsible for its virulence. The treatment of *P. aeruginosa*-associated otitis is challenging due to a high intrinsic resistance of *P. aeruginosa* to several antibiotics.

Attenuation of quorum sensing signals to inhibit bacterial virulence is a novel strategy for the treatment of resistant bacterial pathogens, including *P. aeruginosa*. Therefore, it is important to recognize and define quorum sensing signal molecules in clinical samples. To date, there are no reports on determination of AHLs in the veterinary clinical samples. The purpose of this study was to validate an analytical procedure for determination of the concentration of AHLs in the ear rinses from dogs with *P. aeruginosa*-associated otitis externa.

Samples were obtained with rinsing the ear canals with physiological saline solution. For validation, samples from healthy dogs were spiked with none or different known amounts of the selected AHLs. With the validated procedure, AHLs were analyzed in the samples taken in weekly intervals from two dogs, receiving a standard treatment for *P. aeruginosa*-associated otitis externa.

Results: Validation proved that the procedure enables quantification of AHLs in non-clinical and clinical samples. In addition, a time dependent reduction of AHL concentration was detected for the treated dogs.

Conclusions: Our results indicate that liquid chromatography coupled with tandem mass spectrometry (LC-MS/MS) is superior in detecting AHLs compared to other chromatographic techniques. This is the first report on determination of AHLs in the clinical samples of veterinary importance. The analytical procedure described in this paper is capable of supporting novel antimicrobial strategies, which target quorum sensing.

Keywords: Dogs, Otitis externa, Clinical samples, *Pseudomonas aeruginosa*, Quorum sensing, N-acylhomoserine lactones, Liquid chromatography-tandem mass spectrometry, Validation

* Correspondence: darja.kusar@vf.uni-lj.si
Veterinary Faculty, University of Ljubljana, Gerbičeva 60SI-1115, Ljubljana, Slovenia

Background

Pseudomonas aeruginosa is an important opportunistic pathogen of humans and animals, causing severe infections when the immune system is compromised [1, 2], or after long-lasting antibiotic treatments, injuries and medical procedures [3, 4]. *P. aeruginosa* is a Gram-negative bacterium ubiquitously present in the water and soil. It is naturally resistant to penicillin and amino-penicillins, and to the first and second generations of cephalosporins. It is usually susceptible to aminoglycosides, fluoroquinolones, lipopeptides, ureidopenicillins, carboxypenicillins, carbapenems, and cephalosporins of the third generation [5]. The resistance of *P. aeruginosa*, however, can rapidly develop against any antibiotic [5].

Behavior of bacteria is coordinated, at the level of microbial community, by their gene expression at the intra-species level or less commonly between species. Such coordination of communal behavior is controlled through the production and detection of signal molecules or autoinducers, which is called quorum sensing (QS) [6–10]. The QS system defines the expression of various bacterial phenotypes, depending on the local density of bacterial population, including the virulence factors, biofilm formation and resistance to antibiotics [11]. It is associated with pathogenesis of various diseases in humans and animals, and has a clinically evident effect in human cystic fibrosis (CF) [12], endocarditis and osteomyelitis in rabbits [13, 14], bovine mastitis [15], gastrointestinal diseases [9], and ear canal infections, dermatitis and other secondary infections in dogs [16].

The secondary factors, including *Malassezia* spp. (yeasts), and bacteria of the genera *Staphylococcus*, *Proteus*, *Streptococcus* and *Pseudomonas*, often cause complications to the inflammation of the ear canal (otitis externa, OE) in dogs [17, 18]. Involvement of *P. aeruginosa* in OE (*P. aeruginosa*-associated OE, *Pa*OE) increases the morbidity, prolongs the treatment, and reduces the possibility of a favorable outcome [19, 20]. The ability of *P. aeruginosa* to produce biofilms and synchronize its virulence through QS is very important for the conservation and/or perpetuation of infection [21]. The long and narrow ear canal of dogs represents a very suitable environment for *P. aeruginosa* colonization and the subsequent activation of its QS [7].

One or several signal molecules may be involved in QS. In Gram-negative bacteria, the most common are N-acylhomoserine lactones (AHLs or AI-1) [9, 10, 22, 23]. *P. aeruginosa* QS system shows a hierarchical arrangement with *las* system controlling *rhl* [6–8, 24–28]. It mainly produces N-(3-oxododecanoyl)-L-homoserine lactone (3-oxo-C12-HSL) and N-butanoyl-L-homoserine lactone (C4-HSL), whereas production of N-hexanoyl-L-homoserine lactone (C6-HSL) and shorter 3-oxo-HSLs (3-oxo-C6-HSL, 3-oxo-C8-HSL and 3-oxo-C10-HSL) is less abundant [29, 30]. It was shown that 3-oxo-C12-HSL has the most critical role, as it regulates the expression of several genes involved in activation of the subordinate *rhl* system, where C4-HSL is the most significant autoinducing molecule [6]. In addition to its signalling function, 3-oxo-C12-HSL also exerts antibacterial activities against some other pathogens [31] and a direct immunomodulatory effect on the mammal host [32], itself functioning as a virulence determinant [33] and contributing to the establishment of chronic infections [34]. Under some growth conditions, activation of the *las* system does not precede the activation of *rhl*, but just the opposite, indicating the environmental dependence of their hierarchy [35]. There are various layers of sophistication to *P. aeruginosa* AHL-dependent QS [34, 36] and approximately 10 % of *P. aeruginosa* genome is directly or indirectly regulated by this multi-signal QS system [37]. Some genes are *las* specific, some *rhl*, and others respond to both 3-oxo-C12-HSL and C4-HSL [37]. In addition, at least four QS signalling mechanisms were reported to comprise *P. aeruginosa* QS network, being modulated in accordance to the environmental cues, also of host origin, influencing the virulence phenotypes of *P. aeruginosa* [36].

Detection of signal molecules associated with QS could serve as an indicator for the severity of infection, success of a treatment, and to estimate the outcome of disease [22]. Disruption of QS, called quorum quenching (QQ) [38], could represent a therapeutic tool, complementing or substituting the antibiotic treatment, which would reduce the risk for the development of antibiotic resistance [39]. It was shown that QQ can be achieved through the enzymatic destruction of QS signals, development of antibodies to QS signal molecules, or via agents which block QS [40]. The inhibitors of QS would reduce bacterial pathogenicity, also by increasing the susceptibility of existing biofilms to antibiotics or phagocytosis, and increase effectiveness of the host immune system [39, 41, 42]. Identifying molecules involved in QS in the clinical samples is, therefore, of great importance.

Several reports describing chemical analytical methods for the identification and quantification of selected AHLs are available. The use of a thin layer chromatography [7, 12]; gas chromatography with mass spectrometry (GC-MS) [43, 44]; high-performance liquid chromatography (HPLC) with UV detection [6], mass spectrometry (MS) [12], or coupled with tandem MS (MS/MS) [22, 45]; nuclear magnetic resonance (NMR) [26]; and colorimetry [46] was reported. In addition, a bacterial biosensor system for the detection of AHLs was also described [9]. Although a number of analytical methods were developed, only a few are applicable for determination of low AHL concentrations in clinical samples [22]. Determination of AHLs in physiological samples or complex biological matrices is more complicated than in bacterial culture supernatants due to the interference from matrix, causing most of the analytical problems [7, 9, 12, 22]. The mechanisms behind this phenomenon, commonly referred to as matrix effects and leading to signal suppression or enhancement, are still under investigation due to the great variety of available matrices and the unpredictable effect they might have on the final result [47]. Hence, data defining pathophysiological concentrations of AHLs in the clinical samples have not been often reported. In picomolar to micromolar concentrations, AHLs were discovered in the sputum [7, 12], mucopurulent secretions of respiratory tract [48], lung tissue of patients with CF [49], and saliva and faeces of individuals with gastrointestinal disorders [22]. To the best of our knowledge, no reports were published regarding detection of QS signal molecules in veterinary clinical samples.

In the present work, the analytical procedure for determination of AHLs of *P. aeruginosa* from canine OE clinical samples was introduced and validated. It consisted of the extraction of AHLs (3-oxo-C12-HSL, C4-HSL and C6-HSL) from the ear rinses and their quantification using the liquid chromatography with tandem mass spectrometry (LC-MS/MS).

Methods

Reagents

Solid standard substances C4-HSL, C6-HSL and 3-oxo-C12-HSL with certified purity of 97 % (Sigma-Aldrich, St. Louis, MO, USA) were used. Stock standard solutions of individual AHLs with the concentration of 1 mg/ml (C4-HSL, C6-HSL) and 0.91 mg/ml (3-oxo-C12-HSL) were prepared in methanol. Mixed working standard solutions for preparing the calibration curve containing all the three selected AHL signal molecules, each at the concentration from approx. 1 to 60 ng/ml, were prepared in a mixture of methanol and deionized water (35 + 65). Dichloromethane used for the extraction of AHLs and methanol used for the mobile phase were of analytical and chromatography grade purity, respectively (Merck, Darmstadt, Germany). As the mobile phase, a gradient mixing of methanol and deionized water containing 0.1 % formic acid (Merck) was used. For the rinsing of canine ear canals, saline solution (0.9 % NaCl) was employed.

Sample collection and preparation

Samples were obtained by rinsing the ear canals of dogs with saline solution (30 ml). The collected samples were adjusted to the final volume of 30 ml by sterile saline, centrifuged at 3100 × g for 30 min at 4 °C, and the supernatants were stored at −80 °C till extraction.

For validation, the ear rinses from healthy dogs spiked with known amounts of C4-HSL, C6-HSL and 3-oxo-C12-HSL were used. None of the samples contained AHLs in detectable concentrations prior to spiking. An aliquot of 0.320 ml of the mixed working standard solution containing AHLs in concentrations of approx. 60 ng/ml (61.5 ng/ml of C4-HSL and C6-HSL, 56.9 ng/ml of 3-oxo-C12-HSL) was added to 10 ml of the supernatant, giving the final concentrations of approx. 2 ng/ml (1.97 ng/ml of C4-HSL and C6-HSL, 1.82 ng/ml of 3-oxo-C12-HSL). Thus, a 10-ml sample contained approx. 20 ng of each AHL (19.7 ng of C4-HSL and C6-HSL, 18.2 ng of 3-oxo-C12-HSL).

To test the validated analytical procedure with clinical samples, the ear rinses of two *Pa*OE dogs, collected weekly during the treatment, were used. Samples were taken during a scheduled veterinary checkup at the primary clinic or at the university clinic. As a control, the ear rinse from a healthy dog was employed.

Analytical procedure

For the extraction of AHLs from the ear rinses, a procedure used for determination of AHLs in sputum [7, 12] was modified. One third (10 ml) of a 30-ml sample was extracted three times with 10-ml portions of dichloromethane. The combined extracts were evaporated to dryness at 60 °C using the vacuum evaporator (Syncore Reactor R-48, Büchi, Flawil, Switzerland). The residue was dissolved in 1 ml of the mixture of methanol and deionized water (35 + 65).

The particular AHLs were determined by LC-MS/MS at conditions described elsewhere [22, 45]. In brief, elution of the column was performed with a mixture of methanol–water. The mixing was isocratic for 4 min (35 % methanol, 65 % deionized water), followed by a linear gradient of methanol concentration from 35 to 95 % in 4 min and then back to 35 % in 1 min. The following 2 min, the column was washed again with the mixture of methanol and water (35 + 65). The mobile phase flow rate was 0.25 ml/min, injection volume 10 µl, and column temperature 30 °C. Detection with MS was performed in the positive ion mode. Voltage at the capillary was 0.4 kV. The monitored ions and other parameters are given in Table 1. Measurements were performed with the liquid chromatography system Acquity (Waters, Milford, MA, USA) equipped with an analytical column ZORBAX Eclipse C18, Rapid Resolution HD, 1.8 µm, 2.1 × 100 mm (Agilent, Santa Clara, CA, USA) and mass selective detector Xevo TQ MS (Waters).

Validation procedure

To perform the linearity test, and to determine the limit of detection (LOD) and the limit of quantification (LOQ), the mixed working standard solutions of AHLs

Table 1 LC-MS/MS parameters

AHL	Retention time [min]	Precursor ion m/z[a]	Product ion m/z[a]	Cone voltage [V]	Collision cell voltage [V]
C4-HSL	1.99	172.096	101.980	18	10
		172.096	144.073	18	8
C6-HSL	4.76 (4.77)	200.160	101.984	18	10
		200.160	98.986	18	6
3-oxo-C12-HSL	9.16	298.266	102.038	26	12
		298.266	197.138	26	14

[a]m/z: mass-to-charge ratio

at concentrations from approx. 1 to 60 ng/ml were used, corresponding to AHL concentrations of approx. 0.1 to 6 ng/ml in the ear rinses. The estimation of LOD and LOQ was based on visual evaluation, testing concentrations in the target range expected for AHLs in clinical samples. The LOQ estimate was defined as the lowest amount or concentration of an analyte that is reasonably achievable according to the target range and should be regarded as the reporting limit; LOD was estimated as one third (30 %) of LOQ [50].

The repeatability of results was tested by analyzing five replicates of the ear rinse sample with the addition of C4-HSL, C6-HSL and 3-oxo-C12-HSL at 1.97 ng/ml (C4-HSL, C6-HSL) and 1.82 ng/ml (3-oxo-C12-HSL). The analyses were performed at the same day and by the same operator. For testing the within-laboratory reproducibility, five replicates of the sample were prepared for two more times by two operators at two different days. The results obtained from these experiments were also used for determination of the recovery.

Statistical procedures

The mean ($\overline{x}$) for each AHL was calculated. The repeatability and the within-laboratory reproducibility were expressed by standard deviation (s_r and s_R, respectively) and relative standard deviation (RSD_r and RSD_R, respectively). The RSD_R values were compared to the values calculated from the Horwitz equation ($RSD = 2^{(1-0.5 \log C)}$), taken as a reference. The recovery was calculated according to the equation $rec(\%) = 100\frac{\overline{x}}{a}$, where a represents the spiked concentration of the analyte in the sample [50, 51].

Culture examination

Prior to rinsing the ears of *Pa*OE affected dogs with sterile saline, cotton-swab samples were taken from the ears for bacteriological examination. Samples were inoculated onto blood agar plates (Columbia agar; Oxoid LTD, Basingstoke, Hampshire, England) supplemented with 5 % sheep blood and incubated aerobically at 37 °C for 48 ± 2 h. After 24-h and 48-h incubation, plates were examined for the growth of *Pseudomonas* spp. and other pathogenic bacteria. Colonies morphologically consistent with *P. aeruginosa* were subcultured on fresh blood agar plates for subsequent identification. Bacterial isolates were identified using the methods described by Quinn and colleagues [52]; biochemical characteristics of the isolates were determined using the commercial kit Api 20 NE (BioMérieux, France) according to the manufacturer's instructions.

Results

In Figs. 1, 2 and 3, chromatograms of individual AHL standard solutions C4-HSL (19.7 ng/ml), C6-HSL (19.7 ng/ml) and 3-oxo-C12-HSL (18.2 ng/ml) are presented, respectively. Retention times of C4-HSL, C6-HSL and 3-oxo-C12-HSL were 1.99, 4.76 (4.77) and 9.16 min, respectively (Figs. 1, 2 and 3, Table 1). For each AHL, two transitions of the precursor to product (fragment) ion are shown (e.g., for C4-HSL 172.096 to 101.980 and 172.096 to 144.073). In the figures, the common display of LC-MS/MS chromatograms, with the x-axis showing time and y-axis the relative signal intensity (relative to the highest peak in chromatogram, in %), was adopted.

Equations describing the calibration lines were $y = 2027x + 708$ (C4-HSL), $y = 2603x + 2039$ (C6-HSL) and $y = 1594x + 204$ (3-oxo-C12-HSL). Regression coefficients of the calibration curves were 0.999, 0.998 and 0.999, respectively. Based on the responses obtained, the lowest calibration point (1 ng/ml – or 0.1 ng/ml when referring to 10-ml volumes) was estimated as the lowest quantifiable concentration. Therefore, LOQ for 10-ml samples was estimated to 0.1 ng/ml (1 ng per 10-ml sample) and LOD accordingly lower to 0.03 ng/ml (0.3 ng per 10-ml sample). Expressed in molar concentrations, LOD and LOQ were approx. 175 pM and 584 pM for C4-HSL (with molar mass of 171.2 g/mol), 151 pM and 502 pM for C6-HSL (199.2 g/mol), and 101 pM and 336 pM for 3-oxo-C12-HSL (297.4 g/mol), respectively. Thus, with LOD in the range of 100–200 pM and LOQ in 300–600 pM, LC-MS/MS was confirmed suitable for the purpose as picomolar to micromolar concentrations were reported for clinical samples [7, 12, 22, 48, 49].

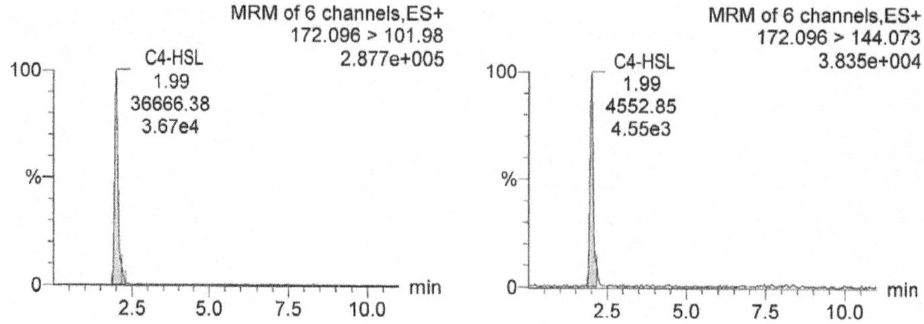

Fig. 1 LC-MS/MS chromatogram of C4-HSL (N-butanoyl-L-homoserine lactone) standard solution with the concentration of 19.7 ng/ml. Transitions 172.096 > 101.98 and 172.096 > 144.073 are shown. The x-axis represents retention time (min) and y-axis the relative intensity of signal (relative to the highest peak in chromatogram, %)

In Tables 2 and 3, parameters of the repeatability and reproducibility test are given. Recoveries, calculated from the results obtained under the within-laboratory reproducibility conditions, were 54 , 89 and 79 % for C4-HSL, C6-HSL and 3-oxo-C12-HSL, respectively. Before calculations, the outliers were excluded using the Grubbs statistical test [50].

When the analytical procedure for determination of C4-HSL, C6-HSL and 3-oxo-C12-HSL was successfully validated, the ear rinses (clinical samples) obtained from a healthy dog (negative control) and two dogs with *Pa*OE (positive samples) were analyzed. In Figs. 4 and 5, a chromatogram of the negative control and an example of C4-HSL chromatogram belonging to a positive sample from the *Pa*OE diseased dog are shown, respectively. The positive-sample chromatogram clearly shows a peak belonging to C4-HSL (Fig. 5), which is missing in the negative-control chromatogram (Fig. 4). It should be recalled that the y-axis scales are in relative units (normalized to the largest peak), resulting in the jagged line reflecting only the background noise in Fig. 4. The largest peak was 7.800×10^2 units in Fig. 4 and 5.161×10^5 units in Fig. 5, therefore the signal was approx. 1000-times higher in the positive sample than in the negative.

In Table 4, the total masses of C4-HSL, C6-HSL and 3-oxo-C12-HSL determined in the ear rinses of two dogs with *Pa*OE collected at weekly intervals during the treatment (week 0, 1, 2, 3, 4, 6 and 8) are given. The contents of C6-HSL and 3-oxo-C12-HSL were distinctly lower than of C4-HSL, making useful only the measurements of C4-HSL contents. In the first dog, the content of C6-HSL was much lower than of C4-HSL, but roughly correlated to fluctuations of C4-HSL; C6-HSL masses were close to LOQ (1 ng per 10-ml sample; week 0–3), but also below LOQ (week 8) or even LOD (0.3 ng per 10-ml sample; week 4 and 6). Surprisingly, the content of 3-oxo-C12-HSL was always below LOD. In the second dog, the contents of C6-HSL and 3-oxo-C12-HSL were below LOD but reached LOQ (C6-HSL) or LOD (3-oxo-C12-HSL) in the third and fourth week, which was in congruence with the increased C4-HSL levels.

In the first dog, the content of C4-HSL decreased in the first month of treatment, but then slightly increased in the sixth week and markedly in the eighth week of treatment (Table 4). At that time (week 6 and 8), a secondary infection of the ear canal was also observed by culture examination, showing the presence of two different *P. aeruginosa* strains. In the second dog, the disease management started with C4-HSL below LOD (day 0),

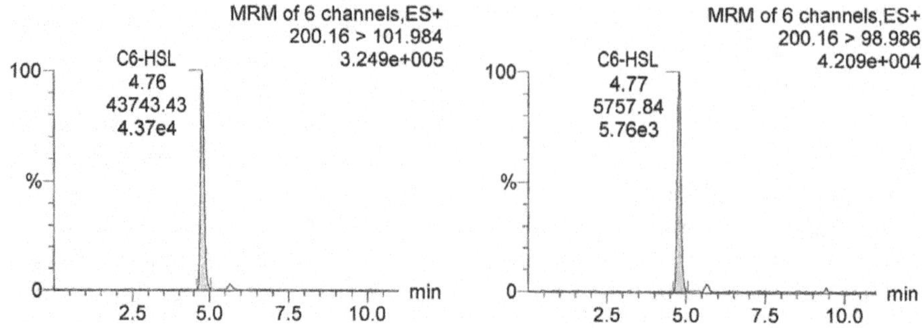

Fig. 2 LC-MS/MS chromatogram of C6-HSL (N-hexanoyl-L-homoserine lactone) standard solution with the concentration of 19.7 ng/ml. Transitions 200.16 > 101.984 and 200.16 > 98.986 are shown. Description of the axes as in Fig. 1

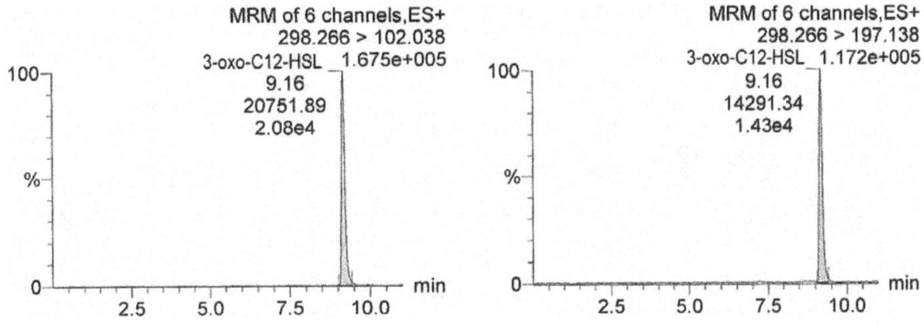

Fig. 3 LC-MS/MS chromatogram of 3-oxo-C12-HSL (N-(3-oxododecanoyl)-L-homoserine lactone) standard solution with the concentration of 18.2 ng/ml. Transitions 298.266 > 102.038 and 298.266 > 197.138 are shown. Description of the axes as in Fig. 1

but its content increased after the first week of treatment (Table 4). The time coincided with isolation of *Proteus mirabilis* from the ear swab. In the second week of treatment, the content of C4-HSL decreased and *P. mirabilis* was no longer detected by culture examination. In the third and fourth week, however, a marked increase of C4-HSL content could be observed, with the appearance of additional *P. aeruginosa* strain (already in week 2) and the reappearance of *P. mirabilis*. Later, in the second month of the treatment, the content of C4-HSL decreased and the secondary infection was resolved (week 6 and 8).

Discussion

The present study demonstrated that AHL signal molecules can be quantified in the ear rinses of *Pa*OE affected dogs using LC-MS/MS. This method proved superior when compared to other chromatographic techniques that were tested in the scope of our preliminary validation experiments: GC-MS [43, 44] and HPLC with UV detection [6]. Namely, of the three methods selected for determination of AHLs in OE clinical samples only LC-MS/MS enabled determination of signal molecules at target concentrations. Two major (3-oxo-C12-HSL, C4-HSL) and one minor (C6-HSL) AHL of *P. aeruginosa* were monitored. Identification of AHLs in clinical samples can have an important diagnostic, therapeutic and prognostic value in human and veterinary medicine.

The detection and quantification limits of the analytical procedure were low enough (LOD: 0.03 ng/ml; LOQ: 0.1 ng/ml) to enable determination of C4-HSL, C6-HSL and 3-oxo-C12-HSL in the ear rinses from dogs with *Pa*OE. The linearity of the procedure was confirmed with the regression coefficient of the calibration curve higher than 0.995. The precision, repeatability and the within-laboratory reproducibility, of the procedure was expressed by standard deviations s [ng] and relative standard deviations RSD [%]. Two outliers were eliminated based on the Grubbs test [50], both belonging to the 3-oxo-C12-HSL measurements from the same day of validation. The resulting RSD_R values for C4-HSL (35 %), C6-HSL (22 %) and 3-oxo-C12-HSL (20 %) were compared to the reference values derived from the Horwitz equation: for the tested concentration of 2 ng/ml, the reference RSD_R value was 41 % [50, 51]. Since the obtained RSD_R values were below 41 %, the reproducibility was considered satisfactory.

The recoveries of C4-HSL, C6-HSL and 3-oxo-C12-HSL at the concentration of 2 ng/ml were 54, 89 and 79 %, respectively. Regarding requirements for the performance of analytical procedures (e.g., Decision 2002/657/EC [51]), the recoveries of C6-HSL and 3-oxo-C12-HSL were considered satisfactory; whereas the recovery of C4-HSL (54 %) was suboptimal (it should be 70–110 %). Similar recovery values were reported previously [7]. The suboptimal recovery of C4-HSL should not be considered a significant limiting factor, because the analytical procedure was primarily used for monitoring the changes in AHL concentrations with time and not to determine their absolute values. However, the obtained recovery values can be used for the correction of results to achieve a good approximation of the actual contents in a sample whenever appropriate.

Table 2 Parameters obtained within the repeatability test

Replicate	C4-HSL	C6-HSL	3-oxo-C12-HSL
Average mass [ng] in 10-ml sample	11.3	19.9	15.6
s_r [ng]	5.7	2.2	2.8
RSD_r [%]	50.2	11	18

Table 3 Parameters obtained within the reproducibility test

Replicate	C4-HSL	C6-HSL	3-oxo-C12-HSL
Average mass [ng] in 10-ml sample	10.6	17.5	14.3
s_R [ng]	3.7	3.8	2.9
RSD_R [%]	35	22	20
Recovery [%]	54	89	79

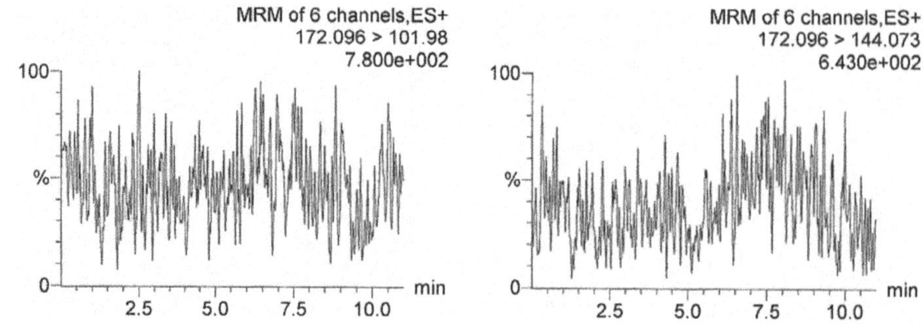

Fig. 4 LC-MS/MS chromatogram of the ear rinse sample from a healthy dog, i.e., the representative chromatogram of a blank matrix. The noisy line reflects only the negative background, as the y-axis scale was normalized to the largest peak of 7.800×10^2 units. Description of the axes as in Fig. 1

Sample sediments, which were obtained after the initial centrifuging of the ear rinses, were tested for residual levels of AHLs prior to validation. This was performed to verify the predominating distribution of analytes into the liquid phase. Sediment analysis was the same as implemented for the supernatants. The quantities of individual AHLs were approximately 20-times lower in the sediments than in their respective supernatants (data not shown), indicating the residual level of less than 5 %. Therefore, only supernatants were used for further analysis.

Samples for the present study were collected from two dogs with *Pa*OE, which was confirmed with the routine bacteriological analyses. The treatment regimen was standard [53–58] and included regular ear irrigations with topical saline flush and local administration of Tris-EDTA/chlorhexidine (0.15 % solution; Otodin, Industria Chimica Fine ICF, Palazzo Pignano, Italy) once daily. Namely, the antiseptic solution Tris-EDTA/chlorhexidine was proven beneficial and safe for the *Pa*OE diseased dogs with unlikely selection for bacterial resistance which would predispose the chronic character of the disease [55–58]. A systemic antibiotic (enrofloxacin) treatment was only employed after clinical condition of dogs deteriorated. To avoid confusion, the state of clinical condition should not be directly deduced from the results of culture examination or AHL content in the samples. Enrofloxacin was administered in the last 14 days of treatment to the first dog and in the first 14 days to the second.

Regarding the total masses of AHLs in the ear lavages of dogs with *Pa*OE, the content of C6-HSL was in general much lower than of C4-HSL, but the fluctuations of these two roughly correlated. The content of C6-HSL was approximating LOQ or even LOD. Moreover, the content of 3-oxo-C12-HSL was always below LOQ or, in most cases, below LOD. According to the results, only C4-HSL measurements showed applicable value. In the first dog, results showed that the content of C4-HSL decreased in the first month of Tris-EDTA/chlorhexidine treatment in accordance to expectations [58], but increased again toward the end of the treatment (slightly in week 6 and markedly in week 8). The increase could be assigned to a secondary infection of the ear canal,

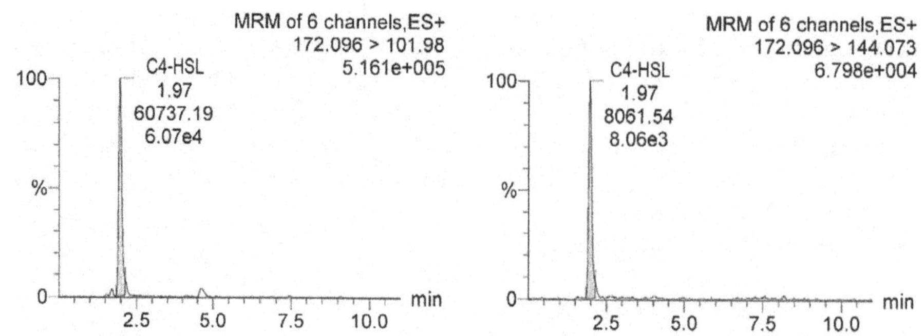

Fig. 5 LC-MS/MS chromatogram of the ear rinse sample from a dog with *Pa*OE (*P. aeruginosa*-associated OE), i.e., the representative chromatogram of a positive sample containing C4-HSL (N-butanoyl-L-homoserine lactone). The y-axis scale was normalized to the peak of 5.161×10^5 units. Chromatograms for other clinical samples appeared similar when regarding detection of individual AHLs, due to the presentation of analyte quantity in relative units and the characteristic analyte retention times. Description of the axes as in Fig. 1

Table 4 Total masses of AHLs in the ear lavages of dogs with *PaOE* (*Pseudomonas aeruginosa*-associated OE), sampled in the course of treatment

Day	Week	1st dog				
		AHL mass [ng]			*Culture examination*[a]	
		C4-HSL	C6-HSL	3-oxo-C12-HSL	*P. aeruginosa*	*Other bacteria*
0	0	33.7	1.1	<0.3	+	–
7	1	26.7	1.1	<0.3	+	–
14	2	29.4	1.2	<0.3	+	–
21	3	15.3	1.2	<0.3	+	–
28	4	1.3	<0.3	<0.3	+	–
42	6	2.7	<0.3	<0.3	+ (two strains[b])	–
56	8	20.7	<1	<0.3	+ (two strains)	–
Day	Week	2nd dog				
		AHL mass [ng]			*Culture examination*	
		C4-HSL	C6-HSL	3-oxo-C12-HSL	*P. aeruginosa*	*Other bacteria*
0	0	<0.3	<0.3	<0.3	+	–
7	1	8.2	<0.3	<0.3	+	*Proteus mirabilis*
14	2	1.9	<0.3	<0.3	+ (two strains)	–
21	3	21.2	1.6	<1	+ (two strains)	*Proteus mirabilis*
28	4	32.4	1.5	<1	+ (two strains)	*Proteus mirabilis*
42	6	3.1	<0.3	<0.3	+ (two strains)	–
56	8	3.4	<0.3	<0.3	+	–

[a]Results of culture examination are given for better understanding and are explained in the text

[b]Indicating a secondary infection with a different *P. aeruginosa* strain, deteriorating the clinical condition of dogs and causing the increase of AHL content in the infected ear canal

which was confirmed by culture examination showing the presence of an additional *P. aeruginosa* strain.

In the second dog, the content of C4-HSL was below LOD at the beginning of the disease management, but increased after the first week of treatment. *P. mirabilis*, a Gram-negative opportunistic pathogen ubiquitously present in the environment and a common secondary factor of OE in dogs [17, 18], was also isolated from the ear canal. Since Gram-negative bacteria employ AHLs for quorum communication, cross-talk communication between the two species cannot be excluded. The inter-species communication was suggested previously between *P. aeruginosa* and *P. mirabilis*, since a variation of AHL QS system was observed in *P. mirabilis* with signaling molecules being structurally similar to AHLs [59]. Namely, in both the cell-free culture supernatants of *P. aeruginosa* and of *P. mirabilis*, compounds capable of activating the AHL biosensor were found, not belonging to AHLs but to structurally similar diketopiperazines (DKPs). In concentration-dependent manner, DKPs were able to activate the AHL biosensor, although their physiological role remains to be discovered, but also suggesting the existence of cross talk among bacterial signaling systems. However, the QS system in *Proteus* sp. is not completely understood and its signaling molecules are not well defined. Although signaling molecules with the structure identical to AHLs are not produced by *P. mirabilis* [60], it was shown that *P. mirabilis* reacts and changes the population features when AHLs produced by other Gram-negative bacteria are added to the culture media [61]. The content of C4-HSL in the second dog decreased in the second week of treatment, which coincided with the disappearance of *P. mirabilis* from the bacteriological sample. The marked increase in C4-HSL was detected in the third and fourth week, which coincided with an additional strain of *P. aeruginosa* and the reappearance of *P. mirabilis* in the bacteriological sample. After the fourth week, the C4-HSL content declined and *P. mirabilis* was no longer present. By the end of the treatment course, the additional strain of *P. aeruginosa* also disappeared.

No AHLs were detected in the negative control sample from a healthy dog. The analytical procedure described and validated in this study is, therefore, capable of monitoring changes in AHL concentration throughout the treatment regimen, reflecting the state of *Pseudomonas* infection.

Concerning 3-oxo-C12-HSL, low concentrations were detected in this study. Similar was observed previously in samples from human patients with CF [7]. Several, interconnected or independent, reasons for this analytical outcome are possible: *i)* 3-oxo-C12-HSL is not a major AHL present in the ear canals of *Pa*OE-diseased dogs or in clinical samples in general; *ii)* deficiency of one or more *P. aeruginosa* QS components leading to reduced synthesis/deployment of 3-oxo-C12-HSL; *iii)* the in-vitro results, which are presently the gold standard for understanding the biology of QS and AHLs, are different from the in-vivo behavior of *P. aeruginosa* QS; and *iv)* limitations of the membrane transport, which are selective to effusion of 3-oxo-C12-HSL from *P. aeruginosa* cytoplasm.

Regarding the results obtained in this study and previously for the samples from human CF patients [7], it is possible that 3-oxo-C12-HSL is not a major AHL present in clinical samples, disease-related or in general. One should not be misled by the terminology that the *rhl* system is 'only' subordinate to *las*, as we can speculate that *rhl* might be more adaptable to current conditions in its milieu or could support greater part of QS communication. A deficiency of one or more QS components of the *rhl* system was previously reported for *P. aeruginosa* canine OE isolates [62], and *P. aeruginosa* mutants with the impaired *las* were also obtained from clinical samples [63]. These QS deficient strains are regularly isolated from clinical or environmental samples and are called the 'cheating' individuals, profiting from the benefits of the cooperating population without contributing to the community [64]. Not all *P. aeruginosa* strains/isolates produce both C4-HSL and 3-oxo-C12-HSL [7, 63]. In addition to the QS deficiencies, the expression of QS is different in *P. aeruginosa* isolates from clinical samples or grown as biofilms when compared to those that are grown in laboratory as broth cultures in nutrient-rich media [12, 65]. Broth cultures are being intensively studied to explain the composition and hierarchy of bacterial QS systems. In the natural environments, however, biofilms are predominating over the planktonic growth [7, 12]. *P. aeruginosa* is notorious for its ability to form biofilms [10]. Isolated from CF sputum of human patients, *P. aeruginosa* produces C4-HSL in excess of 3-oxo-C12-HSL when grown in biofilms but not in broth cultures [65]. If the higher content of C4-HSL over 3-oxo-C12-HSL observed in the present study is due to variation in their production, *P. aeruginosa* from the ear canals of *Pa*OE-diseased dogs is also predominantly present as biofilms. Another reason for low concentrations of 3-oxo-C12-HSL in the studied clinical samples, in addition to QS deficiencies of *P. aeruginosa* strains and differential gene expression in biofilms, could be the fact that 3-oxo-C12-HSL requires an active membrane transport (pump) for its efflux from the cells to the surroundings, whereas C4-HSL diffusion has no such limitation and *P. aeruginosa* cells are freely permeable to C4-HSL [7, 66].

If *P. aeruginosa* is predominately growing in biofilms in the ear canals of *Pa*OE-diseased dogs, another explanation for the low amounts of 3-oxo-C12-HSL can be suggested. Namely, AHLs are restricted in diffusion by the extracellular matrix of biofilms and they reach adequate intracellular concentrations for induction of QS-dependent genes at lower values in comparison to planktonic growth phenotype [67]. Therefore, it is possible that less 3-oxo-C12-HSL is needed in biofilms for the activation of the subordinate *rhl* system, but more with planktonic phenotypes due to diffusion throughout the liquid milieu to reach concentrations high enough for the activation of *rhl*.

P. aeruginosa can adapt to different environments via its regulatory networks and multifunctional signal molecules [34, 36], which can be monitored using the methods such as the one reported in this study. Disrupting QS regulation is a valuable approach to develop new therapeutic strategies. Implementation of alternative therapies (QQ strategies) for *Pa*OE, or other *P. aeruginosa* infections, should have a beneficial impact on patients [68, 69]. Plants, for example, represent a large and unexplored pool of potentially QQ bioactive compounds [70, 71].

Conclusions

The QS system is a defining part of the pathologies caused by *P. aeruginosa* and other bacteria. Detection and quantification of AHLs in clinical samples may provide an important diagnostic and prognostic tool to follow the disease progress, which has already been proven in human CF cases. It would also be possible to initiate and/or terminate, or evaluate, the success of antibiotic treatments in diseases of the *Pa*OE complexity. In this study, the LC-MS/MS analytical procedure for determination of selected *P. aeruginosa* AHLs (C4-HSL, C6-HSL, 3-oxo-C12-HSL) in clinical samples obtained from *Pa*OE-diseased dogs was introduced and successfully validated. For the clinical samples obtained from two *Pa*OE-diseased dogs, low content of 3-oxo-C12-HSL was observed with C4-HSL predominating. To explain the phenomenon, it was suggested, in addition to other hypotheses, that *P. aeruginosa* is growing in the infected ear canals organized in biofilms.

Abbreviations

3-oxo-C12-HSL: N-(3-oxododecanoyl)-L-homoserine lactone; AHLs (or AI-1): N-acylhomoserine lactones; C4-HSL: N-butanoyl-L-homoserine lactone; C6-HSL: N-hexanoyl-L-homoserine lactone; CF: Cystic fibrosis; DKPs: Diketopiperazines; GC-MS: Gas chromatography with mass spectrometry; HPLC: High-performance liquid chromatography; LC-MS/MS: Liquid chromatography with tandem mass spectrometry; LOD: Limit of detection; LOQ: Limit of quantification; MS: Mass spectrometry; MS/MS: Tandem mass spectrometry; NMR: Nuclear magnetic resonance; OE: Otitis externa [inflammation of the external ear canal]; *Pa*OE: *Pseudomonas aeruginosa*-associated OE; QQ: Quorum quenching; QS: Quorum sensing; *rec*: recovery; *RSD*: Relative standard deviation (RSD_r for repeatability, RSD_R for reproducibility); *s*: standard deviation (s_r for repeatability, s_R for reproducibility)

Acknowledgements
This research was conducted in the frame of Research Programs P4-0092 "Animal health, environment and food safety" and P4-0053 "Endocrine, immune and enzyme responses in healthy and sick animals", funded by the Slovenian Research Agency.

Funding
This study was supported by the Slovenian Research Agency grants P4-0053 and P4-0092. The funder had no role in study design, data collection and analyses, decision to publish or preparation of the manuscript.

Authors' contributions
Study conception and design: DK, MV, GTK; Acquisition of samples: JH, TK, MV; Analytical procedures: KŠ, PI, LK, JH, GTK, IZ; Interpretation of data: DK, MV, GTK; Drafting of manuscript: DK, MV, GTK; Critical revision: DK, KŠ, PI, LK, JH, IZ, TK, MV, GTK. All authors read and approved the final manuscript.

Competing interests
The authors declare that they have no competing interests.

Consent for publication
Not applicable.

References

1. Fergie JE, Shema SJ, Lott L, Crawford R, Patrick CC. *Pseudomonas aeruginosa* bacteremia in immunocompromised children: analysis of factors associated with a poor outcome. Clin Infect Dis. 1994;18:390–4.
2. Mendelson MH, Gurtman A, Szabo S, Neibart E, Meyers BR, Policar M, Cheung TW, Lillienfeld D, Hammer G, Reddy S, Choi K, Hirschman SZ. *Pseudomonas aeruginosa* bacteremia in patients with AIDS. Clin Infect Dis. 1994;18:886–95.
3. Brewer SC, Wunderink RG, Jones CB, Leeper KVJ. Ventilator-associated pneumonia due to *Pseudomonas aeruginosa*. Chest. 1996;109:1019–29.
4. Weese JS. A review of multidrug resistant surgical site infections. Vet Comp Orthop Traumatol. 2008;21:1–7.
5. Strateva T, Yordanov D. *Pseudomonas aeruginosa* – a phenomenon of bacterial resistance. J Med Microbiol. 2009;58:1133–48.
6. Reimmann C, Beyeler M, Latifi A, Winteler H, Foglino M, Lazdunski A, Haas D. The global activator GacA of *Pseudomonas aeruginosa* PAO positively controls the production of the autoinducer N-butyryl-homoserine lactone and the formation of the virulence factors pyocyanin, cyanide, and lipase. Mol Microbiol. 1997;24:309–19.
7. Erickson DL, Endersby R, Kirkham A, Stuber K, Vollman DD, Rabin HR, Mitchell I, Storey DG. *Pseudomonas aeruginosa* quorum-sensing systems may control virulence factor expression in the lungs of patients with cystic fibrosis. Infect Immun. 2002;70:1783–90.
8. Waters CM, Bassler BL. Quorum sensing: cell-to-cell communication in bacteria. Annu Rev Cell Dev Biol. 2005;21:319–46.
9. Kumari A, Pasini P, Deo SK, Flomenhoft D, Shashidhar H, Daunert S. Biosensing systems for the detection of bacterial quorum signaling molecules. Anal Chem. 2006;78:7603–9.
10. Boyen F, Eeckhaut V, Van Immerseel F, Pasmans F, Ducatelle R, Haesebrouck F. Quorum sensing in veterinary pathogens: mechanisms, clinical importance and future perspectives. Vet Microbiol. 2009;135:187–95.
11. Miller MB, Bassler BL. Quorum sensing in bacteria. Annu Rev Microbiol. 2001; 55:165–99.
12. Middleton B, Rodgers HC, Cámara M, Knox AJ, Williams P, Hardman A. Direct detection of *N*-acylhomoserine lactones in cystic fibrosis sputum. FEMS Microbiol Lett. 2002;207:1–7.
13. Cheung AL, Eberhardt KJ, Chung E, Yeaman MR, Sullam PM, Ramos M, Bayer AS. Diminished virulence of a sar-/agr- mutant of *Staphylococcus aureus* in the rabbit model of endocarditis. J Clin Invest. 1994;94:1815–22.
14. Gillaspy AF, Hickmon SG, Skinner RA, Thomas JR, Nelson CL, Smeltzer MS. Role of the accessory gene regulator (*agr*) in pathogenesis of staphylococcal osteomyelitis. Infect Immun. 1995;63:3373–80.
15. Buzzola FR, Alvarez LP, Tuchscherr LPN, Barbagelata MS, Lattar SM, Calvinho L, Sordelli DO. Differential abilities of capsulated and noncapsulated *Staphylococcus aureus* isolates from diverse *agr* groups to invade mammary epithelial cells. Infect Immun. 2007;75:886–91.
16. Bannoehr J, Ben Zakour NL, Waller AS, Guardabassi L, Thoday KL, van den Broek AHM, Fitzgerald JR. Population genetic structure of the *Staphylococcus intermedius* group: insights into *agr* diversification and the emergence of methicillin-resistant strains. J Bacteriol. 2007;189:8685–92.
17. August JR. Otitis externa. A disease of multifactorial etiology. Vet Clin North Am Small Anim Pract. 1988;18:731–42.
18. Paterson S. A review of 200 cases of otitis externa in the dog. Vet Dermatol. 2003;14:249. Abstract.
19. Kiss G, Radványi S, Szigeti G. New combination for the therapy of canine otitis externa. Microbiology of otitis externa. J Small Anim Pract. 1997;38:51–6.
20. Carlotti DN, LeRoy ST. Otitis externa in dog: aetiology and clinical findings; literature review and retrospective study of 752 cases. Prat Med Chir Anim Comp. 1997;32:243–57.
21. Kuchma SL, Connolly JP, O'Toole GA. A three-component regulatory system regulates biofilm maturation and type III secretion in *Pseudomonas aeruginosa*. J Bacteriol. 2005;187:1441–54.
22. Kumari A, Pasini P, Daunert S. Detection of bacterial quorum sensing N-acyl homoserine lactones in clinical samples. Anal Bioanal Chem. 2008;391:1619–27.
23. Manefield M, Turner SL. Quorum sensing in context: out of molecular biology and into microbial ecology. Microbiology. 2002;148:3762–4.
24. Gambello MJ, Iglewski BH. Cloning and characterization of the *Pseudomonas aeruginosa lasR* gene, a transcriptional activator of elastase expression. J Bacteriol. 1991;173:3000–9.
25. Ochsner UA, Koch AK, Fiechter A, Reiser J. Isolation and characterization of a regulatory gene affecting rhamnolipid biosurfactant synthesis in *Pseudomonas aeruginosa*. J Bacteriol. 1994;176:2044–54.
26. Pearson JP, Gray KM, Passador L, Tucker KD, Eberhard A, Iglewski BH, Greenberg EP. Structure of the autoinducer required for expression of *Pseudomonas aeruginosa* virulence genes. Proc Natl Acad Sci U S A. 1994;91:197–201.
27. Pearson JP, Passador L, Iglewski BH, Greenberg EP. A second N-acylhomoserine lactone signal produced by *Pseudomonas aeruginosa*. Proc Natl Acad Sci U S A. 1995;92:1490–4.
28. Passador L, Cook JM, Gambrello MJ, Rust L, Iglewski BH. Expression of *Pseudomonas aeruginosa* virulence genes requires cell-to-cell communication. Science. 1993;260:1127–30.
29. Winson MK, Camara M, Latifi A, Foglino M, Chhabra SR, Daykin M, Bally M, Chapon V, Salmond GPC, Bycroft BW, Lazdunski A, Stewart GSAB, Williams P. Multiple N-acyl-L-homoserine lactone signal molecules regulate production of virulence determinants and secondary metabolites in *Pseudomonas aeruginosa*. Proc Natl Acad Sci U S A. 1995;92:9427–31.
30. de Kievit TR, Iglewski BH. Bacterial quorum sensing in pathogenic relationships. Infect Immun. 2000;68:4839–49.
31. Qazi S, Middleton B, Muharram SH, Cockayne A, Hill P, O'Shea P, Chhabra SR, Cámara M, Williams P. N-acylhomoserine lactones antagonize virulence gene expression and quorum sensing in *Staphylococcus aureus*. Infect Immun. 2006;74:910–9.
32. Cooley M, Chhabra SR, Williams P. N-acylhomoserine lactone-mediated quorum sensing: a twist in the tail and a blow for host immunity. Chem Biol. 2008;15:1141–7.
33. Telford G, Wheeler D, Williams P, Tomkins PT, Appleby P, Sewell H, Stewart GSAB, Bycroft BW, Pritchard DI. The *Pseudomonas aeruginosa* quorum-sensing signal molecule *N*-(3-oxododecanoyl)-L-homoserine lactone has immunomodulatory activity. Infect Immun. 1998;66:36–42.
34. Williams P, Cámara M. Quorum sensing and environment adaptation in *Pseudomonas aeruginosa*: a tale of regulatory networks and multifunctional signal molecules. Curr Opin Microbiol. 2009;12:182–91.
35. Duan K, Surette MG. Environmental regulation of *Pseudomonas aeruginosa* PAO1 Las and Rhl quorum-sensing systems. J Bacteriol. 2007;189:4827–36.
36. Lee J, Zhang L. The hierarchy quorum sensing network in *Pseudomonas aeruginosa*. Protein Cell. 2015;6:26–41.
37. Schuster M, Greenberg PE. A network of networks: quorum-sensing gene regulation in *Pseudomonas aeruginosa*. Int J Med Microbiol. 2006;296:73–81.
38. Dong YH, Wang LH, Xu JL, Zhang HB, Zhang XF, Zhang LH. Quenching quorum-sensing dependent bacterial infection by an N-acyl homoserine lactonase. Nature. 2001;411:813–7.
39. Bjarnsholt T, Givskov M. Quorum-sensing blockade as a strategy for enhancing host defences against bacterial pathogens. Philos Trans R Soc Lond B Biol Sci. 2007;362:1213–22.

40. Chan KG, Atkinson S, Mathee K, Sam CK, Chhabra SR, Cámara M, Koh CL, Williams P. Characterization of N-acylhomoserine lactone degrading bacteria associated with the *Zingiber officinale* (ginger) rhizosphere: co-existence of quorum quenching and quorum sensing in *Acinetobacter* and *Burkholderia*. BMC Microbiol. 2011;11:51. doi:10.1186/1471-2180-11-51.
41. Wright III JS, Jin R, Novick RP. Transient interference with staphylococcal quorum sensing blocks abscess formation. Proc Natl Acad Sci U S A. 2005; 102:1691–6.
42. Janssens JC, Steenackers H, Metzger K, Daniels R, Ptacek D, Verhoeven T, Hermans K, Vanderleyden J, De Vos D, De Keersmaecker S. Interference with the quorum sensing systems of *Salmonella enterica* serovar *typhimurium*: possibilities and implications. Commun Agric Appl Biol Sci. 2007;72:35–9.
43. Cataldi TRI, Bianco G, Palazzo L, Quaranta V. Occurrence of N-acyl-L-homoserine lactones in extracts of some Gram-negative bacteria evaluated by gas chromatography-mass spectrometry. Anal Biochem. 2007;361:226–35.
44. Charlton TS, de Nys R, Netting A, Kumar N, Hentzer M, Givskov M, Kjelleberg S. A novel and sensitive method for the quantification of N-3-oxoacyl homoserine lactones using gas chromatography-mass spectrometry: application to a model bacterial biofilm. Environ Microbiol. 2000;2:530–41.
45. Gould TA, Herman J, Krank J, Murphy RC, Churchill MEA. Specificity of acyl-homoserine lactone synthases examined by mass spectrometry. J Bacteriol. 2006;188:773–83.
46. Yang YH, Lee TH, Kim JH, Kim EJ, Joo HS, Lee CS, Kim BG. High-throughput detection method of quorum-sensing molecules by colorimetry and its applications. Anal Biochem. 2006;356:297–9.
47. Trufelli H, Palma P, Famiglini G, Cappiello A. An overview of matrix effects in liquid chromatography–mass spectrometry. Mass Spectrom Rev. 2011;30: 491–509.
48. Chambers CE, Visser MB, Schwab U, Sokol PA. Identification of N-acylhomoserine lactones in mucopurulent respiratory secretions from cystic fibrosis patients. FEMS Microbiol Lett. 2005;244:297–304.
49. Favre-Bonté S, Pache JC, Robert J, Blanc D, Pechère JC, van Delden C. Detection of *Pseudomonas aeruginosa* cell-to-cell signals in lung tissue of cystic fibrosis patients. Microb Pathog. 2002;32:143–7.
50. Miller JN, Miller JC. Statistics and Chemometrics for Analytical Chemistry. 4th ed. Harlow: Prentice; 2000.
51. European Commission. Decision 2002/657/EC of 12 August 2002 implementing Council Directive 96/23/EC concerning the performance of analytical methods and the interpretation of results. Off J. 2002;L221:8–36.
52. Quinn PJ, Carter ME, Markey BK, Carter GR. Clinical Veterinary Microbiology. London: Mosby Wolfe; 1994.
53. Cole LK. Otoscopic evaluation of the ear canal. Vet Clin North Am Small Anim Pract. 2004;34:397–410.
54. Nuttall T, Cole LK. Evidence-based veterinary dermatology: a systemic review of interventions for treatment of *Pseudomonas* otitis in dogs. Vet Dermatol. 2007;18:69–77.
55. Harper WE, Epis JA. Effect of chlorhexidine/EDTA/Tris against bacterial isolates from clinical specimens. Microbios. 1987;51:107–12.
56. Ghibaudo G, Cornegliani L, Martino P. Evaluation of the in vivo effects of Tris-EDTA and chlorhexidine digluconate 0.15% solution in chronic bacterial otitis externa: 11 cases. Vet Dermatol. 2004;15 Suppl 1:65.
57. Guardabassi L, Ghibaudo G, Damborg P. *In vitro* antimicrobial activity of a commercial ear antiseptic containing chlorhexidine and Tris-EDTA. Vet Dermatol. 2009;21:282–6.
58. Hosseini J, Zdovc I, Golob M, Blagus R, Kušar D, Vengušt M, Kotnik T. Effect of treatment with Tris-EDTA/chlorhexidine topical solution on canine *Pseudomonas aeruginosa* otitis externa with or without concomitant treatment with oral fluoroquinolones. Slov Vet Res. 2012;49:133–40.
59. Holden MTG, Chhabra SR, de Nys R, Stead P, Bainton NJ, Hill PJ, Manefield M, Kumar N, Labatte M, England D, Rice S, Givskov M, Salmond GPC, Stewart GSAB, Bycroft BW, Kjelleberg S, Williams P. Quorum-sensing cross talk: isolation and chemical characterization of cyclic dipeptides from *Pseudomonas aeruginosa* and other Gram-negative bacteria. Mol Microbiol. 1999;33:1254–66.
60. Morgenstein RM, Szostek B, Rather PN. Regulation of gene expression during swarmer cell differentiation in *Proteus mirabilis*. FEMS Microbiol Rev. 2010;34:753–63.
61. Stankowska D, Czerwonka G, Rozalska S, Grosicka M, Dziadek J, Kaca W. Influence of quorum sensing signal molecules on biofilm formation in *Proteus mirabilis* O18. Folia Microbiol. 2012;57:53–60.
62. Tron EA, Wilke HL, Petermann SR, Rust L. *Pseudomonas aeruginosa* from canine otitis externa exhibit a quorum sensing deficiency. Vet Microbiol. 2004;99:121–9.
63. Smith EE, Buckley DG, Wu Z, Saenphimmachak C, Hoffman LR, D'Argenio DA, Miller SI, Ramsey BW, Speert DP, Moskowitz SM, Burns JL, Kaul R, Olson MV. Genetic adaptation by *Pseudomonas aeruginosa* to the airways of cystic fibrosis patients. Proc Natl Acad Sci U S A. 2006;103:8487–92.
64. Dunny GM, Brickman TJ, Dworkin M. Multicellular behaviour in bacteria: communication, cooperation, competition and cheating. Bioessays. 2008;30:296–8.
65. Singh PK, Schaefer AL, Parsek MR, Moninger TO, Welsh MJ, Greenberg EP. Quorum-sensing signals indicate that cystic fibrosis lungs are infected with bacterial biofilms. Nature. 2000;407:762–4.
66. Pearson JP, van Delden C, Iglewski BH. Active efflux and diffusion are involved in transport of *Pseudomonas aeruginosa* cell-to-cell signals. J Bacteriol. 1999;181:1203–10.
67. Nilsson P, Olofsson A, Fagerling M, Fagerstrom T, Rice S, Kjelleberg S, Steinberg P. Kinetics of the acyl-homoserine lactone regulatory system in a model biofilm system: how many bacteria constitute a "quorum"? J Mol Biol. 2001;309:631–40.
68. Uroz S, Dessaux Y, Oger P. Quorum sensing and quorum quenching: the yin and yang of bacterial communication. Chem Bio Chem. 2009;10:205–16.
69. Romero M, Acuña L, Otero A. Patents on quorum quenching: interfering with bacterial communication as a strategy to fight infections. Recent Pat Biotechnol. 2012;6:2–12.
70. Kalia VC. Quorum sensing inhibitors: an overview. Biotechnol Adv. 2013;31: 224–45.
71. Truchado P, Larrosa M, Castro-Ibáñez I, Allende A. Plant food extracts and phytochemicals: their role as quorum sensing inhibitors. Trends Food Sci Tech. 2015;43:189–204.

15

Tick- and fly-borne bacteria in ungulates: the prevalence of *Anaplasma phagocytophilum*, haemoplasmas and rickettsiae in water buffalo and deer species in Central Europe, Hungary

Sándor Hornok[1*], László Sugár[2], Isabel G. Fernández de Mera[3], José de la Fuente[3,4], Gábor Horváth[5], Tibor Kovács[6], Attila Micsutka[7], Enikő Gönczi[8], Barbara Flaisz[1], Nóra Takács[1], Róbert Farkas[1], Marina L. Meli[8] and Regina Hofmann-Lehmann[8]

Abstract

Background: Hunting constitutes an important industry in Europe. However, data on the prevalence of vector-borne bacteria in large game animal species are lacking from several countries. Blood or spleen samples (239 and 270, respectively) were taken from red, fallow and roe deer, as well as from water buffaloes, mouflons and wild boars in Hungary, followed by DNA extraction and molecular analyses for *Anaplasma phagocytophilum*, haemoplasmas and rickettsiae.

Results: Based on blood samples, the prevalence rate of *A. phagocytophilum* infection was significantly higher in red deer (97.9%) than in fallow deer (72.7%) and roe deer (60%), and in all these compared to mouflons (6.3%). In addition, 39.2% of the spleen samples from wild boars were PCR positive for *A. phagocytophilum*, but none of the buffalos. Based on blood samples, the prevalence rates of both *Mycoplasma wenyonii* (Mw) and '*Candidatus* M. haemobos' (CMh) infections were significantly higher in buffaloes (Mw: 91.2%; CMh: 73.3%) than in red deer (Mw: 64.6%; CMh: 45.8%), and in both of them compared to fallow deer (Mw: 30.3%; CMh: 9.1%) and roe deer (Mw: 20%; CMh: 1.5%). The prevalence of Mw and CMh infection significantly correlated with the body sizes of these hosts. Furthermore, Mw was significantly more prevalent than CMh in buffaloes, red and roe deer. *Mycoplasma ovis* was detected in mouflons, *M. suis* in wild boars, *R. helvetica* in one fallow deer and one mouflon, and an unidentified *Rickettsia* sp. in a fallow deer.

Conclusions: Forest-dwelling game animal species were found to be important carriers of *A. phagocytophilum*. In contrast, animals grazing grassland (i.e. buffaloes) were less likely to get infected with this *Ixodes ricinus*-borne pathogen. Water buffaloes, deer species, mouflons and wild boars harbored haemoplasmas that may affect domestic ungulates. Evaluated animals with larger body size had significantly higher prevalence of infection with haemoplasmas compared to smaller deer species. The above host species rarely carried rickettsiae.

Keywords: *Anaplasma phagocytophilum*, *Mycoplasma wenyonii*, '*Candidatus* Mycoplasma haemobos', *Mycoplasma suis*, *Rickettsia helvetica*

* Correspondence: Hornok.Sandor@univet.hu
[1]Department of Parasitology and Zoology, University of Veterinary Medicine, Budapest, Hungary
Full list of author information is available at the end of the article

Background

Large game animal species, as exemplified by red deer (*Cervus elaphus*), roe deer (*Capreolus capreolus*) and wild boars (*Sus scrofa*), have increasing populations in Europe [1–3]. Adding to their ecological and economical significance, molecular screening of pathogens they may harbor also deserved special attention during the past decades. Taxonomically, large game animal species are artiodactyls (Mammalia: Cetartiodactyla), therefore it is expectable that they share pathogens with domestic even-toed ungulates [4]. In this context, there are various means of connectivity between game and domestic animals. These include hunting and offal waste disposal, the growing interface between urban and natural habitats, as well as blood-sucking arthropod vectors that may transmit disease agents between wild-living ungulates and livestock. The latter can happen even when they are more distantly separated.

Among arthropods, hard ticks (Acari: Ixodidae) are regarded as the most important vectors in the temperate zone [5]. Large game animal species are the preferred hosts of several tick species (e.g. *Ixodes ricinus* [6]), which have veterinary-medical significance [7]. Therefore, acting as reservoirs, they also play a central role in the maintenance and transmission of tick-borne infections towards humans. In particular, cervids and wild boars are regarded as reservoirs of tick- and/or vector-borne zoonotic pathogens, exemplified by *Anaplasma phagocytophilum* [8], *Mycoplasma suis* [9] and *Rickettsia helvetica* [10]. Accordingly, it was shown that changes in wildlife (especially deer) populations can contribute to the spread tick-borne infections [11].

In such epidemiological scenarios, it is especially important to know the actual prevalence of vector-borne infections in wild-living ungulates, because these infections may pose a risk of spreading to livestock or humans. However, relevant data are lacking from most of Europe. In general, more data are available on *A. phagocytophilum*, but virtually none considering haemotropic *Mycoplasma* spp. (synonymously: haemoplasmas). In Hungary, red deer and roe deer were shown to be important hosts of adults and immature stages of *I. ricinus* [12], and several *I. ricinus*-borne pathogens have been reported, for which game animals are known to be reservoirs (e.g. *A. phagocytophilum* [13] and *R. helvetica* [14]). In addition, haemoplasmas infecting cattle, sheep and pigs were found to be present in Hungary [15–17], but the carrier status of buffaloes, wild ruminants and wild boars has not been evaluated.

Therefore, the aim of this study was to survey and to compare the prevalence rates of selected, important vector-borne pathogens (i.e. *A. phagocytophilum*, haemoplasmas and rickettsiae) among water buffaloes (*Bubalus bubalis*) and five large game species: the red deer (*Cervus elaphus*), the fallow deer (*Dama dama*), the roe deer (*Capreolus capreolus*), the mouflon (*Ovis orientalis*) and the wild boar (*Sus scrofa*) in Hungary. In this country *A. phagocytophilum* and rickettsiae were detected in ticks [13, 14], unlike bovine haemoplasmas [14], which were shown to be fly-borne [15]. Therefore, it was hypothesized that molecular screening of the above hosts might also reveal differences in the prevalence of these infections depending on factors in an eco-epidemiological context (i.e. if the relevant pathogen has predominantly tick-borne or fly-borne transmission).

Methods

Sample collection

Samples were collected from water buffalos in a grassland natural reserve at Mórahalom (46° 13′ 4.5″ N, 19° 53′ 1.3″ E), and from freshly hunted individuals of five large game species in an approx. 3000 km^2 forested region of south-western Hungary (46°15′-46°50′ N, 17°-17° 50′ E), between January 2013 and December, 2014. None of these animals received acaricide or insecticide treatment. From water buffalos, blood samples were drawn from the jugular vein into EDTA tubes. From game animals, blood or spleen samples were collected randomly, depending on conditions allowed by hunters. Blood samples of dead game animals were taken from the heart (using sterile needle and syringe) and transferred into EDTA tubes, whereas spleen samples were cut with sterile scalpel blades and put into plastic vials. Samples included in the study are the following: 60 blood samples of water buffaloes; 48 blood and 96 spleen samples of red deer; 33 blood and 85 spleen samples of fallow deer; 65 blood and 6 spleen samples of roe deer; 16 blood and 4 spleen samples of mouflons; 17 blood and 79 spleen samples of wild boars. All samples were frozen on the day of collection at – 20 °C until processing.

DNA extraction and molecular analyses

The DNA was extracted individually, from 200 μl blood or approx. 10 mg of spleen with the QIAamp DNA Mini Kit (Qiagen, Hilden Germany) according to the manufacturer's instructions, including extraction controls to monitor cross-contamination of samples. PCR methods used for screening in this study are summarized in Table 1. In particular, *A. phagocytophilum* was identified with a species-specific TaqMan real-time PCR; haemoplasmas were first screened with a SYBR Green real-time PCR, then identified with species-specific TaqMan real-time PCRs, also taking into account their host-specificity; *R. helvetica* was screened with a species-specific test, and other rickettsiae with TaqMan real-time PCR. All molecular methods have been published (Table 1), except the following. The *Mycoplasma suis* assay was modified from [18]. Briefly, the 25-μl PCR reaction comprised 12.5 μl of

Table 1 Technical data and references of molecular methods used in this study

Target pathogen categories (target gene)	Oligonucleotides (sequence 5′-3′)	Reference for original method (modified protocol)
Anaplasma phagocytophilum (msp2)	ApMSP2f (ATG GAA GGT AGT GTT GGT TAT GGT ATT) ApMSP2r (TTG GTC TTG AAG CGC TCG TA) ApMSP2p (TGG TGC CAG GGT TGA GCT TGA GAT TG-HEX)	([13]) [35]
haemoplasmas (16S rRNA)	Sybr_For (AGC AAT RCC ATG TGA ACG ATG AA) Sybr_Rev1 (TGG CAC ATA GTT TGC TGT CAC TT) Sybr_Rev2 (GCT GGC ACA TAG TTA GCT GTC ACT)	[36] ([37])
Mycoplasma wenyonii, M. ovis (16S rRNA)	MwenyoniiF (CCA CGT GAA CGA TGA AGG TCT T) MwenyoniiR (GGC ACA TAG TTA GCT GTC ACT TAT TCA A) Mweny_P (FAM-AGT ACC ATC AAG GCG CGC TCA TTT CCT AG-TAMRA)	[38]
'*Candidatus* M. haemobos' (16S rRNA)	Mwen_short.forw (CCA TGT GAA CGA TGA AGG TCT TT) Mwen_short.rev (AGT TTG CTG TCA CTT ATT CAT GAG GTA) Mwen_short.p (VIC-CTA TCA GTT RTT ATC CCT CAT AA-MGB)	[38]
Mycoplasma suis (16S rRNA)	RTsuisF (CCC TGA TTG TAC TAA TTG AAT AAG) RTsuisR (GCG AAC ACT TGT TAA GCA AG) MGBsuis2 (FAM- TGR ATA CAC AYT TCA G -MGBNFQ)	[18]
Rickettsia helvetica (23S rRNA)	Rickhelv.147f (TTT GAA GGA GAC ACG GAA CAC A) Rickhelv.211r (TCC GGT ACT CAA ATC CTC ACG TA) Rickhelv.170p (6FAM-AAC CGT AGC GTA CAC TTA-MGBNFQ)	[39]
other rickettsiae (gltA)	CS-F (TCG CAA ATG TTC ACG GTA CTT T) CS-R (TCG TGC ATT TCT TTC CAT TGT G) CS-P (FAM-TGC AAT AGC AAG AAC CGT AGG CTG GAT G-BHQ)	[39]

2× qPCR Mastermix (Eurogentec, Seraing, Belgium), 900 nM of each primer, 250 nM of probe and 5 µl of DNA. Assays were performed using an ABI PRISM 7500Fast Sequence Detection System (Thermo Fisher Scientific Inc., Waltham, MA, USA). The assay was validated using a ten-fold dilution series of a synthetic DNA containing the target sequence (GeneArt String DNA, Thermo Fisher Scientific Inc).

In addition, amplification and sequencing an approx. 850 bp fragment of the major surface protein 4 (*msp4*) gene of *A. phagocytophilum* was attempted from a representative number of samples (i.e. 4–5 samples with low Ct value per host species). This PCR was performed with the primers MSP4AP5 (5′-ATG AAT TAC AGA GAA TTG CTT GTA GG-. 3′) and MSP4AP3 (5′-TTA ATT GAA AGC AAA TCT TGC TCC TAT G-3′) as reported [19]. The sequences were aligned and compared to reference GenBank sequences by nucleotide BLASTn program (https://blast.ncbi.nlm.nih.gov). Phylogenetic analysis was performed with the Neighbor-Joining method and p-distance model. Sequences were submitted to GenBank (accession numbers: MF974848–60).

Each PCR was run with positive and negative controls (i.e. sequence-verified DNA extract of the relevant agent, and non-template reaction mixture, respectively). Positive controls were always PCR positive, whereas negative controls and extraction controls remained PCR negative.

Data analyses

Exact confidence intervals (CI) of the prevalence rates were calculated at the 95% level. The ratios of positive and negative samples were compared by Fisher's exact test. In the case of host species, of which at least 20 blood samples were available, Spearman rank correlation was used to test the association between the prevalence of haemoplasmas and host body weights. Typical body weight range (i.e. locally characteristic of each species) (Table 2) was assigned according to the local hunting bags, taking into account differences between male and female animals (provided by Prof. L. Sugár). Calculations were performed with both the minimum and maximum body weights. Differences were regarded significant if $P < 0.05$.

Results and discussion

Anaplasma phagocytophilum

Anaplasma phagocytophilum was detected in all evaluated species, except buffaloes (Table 2). These buffaloes are kept in a grassland, which is an unsuitable habitat type for *I. ricinus* as a forest-dwelling tick species [20, 21]. This is the most likely explanation, why buffaloes did not have *A. phagocytophilum* infection, while its prevalence was high in game animal species hunted in forests (Table 2).

Concerning blood samples of game animals (Table 2), the prevalence rate of *A. phagocytophilum* infection was significantly higher in red deer (97.9%, CI: 88.9–100%) than in fallow deer (72.7%, CI: 54.5–86.7%) and roe deer (60%, CI: 47.1–72%) ($P = 0.001$), and in all these compared to mouflons (6.3%, CI: 0.2–30.2%) ($P = 0.0001$). These data confirm the reservoir role of cervids in the epidemiology of *A. phagocytophilum* as known from

Table 2 Results of molecular analyses of DNA samples from water buffalos and large game animal species

Species (body weight range)[a]	Sample type	PCR positives/all tested (percentage)				
		Anaplasma phagocytophilum	haemotropic *Mycoplasma* sp.			*Rickettsia helvetica* [other rickettsiae]
			M. wenyonii [*M. ovis*]	*C. M. haemobos*	*M. suis*	
Water buffalo (300–500 kg)	blood	0/60	55/60 (91.2%)[c, B]	44/60 (73.3%)[c, A]	–	0/60
Red deer (100–200 kg)	blood	47/48 (97.9%)[c]	31/48 (64.6%)[b]	22/48 (45.8%)[b]	–	0/48
	spleen	95/96 (99%)	24/96 (25%)[B] ↑	4/96 (4.2%)[A] ↑	–	0/96
Fallow deer (50–100 kg)	blood	24/33 (72.7%)[b] ↓	10/33 (30.3%)[a]	3/33 (9.1%)[a]	–	0/33
	spleen	81/85 (95.3%)	6/85 (7.1%) ↑	10/85 (11.8%)	–	1/85 (1.2%) [1/85]
Roe deer (25 kg)	blood	39/65 (60%)[b]	13/65 (20%)[a, B]	1/65 (1.5%)[a, A]	–	0/65
	spleen	3/6 (50%)	3/6 (50%)	0/6	–	0/6
Mouflon	blood	1/16 (6.3%)[a] ↓	[1/16 (6.3%)]	0/16	–	1/16 (6.3%)
	spleen	4/4 (100%)	[1/4 (25%)]	0/4	–	0/4
Wild boar	blood	6/17 (35.3%	–	–	8/17 (47.1%)	0/17
	spleen	31/79 (39.2%)	–	–	23/79 (29.1%)	0/79

[a]Estimated body weight range characteristic of the species (i.e. minimum to maximum acc. to females and males) based on local hunting bags (provided by Prof. L. Sugár)
Significance: (1) blood sample-based prevalences, which are significantly different between host species, are marked with different superscript lower case letter within columns, increasing from "a" to "c"; (2) the prevalence of *M. wenyonii* is marked with superscript capital letter "B", if significantly higher than that of *C. M.* haemobos marked with superscript capital letter "A" in the same row; (3) arrows in circle with inverse color point to the significantly higher prevalence, when comparing the two kinds of sampled tissues (blood vs. spleen) for the same host and pathogen

other studies (reviewed in [8]). An important underlying factor to fulfill this reservoir role is that wild ruminants are a preferred host of *I. ricinus*, the vector of *A. phagocytophilum*, as also reported in Hungary [12].

The DNA of *A. phagocytophilum* was detected in 39.2% (CI: 28.4–50.9%) of spleen samples and 35.3% (CI: 14.2–61.7%) of blood samples from wild boars (Table 2). The prevalence of *A. phagocytophilum* in wild boars was shown to be lower in other European countries [8, 22]. Wild boars (as contrasted to cervids) are hosts of the zoonotic variant of *A. phagocytophilum* [23, 24], therefore these preliminary results justify further investigations on the role of wild boars in the epidemiology of human granulocytic anaplasmosis in Hungary.

The *msp4* gene fragment of *A. phagocytophilum* was successfully sequenced from 13 samples (none from mouflons). The highest degree of sequence heterogeneity was observed among samples from red deer, which had up to 3.9% difference (i.e. 96.1% = 816/849 bp similarity). Phylogenetic analysis of *A. phagocytophilum msp4* sequences did not show clustering according to host species (Fig. 1). However, the phylogenetic tree reflected a geographical pattern, because sequences from different host species sampled in Hungary frequently grouped together (Fig. 1).

The DNA of *A. phagocytophilum* was significantly more frequently amplified from spleen than from blood samples of fallow deer and mouflons ($P = 0.001$). This phenomenon is similar to that reported in wild boars in Slovenia [25] and in various game animal species in Poland [26], most likely due to the density of *A. phagocytophilum*-infected granulocytes in the spleen compared to peripheral blood [24].

Haemoplasmas

Haemotropic *Mycoplasma* spp. were detected in all host species evaluated in the study (Table 2). Based on blood samples (Table 2), the prevalence rates of both *Mycoplasma wenyonii* (Mw) and '*Candidatus* M. haemobos' (CMh) infections were significantly higher in buffaloes (Mw: 91.2%, CI: 81.6–97.2%; CMh: 73.3%, CI: 60.3–83.9%) than in red deer (Mw: 64.6%, CI: 49.5–77.8%; CMh: 45.8%, CI: 31.4–60.8%) ($P = 0.0007$ and 0.005, respectively); and in red deer compared to fallow deer (Mw: 30.3%, CI: 15.6–48.7%; CMh: 9.1%, CI: 1.9–24.3%) ($P = 0.003$ and 0.0005, respectively) and roe deer (Mw: 20%, CI: 11.1–31.8%; CMh: 1.5%, CI: 0.1–8.3%) ($P < 0.0001$). In addition, Mw was significantly more prevalent than CMh in buffaloes ($P = 0.015$), in roe deer ($P = 0.001$) and (based on spleen samples) in red deer ($P < 0.0001$) (Table 2). These data prove that cervids and buffaloes are important carriers of haemotropic *Mycoplasma* spp. infecting cattle, to the best of our knowledge, observed for the first time in Europe.

Based on blood samples, there was a highly significant ($r = 1$) positive correlation between the body weights (i.e. body size) of buffaloes and deer species and the prevalence rates of Mw and CMh infections (Table 2). One possible background factor of this observation might be that larger animals (especially if living in an open area, as buffaloes), are more frequently exposed to the bites of blood-sucking vectors of Mw and CMh compared to

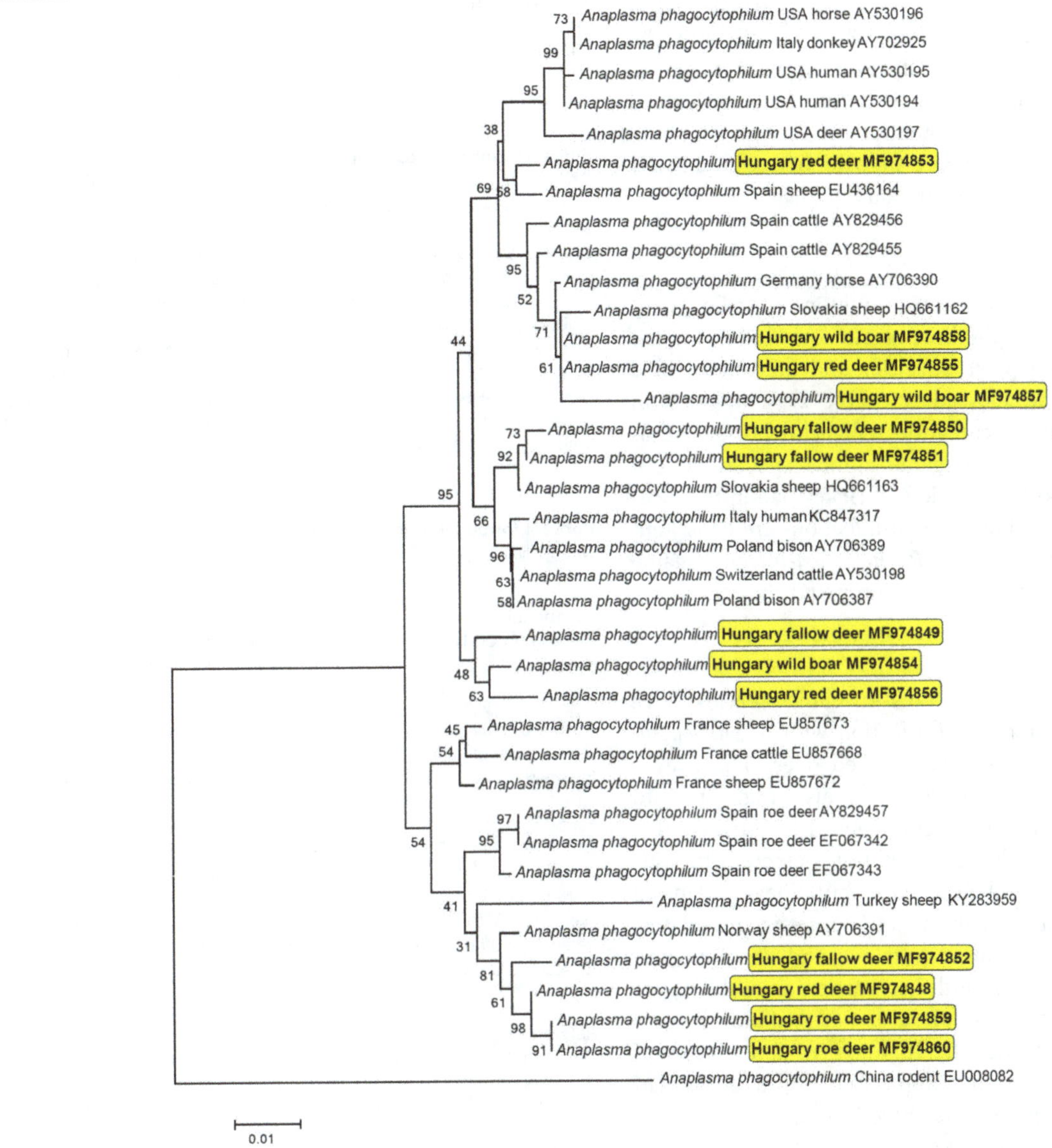

Fig. 1 Neighbor-Joining phylogenetic tree based on the *msp4* gene of *Anaplasma phagocytophilum*, including sequences obtained in this study (indicated with yellow background) and representative sequences from GenBank. Before the accession number, the country and host of origin is shown. Branch lengths represent the number of substitutions per site inferred according to the scale shown

smaller deer species. The most likely vectors of bovine haemoplasmas in Hungary are neither blood-sucking lice (absent from deer and the relevant buffalo herd: [27]) nor ticks [14], but blood-sucking flies [15], which are known to be competent mechanical transmitters of haemoplasmas [28]. Blood-sucking flies were shown to be attracted to their hosts according to body size-dependent stimuli, such as visibility and odor emission [29]. On the other hand, further factors (e.g. host susceptibility, environmental variables) might have also influenced these prevalence rates.

Interestingly, the DNA of bovine haemoplasmas was detected significantly more often in blood than in spleen samples: for Mw in red deer ($P < 0.0001$) and fallow deer ($P = 0.002$), and for CMh in red deer ($P < 0.0001$) (Table 2). This may reflect relatively recent infection in the majority of animals and/or the quick elimination of haemoplasma DNA in the spleen following phagocytosis. Relevant to this, splenic sequestration and phagocytosis of haemoplasmas has been reported [30].

Mycoplasma ovis was detected in mouflons (Table 2). To the best of the authors' knowledge, there are no previous reports on the molecular identification of this haemoplasma in wild-living small ruminants in Europe.

Mycoplasma suis infection was demonstrated in wild boars (Table 2) at a significantly higher prevalence rate (based on blood samples: 47.1%, CI: 23–72.2%) than reported in Germany (i.e. 10%: [31]). This is the first evidence of *M. suis* infection in wild boars in Hungary. The importance of this finding is enhanced by the known zoonotic potential of *M. suis* [32] and recently reported emergence of wild boars in densely populated urban areas of Hungary [33].

Rickettsiae

Rickettsia helvetica was detected only in one fallow deer and one mouflon (to the best of our knowledge, for the first time in these host species), and an unidentified *Rickettsia* sp. in a fallow deer (Table 2). Therefore, in contrast to the above categories of vector-borne pathogens, buffaloes and large game animal species do not appear to be important carriers of rickettsiae in the evaluated region. These low rates of infections are consistent with those in reports of *R. helvetica*-infected game animals in Central and Western Europe [10, 34].

Conclusions

In the evaluated region, forest-dwelling cervids have different prevalence rates of infection with *A. phagocytophilum*, the highest observed in red deer. The prevalence of *A. phagocytophilum* was also high in wild boars compared to other countries. In contrast, this *I. ricinus*-borne pathogen was not detected in animals grazing grassland (i.e. buffaloes). Among haemoplasmas that may affect domestic ungulates, Mw/CMh occur in water buffaloes and deer species, whereas *M. ovis* in mouflons. Larger animals (especially if living in an open area, as buffaloes) were shown to have significantly higher prevalence rates of infection with bovine haemoplasmas. Wild boars had high prevalence of *M. suis* infection, what is important in light of its known zoonotic potential. *Rickettsia helvetica* was detected in fallow deer and mouflon. The rare occurrence of rickettsiae in the evaluated hosts is in line with data reported from other regions of Europe.

Abbreviations

CI: exact confidence interval; CMh: *Candidatus* Mycoplasma haemobos; Mw: *Mycoplasma wenyonii*

Acknowledgements

The study was partly performed using the logistics of the Clinical Laboratory and Center for Clinical Studies, Vetsuisse Faculty, University of Zurich, Zurich, Switzerland.

Funding

This study was financially supported by OTKA115854 (molecular work) and 12190–4/2017/FEKUTSTRAT grant of the Hungarian Ministry of Human Capacities (open access publication). The funders had no role in the study design, data analysis, and decision to publish, or preparation of the manuscript.

Authors' contributions

SH, LS, AM, RF, MLM, RHL conceived and designed the study, worked on methodology. IGFM, JF, GH, TK, EG, BF, NT carried out methodology, analyzed the data. SH wrote the manuscript. All authors read, contributed to and approved the final manuscript.

Ethics approval and consent to participate

On location No. 1 of this study (Mórahalom), buffaloes were sampled for monitoring purposes during regular veterinary care by the vet in charge of this herd (Dr. Tibor Kovács, co-author of this study), therefore no ethical approval was required. Local anesthesia (with 2% lidocaine) was used to alleviate the pain of buffaloes during blood sampling. On location No. 2 of this study (south-western Hungary), game animals were shot by hunters while observing the relevant law (No. LV/1996, on the protection, management and hunting of game animals), in the course of organized hunting activity in the territory of SEFAG Forest Management and Wood Industry Share Co. (permission issued under number 153-1 for 2013/2014) according to the Somogy County Hunting Supervisory Authority. No further ethical approval was required, because on this location no living animals were handled.

Consent for publication

Not applicable.

Competing interests

The authors declare that they have no competing interests. SH is member of the editorial board (Associate Editor) of BMC Veterinary Research.

Author details

[1]Department of Parasitology and Zoology, University of Veterinary Medicine, Budapest, Hungary. [2]Department of Game Management and Ethology, Faculty of Agricultural and Environmental Sciences, University of Kaposvár, Kaposvár, Hungary. [3]SaBio. Instituto de Investigación en Recursos Cinegéticos (IREC-CSIC-UCLM-JCCLM), Ciudad Real, Spain. [4]Department of Veterinary Pathobiology, Center for Veterinary Health Sciences, Oklahoma State University, Stillwater, OK, USA. [5]Veterinary Authority, Csurgó, Hungary. [6]Veterinary Authority, Mórahalom, Hungary. [7]Food Chain Safety and Veterinary Authority, Pásztó, Hungary. [8]Clinical Laboratory and Center for Clinical Studies, Vetsuisse Faculty, University of Zurich, Zurich, Switzerland.

References

1. Burbaitė L, Csányi S. Roe deer population and harvest changes in Europe. Estonian J Ecol. 2009;58:169–80.
2. Burbaitė L, Csányi S. Red deer population and harvest changes in Europe. Acta Zool Lit. 2010;20:179–88.
3. Massei G, Kindberg J, Licoppe A, Gačić D, Šprem N, Kamler J, et al. Wild boar populations up, numbers of hunters down? A review of trends and implications for Europe. Pest Manag Sci. 2015;71:492–500.
4. Martin C, Pastoret PP, Brochier B, Humblet MF, Saegerman C. A survey of the transmission of infectious diseases/infections between wild and domestic ungulates in Europe. Vet Res. 2011;42:70.
5. Jongejan F, Uilenberg G. The global importance of ticks. Parasitology. 2004;129(Suppl):S3–S14.
6. Medlock JM, Hansford KM, Bormane A, Derdakova M, Estrada-Peña A, George JC, et al. Driving forces for changes in geographical distribution of *Ixodes ricinus* ticks in Europe. Parasit Vectors. 2013;6(1)
7. Estrada-Peña A, Jongejan F. Ticks feeding on humans: a review of records on human biting Ixodoidea with special reference to pathogen transmission. Exp Appl Acarol. 1999;23:685–715.
8. Stuen S, Granquist EG, Silaghi C. *Anaplasma phagocytophilum* – a widespread multi-host pathogen with highly adaptive strategies. Front Cell Infect Microbiol. 2013;3:31.
9. Sokoli A, Groebel K, Hoelzle K, Amselgruber WM, Mateos JM, Schneider MK, et al. *Mycoplasma suis* infection results endothelial cell damage and activation: new insight into the cell tropism and pathogenicity of hemotrophic mycoplasma. Vet Res. 2013;44:6.
10. Sprong H, Wielinga PR, Fonville M, Reusken C, Brandenburg AH, Borgsteede F, et al. *Ixodes ricinus* ticks are reservoir hosts for *Rickettsia helvetica* and potentially carry flea-borne *Rickettsia* species. Parasit Vectors. 2009;2:41.

11. Baneth G. Tick-borne infections of animals and humans: a common ground. Int J Parasitol. 2014;44:591–6.
12. Hornok S, Horváth G, Jongejan F, Farkas R. Ixodid ticks on ruminants, with on-host initiated moulting (apolysis) of *Ixodes*, *Haemaphysalis* and *Dermacentor* larvae. Vet Parasitol. 2012;187:350–3.
13. Hornok S, Meli ML, Gönczi E, Halász E, Takács N, Farkas R, et al. Occurrence of ticks and prevalence of *Anaplasma phagocytophilum* and *Borrelia burgdorferi* s.L. in three types of urban biotopes: forests, parks and cemeteries. Ticks Tick Borne Dis. 2014;5:785–9.
14. Hornok S, Meli ML, Perreten A, Farkas R, Willi B, Beugnet F, et al. Molecular investigation of hard ticks (Acari: Ixodidae) and fleas (Siphonaptera: Pulicidae) as potential vectors of rickettsial and mycoplasmal agents. Vet Microbiol. 2010;140:98–104.
15. Hornok S, Micsutka A, Meli ML, Lutz H, Hofmann-Lehmann R. Molecular investigation of transplacental and vector-borne transmission of bovine haemoplasmas. Vet Microbiol. 2011;152:411–4.
16. Hornok S, Meli ML, Erdős A, Hajtós I, Lutz H, Hofmann-Lehmann R. Molecular characterization of two different strains of haemotropic mycoplasmas from a sheep flock with fatal haemolytic anaemia and concomitant *Anaplasma ovis* infection. Vet Microbiol. 2009;136:372–7.
17. Kántás K, Andó P. Eperythrozoonosis in pigs in Hungary. Magyar Allatorvosok Lapja. 1987;42:673–6. (in Hungarian with English abstract)
18. Guimaraes AM, Vieira RF, Poletto R, Vemulapalli R, Santos AP, de Moraes W, et al. A quantitative TaqMan PCR assay for the detection of *Mycoplasma suis*. J Appl Microbiol. 2011;111:417–25.
19. de la Fuente J, Massung RF, Wong SJ, Chu FK, Lutz H, Meli M, von Loewenich FD, Grzeszczuk A, Torina A, Caracappa S, Mangold AJ, Naranjo V, Stuen S, Kocan KM. Sequence analysis of the *msp4* gene of *Anaplasma phagocytophilum* strains. J Clin Microbiol. 2005;43:1309–17.
20. Uspensky I. Preliminary observations on specific adaptations of exophilic ixodid ticks to forests or open country habitats. Exp Appl Acarol. 2002;28:147–54.
21. Hornok S, Farkas R. Influence of biotope on the distribution and peak activity of questing ixodid ticks in Hungary. Med Vet Entomol. 2009;23:41–6.
22. Nahayo A, Bardiau M, Volpe R, Pirson J, Paternostre J, Fett T, et al. Molecular evidence of *Anaplasma phagocytophilum* in wild boar (*Sus scrofa*) in Belgium. BMC Vet Res. 2014;10:80.
23. Michalik J, Stańczak J, Cieniuch S, Racewicz M, Sikora B, Dabert M. Wild boars as hosts of human-pathogenic *Anaplasma phagocytophilum* variants. Emerg Infect Dis. 2012;18:998–1001.
24. de la Fuente J, Gortazar C. Wild boars as hosts of human-pathogenic *Anaplasma phagocytophilum* variants. Emerg Infect Dis. 2012;18:2094–5.
25. Smrdel KS, Bidovec A, Malovrh T, Petrovec M, Duh D, Zupanc TA. Detection of *Anaplasma phagocytophilum* in wild boar in Slovenia. Clin Microbiol Infect. 2008;15(Suppl 2):50–2.
26. Adamska M. Role of some game species and *Ixodes ricinus* ticks in the propagation of *Anaplasma phagocytophilum* in a forest biotope in North-Western Poland. Bull Vet Inst Pulawy. 2010;54:581–4.
27. Egri B, Piszmán R. Prevalence of *Haematopinus tuberculatus* in buffalo stocks. Magyar Allatorvosok Lapja. 2014;136:59–64. (in Hungarian with English abstract)
28. Prullage JB, Williams RE, Gaafar SM. On the transmissibility of *Eperythrozoon suis* by *Stomoxys calcitrans* and *Aedes aegypti*. Vet Parasitol. 1993;50:125–35.
29. Vale GA, Hargrove JW, Solano P, Courtin F, Rayaisse JB, Lehane MJ, Esterhuizen J, Tirados I, Torr SJ. Explaining the host-finding behavior of blood-sucking insects: computerized simulation of the effects of habitat geometry on tsetse fly movement. PLoS Negl Trop Dis. 2014;8:e2901.
30. Maede Y. Sequestration and phagocytosis of *Haemobartonella felis* in the spleen. Am J Vet Res. 1979;40:691–5.
31. Hoelzle K, Engels M, Kramer MM, Wittenbrink MM, Dieckmann SM, Hoelzle LE. Occurrence of *Mycoplasma suis* in wild boars (*Sus scrofa* L.). Vet Microbiol. 2010;143:405–9.
32. Yuan CL, Liang AB, Yao CB, Yang ZB, Zhu JG, Cui L, et al. Prevalence of *Mycoplasma suis* (*Eperythrozoon suis*) infection in swine and swine-farm workers in shanghai, China. Am J Vet Res. 2009;70:890–4.
33. Bogdán O, Heltai M. The occurrence of wild boar in the city of Budapest. Vadbiológia. 2014;16:87–96. (in Hungarian with English abstract)
34. Štefanidesová K, Kocianová E, Boldiš V, Košťanová Z, Kanka P, Némethová D, et al. Evidence of *Anaplasma phagocytophilum* and *Rickettsia helvetica* infection in free-ranging ungulates in Central Slovakia. Eur J Wildl Res. 2008;54:519–24.
35. Courtney JW, Kostelnik LM, Zeidner NS, Massung RF. Multiplex real-time PCR for detection of *Anaplasma phagocytophilum* and *Borrelia burgdorferi*. J Clin Microbiol. 2004;42:3164–8.
36. Willi B, Meli ML, Lüthy R, Honegger H, Wengi N, Hoelzle LE, et al. Development and application of a universal hemoplasma screening assay based on the SYBR green PCR principle. J Clin Microbiol. 2009;47:4049–54.
37. Hornok S, Abichu G, Meli ML, Tánczos B, Sulyok KM, Gyuranecz M, et al. Influence of the biotope on the tick infestation of cattle and on the tick-borne pathogen repertoire of cattle ticks in Ethiopia. PLoS One. 2014;9:e106452.
38. Meli ML, Willi B, Dreher UM, Cattori V, Knubben-Schweizer G, Nuss K, et al. Identification, molecular characterization, and occurrence of two bovine hemoplasma species in Swiss cattle and development of real-time TaqMan quantitative PCR assays for diagnosis of bovine hemoplasma infections. J Clin Microbiol. 2010;48:3563–8.
39. Boretti FS, Perreten A, Meli ML, Cattori V, Willi B, Wengi N, et al. Molecular investigations of *Rickettsia helvetica* infection in dogs, foxes, humans and *Ixodes* spp. ticks. Appl Environ Microbiol. 2009;75:3230–7.

16

Coxiella and *Bartonella* spp. in bats (Chiroptera) captured in the Brazilian Atlantic Forest biome

Michelle Santos Ferreira[1], Alexandro Guterres[1], Tatiana Rozental[1*], Roberto Leonan Morim Novaes[2], Emmanuel Messias Vilar[3], Renata Carvalho de Oliveira[1], Jorlan Fernandes[1], Danielle Forneas[1], Adonai Alvino Junior[1], Martha Lima Brandão[4], José Luis Passos Cordeiro[4], Martín Roberto Del Valle Alvarez[5], Sergio Luiz Althoff[6], Ricardo Moratelli[4], Pedro Cordeiro-Estrela[3], Rui Cerqueira da Silva[7] and Elba Regina Sampaio de Lemos[1*]

Abstract

Background: The role of bats as reservoirs of zoonotic agents, especially pathogenic bacteria such as Bartonella and Coxiella, has been discussed around the world. Recent studies have identified bats as potential hosts of species from the proteobacteria phylum. In Brazil, however, the role of bats in the natural cycle of these agents is poorly investigated and generally neglected. In order to analyze the participation of bats in the epidemiology of diseases caused by *Bartonella*, *Coxiella*, *Rickettsia*, *Anaplasma* and *Ehrlichia*, we conducted a descriptive epidemiological study in three biogeographic regions of the Brazilian Atlantic Forest.

Results: Tissues of 119 bats captured in preserved areas in the states of Rio de Janeiro, Bahia and Santa Catarina from 2014 to 2015 were submitted to molecular analysis using specific primers. *Bartonella* spp. was detected in 22 spleen samples (18.5%, 95% CI: 11.9–26.6), whose phylogenetic analysis revealed the generation of at least two independent clusters, suggesting that these may be new unique genotypes of *Bartonella* species. In addition, four samples (3.4%, 95% CI: 0.9–8.3) were positive for the *htpAB* gene of *C. burnetii* [spleen (2), liver (1) and heart (1)]. *Rickettsia* spp., *Anaplasma* and *Ehrlichia* were not identified. This is the first study reporting *C. burnetii* and *Bartonella* spp. infections in bats from the Atlantic Forest biome.

Conclusions: These findings shed light on potential host range for these bacteria, which are characterized as important zoonotic pathogens.

Keywords: *Coxiella burnetii*, *Bartonella*, Zoonotic bacterial agent, Mammals, Atlantic Forest hotspot, Brazil

Background

Bacteria transmitted by arthropods belonging to the genera *Rickettsia*, *Bartonella*, *Coxiella*, *Ehrlichia* and *Anaplasma* are pathogens of domestic and wild animals as well as humans. These agents cause diseases that may be severe and have a widespread geographic distribution, such as bartonelosis, ehrlichiosis, anaplasmosis, spotted fever, and Coxielosis/Q fever [1–4]. *Bartonella* spp. (proteobacteria $\alpha 2$ group), an intracellular hemotropic bacterium that grows fastidiously, is transmitted mainly by flea bites [4]. *Coxiella burnetii* (proteobacteria γ group), the causative agent of Q fever/Coxiellosis, is a highly infectious zoonotic intracellular bacterium transmitted by inhalation of aerosols or contaminated excreta materials. Ticks are suspected of having a role in the transmission of this pathogen among animals [5]. *Rickettsia* (proteobacteria $\alpha 1$ group) is a representative genus group of pathogenic or non-pathogenic intracellular bacteria transmitted by ticks, mites, lice and fleas [2]. *Ehrlichia* and *Anaplasma* (proteobacteria $\alpha 1$ group), which are known to cause diseases in animals and humans, are kept in the wild in a cycle involving mammals and arthropods

* Correspondence: rozental@ioc.fiocruz.br; elemos@ioc.fiocruz.br
[1]Laboratório de Hantaviroses e Rickettsioses, Pavilhão Helio e Peggy Pereira, 1 Pavimento, Instituto Oswaldo Cruz, Fundação Oswaldo Cruz, Avenida Brasil 4365, Manguinhos, Rio de Janeiro, RJ, Brazil
Full list of author information is available at the end of the article

[6]. In recent years, studies have pointed to bats as hosts of these proteobacteria around the world [7–11]. Their increasing diversity and apparent clade-specific association for *Bartonella* spp. [12] encourages increasing inventory and surveillance efforts, especially in sylvatic environments to better understand their natural transmission cycles.

Bats (order Chiroptera) occur in all continents except Antarctica [13]. Among mammals, they are outnumbered only by rodents in species richness but surpass all other groups in dietary diversity, including fruit eaters, nectar feeders, insectivores, carnivores, blood feeders and omnivores. In biodiversity hotspots such as Brazil's Atlantic Forest, bats are the most diverse and abundant mammals, and they represent wild vertebrates that interact with humans [14] especially in urban areas [15]. The role of bats as important hosts for emerging human diseases has gained the attention of the scientific community. They are recognized for harboring viral infectious agents and, less recognizably, bacterial agents of public health importance [16–18].

In Brazil, the vespertilionid bat species *Histiotus velatus* (tropical big-eared brown bat), and the phyllostomids *Carollia perspicillata* (Seba's short-tailed bat) and *Desmodus rotundus* (common vampire bat) were considered reservoirs of rickettsiae in an experimental study in the 1950s [19]. After more than 50 years, in the city of São Paulo, molossid, vespertilionid and phyllostomid bats were seroreactive to, at least, one rickettsial antigen of the spotted fever group [20]. In Queensland, Australia, in 2014, the DNA of *C. burnetii* was found in bat urine pools of a *Pteropus* (Pteropodidae) [8]. This finding might be indicative of the potential role of these animals as a source of infection for humans and other animal species through the inhalation of contaminated aerosols. Probably related to their sporulation process, *C. burnetii* survives for long periods in the environment, and inhalation is characterized as the main mechanism by which this microorganism is transmitted [21–23].

In addition, there are studies around the world in which from different species of *Bartonella* has been detected in bats for example, in, Peru [24], Kenya [25], United Kingdom [26], Guatemala [27], Nigeria [7], Puerto Rico [28], Vietnam [9], Costa Rica [10] and Taiwan [29]. More recently, strains of *Bartonella mayotimonensis*, a recognized human pathogen, were identified and isolated from bats in the northern hemisphere [30]. In Brazil, up to now, there is one study associating *Bartonella* with bats [11]. However, the real role of bats as hosts and maintainers of the natural cycle of these bacteria in nature remains unknown. Studies proving associations between bats and *C. burnetii*, *Ehrlichia* and *Anaplasma* have not yet been reported.

Considering the growing importance of bats as potential reservoirs and transmitters of different pathogens around the world as well as the paucity of investigations about the role of bats in the dissemination of proteobacteria pathogens, the present study provides information about the circulation of these zoonotic bacteria in bats captured in three Atlantic Forest localities in Brazil where notifications of Brazilian spotted fever, Q fever and bartonelosis have been reported.

Methods

Study areas and sample collection

The study was conducted in three Brazil's Atlantic Forest localities: Oswaldo Cruz Foundation (Fiocruz) Atlantic Forest Biological Station (EFMA; 22°56′22.9"S 43°24′12.2"W), Pedra Branca Massif, Jacarepaguá, which is a metropolitan area of the city of Rio de Janeiro (RJ); city of Igrapiúna, southern region of Bahia (BA), which is within the Environmental Protection Area (APA) of Pratigi (13°50′43.3"S 39°16′17.0"W); Serra do Tabuleiro State Park (PEST; 27°44′30.8"S 48°48′26.7"W), which is located in the central-eastern region of Santa Catarina state (SC) in the metropolitan area of the city Florianópolis (Fig. 1). The vegetation of the three sampling areas are composed by lowland humid forest areas from three different biogeographic regions of the Atlantic Forest biome.

From December 2013 to May 2015, expeditions were carried out and bats were captured using 10 ground-level mist nets (9 × 3 m) each night in forest edges or along pre-existing trails. Permits for field collection were granted by an Brazilian Institute of Environment and Renewable Natural Resources (IBAMA) license under process numbers 19,037–1; Santa Catarina's Environment Foundation (FATMA) no. 043/2014/GERUC/DPEC, Chico Mendes Biodiversity Conservation Institute (ICMBio/SISBIO) no. 26934–1 and no. 17131–4 (ICMBio/SISBIO). Adult males and non-pregnant and non-lactating adult females were euthanized. The euthanasia method consisted of cardiac puncture exsanguination performed after the anesthesia procedure of the animal, according to previously established protocols [31]. Efforts were made to minimize animal suffering following protocols approved by the Institutional Ethics Committee on Animal Research (CEUA) of the Oswaldo Cruz Foundation under process numbers CEUA P.62/11–3 (LW-68/12) and P.42/12–1 (LW-81/12).

The sex, age class and biometry of each bat were registered. Bats tissues (i.e., kidney, liver, spleen, lung and heart) were sampled and preserved in absolute ethanol. Tissue samples were obtained in accordance with recommended safety procedures and followed previously established standard protocols [32]. Bat species was identified following the identification keys available in Gardner [33] and nomenclature in Nogueira et al. [34]. Voucher specimens were deposited at scientific collections from each region where the study was performed: Federal University of Rio de Janeiro, for bats collected in Rio de Janeiro; State University of Santa

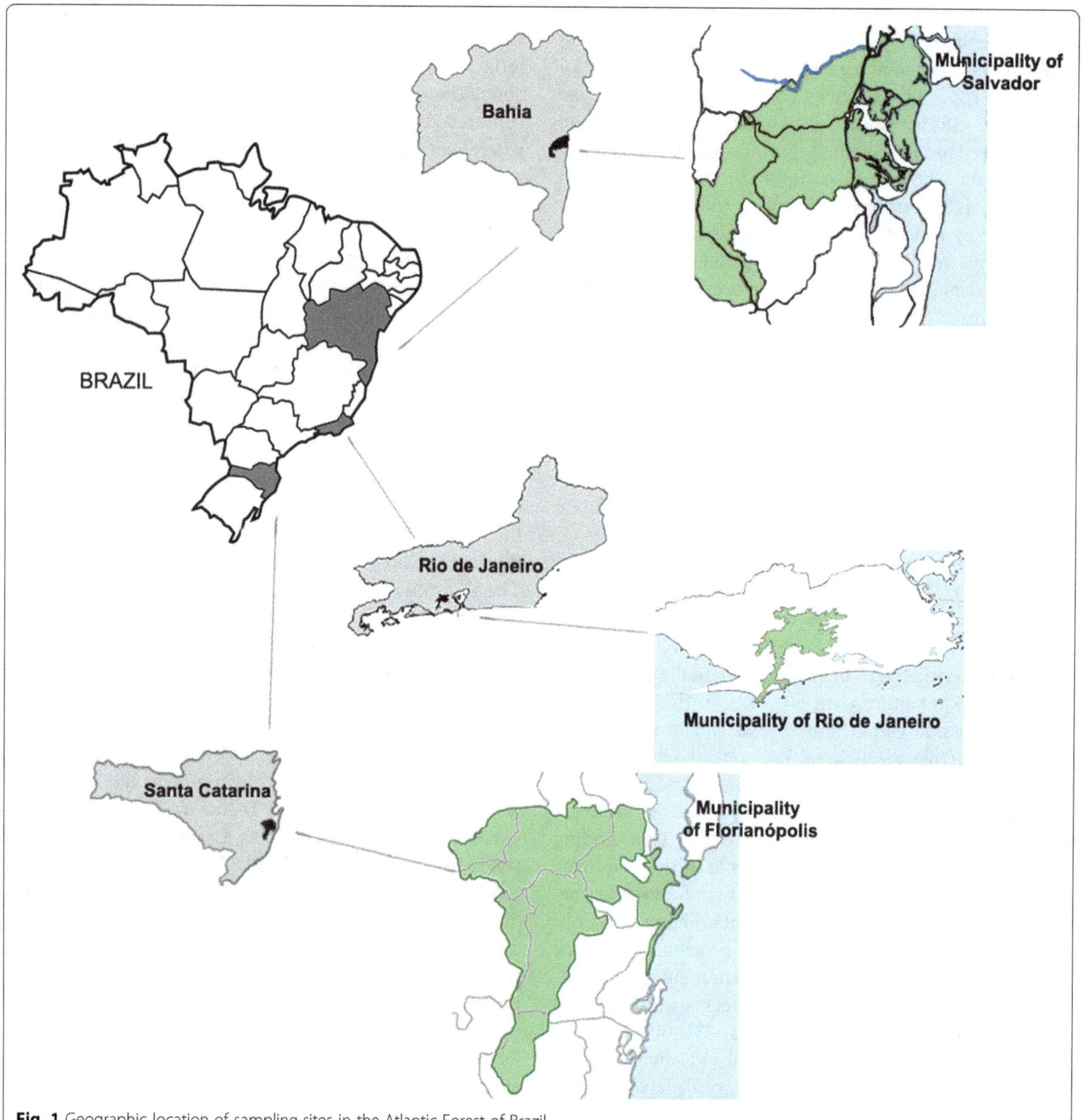

Fig. 1 Geographic location of sampling sites in the Atlantic Forest of Brazil

Cruz, for bats from Bahia; Foundation University of Blumenal and in the Collection of Mammals of the Federal University of Paraíba, for bats collected in Santa Catarina state. Prevalences and approximated confidence intervals (CIs) were calculated using the package "binom". To evaluate the influence of the sex-ratio on the positivity we use a Fisher exact's test.

Nucleic acid extraction

The DNA extraction procedures were performed in laminar flow biosafety cabinet in a Biosafety Level 3 laboratory (Vecobiosafe, Veco, Campinas, SP, Brazil). DNA was extracted from 10 mg of each bat tissue using the commercial QIAamp DNA Mini Kit (QIAGEN, Valencia, CA, USA) according to the manufacturer's instructions. The final volume of 100-μl obtained after elution in AE buffer (QIAGEN, Valencia, CA, USA). Negative controls using nuclease-free water were included in each extraction to check for DNA contamination.

Spleen tissues were investigated for all agents covered in this study; however, in an attempt to identify complementarity of information for *Coxiella burnetii* research, other tissues were tested as well.

PCR amplification

Conventional polymerase chain reaction (PCR) assays was used to detect the target genes. The gene for which each agent investigated in this study was tested is listed below and demonstrated in Table 1. *Bartonella* spp., *gltA* gene [35]. *Coxiella burnetii,* bacterial-specific primers designed to amplify the IS1111 gene [36, 37]. *Rickettsia* spp., a partial sequence of the *gltA* gene [35]. *Ehrlichia* and *Anaplasma* bacterial,16S rRNA gene [38].

The mixture to each reaction contained 2.5 µl of 10X PCR buffer, 0.6 µl of 10 mM of each primer, 0.75–2 µl of 50 mM MgCl2, 0.25 µl deoxynucleotides (20 mM of each deoxynucleotide triphosphate), 0.1 µl Taq Platinum DNA polymerase (5 U/µl Invitrogen, Carlsbad, CA, USA) and nuclease-free water (Promega, Madison, WI, USA) to obtain a final volume of 25 µl. The volumes of the DNA sample varied as a function of the primer used. To *Bartonella* spp. was used 3 µl; to *Rickettsia* spp., 3 µl for PCR 1 and 2 µl for nested PCR; to *C. burnetii,*4 µl for PCR 1 and 2 µl for nested PCR; to *Ehrlichia* and *Anaplasma* spp., 2.5 µl. Volumes pre-established in a previous study [35]. Negative controls using nuclease-free water were included in each PCR assay to check for possible DNA contamination. Genomic DNA extracted from positive clinical samples from the National Reference Laboratory for Rickettsioses were used as positive controls. PCR amplification was subjected to a 1.5% agarose gel, stained with GelRed™ (Biotium, Hayward, CA, USA).

DNA sequencing and phylogenetic analyses

Appropriately sized fragments were purified using Illustra GFX PCR DNA and Gel Band Purification® kit (GE Healthcare, Buckinghamshire, UK), direct nucleotide sequencing amplicon was performed using the BigDye Terminator v3.1 Cycle Sequencing kit, and purification was performed using the BigDye® X-Terminator Purification kit (Applied Biosystems, Foster City, CA, USA), according to the manufacturer's recommendations. The analyses of the amplicons were performed in an ABI Prism 3730XL with 96 capillaries (Applied Biosystems) and the nucleotide sequences were analyzed using MEGA7 software (downloaded from www.megasoftware.net). A consensus sequence for each bacterial genome was derived from contiguous sequences assembled with the same software.

Multiple sequence alignments were done with sequences obtained from this study and sequences from the GenBank using MUSCLE in the SeaView v.4 program [39]. The

Table 1 Oligonucleotide primers used for screening bat samples of *Coxiella burnetii*, *Bartonella* spp., *Rickettsia* spp., *Ehrlichia* spp. and *Anaplasma* spp.

Pathogen	Target gene	Oligonucleotide primer	Primer sequence (5' – 3')	Amplicon size (bp)	Cycling conditions	Reference
Coxiella burnetii	IS1111	Outer primer F Outer primer R Nested primer F Nested primer R	TATGTATCCACCGTAGCCAGC CCCAACAACACCTCCTTATTC AAGCGTGTGGAGGAGCGAA CC CTCGTAATCACCAATCGCT TCGTC	687 bp 440 bp	95 °C for 5 min, 40 cycles of 95 °C for 30s, 60 °C for 30s, 72 °C for 1 min, final extension of 72 °C for 7 min 95 °C for 5 min, 30 cycles of 95 °C for 30 s, 66 °C for 30 s, 72 °C for 30 s, final extension of 72 °C for 5 min	[36] [35, 37]
Bartonella spp.	gltA	Outer primer F Outer primer R	GCTATGTCTGCVTTCT ATCAYGA AGAACAGTAAACATTTCN GTHGG	731 bp	95 °C for 10 min, 35 cycles of 95 °C for 30s, 58 °C for 30s, 72 °C for 1 min, final extension of 72 °C for 8 min	[35]
Rickettsia spp.	gltA	Outer primer F Outer primer R Nested primer F Nested primer R	CATCCTATGGCTATTATGC TTGC TATACTCTCTATG(T/A)AC(A/ G)T(A/G)ACC CTTACCGCTATTAGAATGA TTGC GAGCGA(T/G)AGCTTCAAG(T/ C)TCTAT	885 bp 572 bp	95 °C for 10 min, 30 cycles of 95 °C for 30 s, 55 °C for 40 s, 72 °C for 55 s, final extension of 72 °C for 10 min 95 °C for 7 min, 25 cycles of 95 °C for 30 s, 63 °C for 30 s, 72 °C for 35 s, final extension of 72 °C for 10 min	[35] [35]
Ehrlichia spp. /*Anaplasma* spp.	16 s rRNA	Outer primer F Outer primer R	GGTACCYACAGAAGAAGTCC TGCACTCATCGTTTACAG	345 bp	95 °C for 3 min, 35 cycles of 95 °C for 15 s, 55 °C for 30 s, 72 °C for 30s, final extension of 72 °C for 5 min	[38]

best-fit evolutionary model was determined using MEGA version 7 by the Bayesian Information Criterion [40]. The phylogenetic tree was estimated using two methods: (a) Maximum Likelihood using PhyML implemented in SeaView v.4 [41], where the statistical support of the clades was measured by a heuristic search with 1000 bootstrap replicates; and (b) a Bayesian Markov Chain Monte Carlo (MCMC) method implemented in MrBayes v.3.2.6 [42]. The Bayesian analysis consisted of two simultaneous independent runs of 10 million MCMC generations (burn-in of 25%).

Results

Bat sampling

A total of 119 adult bats belonging to 21 species were sampled; $n = 44$ from EFMA/RJ; $n = 47$ from APA Pratigi/BA and $n = 28$ from PEST/SC (Table 2). The species sampled and their abundances are as follows: *Carollia perspicillata* ($n = 34$), *Desmodus rotundus* (15), *Artibeus lituratus* (14), *Sturnira lilium* (12), *Artibeus fimbriatus* (7), *Rhinophylla pumilio* (7) *Artibeus planirostris* (5), *Dermanura cinerea* (4), *Phyllostomus discolor* (4), *Artibeus obscurus* (2), *Glossophaga soricina* (2), *Myotis nigricans* (2), *Sturnira tildae* (2), *Vampyressa pusilla* (2), *Anoura caudifer* (1), *Chiroderma doriae* (1), *Lonchophylla peracchii* (1), *Micronycteris minuta* (1), *Micronycteris* sp. (1), *Phyllostonus hastatus* (1), and *Trinycteris nicefori* (1).

Detection of *Bartonella* spp.

Bartonella DNA was detected in 22 animals (18.5%, 95% CI: 11.9–26.6) (Table 3) collected from the three regions of this study (Table 2): Jacarepaguá/RJ (10/44; 23.0%, 95% CI: 11.4–37.8); APA Pratigi/BA (7/47; 15%, 95% CI: 6.2–28.3) and PEST/SC (5/28; 18%, 95% CI: 6.0–36.8). Although *S. lilium* (6/22 *Bartonella*-positive bats) and *D. rotundus* (6/22) were the most frequent hosts of *Bartonella*, six other bats species (i.e., *C. perspicillata, A. lituratus, A. fimbriatus, A. obscurus, R. pumilio*and *P. discolor*) were also positive (Table 3). Contrasting the pool of males against the pool of females per locality, in all study areas we found more positive samples for males than females, but only in APA Pratigi/BA this difference was significant (Fisher exact's test $p = 0.0027$). Due to the small sample size per species/locality, we did not run this analysis per species.

However, in this study, we opted to work with sequences that presented fragment sizes that would allow reliable results when submitted to phylogenetic analyses. Thus, of the 22 samples that were positive for the *Bartonella gltA* gene, 11 were included in these analyses. The phylogenetic inference based on the *gltA* gene sequences revealed two different clusters for the new sequences of this study (Fig. 2). In the *gltA* gene tree, the first cluster is composed of two groups; one of them comprised our sequence (EM 209) found in *P. discolor* in the state of Bahia as well as the sequence *Bartonella* sp. clone SJ114 (KJ816690) found in *Carollia sowelli* and the sequence *Bartonella* sp. clone SJ101 (KJ816666) found in *Anoura geoffroyi*, both from Costa Rica (1/ 99). The second group in the same cluster is composed of the sequence of *Bartonella* sp. clone SJ131 (KJ816670) found in *Sturnira lilium* from Costa Rica as a stem lineage in the clade (1/ 85).The next node (1/ 100) within the cluster contained our sequences (EM 805, RM 525) found in *S. lilium* from the states of Santa Catarina and Rio de Janeiro (1/ 83), in a sister relation to the clade of our sequences found in *A. fimbriatus* and *A. obscurus* (RM 524, RM 529) from Rio de Janeiro (0.79/ *).

The second weakly supported cluster comprises two sister groups. One (1/ 99) includes our three sequences (RM 512, RM 534, RM 564) found in *D. rotundus* from the state of Rio de Janeiro, and the other includes the sequence *Bartonella* sp. clone SJ117 (KJ816691) found in *C. perspicillata* from Costa Rica and our two sequences (EM 185, EM 199) found in *C.perspicillata* from Bahia state (0.93/ 95). The other group is composed of the sequence of *Bartonella* sp. clone SJ128 (KJ816692) found in *P. discolor* from Costa Rica as a stem lineage in the group (1/ 94). The next bifurcation within the cluster contained our sequence (EM 819) found in *S. lilium* from Santa Catarina state as well as the sequence of *Bartonella* sp. clone 1 (KY356753) found in an undescribed bat species from Brazil and the sequence *Bartonella* sp. clone SJ130 (KJ816674) found *S. lilium* from Costa Rica (1/ 99).

Detection of *Coxiella burnetii*

Coxiella burnetii DNA was detected in four specimens from two bat species (3.4%, 95% CI: 0.9–8.3), *A. lituratus* (3/4 Coxiella-positive bats) and *A. fimbriatus* (1/4) from two different regions: Jacarepaguá/RJ (3/44; 7%, 95% CI: 1.4–18.6) and PEST/SC (1/28; 4%, 95% CI: 0.1–18.3) (Tables 2 and 3). No differences between positivity in males and females were observed. *Coxiella* DNA sequences showed 100% identity to the complete genome of *C. burnetii* [GenBank CP018005, CP020616, AE 016828, LK 937696]. In our survey, co-infection was detected in one bat sample of *A. fimbriatus* from the Jacarepaguá/RJ region (Table 2). *Rickettsia* spp., *Ehrlichia* spp. and *Anaplasma* spp. DNA was not detected in any of the bat samples tested.

Nucleotide sequence accession numbers

All sequences obtained including 11 for *Bartonella* spp. *gltA* (MH204887-MH204897) and 4 for *Coxiella burnetii* IS1111 (MH229948-MH229951) have been deposited in GenBank.

Table 2 Number of bats collected per locality (n), total number of bats (N), and infected bats (p), 95% confidence intervals of prevalences (CI) by *Bartonella* spp. and *Coxiella burnetii*

Family: Sub-family	Localities				PCR assay		
	Jacarepagua/ RJ n/N(%)	APA Pratigi/BA n/N(%)	PEST/SC n/N(%)	Total bats N(%)	*Bartonella* positive p/N(%;CI)	*Coxiella* positive p/ N(%; CI)	*Bartonella* and *Coxiella* positive p/N(%;CI)
Phyllostomidae: Carolliinae							
Carollia perspicillata	4/34(11.8)	23/34(67.7)	7/34(20.6)	34(28.6)	5/34(14.7; 4.9–31.0)	NS	NA
Rhinophylla pumilio	0/7(0)	7/7(100)	0/7(0)	7(5.9)	1/7(14.3; 0.3–57.8)	NS	NA
Phyllostomidae: Desmodontinae							
Desmodus rotundus	15/15(100)	0/15(0)	0/15(0)	15(12.6)	6/15(40; 16.3–67.7)	NS	NA
Phyllostomidae: Glossophaginae							
Anoura caudifer	0/1(0)	0/1(0)	1/1 (100)	1(0.8)	NS	NS	NA
Glossophaga soricina	2/2(100)	0/2(0)	0/2(0)	2(1.7)	NS	NS	NA
Lonchophylla peracchii	1/1(100)	0/1(0)	0/1(0)	1(0.8)	NS	NS	NA
Phyllostomidae: Glyphonycterinae							
Trinycteris nicefori	0/1(0)	1/1(100)	0/1(0)	1(0.8)	NS	NS	NA
Phyllostomidae: Micronycterinae							
Micronycteris minuta	1/1(100)	0/1(0)	0/1(0)	1(0.8)	NS	NS	NA
Micronycteris sp.	1/1(100)	0/1(0)	0/1(0)	1(0.8)	NS	NS	NA
Phyllostomidae: Phyllostominae							
Phyllostomus discolor	0/4(0)	4/4(100)	0/4(0)	4(3.4)	1/4(25; 0.6–80.5)	NS	NA
Phyllostomus hastatus	0/1(0)	0/1(0)	1/1(100)	1(0.8)	NS	NS	NA
Phyllostomidae: Stenodermatinae							
Artibeus fimbriatus	3/7 (42.9)	0/7(0)	4/7(57.1)	7(5.9)	1/7(14.3; 0.3–57.8)	1/7(14.3; 0.3–57.8)	1/7(14.3; 0.3–57.8)
Artibeus lituratus	4/14(28.6)	2/14(14.3)	8/14(57.1)	14(11.8)	1/14(7.1; 0.1–33.8)	3/14(21.4; 4.6–50.7)	NA
Artibeus obscurus	1/2(50)	0/2(0)	1/2(50)	2(1.7)	1/2(50; 1.2–98.7)	NS	NA
Artibeus planirostris	0/5(0)	5/5(100)	0/5(0)	5(4.2)	NS	NS	NA
Chiroderma doriae	0/1(0)	0/1(0)	1/1(100)	1(0.8)	NS	NS	NA
Dermanura cinerea	0/4(0)	4/4(100)	0/4(0)	4(3.4)	NS	NS	NA
Sturnira lillium	6/12 (50)	0/12(0)	6/12(50)	12(10.1)	6/12(50; 21.0–78.9)	NS	NA
Sturnira tildae	2/2(100)	0/2(0)	0/2(0)	2(1.7)	NS	NS	NA
Vampyressa pusilla	2/2(100)	0/2(0)	0/2(0)	2(1.7)	NS	NS	NA
Vespertilionidae: Myotinae							
Myotis nigricans	2/2(100)	0/2(0)	0/2(0)	2(1.7)	NS	NS	NA
TOTAL	44	47	28	119	22 (18.5; 11.9–26.6)	4 (3.4; 0.9–8.3)	1(0.8; 0.02–4.5)

NS negative sample, *NA* not applicable

Discussion

Considering the growing importance of bats as potential hosts of zoonotic agents of human disease, our findings reveal that bats of different species are infected with *Bartonella* spp. and *C. burnetii* in the Atlantic Forest regions of Rio de Janeiro, Bahia and Santa Catarina. In this study, we found a prevalence of 3.4% of bats positive for *C. burnetii* DNA, all belonging to the genus *Artibeus*. Characteristics of this genus, such as the formation of colonies grouping dozens of individuals of reproductive age [43] can contribute to a rapid and widespread transmission of *C. burnetii* among these animals, especially considering the high resistance of these proteobacteria, which can survive for several weeks in the environment where the

Table 3 Specimens infected by *Bartonella* spp. and *Coxiella burnetii*. Specimens are arranged by species, locality and sex

Field Number	Species	Sex	Locality
Bartonella spp.			
RM 510	*Desmodus rotundus*	Female	Jacarepaguá – RJ
RM 512	*Desmodus rotundus*	Male	Jacarepaguá – RJ
RM 517	*Desmodus rotundus*	Female	Jacarepaguá – RJ
RM 523	*Desmodus rotundus*	Male	Jacarepaguá – RJ
RM 524	*Artibeus fimbriatus*	Male	Jacarepaguá - RJ
RM 525	*Sturnira lilium*	Female	Jacarepaguá - RJ
RM 529	*Artibeus obscurus*	Male	Jacarepaguá - RJ
RM 532	*Sturnira lilium*	Male	Jacarepaguá - RJ
RM 534	*Desmodus rotundus*	Male	Jacarepaguá - RJ
RM 564	*Desmodus rotundus*	Female	Jacarepaguá – RJ
EM 179	*Carollia perspicillata*	Male	APA do Pratigi - BA
EM 185	*Carollia perspicillata*	Male	APA do Pratigi - BA
EM 186	*Artibeus lituratus*	Male	APA do Pratigi - BA
EM 189	*Rhinophylla pumilio*	Male	APA do Pratigi - BA
EM 199	*Carollia perspicillata*	Male	APA do Pratigi - BA
EM 209	*Phyllostomus discolor*	Male	APA do Pratigi - BA
EM 217	*Carollia perspicillata*	Male	APA do Pratigi – BA
EM 795	*Sturnira lilium*	Male	PEST - SC
EM 800	*Carollia perspicillata*	Male	PEST - SC
EM 803	*Sturnira lilium*	Male	PEST - SC
EM 805	*Sturnira lilium*	Male	PEST - SC
EM 819	*Sturnira lilium*	Female	PEST – SC
Coxiella burnetii			
RM 514	*Artibeus lituratus*	Female	Jacarepaguá/RJ
RM 524	*Artibeus fimbriatus*	Male	Jacarepaguá/RJ
RM 557	*Artibeus lituratus*	Male	Jacarepaguá/RJ
EM 817	*Artibeus lituratus*	Female	PEST /SC

animals were present [22]. Our results as well as recently published findings [35, 44] suggest the existence of a complex *C. burnetii* transmission cycle involving a large number of wild and domestic animals in Rio de Janeiro. In addition, the presence of *C. burnetii* DNA in bats captured in the region of Santa Catarina state is the first evidence of the circulation of this agent in the state.

Our prevalence results (18.5%) corroborate other studies worldwide showing the prevalence of *Bartonella* spp. in bats between 18.0–33.3% [10, 24, 27]. In our study, *S. lilium* (27.3%), *D. rotundus* (27.3%) and *C. perspicillata* (22.7%) were the species that presented the highest prevalence of *Bartonella* infection. In South America, similar results were obtained in Peru, with a prevalence of 15% for *C. perspicillata* (4/27), 37% for *D. rotundus*, (10/27) and 4% for *S. lilium* (1/27) [24]. In Brazil, in a study recently carried out in 5 different states, positive samples for *Bartonella* spp. were found in *S. lilium*, *C. perspicillata*, *P. discolor*, *Glossophaga soricina* and *Natalus espiritosantensis* (*Natalusmacrourus* [45]) [11]. Although we have found more positive samples for males than females in all studied areas, the evidence available, including the established knowledge on transmission routes and the role of bats in the circulation of these pathogens, do not allow us to speculate on the pathogen prevalence in males. Further analyses comparing males and females per species are necessary for better understanding the role of sexes in the pathogen circulation.

The phylogenetic tree revealed the formation of independent clades when compared to *Bartonella* species reported in the literature, which may indicate that previously unknown genotypes of *Bartonella* are infecting these bats. This is a common finding with studies of this agent in bats from other regions of the world (e.g., in Guatemala, Nigeria, Costa Rica and China) [7, 10, 27, 46]. Some of our obtained sequences showed a clear separation of the group formed in *Bartonella* sequences found in wild rodents of the Atlantic Forest in the state of Rio de Janeiro (LBCE- Laboratory of Biology and Control of Schistosomiasis), reinforcing that a new genotype may be circulating among bats and that these strains differ between rodents and bats [35]. Interestingly, our sequences were most closely related to others identified in bats from Costa Rica and related only to a single sequence found in a Brazilian bat. Furthermore, positive samples belonging to the *S. lilium* species were grouped into two distinct clades, suggesting that a single bat species is host to two different species of *Bartonella*. Similarly, sequences generated from Bahia, Rio de Janeiro and Santa Catarina states subjected to phylogenetic analyses were divided into two clades and suggested that the circulation of more than one species of *Bartonella* may be associated with bats in each state. Co-infection of different *Bartonella* species in a single bat species was also observed in Kenya, Guatemala, China and Georgia [25, 27, 46, 47]. A recent study demonstrated that *Bartonella* strains tend to cluster according to families, super-families and suborders of bats [48]. In addition, a co-infection with different species of *Bartonella* in a single species of bat may imply a change of bacteria via recombination, as shown by *Bartonella* in rodents [49]. The presence of divergent sequences in the analyzes of this study suggests the presence of more than one *Bartonella* lineage, since the divergence of the sampled sequences of the *gltA* gene varied from 0.0 to 20.9% in sequences of the same clade, the sequence divergence among Bartonella species suggested for this fragment is about 30% [50] (Additional file 1). To characterize the *Bartonella* species, it is necessary to sequencing other housekeeping genes (ie, *rpoB*, *ftsZ*,*groEL* and its) to recognize the diversity of lineages found in bats and to determine the structure of populations and phylogenetic data [51, 52]. Sequencing of the additional genes for improved taxonomic resolution was beyond the scope of this paper.

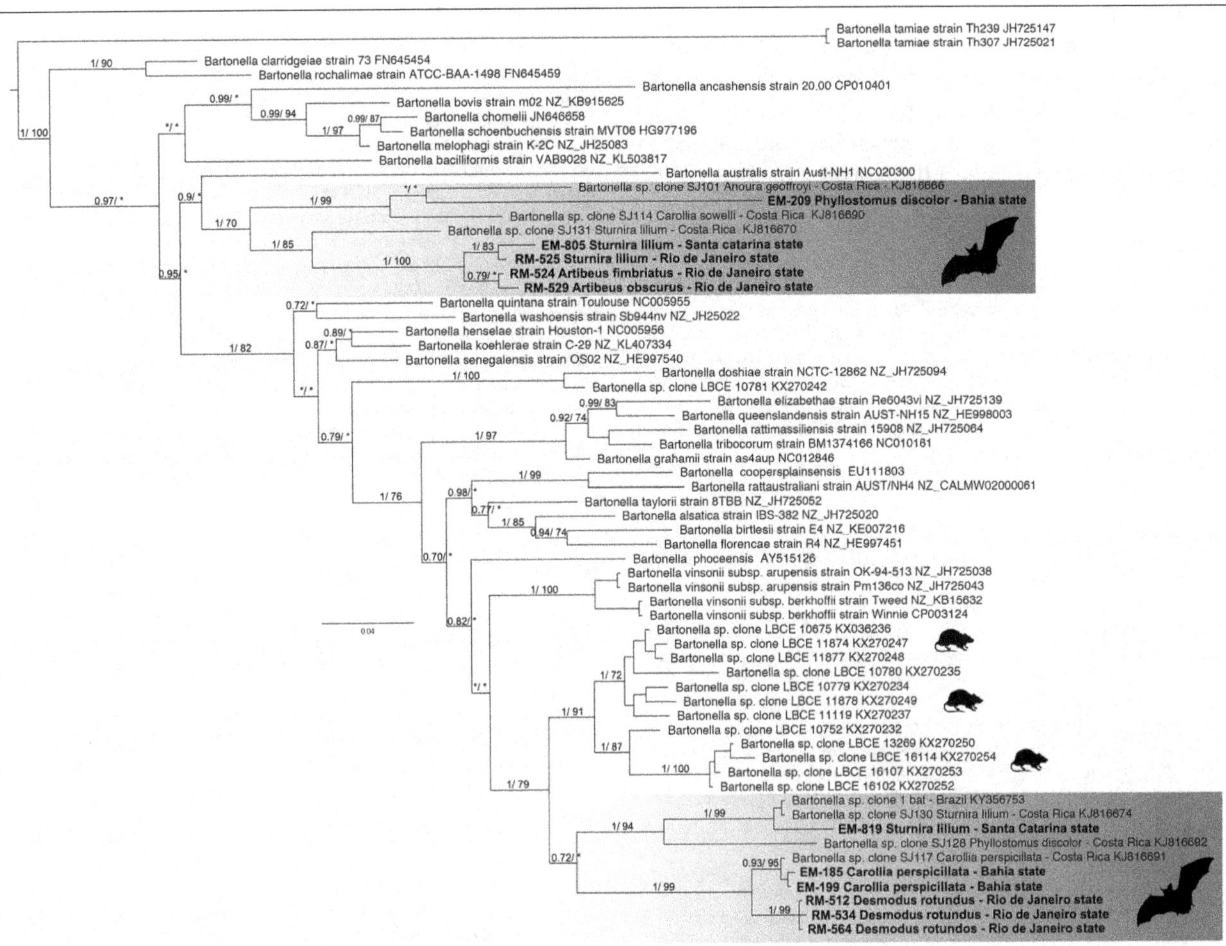

Fig. 2 Phylogenetic relationships based on the *gltA* gene partial (512 nt) sequences of *Bartonella* species. Numbers (≥ 0.7/70%) above branches indicate posterior node probabilities or bootstrap values (Bayesian/ML). *Indicate values below 0.7/70. The Tamura three-parameter model with gamma distributed rate heterogeneity (T92 + G) was selected as the best-fit evolutionary model according to the Bayesian information criterion calculated using MEGA7 [39]. The branch labels include the GenBank accession number and the species or strain

Our study has identified a co-infection with *C. burnetii* and *Bartonella* spp. in an individual of *A. fimbriatus*. Although a pattern cannot be established, dual infection can reinforce the potential of bats to host these bacterial pathogens. Many bat species are gregarious and can form small groups of a few individuals to large colonies of up to 20 million individuals, such as the species *Tadarida brasiliensis* in Bracken Cave in Texas, USA [53]. Furthermore, different bat species can cohabitate in the same shelter, allowing the possibility for interspecific transmission and a high rate of contact within these colonies that can lead to rapid transmission of pathogens [54]. Bats have been identified as potential natural reservoirs of a number of high-impact zoonotic agents. Recently, a study provided evidence that bats are indeed special in hosting more zoonotic viruses and more total viruses per species than rodents [55].

The absence of *Rickettsia* in bat samples corroborate the literature demonstrating that a lack of rickettsial amplification in wild animal is an expected result, since vertebrates act as amplifiers and food sources for ticks, which are in fact the true reservoirs of these proteobacteria in nature [35]. Besides, this reinforces that the role of bats as carriers of *Rickettsia* is still unknown, despite reports in the 1950s that bats harbor pathogenic rickettsial [19, 56, 57]. No samples tested in our study were positive for *Ehrlichia* and *Anaplasma* infections. Although bats have been found infected with proteobacteria of the families Anaplasmataceae [58], there is still no record of DNA amplification of *Ehrlichia* spp. or *Anaplasma* spp. in these mammals. Regardless of which other prior studies have used a similar method, it seems plausible that some negative detections may have resulted from a less sensitive PCR approach (i.e., conventional rather than nested).

Conclusion

This study confirms the presence of infected bats with *C. burnetii* and *Bartonella* spp. in the Brazilian Atlantic Forest. To the best of our knowledge, this is the first study that reports *C. burnetii* infection in Brazilian bats and the first to report *Bartonella* spp. in the Atlantic Forest biome.

Additional file

Additional file 1: Estimates of Evolutionary Divergence between *Bartonella gltA* partial sequences. There were a total of 512 positions in the final dataset. Evolutionary analyses were conducted in MEGA7. Presentation of the PCR positive bats species for *Bartonella* spp. in this study with their respective GenBank accession numbers and the estimated divergence found between *Bartonella gltA* partial sequences of the gene deposited in GenBank.

Abbreviations

APA: Environmental Protection Area; BA: Bahia; CEUA: Ethics Committee on Animal Research; CIs: Confidence intervals; CNPq: Conselho Nacional para o Desenvolvimento Cientifico e Tecnológico; EFMA: Fiocruz Atlantic Forest Biological Station; FAPERJ: Fundação de Amparo à Pesquisa do Estado do Rio de Janeiro; FATMA: Santa Catarina's Environment Foundation; Fiocruz: Oswaldo Cruz Foundation; IBAMA: Brazilian Institute of Environment and Renewable Natural Resources; ICMBio/SISBIO: Chico Mendes Biodiversity Conservation Institute; LBCE: Laboratory of Biology and Control of Schistosomiasis; MCMC: Bayesian Markov Chain Monte Carlo; PAPES: Strategic Health Research Program; PCR: Polymerase chain reaction; PEST: Serra do Tabuleiro State Park; PPBIO: Biodiversity Research Program; RJ: Rio de Janeiro; SC: Santa Catarina

Acknowledgements

The authors would like to thank Phyllis Romijn, Marcelo Pinto, Jairo Barreira, Maria Ogrzewalska, Endiá Almeida, Raphael Gomes and Liana Strecht for assistance with sampling process. We are in debt and very grateful to Dr. Bernardo Rodrigues Teixeira for the assistance in the statistical analysis of this work and MSc Jonathan Gonçalves for reviewing Bartonella subjects. We thank FATMA for their support for collecting licenses. We are deeply indebted to Hotel Plaza Caldas da Imperatriz for their logistic support of this work. We also thank Fernando Maciel Bruggmann for his support during planning, field work and his contagious enthusiasm.

Funding

This study was supported financially by Conselho Nacional para o Desenvolvimento Cientifico e Tecnológico (CNPq) Project 407664/2012-2 APQ, Fundação de Amparo à Pesquisa do Estado do Rio de Janeiro (FAPERJ) project E-26/010.001567/2014 APQ1, Biodiversity Research Program (PPBIO) Mata Atlântica - Rede BioMA (CNPq proc.: 457524/2012-0). RM is supported by Strategic Health Research Program (PAPES VI) Fiocruz/CNPq project 407623/2012-4.

Authors' contributions

All authors substantially contributed to the conception and design of the study. ERSL designed and writing the study protocol. MSF, AG, RLMN, EMV, RCO, AAJ, MLB, JLPC, MRVA, SLA were responsible for bats collection, identification and analysis of the data about bats. MSF, AG, TR, JF, DF were responsible for sample tests. MSF, AG, TR, RM, PCE, ERSL participated in interpretation of results and data analysis, writing and revision of the original manuscript. PCE participated in coordinating the data collection project in the states of Santa Catarina and Bahia. RM and RCS participated in coordinating the project of data collection in the state of Rio de Janeiro. All authors read and approved the final manuscript.

Consent for publication

Not applicable.

Competing interests

The authors declare that they have no competing interests

Author details

[1]Laboratório de Hantaviroses e Rickettsioses, Pavilhão Helio e Peggy Pereira, 1 Pavimento, Instituto Oswaldo Cruz, Fundação Oswaldo Cruz, Avenida Brasil 4365, Manguinhos, Rio de Janeiro, RJ, Brazil. [2]Universidade Federal do Rio de Janeiro, Av. Pedro Calmon, 550, Cidade Universitária, Rio de Janeiro, Rio de Janeiro, RJ, Brazil. [3]Laboratório de Mamíferos, Departamento de Sistemática e Ecologia, Centro de Ciências Exatas e da Natureza, Universidade Federal da Paraíba, Campus I, Castelo Branco, João Pessoa, PB, Brazil. [4]Fundação Oswaldo Cruz, Fiocruz Mata Atlântica, Estrada Rodrigues Caldas, 3400, Taquara, Rio de Janeiro, RJ, Brazil. [5]Departamento de Ciências Biológicas, Universidade Estadual de Santa Cruz, Rodovia Ilhéus - Itabuna, Km. 16 Salobrinho, Ilheus, BA, Brazil. [6]Departamento de Ciências Naturais, Laboratório de Biologia Animal, Fundação Universidade Regional de Blumenau, Ccen, Dcn. FURB - Fundação Universidade Regional de Blumenau Itoupava Seca, Blumenau, SC, Brazil. [7]Laboratório de Vertebrados, Departamento de Ecologia, Instituto de Biologia, Universidade Federal do Rio de Janeiro, Av. Pedro Calmon, 550, Cidade Universitária, Rio de Janeiro, RJ, Brazil.

References

1. Lemos ER, Alvarenga FB, Cintra ML, Ramos MC, Paddock CD, Ferebee TL, Zaki SR, Ferreira FC, Ravagnani RC, Machado RD, Guimaraes MA, Coura JR. Spotted fever in Brazil: a seroepidemiological study and description of clinical cases in an endemic area in the state of Sao Paulo. Am J Trop Med Hyg. 2001;65(4):329–34.
2. Parola P, Paddock CD, Raoult D. Tick-borne rickettsioses around the world: emerging diseases challenging old concepts. Clin Microbiol Rev. 2005;18(4):719–56.
3. Parker NR, Barralet JH, Bell AM. Q fever. Lancet. 2006;367(9511):679–88.
4. Chomel BB, Kasten RW. Bartonellosis, an increasingly recognized zoonosis. J Appl Microbiol. 2010;109(3):743–50.
5. Porter SR, Czaplicki G, Mainil J, Guatteo R, Saegerman C. Q fever: current state of knowledge and perspectives of research of a neglected zoonosis. Int J Microbiol. 2011;2011:248418.
6. Olano JP. Human Ehrlichioses. In: Rickettsial disease, D. Raoult and P. Parola, editors. 2007. New York: Informa healthcare. p. 213–22.
7. Kamani J, Baneth G, Mitchell M, Mumcuoglu KY, Gutierrez R, Harrus S. *Bartonella* species in bats (Chiroptera) and bat flies (Nycteribiidae) from Nigeria, West Africa. Vector Borne Zoonotic Dis. 2014;14(9):625–32.
8. Tozer SJ, Lambert SB, Strong CL, Field HE, Sloots TP, Nissen MD. Potential animal and environmental sources of Q fever infection for humans in Queensland. Zoonoses Public Health. 2014;61(2):105–12.
9. Anh PH, Van Cuong N, Son NT, Tue NT, Kosoy M, Woolhouse ME, Baker S, Bryant JE, Thwaites G, Carrique-Mas JJ, Rabaa MA. Diversity of *Bartonella* spp. in bats, southern Vietnam. Emerg Infect Dis. 2015;21(7):1266–7.
10. Judson SD, Frank HK, Hadly EA. Bartonellae are prevalent and diverse in costa Rican bats and bat flies. Zoonoses Public Health. 2015;62:609–17.
11. Ikeda P, Seki MC, Carrasco AOT, Rudiak LV, Miranda JMD, Goncalves SMM, Hoppe EGL, Albuquerque ACA, Teixeira MMG, Passos CE, Werther K, Machado RZ, Andre MR. Evidence and molecular characterization of *Bartonella* spp. and hemoplasmas in neotropical bats in Brazil. Epidemiol Infect. 2017;145(10):2038–52.
12. McKee CD, Kosoy MY, Bai Y, Osikowicz LM, Franka R, Gilbert AT, Boonmar S, Rupprecht CE, Peruski LF. Diversity and phylogenetic relationships among *Bartonella* strains from Thai bats. PLoS One. 2017;12(7):e0181696.
13. Schipper J, Chanson JS, Chiozza F, Cox NA, Hoffmann M, Katariya V, Lamoreux J, Rodrigues AS, Stuart SN, Temple HJ, et al. The status of the world's land and marine mammals: diversity, threat, and knowledge. Science. 2008;322(5899):225–30.
14. Moratelli R, Calisher CH. Bats and zoonotic viruses: can we confidently link bats with emerging deadly viruses? Mem Inst Oswaldo Cruz. 2015;110(1):1–22.
15. Nunes H, Rocha FL, Cordeiro-Estrela P. Bats in urban areas of Brazil: roosts, food resources and parasites in disturbed environments. Urban Ecosyst. 2017;20(4):953–69.
16. Fenton MB, Davison M, Kunz TH, McCracken GF, Racey PA, Tuttle MD. Linking bats to emerging diseases. Science. 2006;311(5764):1098–9. author reply 1098-9
17. Calisher CH, Childs JE, Field HE, Holmes KV, Schountz T. Bats: important reservoir hosts of emerging viruses. Clin Microbiol Rev. 2006;19(3):531–45.

18. Olival KJ, Hosseini PR, Zambrana-Torrelio C, Ross N, Bogich TL, Daszak P. Host and viral traits predict zoonotic spillover from mammals. Nature. 2017; 546(7660):646–50.
19. Magalhães O. Contribuição ao conhecimento do tifo exantemático neotrópico no Brasil. Mem Inst Oswaldo Cruz. 1953;51:463–73.
20. D'Auria SR, Camargo MC, Pacheco RC, Savani ES, Dias MA, da Rosa AR, de Almeida MF, Labruna MB. Serologic survey for rickettsiosis in bats from Sao Paulo city, Brazil. Vector Borne Zoonotic Dis. 2010;10(5):459–63.
21. Fournier PE, Marrie TJ, Raoult D. Diagnosis of Q fever. J Clin Microbiol. 1998; 36(7):1823–34.
22. Maurin M, Raoult D. Q fever. Clin Microbiol Rev. 1999;12(4):518–53.
23. Angelakis E, Raoult D. Q Fever. Vet Microbiol. 2010;140(3–4):297–309.
24. Bai Y, Recuenco S, Gilbert AT, Osikowicz LM, Gomez J, Rupprecht C, Kosoy MY. Prevalence and diversity of *Bartonella* spp. in bats in Peru. Am J Trop Med Hyg. 2012;87(3):518–23.
25. Kosoy M, Bai Y, Lynch T, Kuzmin IV, Niezgoda M, Franka R, Agwanda B, Breiman RF, Rupprecht CE. *Bartonella* spp. in bats, Kenya. Emerg Infect Dis. 2010;16(12):1875–81.
26. Concannon R, Wynn-Owen K, Simpson VR, Birtles RJ. Molecular characterization of haemoparasites infecting bats (Microchiroptera) in Cornwall. UK Parasitology. 2005;131(Pt 4):489–96.
27. Bai Y, Kosoy M, Recuenco S, Alvarez D, Moran D, Turmelle A, Ellison J, Garcia DL, Estevez A, Lindblade K, Rupprecht C. *Bartonella* spp. in Bats, Guatemala. Emerg Infect Dis. 2011;17(7):1269–72.
28. Olival KJ, Dittmar K, Bai Y, Rostal MK, Lei BR, Daszak P, Kosoy M. *Bartonella* spp. in a Puerto Rican bat community. J Wildl Dis. 2015;51(1):274–8.
29. Lin JW, Hsu YM, Chomel BB, Lin LK, Pei JC, Wu SH, Chang CC. Identification of novel *Bartonella* spp. in bats and evidence of Asian gray shrew as a new potential reservoir of *Bartonella*. Vet Microbiol. 2012;156(1–2):119–26.
30. Veikkolainen V, Vesterinen EJ, Lilley TM, Pulliainen AT. Bats as reservoir hosts of human bacterial pathogen, *Bartonella mayotimonensis*. Emerg Infect Dis. 2014;20(6):960–7.
31. Mills J, Childs J, Ksiazek T, Peters C. Methods for trapping and sampling small mammals for virologic testing. Department of Health and Human Services. Atlanta. 1995;
32. Lemos E, D' APS. Trabalho de campo com animais: procedimentos, riscos e biossegurança. Fiocruz: Rio de Janeiro; 2014. p. 180.
33. Gardner AL. Mammals of South America. Marsupials, xenarthrans, shrews, and bats. Vol. vol. 1. Chicago: University of Chicago Press; 2008.
34. Nogueira M, Lima I, Moratelli R, Tavares V, Gregorin R, Lúcio Peracchi A. Checklist of Brazilian bats, with comments on original records. Check List. 2014;10:808–21.
35. Rozental T, Ferreira MS, Guterres A, Mares-Guia MA, Teixeira BR, Goncalves J, Bonvicino CR, D'Andrea PS, de Lemos ER. Zoonotic pathogens in Atlantic Forest wild rodents in Brazil: *Bartonella* and *Coxiella* infections. Acta Trop. 2017;168:64–73.
36. Hoover TA, Vodkin MH, Williams JC. A *Coxiella burnetti* repeated DNA element resembling a bacterial insertion sequence. J Bacteriol. 1992;174(17):5540–8.
37. Mares-Guia M, Guterres A, Rozental T, Ferreira MDS, Lemos ERS. Clinical and epidemiological use of nested PCR targeting the repetitive element IS1111 associated with the transposase gene from *Coxiella burnetii*. Braz J Microbiol. 2017;
38. Inokuma H, Raoult D, Brouqui P. Detection of Ehrlichia platys DNA in Brown dog ticks (*Rhipicephalus sanguineus*) in Okinawa Island. Japan J Clin Microbiol. 2000;38(11):4219–21.
39. Edgar RC. Muscle: multiple sequence alignment with high accuracy and high throughput. Nucleic Acids Res. 2004;32(5):1792–7.
40. Kumar S, Stecher G, Tamura K. MEGA7: molecular evolutionary genetics analysis version 7.0 for bigger datasets. Mol Biol Evol. 2016;33(7):1870–4.
41. Gouy M, Guindon S, Gascuel O. SeaView version 4: a multiplatform graphical user interface for sequence alignment and phylogenetic tree building. Mol Biol Evol. 2010;27(2):221–4.
42. Ronquist F, Teslenko M, van der Mark P, Ayres DL, Darling A, Hohna S, Larget B, Liu L, Suchard MA, Huelsenbeck JP. MrBayes 3.2: efficient Bayesian phylogenetic inference and model choice across a large model space. Syst Biol. 2012;61(3):539–42.
43. Costa LM, Prata AFD, Moraes D, Conde CFV, Jordão-Nogueira T, Esberard CEL. Deslocamento de *Artibeus fimbriatus* sobre o mar. Chiroptera Neotropical. 2006;12(2):289–90.
44. Mares-Guia MA, Rozental T, Guterres A, Gomes R, Almeida DN, Moreira NS, Barreira JD, Favacho AR, Santana AL, Lemos ER. Molecular identification of the agent of Q fever - *Coxiella burnetii* - in domestic animals in state of Rio de Janeiro, Brazil. Rev Soc Bras Med Trop. 2014;47(2):231–4.
45. Garbino GST, Tejedor A. *Natalus macrourus* (Gervais, 1856) (Chiroptera: Natalidae) is a senior synonym of *Natalus espiritosantensis* (Ruschi, 1951). Mammalia. 2012;77(2):237–40.
46. Han HJ, Wen H, Zhao L, Liu J, Luo LM, Zhou CM, Qin XR, Zhu YL, Zheng XX, Yu XJ. Novel Bartonella species in insectivorous bats, northern China. PLoS One. 2017;12(1)
47. Urushadze L, Bai Y, Osikowicz L, McKee C, Sidamonidze K, Putkaradze D, Imnadze P, Kandaurov A, Kuzmin I, Kosoy M. Prevalence, diversity, and host associations of *Bartonella* strains in bats from Georgia (Caucasus). PLoS Negl Trop Dis. 2017;11(4)
48. McKee CD, Hayman DT, Kosoy MY, Webb CT. Phylogenetic and geographic patterns of bartonella host shifts among bat species. Infect Genet Evol. 2016;44:382–94.
49. Paziewska A, Harris PD, Zwolinska L, Bajer A, Sinski E. Recombination within and between species of the alpha proteobacterium *Bartonella* infecting rodents. Microb Ecol. 2011;61(1):134–45.
50. Norman AF, Regnery R, Jameson P, Greene C, Krause DC. Differentiation of Bartonella-like isolates at the species level by PCR-restriction fragment length polymorphism in the citrate synthase gene. J Clin Microbiol. 1995; 33(7):1797–803.
51. Maiden MC, Bygraves JA, Feil E, Morelli G, Russell JE, Urwin R, Zhang Q, Zhou J, Zurth K, Caugant DA, Feavers IM, Achtman M, Spratt BG. Multilocus sequence typing: a portable approach to the identification of clones within populations of pathogenic microorganisms. Proc Natl Acad Sci U S A. 1998; 95(6):3140–5.
52. La Scola B, Zeaiter Z, Khamis A, Raoult D. Gene-sequence-based criteria for species definition in bacteriology: the *Bartonella* paradigm. Trends Microbiol. 2003;11(7):318–21.
53. Peracchi AL, Lima IP, Reis NR, Nogueira MR, Ortêncio FH, Chiroptera O. In: Reis NR, Peracchi AL, Pedro WA, Lima IP, editors. Mamíferos do Brasil. Londrina: Paraná p; 2006. p. 153–230.
54. Hayman DT, Bowen RA, Cryan PM, McCracken GF, O'Shea TJ, Peel AJ, Gilbert A, Webb CT, Wood JL. Ecology of zoonotic infectious diseases in bats: current knowledge and future directions. Zoonoses Public Health. 2013; 60(1):2–21.
55. Luis AD, Hayman DT, O'Shea TJ, Cryan PM, Gilbert AT, Pulliam JR, Mills JN, Timonin ME, Willis CK, Cunningham AA, Fooks AR, Rupprecht CE, Wood JL, Webb CT. A comparison of bats and rodents as reservoirs of zoonotic viruses: are bats special? Proc Biol Sci. 2013;280(1756):1–9.
56. Magalhães O. Rickettsiasis no Brasil. Bol Oficina Sanit Panam. 1944;23:17–9.
57. Magalhães O, Rocha A. Sensibilidade dos morcegos aos vírus do Tifo Exantemático Neotrópico. no Brasil Brasil-Médico. 1943;57:207–10.
58. Cicuttin GL, Boeri EJ, Beltran FJ, Gury Dohmen FE. Molecular detection of *Neorickettsia risticii* in Brazilian free-tailed bats (*Tadarida brasiliensis*) from Buenos Aires , Argentina. Pesquisa Veterinária Brasileira. 2013;33:648–50.

17

Diagnostic tools of caprine and ovine anaplasmosis

I. I. Shabana[1,2*], N. M. Alhadlag[1] and H. Zaraket[3,4]

Abstract

Background: The diagnosis of anaplasmosis is rather conflicting with other haemoprotozoans. Hence, the study aimed to compare and evaluate the efficiency of competitive ELISA (cELISA), indirect fluorescence antibody (IFA), and Polymerase chain reaction (PCR) for precise diagnosis of *Anaplasma* spp. and to assess their concordance with microscopic examination (ME).

Results: A total of 312 blood samples (189 sheep and 123 goats) were examined for *Anaplasma* infection during a 1 year period. Giemsa-stained blood smears were examined under the microscope. IFA and cELISA were used for the detection of *Anaplasma* spp. antibodies. PCR was used as a standard of truth and for the identification of *Anaplasma* species. Using cELISA assay, 47.4% (148) were positive (93 sheep and 55 goats) with a sensitivity and specificity of 91.9, and 86.9%, respectively. Using IFA, it was found that 57.4% (179) were positive (113 sheep and 66 goats) with a sensitivity and specificity of 100, and 93.3%, respectively. PCR assay identified *A. ovis* in 49 (25.3%) sheep and 30 (15.5%) goats, and *A. phagocytophilum*in 74 (38.1%) sheep and 41 (20.8%) goats.

Conclusions: High sensitivity and specificity values of IFA and ELISA tests compared to microscopic examination strongly support their utility in the diagnosis of *Anaplasma* infection. PCR was a more specific diagnostic tool that allows to discriminate between *Anaplasma* subspecies, which makes it the method of choice for anaplasmosis diagnosis.

Background

Anaplasma are obligate intracellular, Gram-negative, tick-borne rickettsial bacteria that are important animal and human pathogens. Anaplasmosis constitutes a burden to livestock health and production in tropical and sub-tropical regions. It results in great economic losses due to decreased production, mortality, and lowered work efficiency of affected animals [7, 26].There are six recognized *Anaplasma* species: *A. ovis, A. marginale, A. centrale, A. platys, A. bovis,* and *A. phagocytophilum* [48]. *A. ovis* primarily infects sheep and goats, causing ovine and caprine anaplasmosis, respectively [24]. *A. ovis* infection is generally a subclinical or mild condition, while severe infection may involve anemia, abortion, and mortality [43].

* Correspondence: imanibrahim50@yahoo.com
[1]Biology Department, Faculty of Science, Taibah University, Al- madinah Al-munawarah, Saudi Arabia
[2]Faculty of Veterinary Medicine, Department of Bacteriology, Immunology and Mycology, Suez Canal University, Ismailia, Egypt
Full list of author information is available at the end of the article

A. phagocytophilum infects humans and animals and is thought to be zoonotic [38, 49]. The disease is known as tick-borne fever (TBF) in human and ruminants granulocytic anaplasmosis (HGA) in human. Tick-borne fever is characterized by high fever, which may last for one to 2 weeks, followed by a severe neutropenia, which makes the animals susceptible to secondary infections [39, 40]. Ruminants granulocytic anaplasmosis is characterized by fever, myalgia, chills, depression, and headache [47]. Anaplasmosis became a notifiable disease in 1999 [11, 20].

Anaplasmosis diagnosis is usually based on the microscopic examination (ME) of Giemsa-stained blood smears, serological, and molecular diagnostic procedures. Microscopic diagnosis may be difficult in carrier animals, thus various serological techniques have been used for the detection of *Anaplasma*-specific antibodies such as indirect immunofluorescence antibody (IFA), enzyme-linked immunosorbent assay (ELISA), and complement fixation tests (CF) [9, 23].The competitive

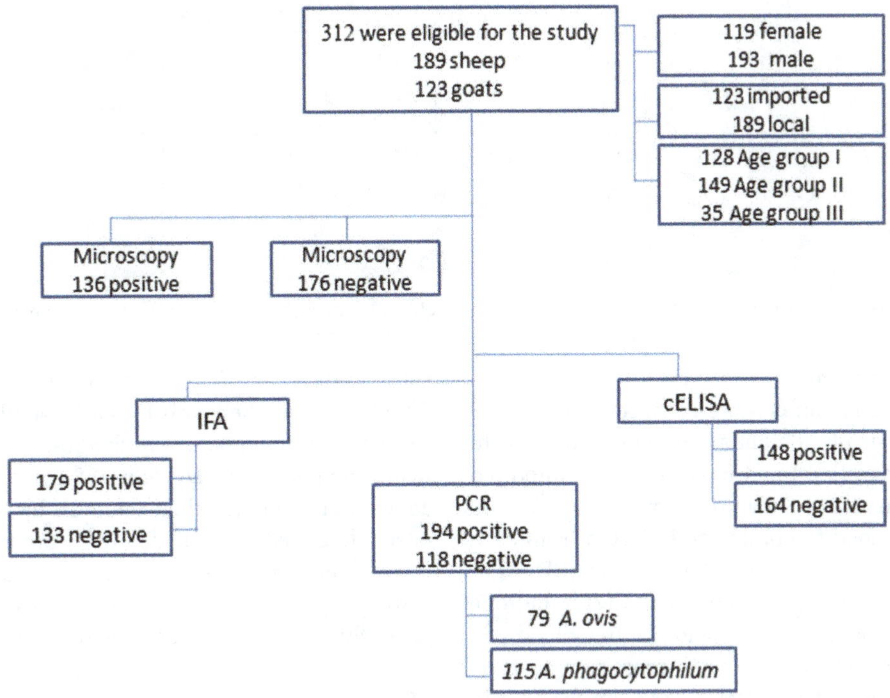

Fig. 1 Study flow chart

ELISA (cELISA) is depending on the use of a monoclonal antibody (Mab) ANAF16C1 that recognizes the conserved (MSP-5) antigen of different *Anaplasma* spp. [28, 46]. cELISA test has high sensitivity and specificity for detection of *Anaplasma* antibodies [27].

The "Gold standard" method for the diagnosis of *Anaplasma* spp. relies on the combination of the microscopic examination and cELISA [22].The indirect immunofluorescence antibody test is widely used for the diagnosis of blood protozoon and Rickettsia [25].The IFA test is commonly used in epidemiological studies because of its low costs [14, 25].

Molecular identification methods such as Polymerase chain reaction (PCR) have several advantages compared to the traditional serologic and blood smear tests [21]. PCR is the most sensitive and reliable diagnostic tool that allows discriminating between *Anaplasma* subspecies [44]. In addition, PCR can detect the coinfections with multiple *Anaplamsa* subspecies [5].

The aim of the study was to assess the sensitivity and specificity of the different diagnostic tools used for detecting anaplasmosis in sheep and goats.

Methods

Study design

This was a prospective study conducted according tothe Standards for Reporting Diagnosis Accuracy Studies (STARD) [13].

Animals

Blood samples were collected from sheep and goats from the local abattoir and different farms in Medina, Kingdom of Saudi Arabia (KSA). Eligibility criteria were suspicion of anaplasmosis among sheep and goats in Medina, which has a subtropical climate and borders on a fully tropical climate. The animals were surveyed for anaplasmosis from September 2011 to November 2012 (Fig. 1). Microscopic examination of blood smears was basically used as a reference diagnosis of anaplasmosis. cELISA and IFA are the most commonly used serological methods to detect antibodies against *Anaplasma*. PCR is the most reliable diagnosis of *Anaplasma* infection.

Table 1 Basic demographics of the sampled animals

Categories		*N* (%)
Gender	Female	119 (38.1%)
	Male	193 (61.9%)
Host	Sheep	189 (60.6%)
	Goat	123 (39.4%)
Source	Imported	123 (39.4%)
	Local	189 (60.6%)
Age	Age group I (2 m-2y)	128 (41.5%)
	Age group II (2y-4y)	149 (47%)
	Age group III (4y-6y)	35 (12%)

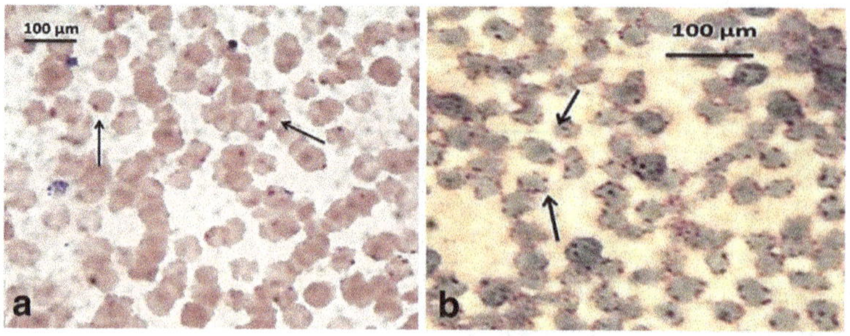

Fig. 2 a, b Anaplasma species under microscope appears as small and roughly spherical intraerythrocytic parasite measuring about 0.2 to 0.5 µm

Blood samples collection

A total of 312 blood samples were collected from 189 sheep and 123 goats of different age groups (2 months to 6 years) and sources (local and imported). The imported animals were either from Sudan, Pakistan, Australia, and Somalia. Venous blood samples were collected from each individual animal in two 4 ml vacutainer tubes (BD vacutainer, BD-Plymouth, UK), one containing EDTA and one additive-free. To separate sera, the additive-free blood was allowed to clot for about 15–30 min at room temperature. The tubes then centrifuged at 1000–2000 rpm for 10 min and serum was collected. The serum specimens were stored at – 20 °C for further use.

Microscopic examination

Thin blood smears were prepared for microscopic examination accordingly the standard protocol [7].The slides were allowed to air-dry before being fixed with absolute methanol. Fixed smears were stained with 10% Giemsa (Cresent diagnostic, KSA) and examined by using compound microscope under oil immersion lens. About 25 fields were examined from each slide for the presence of *Anaplasma* and the number of infected erythrocytes. *Anaplasma* was identified on the basis of its morphology [8].

Competitive ELISA (cELISA) assay

Sera were screened for the presence of *Anaplasma* antibodies by using the VMRD cELISA kit (VMRD Inc., Pullman, WA, USA), according to the manufacturer instructions. The optical density (OD) was measured at 650 nm with an ELISA microplate reader MR-960 (perlong Medical Equipment Co., Ltd., China). The results were calculated according to the formula: 100 [1-(Sample OD ÷ Negative Control OD)]. The positive sample OD must be > 30%.

Immunofluorescence (IFA)assay

Sera were screened for *Anaplasma* immunoglobulin G (IgG) by a semi-quantitative indirect IFA commercial kit (Fuller, USA), according to the manufacturer instructions. Briefly, sera samples were diluted in phosphate-buffer saline (PBS) and 25 µl were transferred to the slide wells. The slides were incubated at 35 °C for 30 min then washed with PBS followed by distilled water to remove the unreacted antibodies. Twenty five µl anti-ovine conjugate with DyLight 488 dye (Fuller, USA) were added and incubated then removed by washing as previously described. The slide was examined by standard fluorescence microscopy (Olympus BX50, Japan) at 400X magnification, the positive reaction appears as green fluorescent small cocci with a red background.

DNA extraction and PCR

DNA extraction was carried out using the G-spinTM Total DNA Extraction Kit (iNtRON Biotechnology, Korea) according to the instructions of the manufacturer. PCR was performed to detect both *Anaplasma phagocytophilum, Anaplasma ovis* using BioinGentech Veterinary PCR Kits (Concepcion, Chile) according to the instructions of the manufacturer. The cycling conditions were initial denaturation at 94 °C for 2 min, 35 cycles (94 °C 30 s, 57 °C30 s, 72 °C 30 sec) and a final extension at 72 °C for 5 min.

Table 2 Microscopic examination

Host	Demographic factor		Positive animals percentage
Sheep (*n* = 189)	Gender	Male (128)	66 (34.9%)[a]
		Female (61)	20 (10.6%)
	Age	Group I (84)	47 (24.9%)[a]
		Group II (89)	36 (19.0%)
		Group III (16)	3 (1.6%)
	Source	imported (82)	53 (28.1%)
		Local (107)	33 (17.5%)
Goat (*n* = 123)	Gender	Male (65)	38 (30.9%)[a]
		Female (58)	12 (9.8%)
	Age	Group I (44)	22 (17.9%)[a]
		Group II (60)	24 (19.5%)
		Group III (19)	4 (3.3%)
	Source	Imported (41)	34 (27.6%)
		Local (82)	16 (13.0%)

Age group I (2 months to 2 years), group II (> 2 -4 years), group III (> 4 - 6 years)
[a]Significant variation

Table 3 Seroprevalence of anaplasma species among sheep and goats

Host	Serological assay	Gender		**Age			Source	
		Female	Male	Group I	Group II	Group III	Imported	Local
Sheep	cELISA	70 (37.0%)	23 (12.2%)	52 (61.1%)	39 (43.8%)	2 (12.5%)	59 (71.1%)	34 (31.7%)
	IFA	82 (43.4%)	31 (16.4%)	60 (31.7%)	45 (23.8%)	8 (4.2%)	69 (36.5%)	44 (23.3%)
Goat	cELISA	39 (60.0%)*	16 (27.6%)	26 (59.1%)	25 (41.7%)	4 (21.1%)	36 (87.8%)	19 (23.1%)
	IFA	45 (36.6%)*	21 (27.6%)	30 (24.4%)	29 (23.6%)	7 (5.7%)	43 (34.9%)	23 (18.7%)

* statistically significant (*P*-value is < 0.05)
**statistically highly significant (*P*-value is < 0.01)

Statistical analysis

Statistical analysis was performed using the Statistical Package for the Social Sciences version 20.0 (SPSS Inc. Chicago, USA). Eta-square and Chi-square were applied to compare the percentage of positive samples by each method. The differences were considered statistically significant when *P*-value is< 0.05.

Results

The examined animals

A total of 189 (60.6%) paired samples were collected from sheep and 123 (39.4%) were obtained from goats. As shown in (Table 1), the animals were classified into three age groups: group I included samples collected from animals aged2 months to 2 years (128; 41.5%), group II included animals > 2 -4 years (149; 47%), and group III included animals > 4 – 6 years (35; 12%). According to the country of origin,189 (60.6%) of the sampled animals were locally bred and included 107 (56.6%) samples collected from sheep and 82 (43.4%) samples of goats, and 123 (39.4%) animals were imported including 82 (66.7%) sheep and 41(33.3%) goats.

Microscopic examination

A total of 312 blood smears were examined for the presence of intra-erythrocytic inclusions using Giemsa stain. *Anaplasma* spp. appeared as small spherical deep purple intraerythrocytic inclusions, measuring about 0.2 to 0.5 μm (Fig. 2a, b). Among the collected specimens, 130 were found positive with an overall prevalence of 43.6%. Among the 130 positive animals, 86 (45.5%)were sheep and 50 (40.7%) were goat (Table 2). The difference in Anapalsma prevalence in sheep and goats was not significant ($P > 0.05$).The highest infection rate of *Anaplasma* spp. was among animals aged 2 m–2y, in sheep (47/86; 54.6%)and goats (22/50; 44%) with a significant correlation ($P < 0.05$). The infection rate was higher albeit not significantly among the imported animals, 64.6% in sheep and 82.9% in goats compared to locally bred animals. Male animals had a higher and significant ($P < 0.05$) infection rate in sheep (66/86; 76.7%) and goats (38/50; 76%) compared to females.

Competitive inhibition ELISA (cELISA) assay

The overall prevalence of *Anaplasma* spp. using cELISA was 47.4% ($n = 148$), including 93 (49.2%) specimens from sheep and 55 (44.7%) from goats. In sheep, the infection rates were higher among males (37%), animals of the age group I (61.1%). and imported animals (71.1%). While in goats, the prevalence was 60% among males, 59.1% among age group I animals, and 87.8% in the imported animals (Table 3). Comparing the data obtained from microscopic examination with cELISA, it was observed that cELISA has high sensitivity (91.9%) and specificity (86.9%) than microscopic examination. The Gold standard of truth for the diagnosis of *Anaplasma* spp. relies on the combination of the microscopic examination and cELISA.

Immunofluorescence (IFA)assay

The presence of the intraerythrocytic *Anaplasma* spp. is indicated by greenish yellow or yellowish fluorescence (Fig. 3a, b). The overall prevalence of *Anaplasma* spp.

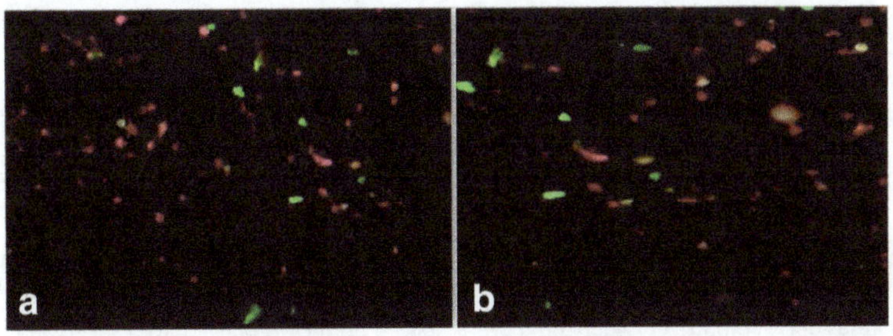

Fig. 3 a, **b** Anaplasma species under fluorescent microscope appears green fluorescent small cocci with a red back ground

Table 4 Sensitivity and specificity of IFA as compared with gold standard (ELISA and ME) of anaplasma spp.

	Gold Standard			
		Positive	Negative	Total
IFA test	positive	125	11	136
	Negative	0	153	153
	Total*	125	164	289

* statistically significant (*P*-value is < 0.05)
**statistically highly significant (*P*-value is < 0.01)

using IFA was 57.4% (179), of which113 (59.8%) were sheep and 66 (53.7%) were goats (Table 3). In sheep, the infection rate was higher among males (43.4%), animals of the age group I (31.7%), and imported animals (36.5%). While in goats, the prevalence was 36.6% among males, 24.4% among age group I animals, and 34.9% in imported animals. The agreement between positive and negative results in cELISA and IFA were 82.7% (148/179). The remainder 17.3% (31 samples) was represented by samples, which were positive in IFA and negative in cELISA. No samples were found to be negative in IFA but positive in cELISA. The Gold Standard for the detection *of Anaplasma* spp. is the concordance of both cELISA and microscopic examination results. The sensitivity and specificity of IFA were 100 and 93.3% respectively, compared with the gold standard (Table 4).

PCR analysis

Molecular identification of *Anaplasma* spp. revealed two distinct species: *Anaplasma ovis* (Fig. 4) and *Anaplasma phagocytophilum* (Fig. 5). *Anaplasma ovis* was detected in 25.3% (25.9% of sheep and 24.4% of goats) of the sampled animals, while *Anaplasma phagocytophilum* was detected in 36.9% (39.2% of sheep and 33.3% of goats). Mixed infections with the two species were detected in18.9% of the animals (20.6% of sheep and 16.3% of goats).The sensitivity and specificity of PCR assay was 73.2 and 89% respectively when compared with microscopic examination (Table 5).

Discussion

Anaplasmosis frequently occurs in tropical and subtropical regions, and it is a major problem to small ruminants [34]. Epidemiologic studies aimed to determine the prevalence of anaplasmosis uses different diagnostic tools, such as microscopic examination of stained blood smears, serological, and molecular tests. The reliability of the diagnostic tests is crucial for accurate diagnosis and estimation of the disease prevalence. Despite microscopic examination and serologic tests are practical and reliable diagnostics to detect *Anaplasma* spp. infection, they have limitations [1, 47]. The accuracy of stained blood smear examination can be hindered by the low number of infected cells, lack of expertise of the examiner, and/or the occurrence of intracellular artifacts [2, 3]. In the early acute phase of infection, serologic assays have limited value, due to the absence of detectable antibodies [5, 42].

Our results showed that the number of infected animals by *Anaplasma* spp. was 43.6% (45.6% in sheep and 40.7% in goats) when examined microscopically compared to 47.4% (49.2% in sheep and 44.7% in goats) using cELISA and 57.4% (59.8% in sheep and 53.7% in goats) by using IFA. On the other hand, the prevalence using PCR was 62.2% (65.1% in sheep and 57.7% in goats), consistent with previous findings [22]. The variability of infection rates determined by different methods maybe attributed to several factors as, age, gender, and species. Previous studies have shown that some cases of anaplasmosis might be missed depending on the detection method used [30, 33].

In this study, sheep had a higher prevalence of anaplasmosis than goats in agreement with previous studies in India and Cyprus [12, 45]. Based on the age factor, it was found that age group I (2 m-2 yrs) had the highest rate of anaplasmosis. Also, gender seemed to play a role whereby anaplasmosis was more prevalent in males than in females. Additionally, *Anaplasma* infection rates were higher among the imported sheep and goats compared with local animals. This could be attributed to the presence of a specific tick vector in the source countries.

Anaplasma is routinely diagnosed by microscopic examination of Giemsa stained blood smears and detection of intraerythrocytic *Anaplasma* inclusions. Microscopic examination is suitable for diagnosis of acute anaplasmosis, but it is not applicable for the detection of pre-symptomatic or

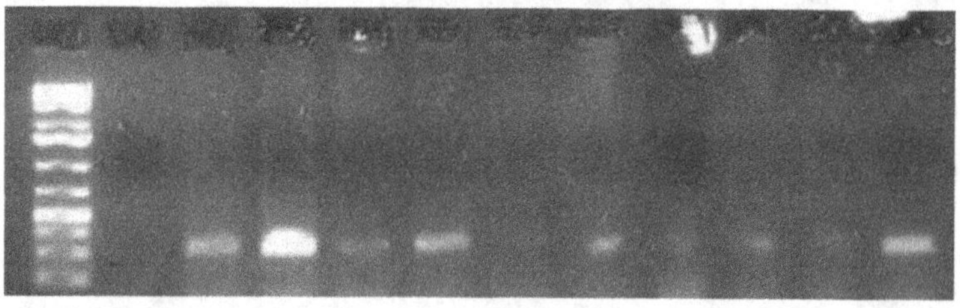

Fig. 4 Agarose gel electrophoreses of PCR products of *Anaplasma ovis* amplified from DNA purified from sheep and goats blood samples. Right arrowhead indicates position of the 271 bp PCR product

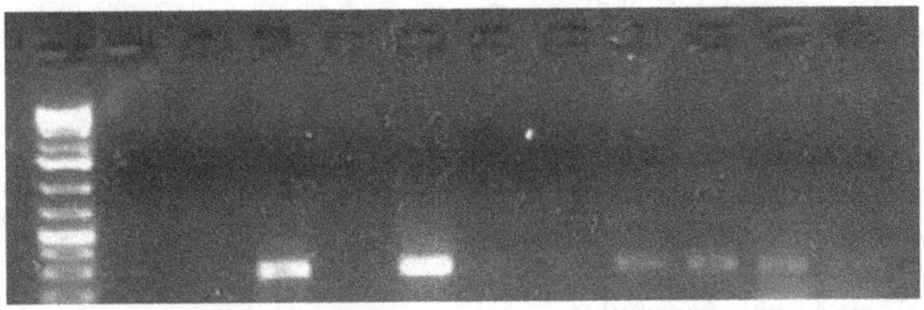

Fig. 5 Agarose gel electrophoreses of PCR products of *Anaplasma phagocytophilum* amplified from DNA purified from sheep and goats blood samples. Right arrowhead indicates position of the 236 bp PCR product

carrier cases due to low numbers of *Anaplasma* infected cells in circulation, which falls below the detection limit [17, 32].The cELISA currently used for diagnosis of anaplasmosis is based on the use of ANAF16C1 Mab that recognizes the MSP5 antigen in *A. marginale, A. central* and *A. ovis*. The MSP-5 antigen is conserved among all known *Anaplasma* spp. [15, 16, 29]. Our results showed that cELISA enabled the detection of more *Anaplasma* cases compared to microscopic examination (62.2% vs. 43.6%, respectively), with 91.9% sensitivity and 86.9% specificity. This was consistent with the findings of Naqid and Zangana [30] who found that the prevalence of *A. ovis* infection in goats was lower (55.9%) using Giemsa stained blood smears compared to cELISA (75.2%).

Indirect fluorescent antibody technique has been recommended and has proven sensitivity for the diagnosis of haemoparasites as *Anaplasma* spp. [35]. Several studies have reported that IFA may be used as an alternative to PCR, CF, and ELISA [10, 23, 38] for the detection of anaplasmosis among sheep and goats [12, 49]. In this study, we found that IFA had high sensitivity (100%) and specificity (91.9%) when compared to the Gold standard (combination of ME and cELISA). A previous study reported a similar level of specificity and sensitivity for IFA when compared with cELISA [22].

Detection of carrier animals is very important, as they play a significant role in the disease epidemiology as reservoirs. Furthermore, it is essential for epidemiologic studies to discriminate between *Anaplasma* species [31]. PCR is reported to be more sensitive than conventional parasitological techniques in different hosts. It also enables the identification of different species [18, 19]. Therefore, we also evaluated PCR for detection of *Anaplasma* species in our animals in comparison with ME, cELISA, and IFA.

The sensitivity of the PCR results was 100% compared to the other diagnostic results. However, in agreement with other studies [30, 32], our results revealed that only 70% of the PCR-positive animals were smear positive. This may be due to animals being examined during the early stage of infection when *Anaplasma*-infected cells are low. Having the ability to detect and differentiate between *Anaplasma* species is important for their accurate diagnosis and better understanding of their burden [11, 42]. Using PCR, we were also able to differentiate between *A. ovis* and *A. phagocytophilum* and to identify animals with mixed infections. In agreement with other studies, our results revealed that 70% of PCR-positive animals were smear positive. This may be due to the animals examined in early stage and there is a low number of *Anaplasma* cells in the circulating blood. Our data and those of others, suggest that PCR may provide a more reliable diagnosis of anaplasmosis particularly during early stages of infection, which would ensure proper management of infected animals and reduction of unnecessary antibiotic use [4, 11].

Comparing the sensitivity of the PCR assay with the cELISA, a lower percentage of animals were seropositive than PCR-positive. A previous study on anaplasmosis seroprevalence using cELISA showed that 88% was seropositive while 76% were positive by using PCR [22]. In our study,47.4% was seropositive while 62.2% were PCR-positive; which means that 14.8% of

Table 5 Molecular identification

	Anaplasma spp.	Gender		**Age			Source	
		Male	Female	Group I	Group II	Group III	Imported	Local
Sheep	*A. ovis*	35 (18.5%)	14 (7.4%)	26 (13.8%)	23 (12.2%)	0	30 (15.9%)	19 (10.0%)
	A. phagocytophylum	50 (26.5%)	24 (12.7%)	37 (19.6%)	31 (16.4%)	6 (4.8%)	38 (20.1%)	36 (19.0%)
Goat	*A. ovis*	*19 (60.0%)	11 (27.6%)	13 (15.4%)	13 (15.4%)	4 (3.3%)	16 (13.0%)	14 (11.4%)
	A. phagocytophylum	20 (16.3%)	21 (17.0%)	23 (18.7%)	16 (13.0%)	2 (1.6%)	15 (12.2%)	26 (21.1%)

* statistically significant (*P*-value is < 0.05)

**statistically highly significant (*P*-value is < 0.01)

PCR-positive sera were seronegative, this may occur in the early stage of infection where antibodies have not yet been produced [5].

The prevalence of *A. phagocytophylum* in sheep was 39. 2%, and in goats it was 33.3%. While, a lower prevalence of *A. ovis* was reported among sheep and goats, 25.9 and 24.3%, respectively, consistent with previous studies in Cyprus, China, Switzerland, and Italy [12, 37, 44, 49].

The zoonotic potential of *A. phagocytophilum* was previously documented [36, 41].The absence of host specificity of *A. phagocytophilum* allows the infection of the human by animal strains and vice versa [6]. Thus, the high prevalence *A. phagocytophilum* detected in the present study constitutes a risk to humans.

Conclusions

Proper disease diagnosis requires reliable tests. Therefore, it is important to evaluate the existing diagnostic methods. The evaluation depends on several factors as; whether the test is suitable for the field and/or the laboratory settings; cost; and time required. Microscopic examination provides reliable results, but it is not suitable to diagnose carrier animals. cELISA is known for its ease of use, low cost, and for being quantitative. IFA is an economical and easy method to perform. In the present study, IFA was highly specific and sensitive, but it requires special laboratory settings such as fluorescent microscope. PCR is the most sensitive and reliable diagnostic tool that achieves simultaneous differentiation between different *Anaplasma* subspecies.

Abbreviations

cELISA: Competitive ELISA; CF: Complement fixation tests; ELISA: Enzyme-linked immunosorbent assay; IFA: Indirect fluorescence antibody; IgG: Immunoglobulin G; Mab: Monoclonal antibody; ME: Microscopic examination; MSP5: A protein epitope of major surface protein 5; OD: The optical density; PBS: Phosphate-buffer saline; PCR: Polymerase chain reaction

Acknowledgements

We thank Dr. Taha, H.A. for her valuable contributions.

Authors' contributions

SII designed the research, established the experiments scheme, analyzed the data, oriented the statistical results, and wrote the manuscript. ANM, collected the sample, and performed laboratory experiments. ZH contributed to the design and wrote the manuscript with SII. All authors read and approved the final manuscript.

Competing interests

The authors declare that they have no competing interests.

Author details

[1]Biology Department, Faculty of Science, Taibah University, Al- madinah Al-munawarah, Saudi Arabia. [2]Faculty of Veterinary Medicine, Department of Bacteriology, Immunology and Mycology, Suez Canal University, Ismailia, Egypt. [3]Department of Experimental Pathology, Immunology & Microbiology, Faculty of Medicine, American University of Beirut, Beirut, Lebanon. [4]Center for Infectious Diseases Research, Faculty of Medicine, American University of Beirut, Beirut, Lebanon.

References

1. Aguero-Rosenfeld ME. Diagnosis of human granulocytic ehrlichiosis: state of the art. Vector Borne Zoonotic Dis. 2002;2:233–9.
2. Bakken JS, Aguero-Rosenfeld ME, Tilden RL, Wormser GP, Horowitz HW, Raffalli JT, Baluch M, Riddell D, Walls JJ, Dumler JS. Serial measurements of hematologic counts during the active phase of human granulocytic ehrlichiosis. Clin Infect Dis. 2001;32:862–70.
3. Bakken JS, Dumler JS. Human granulocytic ehrlichiosis. Clin Infect Dis. 2000; 31:554–60.
4. Bakken JS, Dumler JS. Clinical diagnosis and treatment of human granulocytotropic anaplasmosis. Ann N Y Acad Sci. 2006;1078:236–47.
5. Bakken JS, Haller I, Riddell D, Walls JJ, Dumler JS. The serological response of patients infected with the agent of human granulocytic ehrlichiosis. Clin Infect Dis. 2002;34:22–7.
6. Ben Said M, Belkahia H, Alberti A, Zobba R, Bousrih M, Yahiaoui M. Molecular survey of Anaplasma species in small ruminants reveals the presence of novel strains closely related to *A. phagocytophilum* in Tunisia. Vector Borne Zoonotic Dis. 2015;15(10):580–90.
7. Benjamin MM. Outline of veterinary clinical pathology. III ed. New Delhi: Kalyani Publishers; 2005.
8. Bowmann DD. George's parasitology for veterinarians. 9th ed. Louis: Saunders Elsevier, St; 2009.
9. Bradway DS, Torioni de Echaide S, Knowles DP, Hennager SG, McElwain TF. Sensitivity and specificity of the complement fixation test for detection of cattle persistently infected with *Anaplas mamarginale*. J Vet Diagn Investig. 2001;13(1):79–81.
10. Centers for Disease Control and Prevention (CDC). Anaplasmosis: statistics and epidemiology. 2016. http://www.cdc.gov/anaplasmosis/stats/. Accessed 2016.
11. Chapman AS, Bakken JS, Folk SM, Paddock CD, Bloch KC, Krusell A, Sexton DJ, Buckingham SC, Marshall GS, Storch GA, Dasch GA, McQuiston JH, Swerdlow DL, Dumler SJ, Nicholson WL, Walker DH, Eremeeva ME, Ohl CA, Tickborne Rickettsial Diseases Working Group, CDC. Diagnosis and management of tickborne rickettsial diseases; 2006.
12. Chochlakis D, Ioannou I, Sharif L, Kokkini S, Hristophi N, Dimitriou T, Tselentis Y, Psaroulaki A. Prevalence of Anaplasma sp. in goats and sheep in Cyprus. Vector Borne Zoonotic Dis. 2009;9(5):457–63.
13. Cohen JF, Korevaar DA, Altman DG, Bruns DE, Gatsonis CA, Hooft L, Irwig L, Levine D, Reitsma JB, de Vet HC, Bossuyt PM. STARD 2015 guidelines for reporting diagnostic accuracy studies: explanation and elaboration. Br Med J Open 2016; 6: 012799.
14. De Kroon JF, NM PÃ, Franssen FF, Uilenberg G. The indirect fluorescent antibody test for bovine anaplasmosis. VetQ. 1990;12(2):124–8.
15. de la Fuente J, Lew A, Lutz H, Meli ML, Hofmann-Lehmann R, Shkap V, Molad T, Mangold AJ, Almazán C, Naranjo V, Gortázar C, Torina A, Caracappa S, García-Pérez AL, Barral M, Oporto B, Ceci L, Carelli G, Blouin EF, Kocan KM. Genetic diversity of Anaplasma species major surface proteins and implications for anaplasmosis serodiagnosis and vaccine development. Anim Health Res Rev. 2005;6:75–89.
16. De la Fuente J, Vicente J, Hofle U, Ruiz-Fons F, Fernández de Mera IG, van den Bussche RA, Kocan KM, Gortazar C. Anaplasma infection in free-ranging Iberian red deer in the region of Castilla-La Mancha Spain. Vet Microbiol. 2004;100:163–73.
17. de Waal T. Advances in diagnosis of protozoan diseases. Vet Parasitol. 2012; 189:65–74.
18. Desquesnes M, Davila AMR. Application of PCR-based tools for detection and identification of animal trypanosomes; a review and perspectives. Vet Parasitol. 2002;109(3-4):213–33.
19. Dey A, Singh S. Progress of science from microscopy to microarrays (part 1): diagnosis of parasitic diseases. J Lab Phys. 2009;1:2–6.
20. Dumler JS, Barat NC, Barat CE, Bakken JS. Human granulocytic anaplasmosis and macrophage activation. Clin Infect Dis. 2007;45:199–204.
21. Dumler JS, Brouqui P. Molecular diagnosis of human granulocytic anaplasmosis. Expert Rev Mol Diagn. 2004;4:559–69.

22. Ekici OD, Sevinc F. Comparison of cELISA and IFA tests in the serodiagnosis of anaplasmosis in cattle. Afri J Microbiol Res. 2011;5(10):1188–91.
23. Goff WL, Stiller D, Roeder RA, Johnson LW, Falk D, Gorham JR, McGuire TC. Comparison of a DNA probe, complement fixation and indirect immunofluorescence tests for diagnosing *Anaplasma marginale* in suspected carrier cattle. Vet Microbiol. 1990;24:381–90.
24. Hornok S, Elek V, de la Fuente J, Naranjo V, Farkas R. First serological and molecular evidence on the endemicity of *Anaplasma ovis* and *A. marginale* in Hungary. Vet Microbiol. 2007;122(3-4):316–22.
25. Hungerford LL, Smith RD. Variations in seroprevalence and host factors for bovine Anaplasmosis in Illionis. Vet Res Com. 1997;21:9–18.
26. Jonsson NN, Bock RE, Jorgensen WK. Productivity and health effects of anaplasmosis and babesiosis on Bosindicus cattle and their crosses, and the effects of differing intensity of tick control in Australia. Vet Parasitol. 2008; 155(1-2):1–9.
27. Knowles D, Torioni de Echaide S, Palmer G, McGuire T, Stiller D, McElwain T. Antibody against an *Anaplasma marginale* MSP5 epitope common to tick and erythrocyte stages identifies persistently infected cattle. J Clin Microbiol. 1996;34:2225–30.
28. Mason KL, Gonzalez MV, Chung C, Mousel MR, White SN, Taylor JB, Scoles GA. Validation of an improved Anaplasma antibody competitive ELISA for detection of *Anaplasma ovis* antibody in domestic sheep. J Vet Diagn Investig. 2017;29(5):763–6.
29. McElwain TF. Bovine anaplasmosis. In: Manual of standards for diagnostic tests and vaccines for terrestrial animals. Paris office Int. des.Epizoo; 2004. p. 494–506.
30. Nazifi S, Razavi SM, Mansourian M, Nikahval B, Moghaddam M. Studies on correlations among parasitaemia and some hemolytic indices in two tropical diseases (theileriosis and anaplasmosis) in Fars province of Iran. Trop Anim Health Prod. 2008;40:47–53.
31. Niu QL, Luo JX, Guan GQ, Ma ML, Liu ZJ, Liu AH, et al. Detection and differentiation of ovine Theileria and Babesia by reverse line blotting in China. Parasitol Res. 2009;104(6):1417–23.
32. Noaman V, Shayan P. Comparison of microscopy and PCR-RFLP for detection of *Anaplasma marginale* in carrier cattle. Iran J Microbiol. 2010; 2(2):89–94.
33. Renneker S, Abdo J, Bakheit MA, Kullmann B, Beyer D, Ahmed J. Coinfection of sheep with Anaplasma, Theileria and Babesia species in the Kurdistan region, Iraq. Transbound Emerg Dis. 2013;60(2):113–8.
34. Ros-Garcia A, Barandika JF, Garcia-Perez AL, Juste RA, Hurtado A. Assessment of exposure to piroplasms in sheep grazing in communal mountain pastures by using a multiplex DNA bead-based suspension array. Parasit Vectors. 2013;6(1):277.
35. Salih DA, El Hussein AM, Seitzer U, Ahmed JS. Epidemiological studies on tick-borne diseases of cattle in central Equatoria state, southern Sudan. Parasitol Res. 2007;101(4):1035–44.
36. Scharf W, Schauer S, Freyburger F, Petrovec M, Schaarschmidt-Kiener D, Liebisch G, et al. Distinct host species correlate with *Anaplasma phagocytophilum* ankA gene clusters. J ClinMicrobiol. 2011;49:790–6.
37. Silaghi C1, Scheuerle MC, Friche Passos LM, Thiel C, Pfister K. PCR detection of *Anaplasma phagocytophilum* in goat flocks in an area endemic for tick-borne fever in Switzerland. Parasite. 2011;18(1):57–62.
38. Silva VMG, Araújo FR, Madruga CR, Soares CO, Kessler RH, Almeida MAO, Fragoso SP, Santos LR, Ramos CAN, Bacanelli G, Torres Júnior RAA. Comparison between indirect enzyme-linked immunosorbent assays for *Anaplasma marginale* antibodies with recombinant major surface protein 5 and initial body antigens. Mem Inst Oswaldo Cruz, Rio de Janeiro. 2006; 101(5):511–6.
39. Stuen S, Granquist E, Silaghi C. *Anaplasma phagocytophilum*- a widespread multi-host pathogen with highly adaptive strategies. Front Cell Infect Microbiol. 2013;3:31.
40. Stuen S. *Anaplasma phagocytophilum* – the most widespread tick-borne infection in animals in Europe. Vet Res Commun. 2007;31:79-84.
41. The center of food security and public health2013. http://www.cfsph.iastate.edu/Zoonoses/. Accessed 2013.
42. Thomas RJ, Dumler JS, Carlyon JA. Current management of human granulocytic anaplasmosis, human monocytic ehrlichiosis and Ehrlichia ewingii ehrlichiosis. Expert Rev Anti-Infect Ther. 2009;7:709–22.
43. Torina A, Caracappa S. Tick-borne diseases in sheep and goats: clinical and diagnostic aspects. Small Rumin Res. 2012;106:S6–S11.
40. Stuen S. *Anaplasma phagocytophilum* – the most widespread tick-borne infection in animals in Europe. Vet Res Commun. 2007;31:79-84.
41. The center of food security and public health2013. http://www.cfsph.iastate.edu/Zoonoses/. Accessed 2013.
42. Thomas RJ, Dumler JS, Carlyon JA. Current management of human granulocytic anaplasmosis, human monocytic ehrlichiosis and Ehrlichia ewingii ehrlichiosis. Expert Rev Anti-Infect Ther. 2009;7:709–22.
43. Torina A, Caracappa S. Tick-borne diseases in sheep and goats: clinical and diagnostic aspects. Small Rumin Res. 2012;106:S6–S11.
44. Torina A, Agnone A, Blanda V, Alongi A, D'Agostino R, Caracappa S, Marino AMF, Di Marco V, de la Fuente J. Development and validation of two PCR tests for the detection of and differentiation between *Anaplasma ovis* and *Anaplasma marginale*. Ticks Tick-Borne Dis. 2012;3(5-6):283–7.
45. Velusamy R, Rani N, Ponnudurai G, Anbarasi P. Prevalence of intestinal and haemoprotozoan parasites of small ruminants in Tamil Nadu, India. Vet World. 2015;8(10):1205–9.
46. Visser ES, McGuire TC, Palmer GH, Davis WC, Shkap V, Pipano E, Knowles DP. The *Anaplasma marginale* msp 5 gene encodes a 19-kilodalton protein conserved in all recognized Anaplasma species. Infect Immun. 1992;60: 5139–44.
47. Woldehiwet Z. The natural history of *Anaplasma phagocytophilum*. Vet Parasitol. 2010;167(2-4):108–22.
48. Ybañez AP, Sashika M, Inokuma H. The phylogenetic position of *Anaplasma bovis* and inferences on the phylogeny of the genus Anaplasma. J Vet Med Sci. 2014;76:307.
49. Zhang XC, Zhang LX, Li WH, Wang SW, Sun YL, Wang YY, Guan ZZ, Liu XJ, Yang YS, Zhang SG, Yu HL, Zhang LJ. Ehrlichiosis and zoonotic anaplasmosis in suburban areas of Beijing, China. Vector Borne Zoonotic Dis. 2012;12(11): 932–7.

18

Molecular characterization of fluoroquinolone and/or cephalosporin resistance in *Shigella sonnei* isolates from yaks

Zhen Zhu[1,2†], Yuxiang Shi[2†], Xuzheng Zhou[1], Bing Li[1] and Jiyu Zhang[1*]

Abstract

Background: Members of the genus *Shigella* are intestinal pathogens and a major cause of seasonal outbreaks of bacterial diarrhea worldwide. Although humans are the conventional hosts of *Shigella* species, expansion of the *Shigella* host range to certain animals was recently reported. To investigate the prevalence of *Shigella sonnei* (*S. sonnei*) in yaks and perform molecular characterization, we analyzed 1132 fresh yak diarrheal stool samples and collected a total of 44 S. sonnei isolates.

Results: We performed multilocus sequence typing (MLST) and pulsed-field gel electrophoresis (PFGE) with *XbaI*-digested DNA to study genetic relatedness among the 44 isolates, which were differentiated into 4 sequence types (STs) and 32 PFGE types (PTs). All isolates harbored virulence genes, and 87.36% tested positive for invasion plasmid antigen H (*ipaH*), invasion associated locus (*ial*) and the *Shigella* enterotoxin gene *sen*. According to the results of antimicrobial susceptibility tests, 45.45% (20/44) were resistant to fluoroquinolones and/or cephalosporin. By sequencing the quinolone resistance determining region (QRDR) genes, we identified double mutations in *gyrA* (Ser83-Leu and Asp87-Asn) and a single mutation in *parC* (Ser80-Ile). All 12 fluoroquinolone-resistant *S. sonnei* isolates tested positive for the *aac(6')-Ib-cr* gene but negative for *qepA*. Three isolates harbored *qnr* genes, including two with *qnrS* and one with *qnrB*. In addition, three types of β-lactamase genes, bla_{TEM-1}, bla_{OXA-1} and $bla_{CTX-M-14/79}$, were detected in cephalosporin-resistant isolates.

Conclusions: The findings of this study have enriched our knowledge of fluoroquinolone- and/or cephalosporin-resistant *S. sonnei* isolates from yaks, which has important public health significance.

Keywords: *Shigella sonnei*, MLST, PFGE, Virulence gene, Antimicrobial resistance genes

Background

Bacteria of the genus *Shigella* are important members of the Enterobacteriaceae family and cause acute diarrhea in humans and animals [1–3]. This pathogen has been historically divided into 4 subgroups based on biochemical properties and group-specific O antigens in the outer membrane, specifically subgroups A (*S. dysenteriae*), B (*S. flexneri*), C (*S. boydii*) and D (*S. sonnei*). All four *Shigella* species cause shigellosis and are phylogenetically distinct from *Escherichia coli* [4, 5], with *S. flexneri* and *S. sonnei* being the most prevalent. Notably, *S. sonnei* has become the dominant subgroup in Asian countries in recent years [6, 7].

The specific pathogenicity of a given *Shigella* isolate is derived from the expression of diverse virulence genes that are associated with colonization, invasion/penetration and toxin-mediated disease [8]. The pathogenicity of these virulence genes is often multifactorial, and they are coordinately regulated [9]. An investigation of the virulence determinant genes in *Shigella* would help us

* Correspondence: infzjy@sina.com
†Zhen Zhu and Yuxiang Shi contributed equally to this work.
[1]Key Laboratory of New Animal Drug Project of Gansu Province, Key Laboratory of Veterinary Pharmaceutical Development of the Ministry of Agriculture, Lanzhou Institute of Husbandry and Pharmaceutical Sciences of CAAS, Jiangouyan, Qilihe District, Lanzhou 730050, China
Full list of author information is available at the end of the article

better understand its pathogenicity. However, knowledge regarding the distribution of these genes in *Shigella* isolates from animals is limited.

For *Shigella* infections, prompt therapy with effective antimicrobial agents reduces the duration and severity of illness [10]. However, the progressive increase in resistance to commonly used antimicrobials, especially fluoroquinolones and extended-spectrum cephalosporins, among *Shigella* spp. poses a major therapeutic challenge to the control of diseases caused by these species [10, 11]. In addition, the emergence and global dissemination of multi-drug resistant (MDR) pathogens is increasing rapidly due to the unique ability of bacteria to acquire resistance factors (transmissible genes) from the environment or from other bacteria [12].

Foodborne pathogens are usually carried by the host animal and contaminate the food during the slaughtering process [13]. And food is the main route to human infection with Shigella, including antibiotic-resistant strains [14]. Foods implicated in human cases of shigellosis include fresh fruit and vegetables, raw oysters, deli meats, and unpasteurized milk [15]. Multidrug-resistant *Shigella* has been found in bovine-derived foods such as beef, milk and cheese, which predict potential threats to human [16].

The primary goal of this study was to investigate the incidence of *S. sonnei* in yaks with diarrheal disease in a plateau area. We analyzed the biochemical and serological characteristics, virulence gene profiles, antimicrobial resistance profiles, antimicrobial resistance genes (ARGs) and genotypes and genetic relatedness diversity of *S. sonnei* isolates.

Results

Identification of *S. sonnei* isolates

A total of 44 *S. sonnei* isolates were collected from 1132 fresh diarrheal stool samples from yaks in three Chinese provinces, Gansu, Qinghai and Tibet, from 2014 to 2016. Among these isolates, 24 (54.55%) were collected from Gansu, 15 (34.09%) were collected from Qinghai, and 5 (11.36%) were collected from Tibet. Based on the results of biochemical characterization assays, we observed that all 44 *S. sonnei* isolates possessed the typical biochemical features of *Shigella* species and demonstrated the ability to ferment I-D-galactopyranoside (ONPG), glucose (GLU), mannitol (MAN), melibiose (MEL) and arabinose (ARA). Although both serotypes were isolated in each region, phase I (33/44, 75%) was the predominant serotype, and the detection rate of *S. sonnei* phase I was three times higher than that of phase II (11/44, 25%).

MLST-based genotype analysis

MLST was performed to analyze the genotypic diversity of *S. sonnei* isolates based on 15 housekeeping genes. The 44 isolates were divided into 4 sequence types (STs): ST76, ST116, ST125 and ST155. All four STs were previously reported and belonged to the same clonal complex (CC; CC29). The allele number for each locus and the ST designation are listed in Additional file 1: Table S1 and shared on the EcMLST website. Among these STs, ST116 ($n = 27$) and ST155 ($n = 13$) were the most common, accounting for 90.91% of all STs. ST116 encompassed 16 phase I and 11 phase II serotype isolates; furthermore, all phase II serotype *S. sonnei* isolates in the study were ST116. Interestingly, all four STs were detected in Gansu province, while only ST116 was observed in Qinghai and Tibet provinces (Table 1).

PFGE-based genotype analysis

The genotypes and genetic relatedness diversity of the 44 *S. sonnei* isolates were assessed by PFGE. At 80% similarity, *Xba*I-digested *S. sonnei* DNA generated 32 reproducible unique PFGE banding patterns (PT), yielding three major groups: A ($n = 17$), B ($n = 25$), and C ($n = 2$) (Fig. 1). Most isolates contained in PT group A were collected from the same geographical region (Gansu province) with the exception of one Tibet isolate (SS036). Group B contained the highest number of isolates, accounting for 56.82% of total isolates. In addition, almost all Qinghai isolates were clustered in group B2, with the exception of SS017. Interestingly, we also observed that different serotypes affect the PT cluster. In this study, all 17 group A isolates belonged to the phase I serotype, while all of the phase II isolates clustered into group B. The large number of PT types suggested a capricious genotypic and genetic diversity among *S. sonnei* strains, which adapt to different environments.

Table 1 Statistical analysis of the distribution of 4 MLST types among 44 *S. sonnei* isolates in different provinces

MLST types	Total ($n = 44$)		Gansu ($n = 24$)		Qinghai ($n = 15$)		Tibet ($n = 5$)	
	phase I ($n = 33$)	phase II ($n = 11$)	phase I ($n = 20$)	phase II ($n = 4$)	phase I ($n = 10$)	phase II ($n = 5$)	phase I ($n = 3$)	phase II ($n = 2$)
ST76	1 (3.03%)	0	1 (5%)	0	0	0	0	0
ST116	16 (48.48%)	11 (100%)	3 (15%)	4 (100%)	10 (100%)	5 (100%)	3 (100%)	2 (100%)
ST123	3 (9.09%)	0	3 (15%)	0	0	0	0	0
ST155	13 (39.39%)	0	13 (65%)	0	0	0	0	0

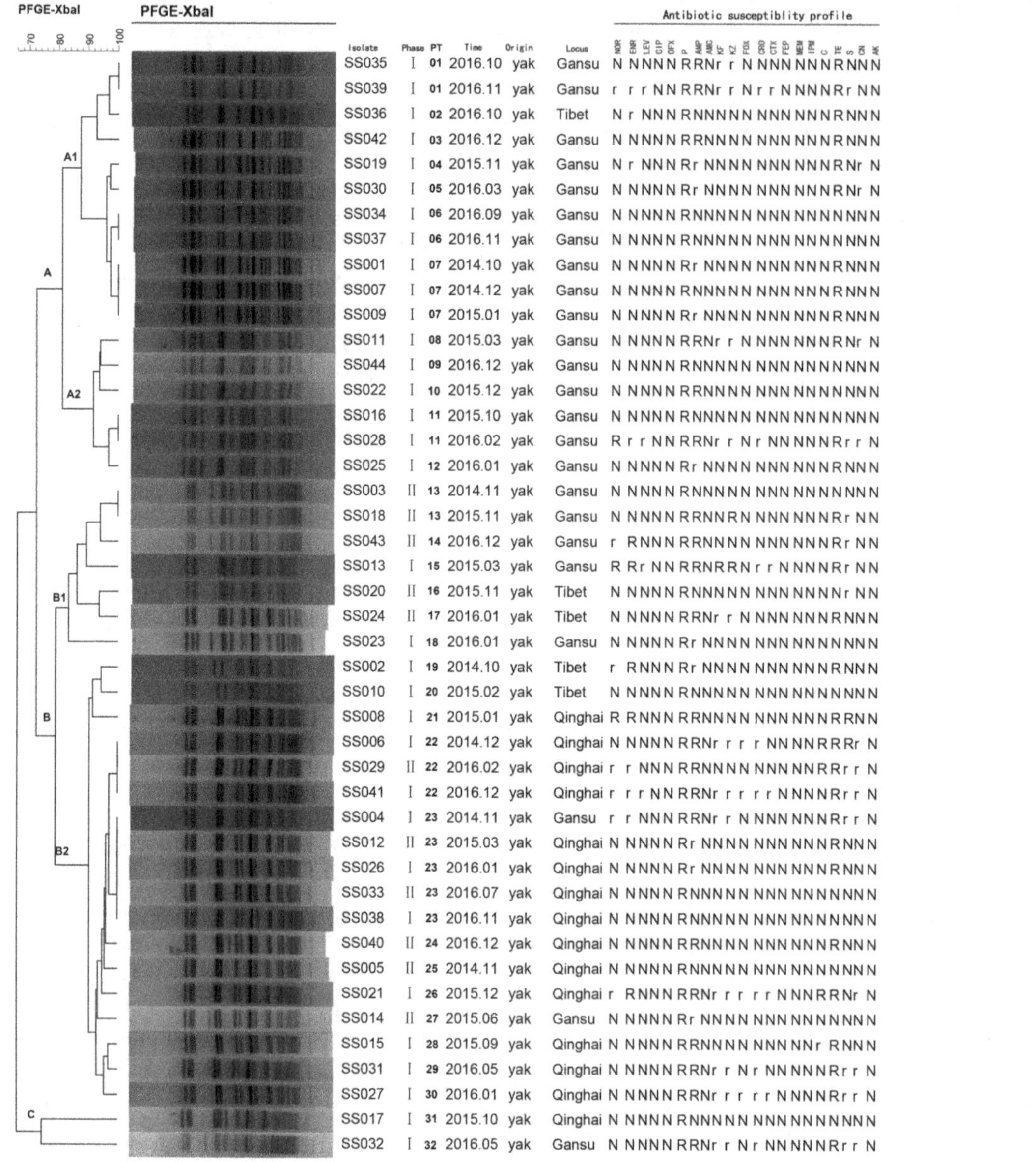

Fig. 1 Dendrogram of 44 *Xba*I-digested *S. sonnei* isolates based on the cluster analysis of PFGE patterns. The dendrogram was constructed using the UPGMA clustering method. The corresponding antibiotic resistance profile, PFGE pattern and background information for each strain is listed on the right side of the dendrogram. R = resistance and no bacteriostatic ring; r = resistance and positive bacteriostatic ring; N = sensitive and intermediary bacteriostatic ring

Virulence genes

The virulence gene profiles of the isolates are listed in Additional file 2: Table S2. Only 3 virulence genes (*ipaH*, *ial* and *sen*) were observed in this study. Among them, the invasive plasmid gene *ipaH* was observed in all isolates, followed by *ial* (38/44, 86.36%) and *sen* (37/44, 84.09%). All isolates tested negative for *set1A*, *set1B* and *stx*.

According to their virulence gene distribution, the 44 *S. sonnei* isolates formed 3 gene profile patterns (Additional file 3: Table S3). VT3, which was positive for *ipaH*, *ial* and *sen*, contained the highest number of isolates (37, 87.36%) and was the major VT present in each province. VT2, which was positive for ipaH and ial, was only detected in one Qinghai isolate (SS005). Six isolates (13.64%), one in Gansu and five in Qinghai, belonged to VT1, which was only positive for *ipaH*.

Antimicrobial susceptibility profiles

The antimicrobial resistance profiles of the 44 *S. sonnei* isolates to 21 antimicrobials are listed in Fig. 1 and Table 2. The antimicrobial susceptibility results showed that all *S. sonnei* isolates were sensitive to ciprofloxacin,

Table 2 Statistical analysis of the results of antimicrobial susceptibility testing of 21 antibiotics for 44 *S. sonnei* isolates

Antimicrobial	Antimicrobial resistance rate [No. (%)]						
	Total ($n = 44$)	Gansu ($n = 24$)		Qinghai ($n = 15$)		Tibet ($n = 5$)	
		phase I ($n = 20$)	phase II ($n = 4$)	phase I ($n = 10$)	phase II ($n = 5$)	phase I ($n = 3$)	phase II ($n = 2$)
Norfloxacin	10 (22.73%)	4 (20%)	1 (25%)	3 (30%)	1 (20%)	1 (33.33%)	0
Enrofloxacin	12 (27.27%)	5 (25%)	1 (25%)	3 (30%)	1 (20%)	2 (66.67%)	0
Levofloxacin	4 (9.09%)	3 (15%)	0	1 (10%)	0	0	0
Ciprofloxacin	0	0	0	0	0	0	0
Ofloxacin	0	0	0	0	0	0	0
Penicillin G	44 (100%)	20 (100%)	4 (100%)	10 (100%)	5 (100%)	3 (100%)	2 (100%)
Ampicillin	31 (70.45%)	15 (75%)	3 (75%)	8 (80%)	3 (60%)	1 (33.33%)	1 (50%)
Amoxicillin/clavulanic acid	0	0	0	0	0	0	0
Cephalothin	13 (29.55%)	7 (35%)	0	5 (50%)	0	0	1 (50%)
Cephazolin	14 (31.82%)	7 (35%)	1 (25%)	5 (50%)	0	0	1 (50%)
Cefoxitin	4 (9.09%)	0	0	4 (40%)	0	0	0
Ceftriaxone	9 (20.45%)	4 (20%)	0	5 (50%)	0	0	0
Cefotaxime	5 (11.36%)	2 (10%)	0	3 (30%)	0	0	0
Cefepime	0	0	0	0	0	0	0
Meropenem	0	0	0	0	0	0	0
Imipenem	0	0	0	0	0	0	0
Chloramphenicol	4 (9.09%)	0	0	3 (30%)	1 (20%)	0	0
Tetracycline	30 (68.18%)	14 (70%)	2 (50%)	8 (80%)	3 (60%)	2 (66.67%)	1 (50%)
Streptomycin	14 (31.82%)	5 (25%)	2 (50%)	5 (50%)	1 (20%)	0	1 (50%)
Gentamicin	12 (27.27%)	6 (30%)	0	5 (50%)	1 (20%)	0	0
Amikacin	0	0	0	0	0	0	0

ofloxacin, amoxicillin/clavulanic acid, cefepime, meropenem, imipenem, and amikacin but resistant to penicillin G. The resistance rates to other antimicrobials are as follows: ampicillin (31/44, 70.45%), tetracycline (30/44, 68.18%), cephazolin (14/44, 31.82%), streptomycin (14/44, 31.82%), cephalothin (13/44, 29.55%), enrofloxacin (12/44, 27.27%), gentamicin (12/44, 27.27%), norfloxacin (10/44, 22.73%), ceftriaxone (9/44, 20.45%), cefotaxime (5/44, 11.36%), levofloxacin (4/44, 9.09%), cefoxitin (4/44, 9.09%), and chloramphenicol (4/44, 9.09%). Although the observed resistance to most antimicrobials (with the exception of penicillin G, ampicillin and tetracycline) was less than 50%, multidrug-resistant (MDR) *S. sonnei* isolates, which were defined as being resistant to 3 or more antimicrobial agent subclasses, accounted for 43.18% of isolates (19/44).

Remarkably, the rates of resistance to fluoroquinolones and cephalosporin were 27.275% (12/44) and 31.82% (14/44), respectively, and 13.64% (6/44) of isolates were resistant to both fluoroquinolones and cephalosporin. Moreover, all fluoroquinolone-resistant isolates belonged to the MDR group. Interestingly, the fluoroquinolone- and/or cephalosporin-resistant isolates demonstrated diverse antimicrobial resistance profiles, and no isolates had the same resistance profile (Table 3 and Fig. 1).

Molecular analysis of antimicrobial resistance determinants

In the present study, all four QRDR genes (*gyrA*, *gyrB*, *parC*, and *parE*) were sequenced and compared with reference sequences. According to the results, double mutations in *gyrA* (Ser83-Leu and Asp87-Asn) and a single mutation in *parC* (Ser80-Ile) were associated with fluoroquinolone resistance in *S. sonnei* isolates (Table 3). The encoded Ser83-Leu amino acid substitution in *gyrA* was observed in every fluoroquinolone-resistant isolate, and 66.67% (8/12) of fluoroquinolone-resistant isolates possessed the Asp87-Asn mutation in *gyrA*. Only four isolates harbored all three amino acid substitutions. Interestingly, all four of these isolates belonged to the phase I serotype.

In addition to the identification of substitutions in QRDR genes, PMQR genes were amplified and sequenced. According to the results, all fluoroquinolone-resistant isolates harbored the *aac(6′)-Ib-cr* gene. The *qepA* gene, which encodes an efflux pump, was not observed in the

Table 3 Analysis of amino acid types in QRDRs and ARGs in *S. sonnei* isolates with resistance to fluoroquinolones and/or cephalosporin

Strain name	Antimicrobial resistance profiles	Fluoroquinolone resistance genes					Cephalosporin resistance genes		
		QRDR			PMQR genes		*TEM*	*OXA*	*CTX-M*
		gyrA		*parC*	*aac(6')-Ib-cr*	*qnr*			
		83 (S)	87 (D)	80 (S)					
SS036	ENR/TE	L	D	S	*aac(6')-Ib-cr*	NA	—	—	—
SS019	ENR/AMP/TE/CN	L	D	S	*aac(6')-Ib-cr*	NA	—	—	—
SS002	NOR/ENR/AMP/TE	L	D	S	*aac(6')-Ib-cr*	NA	—	—	—
SS008	NOR/ENR/AMP/TE/S	L	N	S	*aac(6')-Ib-cr*	qnrB	—	—	—
SS043	NOR/ENR/AMP/TE/S	L	D	I	*aac(6')-Ib-cr*	NA	—	—	—
SS029	NOR/ENR/AMP/C/TE/S/CN	L	N	S	*aac(6')-Ib-cr*	NA	—	—	—
SS018	AMP/KZ/TE/S	—	—	—	—	—	*TEM-1*	NA	NA
SS024	AMP/KF/KZ/TE	—	—	—	—	—	*TEM-1*	NA	NA
SS035	AMP/KF/KZ/TE	—	—	—	—	—	*TEM-1*	NA	NA
SS011	AMP/KF/KZ/TE/CN	—	—	—	—	—	*TEM-1*	NA	NA
SS031	AMP/KF/KZ/CRO/TE/S/CN	—	—	—	—	—	*TEM-1*	*OXA-1*	NA
SS032	AMP/KF/KZ/CRO/TE/S/CN	—	—	—	—	—	*TEM-1*	*OXA-1*	NA
SS006	AMP/KF/KZ/FOX/CRO/C/TE/S/CN	—	—	—	—	—	*TEM-1*	*OXA-1*	NA
SS027	AMP/KF/KZ/FOX/CRO/CTX/TE/S/CN	—	—	—	—	—	*TEM-1*	NA	*CTX-M-79*
SS004	NOR/ENR/AMP/KF/KZ/TE/S/CN	L	N	S	*aac(6')-Ib-cr*	NA	*TEM-1*	*OXA-1*	NA
SS028	NOR/ENR/LEV/AMP/KF/KZ/CRO/TE/S/CN	L	N	I	*aac(6')-Ib-cr*	NA	*TEM-1*	*OXA-1*	NA
SS013	NOR/ENR/LEV/AMP/KF/KZ/CRO/CTX/TE/S	L	N	I	*aac(6')-Ib-cr*	NA	*TEM-1*	*OXA-1*	*CTX-M-14*
SS039	NOR/ENR/LEV/AMP/KF/KZ/CRO/CTX/TE/S	L	N	I	*aac(6')-Ib-cr*	NA	*TEM-1*	*OXA-1*	*CTX-M-14*
SS021	NOR/ENR/AMP/KF/KZ/FOX/CRO/CTX/C/TE/CN	L	N	S	*aac(6')-Ib-cr*	*qnrS*	*TEM-1*	*OXA-1*	*CTX-M-14*
SS041	NOR/ENR/LEV/AMP/KF/KZ/FOX/CRO/CTX/TE/S/CN	L	N	I	*aac(6')-Ib-cr*	*qnrS*	*TEM-1*	*OXA-1*	*CTX-M-14*

S Ser, *L* Leu, *D* Asp, *N* Asn, *I* Ile, *NA* not available; "—": not detected

studied isolates. Only three Qinghai isolates tested positive for the *qnr* gene, with two having *qnrS* and one having *qnrB* (Table 3).

For the 14 cephalosporin-resistant isolates, only three β-lactamase gene types (bla_{TEM}, bla_{OXA} and $bla_{CTX\text{-}M}$) were observed. All isolates tested positive for the bla_{TEM} gene and showed 100% identity with the bla_{TEM-1} subtype. And all the third-cephalosporin resistant isolates were positive for bla_{OXA} ($bla_{OXA\text{-}1}$), except SS027. Five out of the fourteen cephalosporin-resistant isolates tested positive for $bla_{CTX\text{-}M}$, 4 of which had the $bla_{CTX\text{-}M\text{-}14}$ gene, and 1 had the $bla_{CTX\text{-}M\text{-}79}$ gene.

Discussion

Bacillary dysentery caused by *Shigella* is endemic throughout the world. Humans are the natural hosts of *Shigella*, although reports of *Shigella* infections in animals (fish, calves, piglets, and chickens) have emerged [2, 17–19]. We previously confirmed the existence of diverse *S. sonnei* isolates in yak in local epidemiological studies. The rate of *S. sonnei* isolation from the diarrhea of yaks was 3.89% (44/1132), and the predominant serotype was phase I, which was isolated three times more frequently than phase II. In addition, 54 *S. flexneri* isolates with diverse serotypes were reported in our previous study [19].

MLST and PFGE have shown comparable discrimination in terms of their ability to subtype *S. sonnei*. In this study, 44 *S. sonnei* isolates from yaks were grouped into 4 STs based on 15 housekeeping genes. Comparison of these genes with the standard gene types on the EcMLST website revealed that the different STs of these isolates were primarily attributable to three genes, *aspC*, *mutS*, and *ropS*. In addition, all isolates belonged to the same clonal complex, suggesting a relatively close genetic relationship among them. In our study, the majority of isolates ($n = 27$ and $n = 13$) belonged to ST116 and ST155, respectively. However, ST76, ST116, and ST114 were previously reported in human isolates [20, 21]. PFGE is a broadly applicable typing method that has high resolution for the molecular characterization of several enteric bacteria, including *Shigella* [20]. Based on our PFGE analysis, the *S. sonnei* isolates in the present study were heterogeneous and distributed into 32 PTs.

The clustering of these diverse PTs allows us to learn more about the epidemiological characteristics of *S. sonnei* in specific geographical regions. PFGE appeared to have a higher discriminatory power for genotypes and genetic relatedness diversity analysis than MLST.

Virulence genes are responsible for the invasion of virulent *Shigella* strains into intestinal epithelial cells, resulting in dysentery in hosts [22]. *ipaH*, which is typically used as a marker of *Shigella*, was harbored by all isolates. Additionally, in this study, most isolates simultaneously harbored the *ial* and *sen* genes. The diversity of the observed virulence genes suggested the isolates were pathogenic. Moreover, virulence genes were frequently located in megaplasmids, which allow *Shigella* to acquire and disseminate bacterial invasion genes through mobile genetic elements [23].

Recently, antimicrobial-resistant and MDR *S. sonnei* isolates have been widely isolated [20, 23]. In this study, we isolated MDR *S. sonnei* isolates from yaks. More than half of the isolates were resistant to conventional and commonly used antimicrobials: penicillin G (100%), ampicillin (70.45%), and tetracycline (68.18%). Fortunately, for most antimicrobials, the rates and levels of resistance of *Shigella* isolates from yaks were less than those from isolates from livestock [24]. Notably, although only low rates of resistance and MIC values to fluoroquinolones and/or cephalosporin were observed, some *S. sonnei* had acquired the ability to survive the selective pressures of these antimicrobials, which will limit the control and treatment of shigellosis.

Fluoroquinolone resistance is primarily mediated by the accumulation of sequential mutations in four QRDR genes: *gyrA* and *gyrB*, which encode DNA gyrase, and *parC* and *parE*, which encode and topoisomerase IV [25]. The primary mutations are located in *gyrA* and *parC*. According to a previous study, the major mutations in *gyrA* codons 81 (Gly → Ser), 83 (Ser → Leu), 87 (Asp→Asn/Gly/Tyr), and 211 (His→Tyr) and *parC* codons 80 (Ser → Ile), 83 (Ser → Leu), and 129 (Ser → Pro) are associated with quinolone and/or fluoroquinolone resistance in *Shigella* [11, 24, 26, 27]. Furthermore, the continuous accumulation of mutations at multiple positions and different mutations at the same position may lead to diverse levels of resistance [23]. In this study, we identified QRDR mutations in all fluoroquinolone-resistant *S. sonnei*, observing only a few classic amino acid substitutions in *gyrA* and *parC*.

The PMQR determinants are typically located on mobile or transposable genetic elements, which may facilitate dissemination among *Shigella* species and other members of the Enterobacteriaceae family [28, 29]. Recently, the diversity of PMQR determinants has emerged as an important issue worldwide [27]. Among the PMQR genes, *aac(6′)-Ib-cr*, which encodes aminoglycoside acetyl transferase and is responsible for reduced fluoroquinolone activity, was the most prevalent in our study. The *qnr*-encoded family of proteins protects DNA gyrase from quinolones and confers low-level resistance [30]. *QnrS* were majority prevalence in *Shigella* (*S.sonnei* and *S.flexneri*) in China, while *qnrB* previously in India [23, 26]. In addition, the plasmid-mediated efflux pump-encoding gene *qepA* was detected at lower frequencies [27]. The presence of PMQR genes may help microorganisms develop resistance by conferring mutations and facilitating the selection of higher-level quinolone resistance [31].

ESBLs continue to be the major defense mechanism against cephalosporins among Gram-negative bacteria [32]. Since first being identified in the 1980s, different types of ESBLs belonging to the *TEM*, *OXA*, *SHV* and *CTX-M* families have been widely reported in Enterobacteriaceae, including *Shigella* species [33, 34]. The global spread of ESBL-producing *Shigella* is difficult to control and eradicate because these bacteria reside in the intestines of humans and animals and harbor epidemic resistance plasmids. Therefore, the prevalence of ESBL-producing *S. sonnei* in yaks represents a substantial threat.

Conclusion

Antimicrobial-resistant *Shigella* remains a serious threat to humans and animals; however, knowledge of the molecular epidemiology of this pathogen in yaks is limited. *Shigella* species typically harbor various plasmids that are associated with invasion into host intestinal epithelial cells and antimicrobial resistance and may be transferred between different bacteria. In the present study the *S. sonnei* strains isolated from yaks that tested positive for diverse virulence genes and ARGs represent a potential threat to hosts, including humans. Therefore, continuous and extensive surveillance will be necessary to control and reduce the threat of foodborne pathogens, such as *Shigella*, *Salmonella* and *E. coli*.

Methods

Bacterial isolates and serological confirmation

A total of 44 *S. sonnei* isolates were obtained from yaks with diarrhea from October 2014 to December 2016. All yaks have hardly been exposed to any antibiotic except for a few of penicillin to against the disease. All isolates were collected directly from fresh stool samples, plated on Salmonella-Shigella (SS) selective agar and confirmed on MacConkey (MAC) agar at 37 °C for 18 to 24 h. Colorless, semitransparent, smooth, and moist circular plaques were considered presumptive *Shigella* isolates and were selected for further confirmation [34]. The presumptive positive *Shigella* isolates were identified using API 20 E kits (bioMerieux, Marcy-l'Etoile, France), and serotypes were tested with a commercially available kit

(Denka Seiken; Tokyo, Japan) according to the manufacturer's recommendations.

Multilocus sequence typing (MLST)

MLST was performed for each isolate according to the protocols described on the EcMLST website (http://www.shigatox.net/ecmlst). The following PCR amplification conditions were used for 15 housekeeping genes: 94 °C for 5 min, followed by 30 cycles of 94 °C for 30 s, 55 °C for 30 s, and 72 °C for 1 min, with incubation for 10 min at 72 °C with ExTaq DNA polymerase (Takara; Dalian, China). The PCR products were sequenced bi-directionally, and sequences of the 15 housekeeping genes were edited using SeqMan 7.0. Finally, the sequences were uploaded to the EcMLST website for comparison, which allowed us to determine the gene and ST type [35].

Pulsed-field gel electrophoresis (PFGE)

All *S. sonnei* isolates were analyzed for genetic relatedness by PFGE after digestion with the restriction enzyme *Xba*I (TaKaRa; Japan) according to the recommendations of a previous study [36]. *Salmonella enterica* serotype Braenderup strain H9812 was used as a molecular size maker. Electrophoresis was performed with a Bio-Rad CHEF Mapper XA system (Bio-Rad; USA) in a 1% SeaKem Gold agarose gel (Lonza; USA) in 0.5X TBE buffer with a size range of 30–700 kb. The PFGE run conditions were 6 V/cm with a switch from 2.16 to 54.17 s for 21 h at 14 °C.

After gel electrophoresis, gels were stained with ethidium bromide, rinsed, and photographed with a Universal Hood II (Bio-Rad; USA). The PFGE patterns were analyzed with BioNumerics using the Dice similarity coefficient, unweighted pair-group method with arithmetic mean (UPGMA) and 1.0% tolerance.

Detection of virulence genes by PCR

All *S. sonnei* isolates were examined for the presence of six virulence genes, invasion plasmid antigen H (*ipaH*), invasion associated locus (*ial*), Shiga toxin gene (*stx*), and *Shigella* enterotoxin genes (*set1A*, *set1B*, and *sen*), by PCR according to published procedures [23, 37]. The primers for these virulence genes are listed in Additional file 4: Table S4. Amplification products were separated by 1% agarose gel electrophoresis and stained with ethidium bromide.

Antimicrobial susceptibility

Antimicrobial susceptibility testing was performed by the Kirby-Bauer disc diffusion method on Muller-Hinton agar (MHA) plates following the guidelines of the Clinical and Laboratory Standards Institute (CLSI) using commercially available antimicrobial discs (Oxoid, UK). Twenty-one antimicrobial discs were used in this study: norfloxacin (NOR, 10 μg), enrofloxacin (ENR, 5 μg), levofloxacin (LEV, 5 μg), ciprofloxacin (CIP, 5 μg), ofloxacin (OFX, 5 μg), penicillin G (P, 10 μg), ampicillin (AMP, 10 μg), amoxicillin/clavulanic acid (AMC, 30 μg), cephalothin (KF, 30 μg), cephazolin (KZ, 30 μg), cefoxitin (FOX, 30 μg), ceftriaxone (CRO, 30 μg), cefotaxime (CTX, 30 μg), cefepime (FEP, 30 μg), imipenem (IPM, 10 μg), meropenem (MEM, 10 μg), chloramphenicol (C, 30 μg), tetracycline (TE, 30 μg), streptomycin (S, 10 μg), gentamicin (CN, 10 μg), and amikacin (AK, 30 μg). *E. coli* ATCC 25922 was used as a control strain. The standard of antibiotic susceptibility for CLSI were list in Additional file 5: Table S5.

Detection of β-lactamase and quinolone resistance genes

Cephalosporin- and/or fluoroquinolone-resistant *S. sonnei* isolates were assayed by PCR using 24 primer panels to determine the underlying mechanism conferring resistance (Additional file 6: Table S6). Specifically, 6 plasmid-mediated quinolone resistance (PMQRs) determinant genes (*qnrA*, *qnrB*, *qnrD*, *qnrS*, *qepA* and *aac(6′)-Ib-cr*) and 4 quinolone resistance determining region (QRDR) genes (*gyrA*, *gyrB*, *parC* and *parE*) were amplified to clarify the underlying mechanism conferring resistance to quinolones [38–40]. Extended-spectrum β-lactamase (ESBL) genes ($bla_{CTX\text{-}M}$, bla_{SHV}, bla_{TEM}, and bla_{OXA}) were detected in cephalosporin-resistant isolates [39, 41, 42].

Additional files

Additional file 1: Table S1. MLST allelic profiles and ST designations of 44 *S. sonnei* isolates from this study.

Additional file 2: Table S2. Statistical analysis of the presence of virulence genes in each S. sonnei isolate.

Additional file 3: Table S3. Statistical analysis of the occurrence of each virulence gene profile in different provinces.

Additional file 4: Table S4. Primers used to detect virulence genes.

Additional file 5: Table S5. The standard of antibiotic susceptibility for K-B disc-diffusion method.

Additional file 6: Table S6. Primers used to detect antibiotic resistance determinant genes.

Abbreviations

ESBL: Extended-spectrum β-lactamase; MLST: Multilocus sequence typing; PFGE: Pulsed-field gel electrophoresis; PMQRs: Plasmid-mediated quinolone resistance; QRDR: Quinolone resistance determining region; VT: Virulence gene profile types

Acknowledgments

The authors warmly thank to all veterinarians and personnel of the farms that provided the samples for this study.

Funding

This work was financed by grants from the National Natural Science Foundation of China (31272603, 31101836).

Authors' contributions

ZZ and YXS contributed equally to first author in this work. ZZ conceived, designed, performed the experiments and drafted the manuscript the study. YXS collected the samples from Qinghai, performed PFGE and MLST work. XZZ collected the samples from Gansu and isolated Shigella sonneri. BL participated in PCR and sequencing experiments. JYZ designed the study, helped with and supervised the execution of laboratory work, as well as the statistical interpretation of the data and reviewed the final paper. All authors read and approved the final manuscript.

Competing interests

The authors declare that they have no competing interests.

Author details

[1]Key Laboratory of New Animal Drug Project of Gansu Province, Key Laboratory of Veterinary Pharmaceutical Development of the Ministry of Agriculture, Lanzhou Institute of Husbandry and Pharmaceutical Sciences of CAAS, Jiangouyan, Qilihe District, Lanzhou 730050, China. [2]College of Life Science and Food Engineering, Hebei University of Engineering, Hanshan District, Handan 056038, China.

References

1. Stirling J, Griffith M, Blair I, Cormican M, Dooley JS, Goldsmith CE, Glover SG, Loughrey A, Lowery CJ, Matsuda M, McClurg R, McCorry K, McDowell D, McMahon A, Cherie Millar B, Nagano Y, Rao JR, Rooney PJ, Smyth M, Snelling WJ, Xu J, Moore JE. Prevalence of gastrointestinal bacterial pathogens in a population of zoo animals. Zoonoses Public Health. 2008; 55(3):166–72.
2. Shi R, Yang X, Chen L, Chang HT, Liu HY, Zhao J, Wang XW, Wang CQ. Pathogenicity of Shigella in chickens. PLoS One. 2014;9(6):e100264.
3. Parajuli P, Adamski M, Verma NK. Bacteriophages are the major drivers of Shigella flexneri serotype 1c genome plasticity: a complete genome analysis. BMC Genomics. 2017;18(1):722.
4. Pupo GM, Lan R, Reeves PR. Multiple independent origins of Shigella clones of Escherichia coli and convergent evolution of many of their characteristics. Proc Natl Acad Sci U S. 2000;7(19):10567–72.
5. Xia S, Xu B, Huang L, Zhao JY, Ran L, Zhang J, Chen H, Pulsrikarn C, Pornruangwong S, Aarestrup FM, Hendriksen RS. Prevalence and characterization of human Shigella infections in Henan Province, China, in 2006. J Clin Microbiol. 2011;49(1):232–42.
6. Bangtrakulnonth A, Vieira AR, Lo Fo Wong DM, Pornreongwong S, Pulsrikarn C, Sawanpanyalert P, Hendriksen RS, Aarestrup FM. Shigella from humans in Thailand during 1993 to 2006: spatial-time trends in species and serotype distribution. Foodborne Pathog Dis. 2008;5(6):773–84.
7. Qu F, Bao C, Chen S, Cui E, Guo T, Wang H, Zhang J, Wang H, Tang YW, Mao Y. Genotypes and antimicrobial profiles of Shigella sonnei isolates from diarrheal patients circulating in Beijing between 2002 and 2007. Diagn Microbiol Infect Dis. 2012;74(2):166–70.
8. Zhang CL, Liu QZ, Wang J, Chu X, Shen LM, Guo YY. Epidemic and virulence characteristic of Shigella spp. with extended-spectrum cephalosporin resistance in Xiaoshan District, Hangzhou, China. BMC Infect Dis. 2014;14:260.
9. Qu M, Zhang X, Liu G, Huang Y, Jia L, Liang W, Li X, Wu X, Li J, Yan H, Kan B, Wang Q. An eight-year study of Shigella species in Beijing, China: serodiversity, virulence genes, and antimicrobial resistance. J Infect Dev Ctries. 2014;8(7):904–8.
10. Azmi IJ, Khajanchi BK, Akter F, Hasan TN, Shahnaij M, Akter M, Banik A, Sultana H, Hossain MA, Ahmed MK, Faruque SM, Talukder KA. Fluoroquinolone resistance mechanisms of Shigella flexneri isolated in Bangladesh. PLoS One. 2014;9(7):e102533.
11. Sabra AH, Araj GF, Kattar MM, Abi-Rached RY, Khairallah MT, Klena JD, Matar GM. Molecular characterization of ESBL-producing Shigella sonnei isolates from patients with bacilliary dysentery in Lebanon. J Infect Dev Ctries. 2009; 3(4):300–5.
12. Ud-Din AI, Wahid SU, Latif HA, Shahnaij M, Akter M, Azmi IJ, Hasan TN, Ahmed D, Hossain MA, Faruque AS, Faruque SM, Talukder KA. Changing trends in the prevalence of Shigella species: emergence of multi-drug resistant Shigella sonnei biotype g in Bangladesh. PLoS One. 2013;8(12):e82601.
13. Schlundt J. Emerging food-borne pathogens. Biomed Environ Sci. 2001; 14(1–2):44–52.
14. Newell DG, Koopmans M, Verhoef L, Duizer E, Aidara-Kane A, Sprong H, Opsteegh M, Langelaar M, Threfall J, Scheutz F, van der Giessen J, Kruse H. Food-borne diseases - the challenges of 20 years ago still persist while new ones continue to emerge. Int J Food Microbiol. 2010;139(Suppl 1):S3–15.
15. EFSA (European Food Safety Authority). Scientific opinion of the panel on biological hazards on a request from the European food safety authority on foodborne antimicrobial resistance as a biological hazard. EFSA J. 2008;765:1–87.
16. Ahmed AM, Shimamoto T. Molecular characterization of multidrug-resistant Shigella spp. of food origin. Int J Food Microbiol. 2015;194:78–82.
17. Onyango DM, Wandili S, Kakai R, Waindi EN. Isolation of Salmonella and Shigella from fish harvested from the Winam gulf of Lake Victoria. Kenya J Infect Dev Ctries. 2009;3(2):99–104.
18. Priamukhina NS, Kilesso VA, Tikhomirov ED. Animal carriers of Shigella and their possible epidemiological importance. Zh Mikrobiol Epidemiol Immunobiol. 1984;11:20–4.
19. Maurelli AT, Routh PR, Dillman RC, Ficken MD, Weinstock DM, Almond GW, Orndorff PE. Shigella infection as observed in the experimentally inoculated domestic pig, Sus scrofa domestica. Microb Pathog. 1998;25(4):189–96.
20. Li S, Wang J, Wei X, Liu Y, You L, Luo X, Tang G, Sun Q, Ye C, Xu J, Wang D. Molecular characterization of Shigella sonnei: an increasingly prevalent etiologic agent of shigellosis in Guizhou Province, Southwest of China. PLoS One. 2016;11(5):e0156020.
21. Cheng T, Shi X, Yong W, Wang J, Xie G, Ding J. Molecular typing of Shigella sonnei isolates circulating in Nanjing, China, 2007-2011. J Infect Dev Ctries. 2014;8(12):1525–32.
22. Ashida H, Ogawa M, Mimuro H, Kobayashi T, Sanada T, Sasakawa C. Shigella are versatile mucosal pathogens that circumvent the host innate immune system. Curr Opin Immunol. 2011;23(4):448–55.
23. Das A, Natarajan M, Mandal J. The emergence of quinolone resistant *Shigella sonnei*, Pondicherry, India. PLoS One. 2016;11(8):e0160290.
24. Zhu Z, Cao M, Zhou X, Li B, Zhang J. Epidemic characterization and molecular genotyping of Shigella flexneri isolated from calves with diarrhea in Northwest China. Antimicrob Resist Infect Control. 2017;6:92.
25. Taneja N, Kumar A, Appannanavar S, Verma G, Sharma M. Plasmid-mediated quinolone resistance in Shigella isolates over a decade in India. J Glob Antimicrob Resist. 2014;2(1):59–60.
26. Cui X, Wang J, Yang C, Liang B, Ma Q, Yi S, Li H, Liu H, Li P, Wu Z, Xie J, Jia L, Hao R, Wang L, Hua Y, Qiu S, Song H. Prevalence and antimicrobial resistance of Shigella flexneri serotype 2 variant in China. Front Microbiol. 2015;6:435.
27. Gu B, Qin TT, Fan WT, Bi RR, Chen Y, Li Y, Ma P. Novel mutations in gyrA and parC among Shigella sonnei strains from Jiangsu Province of China, 2002-2011. Int J Infect Dis. 2017;59:44–9.
28. Folster JP, Pecic G, Bowen A, Rickert R, Carattoli A, Whichard JM. Decreased susceptibility to ciprofloxacin among Shigella isolates in the United States, 2006 to 2009. Antimicrob Agents Chemother. 2011;55(4):1758–60.
29. Rodríguez-Martínez JM, Machuca J, Cano ME, Calvo J, Martínez-Martínez L, Pascual A. Plasmid-mediated quinolone resistance: two decades on. Drug Resist Updat. 2016;29:13–29.
30. Jacoby GA, Gacharna N, Black TA, Miller GH, Hooper DC. Temporal appearance of plasmid-mediated quinolone resistance genes. Antimicrob Agents Chemother. 2009;53(4):1665–6.
31. Yang H, Duan G, Zhu J, Zhang W, Xi Y, Fan Q. Prevalence and characterisation of plasmid-mediated quinolone resistance and mutations in the gyrase and topoisomerase IV genes among Shigella isolates from Henan, China, between 2001 and 2008. Int J Antimicrob Agents. 2013;42(2):173–7.
32. Li J, Li B, Ni Y, Sun J. Molecular characterization of the extended-spectrum beta-lactamase (ESBL)-producing Shigella spp. in Shanghai. Eur J Clin Microbiol Infect Dis. 2015;34(3):447–51.
33. Robin F, Beyrouthy R, Bonacorsi S, Aissa N, Bret L, Brieu N, Cattoir V, Chapuis A, Chardon H, Degand N, Doucet-Populaire F, Dubois V, Fortineau N, Grillon A, Lanotte P, Leyssene D, Patry I, Podglajen I, Recule C, Ros A, Colomb-Cotinat M, Ponties V, Ploy MC, Bonnet R. Inventory of Extended-Spectrum-β-Lactamase-Producing Enterobacteriaceae in France as assessed by a multicenter study. Antimicrob Agents Chemother. 2017;61(3):e01911–16.
34. Tajbakhsh M, García Migura L, Rahbar M, Svendsen CA, Mohammadzadeh M, Zali MR, Aarestrup FM, Hendriksen RS. Antimicrobial-resistant Shigella infections from Iran: an overlooked problem? J Antimicrob Chemother. 2012;67(5):1128–33.
35. Yang C, Li P, Zhang X, Ma Q, Cui X, Li H, Liu H, Wang J, Xie J, Wu F, Sheng C, Du X, Qi L, Su W, Jia L, Xu X, Zhao J, Xia S, Zhou N, Ma H, Qiu S, Song H.

Molecular characterization and analysis of high-level multidrug-resistance of Shigella flexneri serotype 4s strains from China. Sci Rep. 2016;6:29124.
36. Qu F, Cui E, Guo T, Li H, Chen S, Liu L, Han W, Bao C, Mao Y, Tang YW. Nasal colonization of and clonal transmission of methicillin-susceptible Staphylococcus aureus among Chinese military volunteers. J Clin Microbiol. 2010;48(1):64–9.
37. Talukder KA, Mondol AS, Islam MA, Islam Z, Dutta DK, Khajanchi BK, Azmi IJ, Hossain MA, Rahman M, Cheasty T, Cravioto A, Nair GB, Sack DA. A novel serovar of Shigella dysenteriae from patients with diarrhoea in Bangladesh. J Med Microbiol. 2007;56(Pt 5):654–8.
38. Hu LF, Li JB, Ye Y, Li X. Mutations in the GyrA subunit of DNA gyrase and the ParC subunit of topoisomerase IV in clinical strains of fluoroquinolone-resistant *Shigella* in Anhui. China J Microbiol. 2007;45(2):168–70.
39. Tariq A, Haque A, Ali A, Bashir S, Habeeb MA, Salman M, Sarwar Y. Molecular profiling of antimicrobial resistance and integron association of multidrug-resistant clinical isolates of Shigella species from Faisalabad, Pakistan. Can J Microbiol. 2012;58(9):1047–54.
40. Colobatiu L, Tabaran A, Flonta M, Oniga O, Mirel S, Mihaiu M. First description of plasmid-mediated quinolone resistance determinants and β-lactamase encoding genes in non-typhoidal Salmonella isolated from humans, one companion animal and food in Romania. Gut Pathog. 2015;7:16.
41. Zong Z, Partridge SR, Thomas L, Iredell JR. Dominance of blaCTX-M within an Australian extended-spectrum beta-lactamase gene pool. Antimicrob Agents Chemother. 2008;52(11):4198–202.
42. Liu J, Zeng T, Su G, Lin LY, Zhao Y, Yang WQ, Xie WX, Zhao ZG, Li GM. The dissemination mode of drug-resistant genes in Enterobacter cloacae. Indian J Med Microbiol. 2015;33(Suppl):87–92.

19

A novel approach to identifying and quantifying neutrophil extracellular trap formation in septic dogs using immunofluorescence microscopy

Ronald H. L. Li[1*], Lynelle R. Johnson[2], Casey Kohen[3] and Fern Tablin[4]

Abstract

Background: Canine neutrophils release neutrophil extracellular traps (NETs) in response to lipopolysaccharide but NETs from clinical septic dogs had not been identified. The primary aim is to describe the methodology of identifying and quantifying neutrophil extracellular traps (NETs) in cytology samples of septic foci in dogs with sepsis using immunofluorescence microscopy. Cytology samples including endotracheal tracheal wash (ETW), bronchoalveolar lavage (BAL), abdominal and pleural effusion collected from 5 dogs (3 septic, 2 non-septic) were fixed, permeabilized and stained for myeloperoxidase (MPO), citrullinated histone H3 (citH3) and cell-free DNA (cfDNA). Fluorescence microscopy was used to identify and quantify NETs in 10 random views at 40× magnification. NETs were identified based on co-localization of MPO, citH3 and cfDNA. NETs were quantified as a ratio (number of NETs: number of neutrophils). Neutrophils were identified based on cytoplasmic MPO, cellular diameter and nuclear morphology.

Results: NETs were identified and quantified in all cytology samples collected from septic dogs. A small number of NETs was documented in one dog with sterile chronic bronchitis. No NETs were found in sterile abdominal effusion collected from one dog with congestive heart failure.

Conclusions: Immunofluorescence microscopy could be a useful tool for the study of NETs in dogs with clinical sepsis.

Keywords: Peptidylarginine deiminase, Citrullinated histones, Cell-free DNA, Sepsis

Background

In response to bacterial infection, neutrophils release neutrophil extracellular traps (NETs), which are web-like scaffolds of extracellular DNA decorated with histones and neutrophil granular proteins such as myeloperoxidase (MPO) and neutrophil elastase [1]. Bacteria, entrapped within NETs, are either phagocytosed by adjacent neutrophils or killed by high concentrations of extracellular antimicrobial proteins [2]. Although NETs are found to limit bacterial dissemination in septic mice, overzealous NET production (NETosis) is associated with sepsis-associated organ dysfunction such as acute lung injury, acute kidney injury and mortality [3, 4]. This paradox highlights the fact that dysregulation of NETosis likely plays a key role in perpetuating tissue damage and organ dysfunction. NET components such as histones, once released extracellularly, can function as a damage-associated molecular pattern resulting in cytotoxicity, inflammation and microvascular dysfunction [5]. In human septic patients, elevated intravascular NET components such as cell-free DNA (cfDNA) and citrullinated histones are associated with mortality [6, 7].

To date, NETs have not been documented in dogs with bacterial sepsis. Isolated canine neutrophils have been shown to release NETs in response to *E. coli* lipopolysaccharide and the chemical, phorbol 12-myristate

* Correspondence: rhli@ucdavis.edu
[1]Department of Veterinary Surgical and Radiological Sciences, School of Veterinary Medicine, University of California, One Shield Avenue, Davis, California 95161, USA
Full list of author information is available at the end of the article

13-acetate [8, 9]. Several methods of plasma cfDNA quantification have been described in dogs with sepsis, neoplasia and immune-mediated haemolytic anemia [8, 10]. However, the use of cfDNA as a NETosis biomarker is controversial as there is evidence suggesting that cfDNA does not originate specifically from NET-producing neutrophils [11]. Citrullinated histones and myeloperoxidase (MPO), other NET biomarkers, have not been identified in septic dogs. Because NETs may contribute to the pathophysiology of sepsis in dogs, a method allowing specific and objective identification and quantification of NETs in septic dogs is needed.

In this methodology manuscript, we sought to describe a novel technique to visualize and quantify NETs in cytological samples of septic foci in dogs using immunofluorescence microscopy.

Methods

The study protocol was approved by the Institutional Animal Care and Use Committee at the University of California, Davis. Client-owned dogs admitted to the William R. Pritchard Veterinary Medical Teaching Hospital of University of California, Davis and diagnosed with sepsis were eligible for enrolment. Sepsis was diagnosed based on the presence of systemic or local bacterial infection and systemic inflammatory response syndrome (SIRS). SIRS was identified based on previously published criteria [12]. Only dogs with cytological samples collected from their respective septic foci were enrolled. Clinical management of patients was determined by the primary attending clinicians. Bacterial infection was diagnosed based on cytologic identification of intracellular bacteria and positive bacterial cultures from patient samples. Non-septic dogs with matched cytology samples were included as controls. Medical records were reviewed for patients' signalment including age, breed and sex as well as outcome and bacterial culture results.

In Dog 1, an ETW was performed by passing an infant feeding tube down a sterile endotracheal tube to approximately the level of the carina. In Dog 4, bronchoalveolar lavage (BAL) at multiple sites (right cranial, left and right caudal bronchi) was performed through the biopsy channel of the endoscope after bronchoscopic examination. Abdominal and pleural effusion were collected via ultrasound-guided needle aspiration.

Cytology samples were immediately placed on ice and diluted (1-fold) in Dulbecco's phosphate buffered saline (DPBS) with 1% bovine serum albumin. Samples were further diluted (2 to 3-fold) before concentrated onto microscope slides using a cytocentrifuge (Cytospin 4, ThermoScientific Inc., Grand Island, NY) (1500 rpm, 5 min), air dried, and stored at -20 °C until further analysis. The residual samples were submitted to the University of California Veterinary Medical Teaching Hospital clinical diagnostic laboratory for culture and susceptibility, total nucleated cell counts (Advia 120, Siemens, Deerfield, IL) and cytologic assessment by board-certified clinical pathologists.

Immunofluorescence microscopy

Cells were first fixed in 4% paraformaldehyde then permeabilized using 1% NP-40 (Surfact-AMPs™ NP-40, Pierce, Rockford, IL) before washing 3 times with DPBS. A modified double immunolabeling protocol was utilized because the primary antibodies used to detect MPO and citrullinated histone H3 (citH3) were produced in the same species [13]. In brief, cells were first blocked with 5% goat serum (1 h, 37 °C) before incubating with 1:400 (2.5 μg/ml) rabbit polyclonal anti-citH3 antibodies (ab5103,

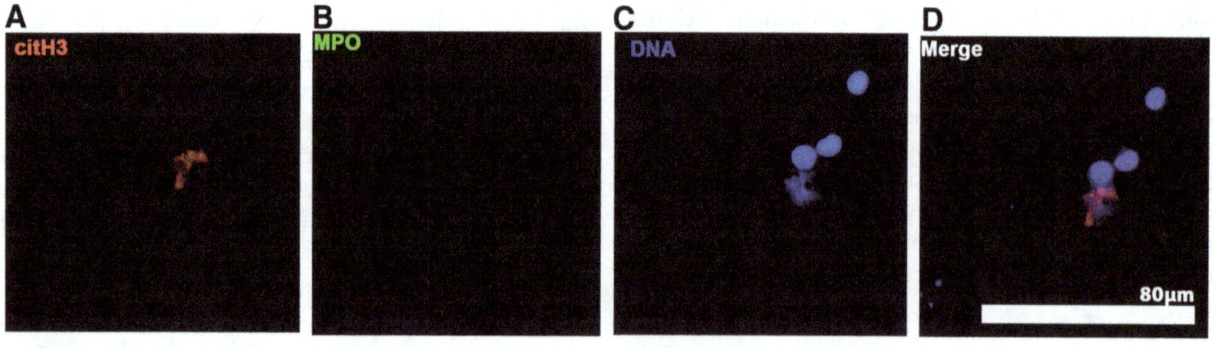

Fig. 1 Representative immunofluorescent images of cytology samples of bronchoalveolar lavage from a dog demonstrating the use of interference controls. Cells were fixed, permeabilized, and incubated with rabbit anti-human citrullinated histone H3 (citH3) antibody, followed by secondary goat anti-rabbit antibody conjugated with Alexa Fluor 568. After blocking with rabbit serum and unconjugated goat anti-rabbit Fab fragments, cells were incubated with goat anti-rabbit antibody conjugated with Alexa Fluor 488 without the second primary antibody against myeloperoxidase (MPO). Cells analysed under the TEXAS RED channel demonstrated presence of citH3 (red) (**a**), while no non-specific binding of secondary body conjugated to Alexa Fluor 488 was detected (**b**). DNA was stained with DAPI (**c**) to ensure the colocalization of citH3 and DNA (**d**). Original 40× magnification

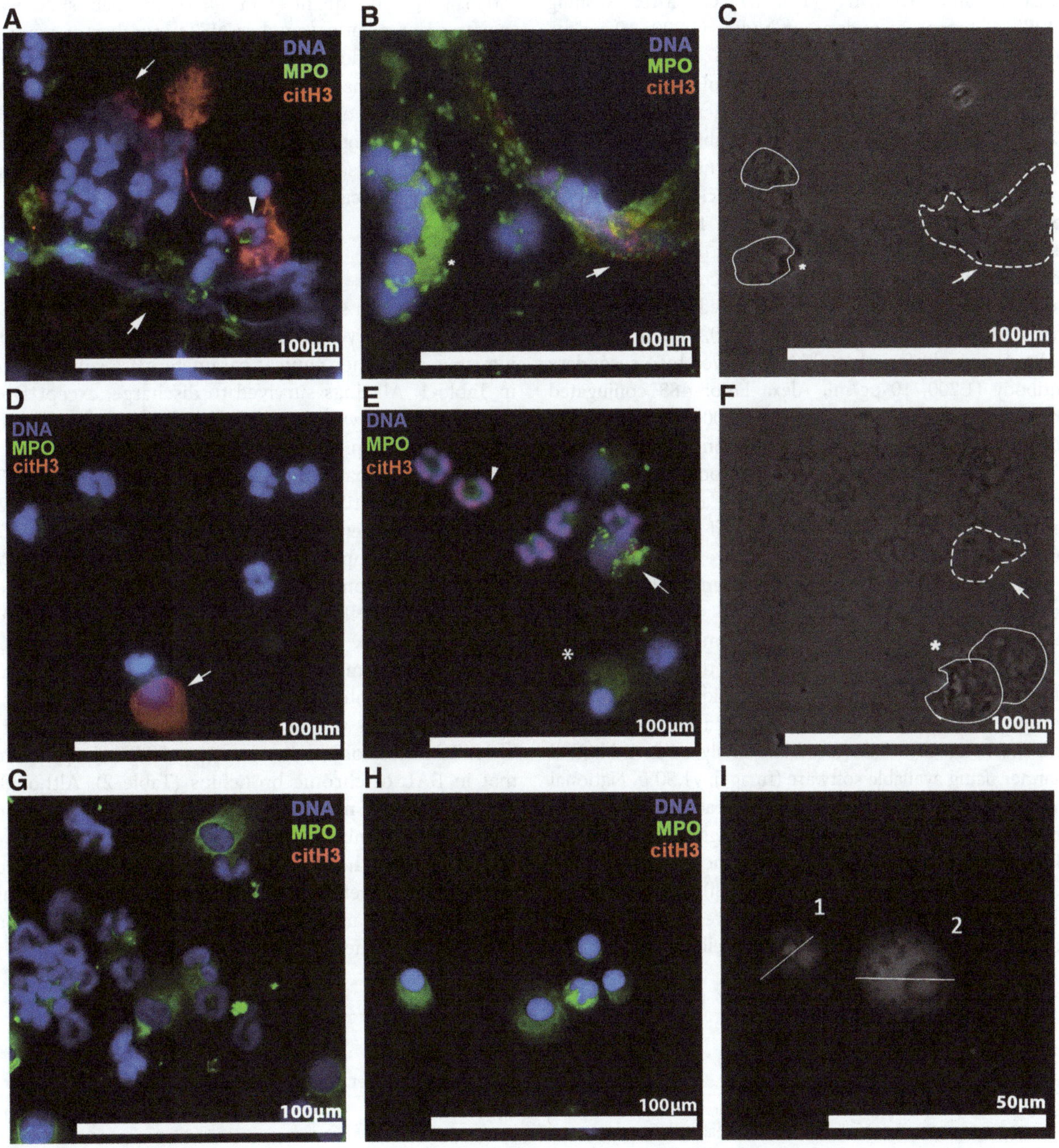

Fig. 2 Representative immunofluorescent images of cytology samples from 3 septic and 2 non-septic dogs. Cells were fixed, permeabilized and stained for citrullinated histone H3 (citH3, red), myeloperoxidase (MPO, green) and DNA (blue). NETs were identified by co-localization of decondensed cell-free DNA (cfDNA), citH3 and MPO. **a**, **b** Endotracheal wash from a dog with aspiration pneumonia. Note the vast amount of decondensed DNA decorated with extracellular citH3 and MPO surrounding nearby neutrophils (dotted outline). Activated pulmonary macrophages also were identified (*). **c** In the respective phase contrast image, phagocytized bacteria within activated pulmonary macrophages (*) and bacteria (arrow) within a NET (dash outline) were detected. NETs (dotted outline) were identified in septic abdominal (**d**) and pleural fluid (**e**). **e**, **f** The respective phase contrast image showed bacteria within a NET (dotted outline) and phagocytized bacteria within macrophages (*). Some neutrophils in septic effusion (**a**, **e**) had chromatin stained positive for citH3 (arrow heads). Non-degenerate neutrophils and activated macrophages were seen in abdominal fluid acquired from a dog with congestive heart failure (**g**) and a dog with chronic bronchitis (**h**); no NETs were identified. **i** A grayscale image stained for MPO and DNA demonstrating the measurement of cell diameter and nuclear morphology. Diameter of cell 1 was measured to be 8 μm. Cell 1 was identified to be a neutrophil based on its lobulated nuclei. Cell 2 was identified to be an activated pulmonary macrophage with a cell diameter of 18.5 μm, with rounded non-lobulated nuclei and presence of cytoplasmic vacuoles. Original 40× magnification. **a**–**h** Scale bar = 100 μm; (**i**) Scale bar = 50 μm

Abcam, Cambridge, MA) (1 h, 37 °C). After washing (DPBS, 3 times), secondary antibodies (1:200, 10 μg/ml, polyclonal goat anti-rabbit antibodies conjugated with Alexa Fluor 568, A-11011, ThermoFisher Scientific, Rockford, IL) was added to cells and incubated for 1 h at 37 °C. Blocking steps utilizing 10% rabbit serum (4 °C, overnight) followed by incubation with unconjugated goat anti-rabbit Fab fragments (50 μg/mL, Jackson ImmunoResearch Laboratories, West Grove, PA) for 2 h at room temperature were performed to prevent the MPO primary antibody from binding to the first secondary antibody. To identify MPO, samples were labelled with polyclonal rabbit anti-human MPO antibody (1:200, 2 μg/ml, A 0398, Dako, Denmark) for 1 h at 37 °C followed by a secondary antibody (1:200, 10 μg/ml, Alexa Fluor 488 conjugated polyclonal goat anti-rabbit IgG, A-11008, ThermoFisher Scientific, Rockford, IL). DNA was stained with 300 nM 4′,6-Diamidino-2-Phenylindole, Dihydrochloride. Interference controls without either primary antibodies in the second immunolabeling step (Type II inference) were demonstrated in Fig. 1 [13].

An EVOS FL Cell Imaging System (ThermoFisher Scientific, Rockford, IL) was used to acquire the immunofluorescent images. Prior to image capture and analysis, the authors were blinded to the conditions by randomly assigning a number to each slide. At 40× magnification, 10 random fields were captured for each sample and the images were acquired and analyzed in a blinded manner using available software (ImageJ, v1.50 g, National Institute of Health). Exposure times of each channel (blue, green or red) were kept constant throughout the analysis. Neutrophils were identified based on nuclear morphology, cell diameter of less than 15 μm (Fig. 2i) and presence of MPO within the cytoplasm. NETs were identified based on co-localization of cfDNA, extracellular MPO, and citH3 [14]. The quantity of NETs in each slide was expressed as a ratio (number NETs: number of neutrophils) in 10 random fields. Cells with citH3 expression were quantified as a ratio (Cells $_{\text{CitH3}}$: Cells $_{\text{no CitH3}}$) by dividing the total of number of cells expressing intracellular citH3 by the total number of cells without intracellular citH3. For septic samples, phase-contrast microscopy was used to visualize bacteria.

Results

Five dogs (3 with sepsis, 2 without sepsis) were enrolled between February and December 2016. Initial presenting signs and other clinical parameters are summarized in Table 1. All dogs survived to discharge, except Dog 3, which underwent cardiopulmonary arrest shortly after presentation.

Cytology and bacterial culture results, as well as NET and citH3 quantification are summarized in Table 2. Immunofluorescent images revealed the presence of NETs in the samples from septic dogs including ETW (Fig. 2a, b), abdominal fluid (Fig. 2d) and pleural effusion (Fig. 2e). NETs consisted of extracellular DNA, MPO and citH3. Using phase contrast microscopy of the respective immunofluorescent views, intracellular bacteria were noted within neutrophils and/or macrophages as well as within NETs (Fig. 2c, f). The quantity of NETs was 3-fold higher in septic ETW compared to that in BAL of chronic bronchitis (Table 2). Although an abundance of non-degenerate neutrophils was found in sterile abdominal effusion obtained from the dog with congestive heart failure, no NETs were identified (Fig. 2g). A subset of neutrophils from septic effusions also underwent intracellular histone H3 citrullination (Fig. 2a, e), whereas intracellular citH3 was rarely

Table 1 Summary of demographic variables, presenting signs and clinical parameters

Dog	Age	Breed	Presenting Signs	SIRS criteria				Diagnosis
				HR (per min)	RR (per minute)	Body temperature (°C)	WBC (× 10^3/μL)	
1	11	Pug	Acute onset of respiratory distress following 24 h of treatment for presumed aspiration pneumonia	60	60	37.2	27.3	Respiratory failure secondary to aspiration pneumonia
2	2	Mixed	Acute onset of respiratory distress with right-sided pneumothorax and small-volume pleural effusion	84	60	39.4	22.0	Bacterial pyothorax
3	9	German Shepherd Dog	Chronic lethargy, inappetence and abdominal pain	150	36	43.5	9.72	Septic peritonitis due to gastric wall necrosis
4	8	Brittany Spaniel	Intermittent productive cough	114	30	38.9	18.3	Chronic bronchitis
5	14	Newfoundland	1-week history of cough and abdominal swelling Atrial fibrillation	240	40	38.1	N/A	Congestive heart failure

HR heart rate
RR respiratory rate
WBC white blood count
N/A not available

Table 2 Summary of cytology, bacteriology results and NET quantification

	Differential cytology	Cytological diagnosis	Bacteriology	NET (NET:cells)	Ratio of intracellular citH3
Endotracheal Tracheal Lavage					
Dog 1	TNCC: $10.36 \times 10^3/\mu L$ Neutrophils: 85% Lymphocytes: 0% Macrophages: 15% Eosinophils: 0%	Marked suppurative inflammation	*Staphylococcus intermedius, Corynebacterium sp., Mycoplasma sp.*	0.070	0.093
Pleural effusion					
Dog 2	TNCC: 482×10^3 /μL Neutrophils: 78% Macrophages: 20% Others: 2%	Marked septic suppurative inflammation	*Streptococcus Viridans* *Fusobacterium nucleatum*	0.26	0.67
Abdominal Fluid					
Dog 3	TNCC: $21.6 \times 10^3/\mu L$ Neutrophils: 84% Lymphocytes:12% Macrophages: 4% Eosinophils: 0%	Moderate septic suppurative inflammation	*Enterococcus faecalis* *Enterococcus faecium*	0.14	0.24
Bronchoalveolar Lavage					
Dog 4	TNCC: $0.54 \times 10^3/\mu L$ Neutrophils: 17% Lymphocytes: 18% Macrophages: 41% Eosinophils: 24%	Mild mixed inflammation	*Negative*	0.016	0.032
Pleural Effusion					
Dog 5	TNCC: $2.5 \times 10^3/\mu L$ Neutrophils: 28% Lymphocytes: 1% Macrophages: 69% Others: 2%	Mild mixed inflammation	*Negative*	0	0.0032

TNCC total nucleated cell count
NET neutrophil extracellular trap
CitH3 citrullinated histone H3

observed in cytology obtained from dogs without bacterial infections (Fig. 2g, h) (Table 2).

Discussion

By utilizing double immunolabelling and 3-channel fluorescence microscopy, we identified, for the time first, NET formation in dogs with clinical sepsis. We also developed a protocol for quantifying NETs and intracellular citH3 expression in clinical cytology samples using accessible public domain software.

In this study, NETs from cytology samples were quantified based on co-localization of NET components: cfDNA, MPO and citH3. MPO, which resides within neutrophil primary granules, catalyzes the formation of hypochlorite and is released into phagosomes where bacteria are killed by high concentrations of hypochlorite and peroxides [15]. During NETosis, granular proteins including MPO along with cfDNA, are released into the extracellular space [16]. However, since leakage of MPO and DNA also occurs in necrosis, cfDNA and extracellular MPO are not specific markers of NETosis. Histone citrullination or deimination, which converts the N-terminus arginine to citrulline, is a unique process occurring in neutrophils undergoing NETosis [17]. Histone citrullination, catalzyed by the enzyme, peptidylarginine deiminase 4 (PAD4), alters the electrostatic interactions between DNA and histones causing chromatin decondensation and release of cfDNA during NETosis [18]. We have recently shown that lipopolysaccharide-mediated NETosis in vitro requires histone H3 hypercitrullination by PAD in canine neutrophils [9]. The substantial number of citH3 positive cells identified in culture-positive samples suggests that a similar cellular process also occurs in vivo. Thus, citH3 within canine NETs may serve as diagnostic marker of bacterial infection in dogs.

The discovery of NETs in septic foci highlights that NETosis is likely a highly-conserved component of innate immunity during bacterial infections in dogs as in other species. We provided, for the first time, direct imaging evidence for the binding of bacteria within the structural elements of canine NETs. This, however, does not definitively indicate that NETs in dogs can entrap bacteria and prevent systemic dissemination of bacteria in vivo. Based on other in vitro and in vivo experiments, bacteria like *Staphylococcus aureus* can acquire resistance to the bactericidal properties of NETs over time [19]. An added level of complexity in the study of NETs is that while NETs possess important antimicrobial properties, overzealous production of NETs can be detrimental to the host [4]. MPO can augment tissue inflammation by activating nearby neutrophils and inducing further NETosis [16, 20]. Free histones have been shown to act as damage-associated molecular patterns impairing endothelial function and initiating inflammation, cytotoxicity and coagulation in mice [5, 21]. It is unknown if citH3 released via NETosis within body compartments could lead to elevated circulating levels of citH3 in dogs. CitH3 as a biomarker of canine sepsis requires further investigation.

The abundance of NETs found in septic tracheal wash fluid from Dog 1 suggests that canine neutrophils release NETs into the airways in response to acute bacterial infection. However, a small quantity of NETs also was found in BAL from Dog 4 with sterile chronic pulmonary inflammation. In human beings, NETosis is commonly associated with chronic bronchitis and chronic obstructive pulmonary disease. The degree of NETosis correlates with the presence of neutrophils in the airways, and it is conceivable that NETosis also occurs in cases of canine chronic bronchitis with progressively severe neutrophilic inflammation [22]. This requires further investigation in a larger number of dogs.

This study has several limitations. Direct visualization and quantification of NETs in cytology samples can be challenging due to the lack of standardized cell counts and variable cell types. Because the number of NETs is dependent on the number of neutrophils in each sample, we measured NETs and citH3 positive neutrophils relative to the number of neutrophils. Due to the presence of various cell types, we also employed robust criteria to classify and quantify neutrophils. However, canine neutrophils that have not yet released NETs but have undergone chromatin decondensation may have non-lobulated and rounded nuclei [17]. These changes in chromatin morphology might have affected our ability to accurately identify neutrophils and hence under- or overestimated the quantity of NETs produced. Co-immunostaining of a canine-specific neutrophil surface marker with a different fluorophore could allow for more accurate cell enumeration. Because microscopic evaluation is subjected to observer bias, we utilized a standardized protocol to acquire and analyze images in a randomized and blinded manner. A major drawback of this technique is that it is labor intensive, requiring multiple incubation steps and advanced training in microscopy. Lastly, the small number of dogs included in this study represent a limitation. Further studies are needed to validate this technique in a larger population of clinical dogs and to determine its diagnostic and prognostic value in dogs with sepsis.

Conclusion

NETs can be identified in septic fluids collected from clinical patients. The technique presented here can be a useful tool for the research of NETs and canine sepsis.

Abbreviations

BAL: Bronchoalveolar lavage; cfDNA: Cell-free DNA; citH3: Citrullinated Histone H3; DPBS: Dulbecco's phosphate buffered saline; ETW: Endotracheal wash; MPO: Myeloperoxidase; NETs: Neutrophil extracellular traps

Acknowledgements

The authors would like to thank Dr. Kevin Woolard for assistance with fluorescence microscopy.

Funding

The corresponding author is funded by the Morris Animal Foundation (D15CA-907) and the study is supported by Center for Companion Animal Health (2016–24-F), the Oak Tree Racing Association, the State of California Pari-Mutual Fund, and contributions by private donors (University of California Davis, Center for Equine Health). The funding bodies did not take part in the design of the study, collection, analysis and interpretation of the data and the preparation of this manuscript.

Authors' contributions

RHLL, LRJ and FT contributed to the study design, collection of samples, interpretation of the data and editing of the manuscript. CK contributed to collection of samples, interpretation of data and edition of the manuscript. RHLL performed the immunofluorescence microscopy and was a major contributor in writing the manuscript. All authors read and approved the final manuscript.

Consent for publication

Not applicable.

Competing interests

The authors declare that they have no competing interests.

Author details

[1]Department of Veterinary Surgical and Radiological Sciences, School of Veterinary Medicine, University of California, One Shield Avenue, Davis, California 95161, USA. [2]Department of Medicine and Epidemiology, School of Veterinary Medicine, University of California, Davis, California, USA. [3]William Pritchard Veterinary Medical Teach Hospital, University of California, Davis, California, USA. [4]Department of Anatomy, Physiology and Cell Biology, School of Veterinary Medicine, University of California, Davis, California, USA.

References

1. Brinkmann V, Reichard U, Goosmann C, Fauler B, Uhlemann Y, Weiss DS, Weinrauch Y, Zychlinsky A. Neutrophil extracellular traps kill bacteria. Science. 2004;303(5663):1532–5.
2. Brinkmann V, Zychlinsky A. Beneficial suicide: why neutrophils die to make NETs. Nat Rev Microbiol. 2007;5(8):577–82.
3. McDonald B, Urrutia R, Yipp BG, Jenne CN, Kubes P. Intravascular neutrophil extracellular traps capture bacteria from the bloodstream during sepsis. Cell Host Microbe. 2012;12(3):324–33.
4. Czaikoski PG, Mota JM, Nascimento DC, Sonego F, Castanheira FV, Melo PH, Scortegagna GT, Silva RL, Barroso-Sousa R, Souto FO, et al. Neutrophil

extracellular traps induce organ damage during experimental and clinical Sepsis. PLoS One. 2016;11(2):e0148142.

5. Chen R, Kang R, Fan XG, Tang D. Release and activity of histone in diseases. Cell Death Dis. 2014;5:e1370.
6. Dwivedi DJ, Toltl LJ, Swystun LL, Pogue J, Liaw KL, Weitz JI, Cook DJ, Fox-Robichaud AE, Liaw PC, Canadian Critical Care Translational Biology G. Prognostic utility and characterization of cell-free DNA in patients with severe sepsis. Crit Care. 2012;16(4):R151.
7. Kawai C, Kotani H, Miyao M, Ishida T, Jemail L, Abiru H, Tamaki K. Circulating extracellular histones are clinically relevant mediators of multiple organ injury. Am J Pathol. 2016;186(4):829–43.
8. Jeffery U, Kimura K, Gray R, Lueth P, Bellaire B, LeVine D. Dogs cast NETs too: canine neutrophil extracellular traps in health and immune-mediated hemolytic anemia. Vet Immunol Immunopathol. 2015;168(3–4):262–8.
9. Li RHL, Ng G, Tablin F. Lipopolysaccharide-induced neutrophil extracellular trap formation in canine neutrophils is dependent on histone H3 citrullination by peptidylarginine deiminase. Vet Immunol Immunopathol. 2017;193-194:29–37.
10. Letendre JA, Goggs R. Measurement of plasma cell-free DNA concentrations in dogs with sepsis, trauma, and neoplasia. J Vet Emerg Crit Care (San Antonio). 2017;27(3):307–14.
11. Hamaguchi S, Akeda Y, Yamamoto N, Seki M, Yamamoto K, Oishi K, Tomono K. Origin of circulating free DNA in Sepsis: analysis of the CLP mouse model. Mediat Inflamm. 2015;2015:614518.
12. Hauptman JG, Walshaw R, Olivier NB. Evaluation of the sensitivity and specificity of diagnostic criteria for sepsis in dogs. Vet Surg. 1997;26(5):393–7.
13. Negoescu A, Labat-Moleur F, Lorimier P, Lamarcq L, Guillermet C, Chambaz E, Brambilla E. F(ab) secondary antibodies: a general method for double immunolabeling with primary antisera from the same species. Efficiency control by chemiluminescence. J Histochem Cytochem. 1994;42(3):433–7.
14. Narasaraju T, Yang E, Samy RP, Ng HH, Poh WP, Liew AA, Phoon MC, van Rooijen N, Chow VT. Excessive neutrophils and neutrophil extracellular traps contribute to acute lung injury of influenza pneumonitis. Am J Pathol. 2011; 179(1):199–210.
15. Stelmaszynska T, Zgliczynski JM. Myeloperoxidase of human neutrophilic granulocytes as chlorinating enzyme. Eur J Biochem. 1974;45(1):305–12.
16. Papayannopoulos V, Metzler KD, Hakkim A, Zychlinsky A. Neutrophil elastase and myeloperoxidase regulate the formation of neutrophil extracellular traps. J Cell Biol. 2010;191(3):677–91.
17. Wang Y, Li M, Stadler S, Correll S, Li P, Wang D, Hayama R, Leonelli L, Han H, Grigoryev SA, et al. Histone hypercitrullination mediates chromatin decondensation and neutrophil extracellular trap formation. J Cell Biol. 2009;184(2):205–13.
18. Leshner M, Wang S, Lewis C, Zheng H, Chen XA, Santy L, Wang Y. PAD4 mediated histone hypercitrullination induces heterochromatin decondensation and chromatin unfolding to form neutrophil extracellular trap-like structures. Front Immunol. 2012;3:307.
19. Thammavongsa V, Missiakas DM, Schneewind O. Staphylococcus aureus degrades neutrophil extracellular traps to promote immune cell death. Science. 2013;342(6160):863–6.
20. Matthijsen RA, Huugen D, Hoebers NT, De Vries B, Peutz-Kootstra CJ, Aratani Y, Daha MR, Tervaert JWC, Buurman WA, Heeringa P. Myeloperoxidase is critically involved in the induction of organ damage after renal ischemia reperfusion. Am J Pathol. 2007;171(6):1743–52.
21. Gould TJ, Vu TT, Swystun LL, Dwivedi DJ, Mai SH, Weitz JI, Liaw PC. Neutrophil extracellular traps promote thrombin generation through platelet-dependent and platelet-independent mechanisms. Arterioscler Thromb Vasc Biol. 2014;34(9):1977–84.
22. Wright TK, Gibson PG, Simpson JL, McDonald VM, Wood LG, Baines KJ. Neutrophil extracellular traps are associated with inflammation in chronic airway disease. Respirology. 2016;21(3):467–75.

20

Invasion and replication of *Yersinia ruckeri* in fish cell cultures

Simon Menanteau-Ledouble[1*], Mark L. Lawrence[2] and Mansour El-Matbouli[1]

Abstract

Background: Like many members of the *Enterobacteriaceae* family, *Yersinia ruckeri* has the ability to invade non professional phagocytic cells. Intracellular location is advantageous for the bacterium because it shields it from the immune system and can help it cross epithelial membranes and gain entry into the host. In the present manuscript, we report on our investigation regarding the mechanisms of *Y. ruckeri*'s invasion of host cells.

Results: A gentamycin assay was applied to two isolates, belonging to both the biotype 1 (ATCC 29473) and biotype 2 (A7959–11) and using several cell culture types: Atlantic Salmon Kidney, Salmon Head Kidney and, Chinook salmon embryos cells at both low and high passage numbers. Varying degrees of sensitivity to *Y. ruckeri* infection were found between the cell types and the biotype 1 strain was found to be more invasive than the non-motile biotype 2 isolate. Furthermore, the effect of six chemical compounds (Cytochalasin D, TAE 226, vinblastine, genistein, colchicine and, N-acetylcysteine), known to interfere with bacterial invasion strategies, were investigated. All of these compounds had a significant impact on the ability of the bacterium to invade host cells. Changes in the concentration of bacterial cells over time were investigated and the results suggested that neither isolate could survive intracellularly for sustained periods.

Conclusions: These results suggest that *Y. ruckeri* can gain entrance into host cells through several mechanisms, and might take advantage of both the actin and microtubule cytoskeletal systems.

Keywords: Intracellular invasion, Gentamycin assay, Atlantic Salmon kidney cells, Chinook Salmon embryo cells, Salmon head kidney cells

Background

Yersinia ruckeri [1] is a member of the *Enterobacteriaceae* family [2]. It is mostly known as a disease agent in salmonid fish even if many more species are susceptible to the disease [3]. Infections have been associated with a generalized bacteraemia and septicaemia as well as petechial and hemorrhagic lesions, particularly in the oral region [4]. While efficient bacterin-based vaccination has been introduced and has been widely adopted to control the bacterium [2], non-motile isolates belonging to the biotype 2 have been reported that are able to cause disease even in vaccinated fish [5, 6]. More recently, new vaccines have been made commercially available that contain both the biotype 1 and the biotype 2 and aim at protecting the fish against either biotypes of the bacterium [7].

Several *Enterobacteriaceae*, such as the fish bacterial pathogens *Edwardsiella ictaluri*, have demonstrated the ability to invade non professional phagocytic cells [8]. Not only can such intracellular location shield bacteria from the immune system [9], it can provide an environment richer in limited compounds such as iron.

Y. ruckeri was also shown to invade epithelial cells [10–12]; however, this ability has received limited scrutiny. Most notably, Tobback et al. [12] used a variety of techniques to demonstrate the ability of several isolates of *Y. ruckeri* to invade Chinook salmon embryo cell line (CHSE-214), fathead minnow epithelial cell line (FHM) and rainbow trout liver cell line (R1). The present study is a continuation of their work. In other members of the *Enterobacteriaceae* family, several strategies have been described that allow the bacterium to take advantage of host mechanisms to gain entry into the eukaryotic cells.

* Correspondence: simon.menanteau-ledouble@vetmeduni.ac.at
[1]Clinical Division of Fish Medicine, University of Veterinary Medicine, Veterinärplatz 1, 1210 Vienna, Austria
Full list of author information is available at the end of the article

One of these strategies is termed the "zipper mechanism" and has been described in *Yersinia enterocolitica* and *Yersinia pseudotuberculosis*. In these species, adhesin molecules on the surface of the bacteria interact with receptors on the surface of the host cell. For example, both *Yersinia* invasins [13] and adhesin A (YadA) [14, 15] proteins targets the β1-integrins. The interactions between these molecules initiate a signalling cascade that includes the signalling proteins Racl and CDC42 as key components. This signalling cascade results in the recruitment of additional receptors, in particular focal adhesion kinase (FAK), to the area [16, 17] and these additional receptors bind to the surface of the bacterium, folding the host cell's membrane to engulf the bacterium [17].

The other main mechanism of entry described in *Enterobacteriaceae* is the trigger mechanism, which relies on the type III secretion system (T3SS) to inject effector proteins into the cytoplasm of the host cell where they activate various proteins belonging to the Rho family, including CDC42 and Racl. These proteins regulate the activity of actin filaments and the formation of filopodial and lamellipodial structures that allow for cell migration as well as the cytoskeletal deformation required for phagocytosis. Effector proteins secreted through the T3SS can therefore trigger the uptake of the bacterial pathogen by the host cells [18].

An example of the trigger mechanism has been described for the Ssa-Esc family of T3SS. The Ssa-Esc family is one of the major families of T3SS, and it has been most studied in *Salmonella* and enterohaemorrhagic *Escherichia coli* [19]. About 30 effector proteins are known to be secreted through T3SSs belonging to the Ssa-Esc family, and five of these proteins (SopE/E2, SopB, SipA, SipC and SptP) play a role in the internalisation of *Salmonella* by non phagocytic cells. SopE/E2 and SopB activate Rho GTPase, which leads to the activation of Cdc42 and Racl [20], resulting to the remodelling of actin and the formation of filopodial structures. SipA and SipC induce polymerization and bundling of actin, and SopB causes the generation of macropinosomes and *Salmonella* containing vacuoles (SCVs). The role of SptP is to revert these changes and restore a normal state in the host cell [21, 22].

Interestingly, T3SSs belonging to the Ssa-Esc family have also been described in members of the *Yersinia* genus [23], although in *Yersinia pestis* several genes appear missing from the bacterial genome rendering this secretion system non-functional [24]. A T3SS belonging to the Ssa-Esc family has also been identified in several *Y. ruckeri* [25, 26], which suggests that the trigger mechanism could possibly play a role in the invasiveness of *Y. ruckeri*. However, very little is known about *Y. ruckeri*'s T3SS and its repertoire of effector proteins.

The present study was designed to investigate the targets of *Y. ruckeri*'s invasion mechanisms and expend on the work previously reported by Tobback et al. [12], in particular by confirming that their results applied to other cell lines beyond the ones they tested as well as by investigating if the non-motile biotype 2 isolate showed the same ability to invade host cells. Consequently, we measured the ability of two *Y. ruckeri* isolates, ATCC 29473 (biotype 1) and A7959–11 (biotype 2), to adhere to Chinook Salmon Embryo 214 (CHSE-214) cell cultures as well as to invade CHSE-214 cells at both a low and high passage number and Atlantic Salmon Kidney ATCC® CRL-2747 (ASK) and Salmon Head Kidney (SHK) cell cultures. Furthermore, the effects of several chemical compounds known to interfere with bacterial invasion strategies were also studied to improve our understanding of the host mechanisms targeted by *Y. ruckeri*. Finally, changes in the intracellular survival of bacteria over time were also investigated to assess the ability of the bacteria to survive intracellularly over prolonged periods of time.

Methods

Bacterial isolates and cell strains

Two *Y. ruckeri* isolates were used in this study: ATCC 29473 is a type strain and a motile isolate that belongs to the biotype 1. A7959–11 is a non-motile clinical isolate that originated from an outbreak in rainbow trout (*Oncorhynchus mykiss*) in Austria and belongs to the biotype 2. In our experience, the virulence of ATCC 29473 is much lower than that of A7959–11 in rainbow trout (*O. mykiss*), with LD50 by immersion of 10^{10} and $< 6.5 \times 10^5$, respectively.

To confirm that spectrophotometry was an accurate way to measure and normalize the concentration of both isolates, both *Y. ruckeri* ATCC 29473 and A7959–11 were cultivated overnight in brain heart infusion (BHI, Oxoid). Afterwards, the optical densities (OD) in the cultures were measured by spectrophotometry at 600 nm, and both cultures were diluted to the same OD of 0.5 at 600 nm. Both cultures were serially diluted, spread on BHI-agar, and incubated overnight at 22 °C. The number of colony forming units (CFU) on the plates were quantified and compared.

ASK and CHSE-214 cells originated from the American Type Culture Collection (ATCC) while SHK originated from the National Collection of Type Cultures Culture Collections subdivision from the Health Protection Agency (HPA). All cell lines were obtained through Sigma-Aldrich (Austria) except for ASK that was obtained directly from the ATCC.

Invasion assay

Assays were conducted in 24 well plates following the procedure described by Skirpstunas and Baldwin [8] with some minor modifications: because of *Y. ruckeri*'s lower optimal temperature, all assays were performed at room temperature rather than 26 °C. Moreover, because of this lower temperature, the duration of the first incubation time was increased to five hours.

These assays were performed on ASK, SHK, and two strains of CHSE-214 cells with a different passage number: Earlier work in our laboratory had indicated that the older CHSE-214 cells showed different sensitivity to viral infection than the younger ones. Furthermore they adhered less strongly to the culture flasks suggesting that they might express surface adhesion molecules differently. Because of the important role that such adhesion molecules can play in the adherence and invasiveness of bacterial pathogens, including within the genus *Yersinia* [27, 28], it was decided to compare both old and young CHSE-214 strains.

Two cell types were used at a time: CHSE-214 cells with a low passage number were cultivated in the 12 leftmost wells of a 24 well plate while another cell type was cultivated in the remaining 12 wells. The cells were cultivated in minimum essential medium (MEM, Gibco) until they reached confluence. At the same time, both bacterial isolates were grown overnight in BHI at 20 °C. Their concentration was assessed by spectrometry at 600 nm, and the cultures were diluted in broth to the same optical density of 0.5. The bacteria were centrifuged at 4000 g for 10 min and resuspended in an equal volume of MEM before being diluted 10 times in MEM. The culture medium was replaced in each well with 1 ml of the bacterial suspension, and the bacteria were left to interact with the cells for five hours at room temperature. Afterwards, the solution was removed, the cells were washed twice with un-inoculated medium, and the supernatant was replaced with medium containing the antibiotic gentamycin (Sigma-Aldrich) at a concentration of 100 μg ml^{-1}. The antibiotic was left to act for four hours, after which the cells were washed twice with culture medium before replacing the medium with medium containing 1% of the detergent Triton-X (Sigma-Aldrich). The cells were incubated in the detergent for 10 min before being triturated with a micropipette, serially diluted from 10^{-1} to 10^{-4}, and spread on brain heart infusion agar (BHI agar, Oxoid) in quadruplicate. Each assay was performed at least four times.

To confirm the efficacy of the gentamycin selection, both isolates were cultivated to the OD600 of 0.5. Both cultures were centrifuged at 4000 g for 10 min and resuspended in an equal volume of MEM before being diluted 10 times in gentamycin-containing MEM (100 μg ml^{-1}). After four hours of incubation, the bacteria were serially diluted and the 10^{0}, 10^{-1}, 10^{-2} and 10^{-3} dilution were plated on LB agar plate and incubated overnight at 25 °C. The absence of any bacterial growth confirmed that the bacteria needed to invade and take shelter into eukaryotic cells to survive the gentamycin assay.

Conversely, an experiment was performed using CHSE-214 cells. The procedure was similar to the gentamycin assay except that no gentamycin was added to the medium during the second incubation. Because it was estimated that the bacterial count would be higher in the absence of gentamycin, serial dilution was performed up to 10^{8}. This resulted in 5.62×10^{8} and 8.43×10^{8} CFU per ml for the ATCC 29473 and the A7959–11 isolates, respectively. No significant difference was found between these two isolates ($P = 0.309$), however a significant effect was found for the gentamycin ($P < 0.05$) for both cell types confirming that this antibiotic was highly efficacious at killing extracellular *Y. ruckeri*.

Moreover, for each assay, cells were left uninfected to use as a negative control to confirm that no bacteria could be recovered from the uninfected plates and confirm the absence of bacterial contamination.

In addition, another control assay was performed during which uninfected cells were exposed to Triton X and triturated in the manner previously mentioned. The cells were then stained with Trypan blue and observed using inverted microscopy to confirm that this procedure resulted in the lysis of the cultured cells.

Conversely, another control was performed in which the infection procedure was performed as usual save that no Triton-X was added at the end and not trituration took place. No bacteria could be recovered from the supernatant confirming that these steps were necessary to the release of the bacteria.

Blocker assay

The next step of the experiment was designed to investigate the effectiveness of various chemical blockers to interfere with the bacterium's ability to invade host cells. To simplify and streamline the investigation and because it was felt that the mechanisms of infection did not vary qualitatively between cell types and isolates, the research focussed on the CHSE-214 cell line with a low passage number and the *Y. ruckeri* isolate ATCC 29473. The bacteria were resuspended to an optical density of 0.5 nm in culture medium (MEM, Gibco) into which a working solution of one of the blockers was added (Table 1) and incubated alongside the cells for five hours. Afterwards, the cells were rinsed three times with PBS and the same working solutions were added to MEM supplemented with gentamycin (100 μg ml^{-1}). After four hours, the cells were lysed by 10 min incubation in medium supplemented with Triton-X (1%) followed by trituration before being serially diluted from 10^{-1} to 10^{-4}, and spread on BHI agar. Each assay was performed five times.

Six blockers were investigated: Cytochalasin D, TAE 226, vinblastine, genistein, colchicine and, N-acetylcysteine (all

Table 1 Effect of the chemical blockers on the intracellular invasion of *Yersinia ruckeri*

Blocker	Working concentration	Average CFU/ml	Standard deviation	Significance	Percentage inhibition
Control	–	3.9×10^4	2.35×10^4	–	–
Cytochalasin D	2 µM	4.8×10^2	1.7×10^2	$P < 0.05$	98.8%
TAE 226	10 µM	2.4×10^4	1.6×10^4	$P < 0.05$	39.0%
Vinblastine	10 µM	3.4×10^3	1.1×10^3	$P < 0.05$	91.5%
Genistein	1 mM	4.9×10^3	2.2×10^3	$P < 0.05$	87.5%
Colchicine	2 µM	1.7×10^3	1.3×10^3	$P < 0.05$	95.8%
N-acetylcysteine	5 mM	0.0	0.0	$P < 0.05$	100.0%

The numbers presented are based on *Y. ruckeri* strain ATCC 29473 infection a Chinook Salmon Embryo cell culture

blockers were obtained from Sigma Aldrich except TAE 226, which was acquired from Apexbio technology). Each blocker was assayed in quadruplicate.

To investigate any potential toxic effect of the blockers on the survival of both bacteria and host cells, control tests were performed in which bacteria were incubated alongside the blockers for five hours before being serially diluted and plated. Another control exposed the cell cultures to the blockers. Afterwards, a solution of Trypan Blue was added to the cells and incubated for one minute. The cells were then fixed by addition of formalin to a concentration of 4%. After ten minutes, the formalin was removed and the cells were rinsed 3 times in PBS. The cells were then observed using an inverted microscope. Each cell types was observed five times and each time a hundred cells were counted and the number of blue cells counted in order to obtain the percentage of live versus dead cells. The results showed that N-acetylcysteine had a negative impact on the survival of the host cells ($P = 0.02$).

Adhesion assay

An adhesion assay was performed based on a modified version of the protocol designed by Kotzamanidis et al. [29]: Bacterial cells belonging to both the isolate A7959–11 and ATCC 29473 were used in parallel. The bacterial cultures were grown overnight and their concentration was adjusted to an O.D of 0.5. After that, they were added to the CHSE-214 cell cultures as previously described. Because this section of the experiment aimed at investigating the initial adhesion on the cells and not the bacterial multiplication, a shorter incubation time of 90 min at room temperature was chosen. Afterwards, the cells were fixed by addition of formalin to a concentration of 4%. The medium was removed and the cells were washed three times with PBS to rinse away the bacterial cells that were not attached. The cells and bacteria were stained using Giemsa before being imaged by inverted microscopy (Leica DM IRB). 100 CHSE-214 cells were observed and the number of attached bacteria was counted. This was performed five times for both isolates to determine the number of attached bacteria per hundred cells. Based on Kotzamanidis et al. [29], it was determined that the bacteria were strongly adhesive if more than 40 bacterial cells were found per hundred CHSE-214 cells.

Intracellular replication assay

To assess the ability of the bacterium to survive and multiply inside host cells, another gentamycin assay was performed using CHSE-214 cells and both *Y. ruckeri* isolates.

In this assay too, incubation times varied in order to capture the change in bacterial concentration overtime: the bacteria were left to interact with the cells for one hour, after which the medium was replaced with one containing gentamycin (100 µg ml^{-1}). The antibiotic was left to interact with the cells for two, six, or fifteen hours (for a total infection time of three, seven, and sixteen hours). At the end of the incubation period, the blocker containing medium was removed, and the cultures were rinsed twice before being lysed with Triton X and plated. Each combination of isolate and time point was assayed in triplicate.

Moreover, the same protocol was repeated a second time with the exception that MEM supplemented with 10% formalin was added at the end of each incubation period rather than MEM supplemented with Triton X. The cells were incubated with formalin for 10 min, afterwards the medium was removed and the cells were washed twice with phosphate buffered saline (PBS). Once all the stain had been fixed a solution of GIEMSA was added on top of the cells, left to incubate for 5 min then rinsed three times in PBS. Afterwards, the cell cultures were examined using an inverted microscope to assess damage to the cell tissue visually.

Statistical analysis

The number of colony forming units was determined on each plate, and the corresponding number of surviving bacteria per ml was calculated. The distributions of these numbers were checked for normality using Levene's test. When the distribution was normal, analysis of variance was performed. Because normality could not be assumed in many cases, a non-parametric test was then performed using a Dunnet's T-test. All statistics were performed using SPSS 24 (IBM).

Results

Susceptibility of the various strains and invasiveness of the two isolates

Initial serial dilution showed comparable bacterial concentrations between both isolates cultivated at an identical OD of 0.5 at 600 nm: 1.5×10^{09} CFU/ml for *Y. ruckeri* ATCC 29473 and 8.4×10^{08} CFU/ml for *Y. ruckeri* A7959–11 ($P = 0.748$).

CHSE-214 cells with a low passage number were more susceptible than both CHSE-214 cells with a high passage number (Fig. 1) and ASK ($P < 0.05$) but not significantly different compared to SHK ($P = 0.44$). Similarly, SHK was significantly more susceptible than all cell type ($P < 0.05$) with the exception of CHSE-214 with a low passage number.

Overall, the ATCC 29473 strain was significantly more infectious than isolate A7959–11 in most cell types: The average number of surviving bacteria across all cell types was 1.89×10^4 CFU/ml for the ATCC 29473 strain and 1.38×10^4 CFU/ml for the isolate A7959–11 ($P < 0.05$). However, this difference was not as strong when only considering the CHSE-214 cells: while more *Y. ruckeri* of the ATCC 29473 strain were recovered (1.6×10^4 CFU/ml compared to 1.1×10^4 CFU/ml), this difference was not significant ($P = 0.133$).

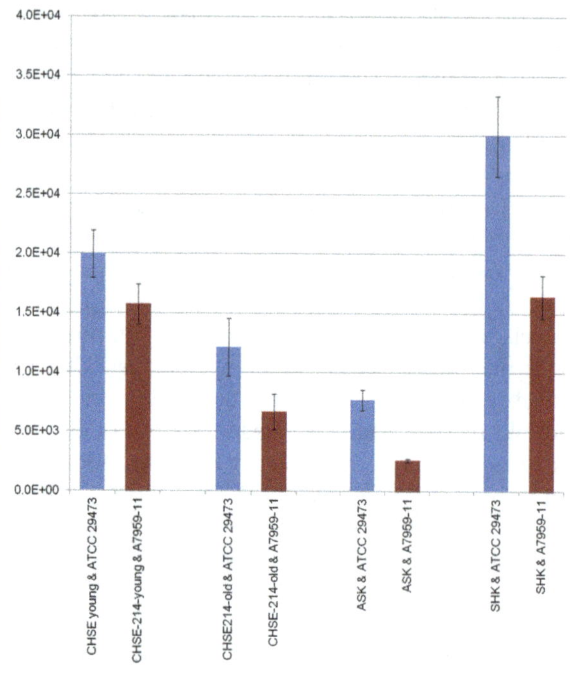

Fig. 1 Susceptibility of the various cell types tested to ATCC 29473 and A7959–11. The number represents the average number of attached bacterial cells per ml. Error bars represent the standard errors values

Blocker activity

In all cases, addition of the chemical blockers was associated with a significantly reduced bacterial concentrations (Fig. 2; $P < 0.05$), indicating that the blockers interfered with bacterial invasion. The blocker that had the least impact was TAE226, a compound that interferes with the activation of FAK on the surface of the host cells. The concentration of bacteria isolated at the end of the gentamycin assay was found to be 2.4×10^4 CFU/ml, compared to 3.9×10^4 CFU/ml in the untreated control cultures ($P = 0.004$). On the other hand, the blocker that had the most impact was the Rac1 inhibitor N-acetylcysteine, which totally blocked bacterial invasion (no bacteria were isolated) (Fig. 2, $P < 0.001$).

The controls showed no toxic effect of the blockers on the bacteria ($P = 0.577$). Interestingly, while most of the blockers did not affect the viability of the cells ($P = 0.304$), N-acetylcysteine did reduce the viability of the cells from 95.8% to 88.4% in the controls and N-acetylcysteine treated cells, respectively ($P = 0.02$).

Intracellular replication assay

Both isolate were found to be strongly adhesive, based on the criterion by Kotzamanidis et al. [29]: 163 bacterial cells were found attached per hundred CHSE-214 cells for isolate ATCC 29473 and 127 were found for isolate A7959–11 (Fig. 3). Moreover, isolate ATCC 29473 was found to be significantly more adhesive than isolate A7959–11 ($P = 0.044$).

Intracellular replication assay

For both isolates, the amount of bacteria surviving intracellularly decreased as the incubation time increased (Fig. 4). This was most evident for the biotype 2 isolate (A7959–11) where the number of bacteria was reduced from an average of 0.4×10^3 CFU/ml after 3 h of incubation to 0.2×10^3 CFU/ml after 7 h ($P = 0.024$) and 0.05×10^3 CFU/ml after 16 h. Conversely, while the number of CFUs in the biotype 1 isolate (ATCC 29473) decreased between 3 and 7 h post-infection, from 1.7×10^3 CFU/ml to 0.7×10^3 CFU/ml ($P = 0.036$), this number appeared to stabilize after that point and did not differ significantly at 16 h (0.7×10^3 CFU/ml; $P = 0.935$).

Upon microscopic examination, the tissue culture showed progressive deterioration as the bacteria damaged the cells. Tears appeared in the monolayer and cells became detached within 1 h post infection (Fig. 5). These changes were more marked at 6 h post infection, in particular in the cells infected with the

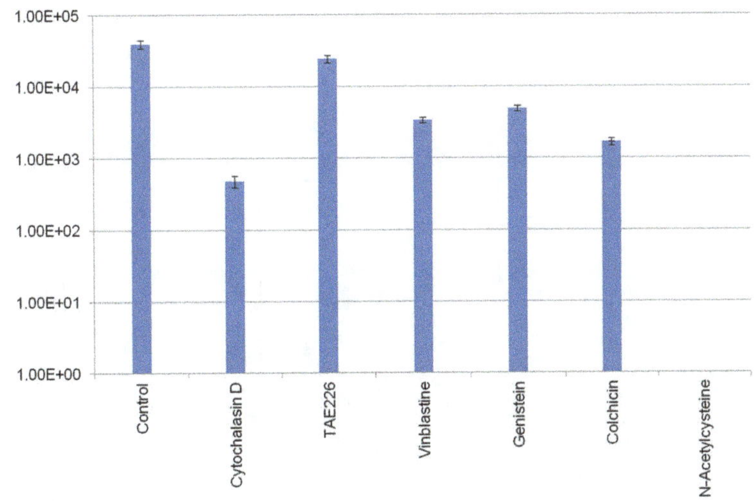

Fig. 2 Effect of the chemical blockers on the intracellular invasion of *Yersinia ruckeri* ATCC 29473 on CHSE-214 cells. Error bars represent the standard errors values

A7959–11 isolate. By the 16 h time-point, most of the cell monolayer had been destroyed.

Discussion

The various cell types displayed differing sensitivity to bacterial infection. This has been previously reported for several intracellular bacterial pathogens: for example, Elkamel and Thune [30] demonstrated than the number of *Photobacterium damselae* subsp. *piscicida* to survive a gentamycin assay was ten time higher in Fathead minnow (FHM) than in channel catfish ovary (CCO), or *Epithelioma papillosum cyprini* (EPC) cell cultures. Similarly, Skirpstunas and Baldwin [8] investigated the propensity of intestinal epithelial cells-6 (IEC-6), Henle 407, FHM, and trypsin/pepsin-harvested channel catfish enteric epithelial cells to invasion by *E. ictaluri* isolate LA89–9 and reported that the invasion efficiencies was lower in IEC-6 and Henle 407 than in FHM cells. Furthermore, the invasion efficiency was even lower in the trypsin/pepsin-harvested channel catfish cells, possibly because the harvesting process had damaged some surface receptors [8]. Finally, Tobback et al. investigated the ability of three *Y. ruckeri* isolate to invade several cell lines (CHSE-214, FHM and R1) [12]. These authors reported difference between the susceptibility of the various cell lines with CHSE-214 being the most susceptible. This is similar to our present results were both isolates were able to infect multiple cell line and where CHSE-214 was very susceptible to both isolates. In the present study we analysed two additional cell types beside CHSE-214 and confirmed that *Y. ruckeri* could also infect them. This appears to confirm that *Y. ruckeri* can infect a wide range of cell lines and that the mechanisms it targets as part of the invasion process are well conserved.

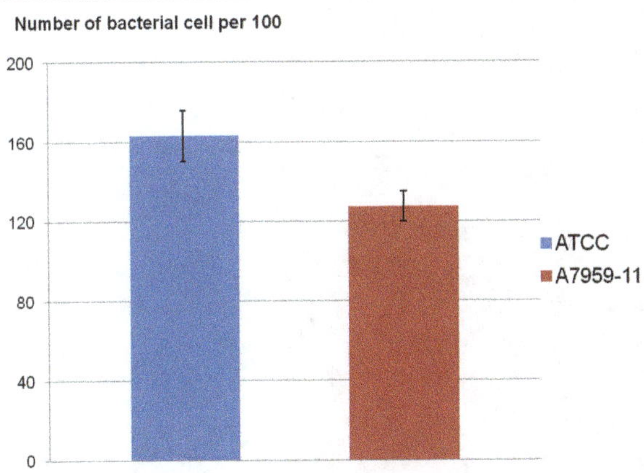

Fig. 3 Adhesion of both isolates ATCC 29473 and A7959–11 during the adhesion assay. The number represents the average number of attached bacterial cells per hundred CHSE-214 cells after 90 min incubation at room temperature. Error bars represent the standard errors values

Interestingly, we observed a significant difference in sensitivity between CHSE-214 cell cultures with different passage numbers ($P < 0.05$). Effects of passage number on CHSE-214 phenotype had previously been noted in our laboratory with the younger cell CHSE-214 adhering more tightly to the culture flask than CHSE-214 with a higher passage number. Moreover, susceptibility to viral infection also varied between both cultures. This prompted determination of the effect of passage number in our study as adhesion molecules often play an important role as targets for entry of several members of the *Yersinia* genus [14–17]. Our findings suggest that adhesion molecules on the surface of the host cells might be targeted by *Y. ruckeri* invasion mechanisms. This would be consistent with *Y. ruckeri*'s ability to infect a wide-range of cells as adhesion

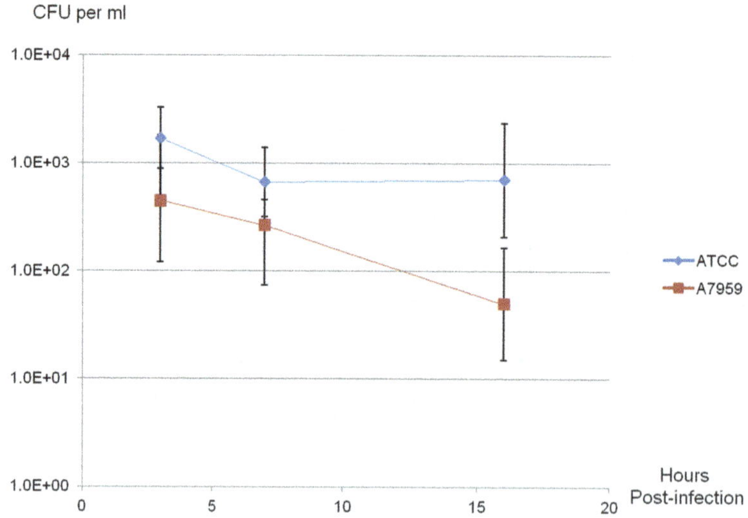

Fig. 4 Concentrations from both isolate ATCC 29473 and A7959–11 at several time-points post-inoculation. The concentrations represent the mean bacterial numbers in CFU per ml at 1, 7 and 16 h during the gentamycin assay. Error bars represent standard deviations

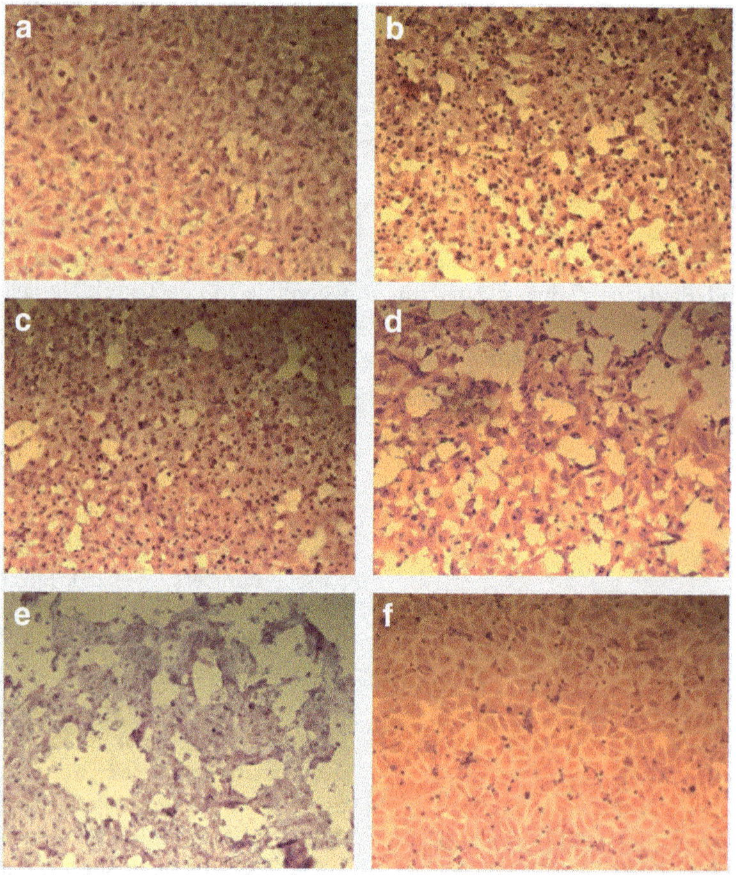

Fig. 5 Inverted microscopy of cell layers infected with isolates ATCC 29473 and A7959–11 at several time-points post-inoculation. **a** Isolate ATCC 29470, 1 h post-infection; **b** Isolate A7959–11, 1 h post-infection; **c** Isolate ATCC 29470, 6 h post-infection; **d** Isolate A7959–11, 6 h post-infection; **e** Isolate ATCC 29470, 12 h post-infection; **f** Uninfected control, s post-infection

molecules are well conserved [31]. Further studies will be required to confirm these results and identify the specific molecules targeted on the host cell surface.

ATCC 29473 was significantly more infectious than the non-motile isolate A7959–11 ($P < 0.05$), despite the latter originating from a clinical case and ATCC 29473 being less virulent in vivo in *O. mykiss*. Similarly, the type strain ATCC 29473 was significantly more infectious in most cell lines. Interestingly, it has been shown in *Y. enterocolitica* that motility contributed to bringing the bacteria in contact with the cells [32] and that non-motile isolates are less able to invade Human epithelial type 2 (HEp-2) cells. Based on the present findings, it is therefore possible that a similar situation exists in *Y. ruckeri*. This is consistent with findings reported by Kim in 2000 that suggested that the flagellum of *Y. ruckeri* plays a critical role in the early stages the bacterium's attachment and entry into the host (Kim 2000, as quoted by Barnes in 2011 [2]).

We tested several chemical compounds that are known to interfere with aspects of the host cell's physiology and hinder bacterial invasion. Because these various chemical compounds target different aspects of this physiology, comparing their effectiveness at hindering bacterial invasion can highlight which of the host's mechanisms are taken advantage of by the bacterium.

Cytochalasin D, a mycotoxin interferes with actin filaments [33], prevents actin polymerization [34, 35] and inhibits membrane ruffling and blebbing [33]. In the present study, cytochalasin D reduced the ability of *Y. ruckeri* isolate ATCC 29473 to survive the gentamycin assay almost 100 fold ($P < 0.05$). This is similar with the results previously reported by Tobback et al. [12]. Colchicine hinders the microtubule cytoskeletal network as it depolymerises and destabilizes microtubules [36, 37]. Colchicine has previously been shown to hinder the invasion of Caco-2 (colonic carcinoma) cell lines by *Listeria monocytogenes* [36] as well as the invasion of HeLa by *Pseudomonas aeruginosa* [37]. Similar results were previously reported in *Y. ruckeri* by Tobback et al. [12] as well as in the present experiment (Table 1; Fig. 2.). TAE226 inhibits the extracellular matrix-dependent phosphorylation of the FAK integrin [38]. FAK is the target of *Campylobacter jejuni*'s fibronectin binding protein [38, 39]. In the present study, TAE226 appeared to have the least effect on the invasiveness of *Y. ruckeri* ($P < 0.05$; inhibition rate of 39.0%). This suggests that, while FAK might be involved in *Y. ruckeri*'s invasion of the host cells, this is not the only protein targeted by the bacterium. Vinblastine has the ability to react with microtubules, crystallizing them into helical structures [40] and addition of vinblastine has been shown to inhibit the invasion of intestine-derived epithelial cells (INT407) by *Enterobacter sakazakii* [41]. Here, vinblastine similarly hindered *Y. ruckeri*'s invasion of CHSE-214 ($P < 0.05$). Genistein blocks the binding of ATP to tyrosine phosphate kinase [42] and interferes with the phosphorylation of p38, p42/44, and, p-JNK, preventing polymerization of tubulin [43, 44]. Previously, genistein has been shown to strongly inhibit the invasion of HeLA cells by *E. coli* expressing the invasin protein cloned from *Y. enterocolitica* [9, 45]. In the present study, our results showed that genistein could also hinder invasion of *Y. ruckeri* into CHSE-214 cells. Interestingly, the inhibition rate in our experiment was lower than the one reported by Rosenshine et al. [9]: 87.5% compared to 98.5%. Because Rosenshine et al. [9] cloned one specific invasion molecule from *Y. enterolitica*; the lower inhibition rate observed in the present study could possibly be explained by *Y. ruckeri* having multiple redundant mechanisms to invade host cells. Finally, N-acetylcysteine has been shown to inhibit the activation of Rac1 by *Fusobacterium nucleatum* [46]. It plays as a regulator of both the actin [47, 48] and the microtubule cytoskeleton. Rac1 regulates the formation of lamellipodia at the edge of fibroblasts [49–51] and members of the *Enterobacteriacea* can activate Rac1 using proteins secreted via the T3SS, triggering membrane ruffling and phagocytic independent internalization of the bacterium [52]. In the present study, addition of N-acetylcysteine to a final concentration of 5 mM appeared to totally inhibit the ability of *Y. ruckeri* to invade cell cultures ($P < 0.05$). Controls have shown that N-acetylcysteine had a significant toxic effect on CHSE cells. This most likely contributed to its disruptive effect; however, it seems unlikely that the comparatively limited toxic effect accounts for the entirety of the invasion inhibition. Despite these chemicals affecting several different aspects of the host physiology, all blockers were efficacious at hindering *Y. ruckeri*'s invasion. Notably, some of the chemicals affect the actin filaments, and others inhibit the microtubule network. These results are consistent with that previously reported by Tobback et al. [12], however, additional blockers were tested in the present study alongside Cytochalasin D and colchicine. Our present results suggest that *Y. ruckeri* targets multiple host mechanisms to gain intracellular entry. This would be similar to what has already been described for other members of the genus *Yersinia*. The fact that N-acetylcysteine was the most efficacious of the chemical compounds tested would be consistent with this hypothesis as both the actin and microtubule cytoskeleton apparatus are regulated by Rac1, the target of N-acetylcysteine [53].

Bacterial survival decreased as the duration of the infection period increased (Fig. 3), again, this is consistent to what has been reported by Tobback et al. [12]. In the present study, we found that intracellular invasion destroyed the infected cells which would explain their inability to shield the bacteria for a sustained duration.

Ohtani et al. [11] have shown that *Y. ruckeri* was able to invade the gill epithelial cells intracellularly and have suggested that the gill epithelium might constitute the bacterium's main route of entry into the host. Our present findings are compatible with this proposition because sustained intracellular survival would not be required to cross-the epithelium. Indeed, Ohtani et al. [11] reported presence of *Y. ruckeri* in the blood as early as one minute after infecting the fish by immersion.

Conclusion

In the present study, we build up on the experiments by Tobback et al. [12] and applied a series of gentamycin assays to investigate the ability of two isolates of *Y. ruckeri* to invade epithelial cells and found that all four of the cell types investigated (ASK, SHK and CHSE-214 with either a low or a high passage number) were susceptible to invasion. Furthermore the biotype 1 isolate (ATCC 29473) was significantly more infectious than our non-motile biotype 2 isolate (A7959–11), despite the fact that A7959–11 originated from a clinical case and was more virulent in vivo. This is reminiscent of what has been previously reported in *Y. enterocolitica* where non-motile isolates appeared less capable of intracellular invasion.

Chemical blockers targeting either the actin or microtubule cytoskeletal apparatus all reduced the susceptibility of CHSE-214 cells to invasion by the isolate ATCC 29473. This suggests that *Y. ruckeri* is able to initiate intracellular uptake through several host mechanisms. This hypothesis would be consistent with the fact that N-acetylcysteine, a compound that targets the regulator Racl, appeared to completely prevent intracellular invasion as Racl is involved with the regulation of both the actin and microtubules cytoskeletons. Finally, it was shown that increasing the incubation time reduced bacterial survival, indicating that the bacterium is unable to survive intracellularly for long periods of time. This finding is likely explained by the bacteria quickly destroying the infected cells and would be consistent with the hypothesis that intracellular invasion plays a very specific role in the development of disease, for example as a mean of crossing the epithelium and gain entry into the host. To conclude, the present study confirms the ability of *Y. ruckeri* to facultatively invade a variety of host-cell lines. Interestingly, a difference was found between isolates belonging to the two biotypes.

Abbreviations

ASK: Atlantic Salmon Kidney; ATCC: American Type Culture Collection; BHI: Brain Heart Infusion; CCO: Channel Catfish Ovary; CDC42: Cell division control protein 42 homolog; CFU: Colony Forming Units; CHSE-214: Chinook salmon embryos cells; EPC: Epithelioma papillosum cyprini; FAK: Focal Adhesion Kinase; FHM: Fathead minnow; GTP: Guanosine triphosphate; HeLA cells: Henrietta Lacks cell culture; Hep-2: Human epithelial type 2; HOK-16B: Human Oral Keratinocytes-16B; HPA: Health Protection Agency; MAPK: Mitogen Activated Protein Kinase; MEM: Minimum Essential Medium; PBS: Phosphate Buffered Saline

Acknowledgments

The authors wish to thank Dr. Andrea Dressler for her assistance with the microbiology section of the manuscript as well as Prof. Oskar Schachner for his invaluable assistance with the cell culture.

Funding

This research was financed by the Austrian Science Funds (Fonds zur Förderung der wissenschaftlichen Forschung), project P28837-B22. This funding body played no role in the design of the study or interpretation of data.

Authors' contributions

SML conceived this project, carried out the research and drafted the manuscript. MLL and MEL participated in the study design and helped to draft the manuscript. All authors read and approved the final manuscript.

Consent for publication

Not applicable.

Competing interests

The authors declare that they have no competing interests.

Author details

[1]Clinical Division of Fish Medicine, University of Veterinary Medicine, Veterinärplatz 1, 1210 Vienna, Austria. [2]Department of Basic Sciences, College of Veterinary Medicine, Mississippi State University, Mississippi State, MS, USA.

References

1. Ewing WH, Ross AJ, Brenner DJ, Fanning GR. *Yersinia ruckeri* sp. nov., the Redmouth (RM) bacterium. J Syst Bacteriol. 1978;28:37–44.
2. Barnes AC. Enteric redmouth disease (ERM) (*Yersinia ruckeri*). Fish Dis. Disord. Vol. 3 viral, Bact. fungal Infect. [Internet]. Wallingford: CABI; 2011. p. 484–511. Available from: http://www.cabi.org/cabebooks/ebook/20113056583
3. Kumar G, Menanteau-Ledouble S, Saleh M, El-Matbouli M. *Yersinia ruckeri*, the causative agent of enteric redmouth disease in fish. Vet. Res. [Internet]. 2015;46:103. Available from: http://www.veterinaryresearch.org/content/46/1/103
4. Roberts RJ. The bacteriology of Teleosts. In: Roberts RJ, editor. Fish Pathol. 4th ed. Wiley-Blackwell; 2012. p. 339–82.
5. Fouz B, Zarza C, Amaro C. First description of non-motile *Yersinia ruckeri* serovar I strains causing disease in rainbow trout, *Oncorhynchus mykiss* (Walbaum), cultured in Spain. J. Fish dis. [internet]. Blackwell Publishing Ltd; 2006;29:339–346. Available from: https://doi.org/10.1111/j.1365-2761.2006.00723.x
6. Arias CR, Olivares-Fuster O, Hayden K, Shoemaker CA, Grizzle JM, Klesius PH. First report of *Yersinia ruckeri* biotype 2 in the USA. J Aquat Anim Health. 2007;19:35–40.
7. Deshmukh S, Raida MK, Dalsgaard I, Chettri JK, Kania PW, Buchmann K. Comparative protection of two different commercial vaccines against *Yersinia ruckeri* serotype O1 and biotype 2 in rainbow trout (*Oncorhynchus mykiss*). Vet. Immunol. Immunopathol [Internet]. Elsevier B.V.; 2012;145:379–385. Available from: https://doi.org/10.1016/j.vetimm.2011.12.014
8. Skirpstunas RT, Baldwin TJ. *Edwardsiella ictaluri* invasions of IEC-6, Henle 407, fathead minnow and channel catfish enteric epithelial cells. Dis. Aquat. Organ. [internet]. 2002;51:161–167. Available from: http://www.ncbi.nlm.nih.gov/pubmed/12465874

9. Rosenshine I, Duronio V, Finlay BB. Tyrosine protein kinase inhibitors block Invasin-promoted bacterial uptake by epithelial cells. Infect Immun. 1992;60:2211–7.
10. McIntosh D, Austin B, Flaño E, Villena A, Martínez-Pereda JA, Tarazona JV. Lack of uptake of *Renibacterium salmoninarum* by gill epithelia of rainbow trout. J Fish Biol [Internet]. 2000;56:1053–61. Available from: http://onlinelibrary.wiley.com/doi/10.1111/j.1095-8649.2000.tb02122.x/full.
11. Ohtani M, Villumsen KR, Strom HK, Raida MK. 3D visualization of the initial *Yersinia ruckeri* infection route in rainbow trout (*Oncorhynchus mykiss*) by optical projection tomography. PLoS One. 2014;9(2)
12. Tobback E, Decostere A, Hermans K, Van den Broeck W, Haesebrouck F, Chiers K. In vitro markers for virulence in *Yersinia ruckeri*. J. Fish dis. [internet]. Blackwell Publishing Ltd; 2010;33:197–209. Available from: https://doi.org/10.1111/j.1365-2761.2009.01106.x
13. Leong JM, Fournier RS, Isberg RR. Identification of the integrin binding domain of the *Yersinia pseudotuberculosis* invasin protein. EMBO J [Internet]. 1990;9:1979–89. Available from: http://www.pubmedcentral.nih.gov/articlerender.fcgi?artid=551907&tool=pmcentrez&rendertype=abstract
14. Eitel J, Dersch P. The YadA protein of *Yersinia pseudotuberculosis* mediates high-efficiency uptake into human cells under environmental conditions in which Invasin is repressed. Infect Immun [Internet]. 2002;70:4880–91. Available from: http://iai.asm.org/content/70/9/4880.abstract
15. Eitel J, Heise T, Thiesen U, Dersch P. Cell invasion and IL-8 production pathways initiated by YadA of *Yersinia pseudotuberculosis* require common signalling molecules (FAK, c-Src, Ras) and distinct cell factors. Cell Microbiol. 2005;7:63–77.
16. Grassl GA, Bohn E, Müller Y, Bühler OT, Autenrieth IB. Interaction of *Yersinia enterocolitica* with epithelial cells: invasin beyond invasion. Int J Med Microbiol. 2003;293:41–54.
17. Cossart P, Invasion SPJB. The paradigms of Enteroinvasive pathogens. Science (80-.). 2004;304:242–8.
18. Van Nhieu TG, Sansonetti P. Mechanism of *Shigella* entry into epithelial cells. Curr Opin Microbiol. 1999;2:51–5.
19. Troisfontaines P, Type III. Secretion: more systems than you think. Physiology [Internet]. 2005;20:326–39. Available from: http://physiologyonline.physiology.org/cgi/doi/10.1152/physiol.00011.2005
20. Patel JC, Galán JE. Manipulation of the host actin cytoskeleton by *Salmonella* — all in the name of entry. Curr Opin Microbiol [Internet]. 2005; 8:10–5. Available from: http://linkinghub.elsevier.com/retrieve/pii/S1369527404001547
21. Fu Y, Galán JE. A *salmonella* protein antagonizes Rac-1 and Cdc42 to mediate host-cell recovery after bacterial invasion. Nature [Internet]. 1999; 401:293–7. Available from: http://www.nature.com/doifinder/10.1038/45829.
22. Johnson R, Byrne A, Berger CN, Klemm E, Crepin VF, Dougan G, et al. The Type III Secretion System Effector SptP of *Salmonella enterica* Serovar Typhi. Silhavy TJ, editor. J. Bacteriol. [Internet]. 2017;199:e00647-16. Available from: http://jb.asm.org/lookup/doi/10.1128/JB.00647-16
23. Parkhill J, Wren BW, Thomson NR, Titball RW, Holden MT, Prentice MB, et al. Genome sequence of *Yersinia pestis*, the causative agent of plague. Nature. 2001/10/05 2001;413:523–527.
24. Pallen MJ, Beatson S a, Bioinformatics BCM. Genomics and evolution of non-flagellar type-III secretion systems: a Darwinian perpective. FEMS Microbiol Rev. 2005;29:201–29.
25. Gunasena DK, Komrower JR, Macintyre S. The fish pathogen *Yersinia ruckeri* possesses a TTS system. In: Skurnik M, Bengoechea J, Granfors K, editors. The genus Yersinia [internet]. Boston: Kluwer Academic Publishers; 2003. p. 105–107. Available from: https://doi.org/10.1007/0-306-48416-1_19
26. Liu T, Wang K-Y, Wang J, Chen D-F, Huang X-L, Ouyang P, et al. Genome Sequence of the Fish Pathogen *Yersinia ruckeri* SC09 Provides Insights into Niche Adaptation and Pathogenic Mechanism. Int. J. Mol. Sci. [Internet]. 2016;17:557. Available from: http://www.mdpi.com/1422-0067/17/4/557
27. Barnhart MM, Schilling JD, Backhed F, Dahlfors AR, Normark S, Host-Pathogen Interactions HSJ. Structure and function of pili. In: Sansonetti P, Zychlinsky A, editors. Mol. Cell. Microbiol. San Diego: Academic Press; 2002. p. 133–59.
28. Boyle EC, Finlay BB. Bacterial pathogenesis: exploiting cellular adherence. Curr Opin Cell Biol. 2003;15:633–9.
29. Kotzamanidis C, Kourelis A, Litopoulou-Tzanetaki E, Tzanetakis N, Yiangou M. Evaluation of adhesion capacity, cell surface traits and immunomodulatory activity of presumptive probiotic *Lactobacillus* strains. Int. J. Food Microbiol. [Internet]. Elsevier B.V. 2010;140:154–163. Available from: https://doi.org/10.1016/j.ijfoodmicro.2010.04.004
30. Elkamel A, Thune R. Invasion and Replication of *Photobacterium damselae* subsp. *piscicida* in Fish Cell Lines. J. Aquat. Anim. Health [Internet]. 2003;15: 167–74. Available from: http://onlinelibrary.wiley.com/doi/10.1577/03-010/abstract
31. Hynes RO, Zhaot Q. The evolution of cell adhesion. J Cell Biol. 2000; 150:89–96.
32. Young GM, Badger JL, Miller VL. Motility is required to initiate host cell invasion by *Yersinia enterocolitica* Motility Is Required To Initiate Host Cell Invasion by *Yersinia enterocolitica*. Infection. 2000;68:4323–6.
33. Schliwa M. Action of cytochalasin D on cytoskeletal networks. J Cell Biol. 1982;92:79–91.
34. May J a, Ratan H, Glenn JR, Lösche W, Spangenberg P, Heptinstall S. GPIIb-IIIa antagonists cause rapid disaggregation of platelets pre-treated with cytochalasin D. Evidence that the stability of platelet aggregates depends on normal cytoskeletal assembly. Platelets [internet]. 1998;9:227–32. Available from: http://www.ncbi.nlm.nih.gov/pubmed/16793707
35. Richard JF, Petit L, Gibert M, Marvaud JC, Bouchaud C, Popoff MR. Bacterial toxins modifying the actin cytoskeleton. Int. Microbiol. [internet]. 1999;2:185–94. Available from: http://www.ncbi.nlm.nih.gov/pubmed/10943412
36. Kuhn M. The microtubule depolymerizing drugs nocodazole and colchicine inhibit the uptake of *Listeria monocytogenes* by P388D1 macrophages. FEMS Microbiol Lett [Internet]. 1998;160:87–90. Available from: https://www.ncbi.nlm.nih.gov/pubmed/9495017.
37. Sana TG, Baumann C, Merdes A, Soscia C, Rattei T, Hachani A, et al. Internalization of *Pseudomonas aeruginosa* Strain PAO1 into Epithelial Cells Is Promoted by Interaction of a T6SS Effector with the Microtubule Network. MBio [Internet]. 2015;6:e00712. Available from: http://mbio.asm.org/lookup/doi/10.1128/mBio.00712-15
38. Eucker TP, Konkel ME. The cooperative action of bacterial fibronectin-binding proteins and secreted proteins promote maximal *Campylobacter jejuni* invasion of host cells by stimulating membrane ruffling. Cell Microbiol. 2012;14:226–38.
39. Neal-McKinney JM, Konkel ME. The *Campylobacter jejuni* CiaC virulence protein is secreted from the flagellum and delivered to the cytosol of host cells. Front. Cell. Infect. Microbiol. [Internet]. 2012;2:1–15. Available from: http://journal.frontiersin.org/article/10.3389/fcimb.2012.00031/abstract
40. Behnke O, Forer A. Vinblastine as a cause of direct transformation of some microtubules into helical structures. Exp. cell res. [internet]. 1972;73:506–9. Available from: http://www.ncbi.nlm.nih.gov/pubmed/5054343
41. Mohan Nair MK, Venkitanarayanan K. Role of bacterial OmpA and host cytoskeleton in the invasion of human intestinal epithelial cells by *Enterobacter sakazakii*. Pediatr. Res. [internet]. 2007;62:664–9. Available from: http://www.ncbi.nlm.nih.gov/pubmed/17957161
42. Akiyama T, Ishida J, Nakagawa S, Ogawara H, Watanabe S, Itoh N, et al. Genistein, a specific inhibitor of tyrosine-specific protein kinases. J Biol Chem. 1987;262:5592–5.
43. Mukherjee S, Acharya BR, Bhattacharyya B, Chakrabarti G. Genistein arrests cell cycle progression of A549 cells at the G(2)/M phase and depolymerizes interphase microtubules through binding to a unique site of tubulin. Biochem Int. 2010;49:1702–12. Available from: http://pubs.acs.org/doi/abs/10.1021/bi901760d
44. Cui S, Wang J, Wu Q, Qian J, Yang C, Bo P. Genistein inhibits the growth and regulates the migration and invasion abilities of melanoma cells via the FAK/paxillin and MAPK pathways. Oncotarget [Internet] 2017;8:21674–21691. Available from: http://www.ncbi.nlm.nih.gov/pubmed/28423510%0A; http://www.oncotarget.com/abstract/15535.
45. Pepe JC, Miller VL. The *Yersinia enterocolitica*-Inv gene product is an outer membrane protein that shares epitopes with *Yersinia pseudotuberculosis* Invasin. J Bacteriol. 1990;172:3780–9.
46. Alam J, Baek KJ, Choi YS, Kim YC, Choi Y. N-acetylcysteine and the human serum components that inhibit bacterial invasion of gingival epithelial cells prevent experimental periodontitis in mice. J. Periodontal Implant Sci. [Internet]. 2014;44:266. Available from: http://synapse.koreamed.org/DOIx.php?id=10.5051/jpis.2014.44.6.266
47. Guo F, Debidda M, Yang L, Williams DA, Zheng Y. Genetic deletion of Rac1 GTPase reveals its critical role in actin stress fiber formation and focal adhesion complex assembly. J Biol Chem [Internet]. 2006;281: 18652–9. Available from: http://www.jbc.org/cgi/doi/10.1074/jbc.M603508200

48. Ntantie E, Fletcher J, Amissah F, Salako OO, Nkembo AT, Poku RA, et al. Polyisoprenylated cysteinyl amide inhibitors disrupt actin cytoskeleton organization, induce cell rounding and block migration of non-small cell lung cancer. Oncotarget [Internet]. 2017; Available from: http://www.oncotarget.com/abstract/15956.
49. Ridley AJ, Paterson HF, Johnston CL, Diekmann D, Hall A. The small GTP-binding protein rac regulates growth factor-induced membrane ruffling. Cell [Internet]. 1992;70:401–10. Available from: http://linkinghub.elsevier.com/retrieve/pii/0092867492901648
50. Takai Y, Sasaki T, Matozaki T. Small GTP-binding proteins. Physiol Rev. 2001;81:153–208.
51. Chen QY, Xu LQ, Jiao DM, Yao QH, Wang YY, Hu HZ, et al. Silencing of Rac1 modifies lung cancer cell migration, invasion and actin cytoskeleton rearrangements and enhances chemosensitivity to antitumor drugs. Int J Mol Med. 2011;28:769–76.
52. Bulgin R, Arbeloa A, Goulding D, Dougan G, Crepin VF, Raymond B, et al. The T3SS effector EspT defines a new category of invasive Enteropathogenic *E. coli* (EPEC) which form intracellular actin pedestals. Van Nhieu GT, editor. PLoS Pathog. [internet]. 2009;5:e1000683. Available from: http://www.ncbi.nlm.nih.gov/pubmed/20011125
53. Wittmann T, Bokoch GM, Waterman-Storer CM. Regulation of leading edge microtubule and actin dynamics downstream of Rac1. J Cell Biol. 2003;161:845–51.

21

Bacteria and parasites in *Podarcis sicula* and *P. sicula klemmerii*

Ludovico Dipineto[1*], Pasquale Raia[2], Lorena Varriale[1], Luca Borrelli[1], Vittorio Botta[1], Carmela Serio[2], Michele Capasso[1] and Laura Rinaldi[1]

Abstract

Background: New epidemiological data on bacterial and parasitic infections in 24 Italian wall lizards, namely *Podarcis sicula* (mainland population) and *P. sicula klemmerii* (insular population) in southern Italy were provided. To achieve this goal, samples were collected from individuals belonging to the two populations and analysed by microbiological and parasitological methods.

Results: A wide range of bacteria (e.g. *Pantoea* spp., *Citrobacter* spp., *Morganella* spp., *Pseudomonas*, *Enterobacter* spp., *Staphylococcus* spp. and *Escherichia coli*) and parasites (e.g. *Ophionyssus natricis*, coccidia, Dicrocoelidae) were detected in both *P. sicula* and *P. sicula klemmerii* individuals. Insular population presented similar bacterial and parasitic diversity to its mainland counterpart. Ampicillin was the antimicrobial with the highest resistance rate.

Conclusion: This study highlighted various bacteria and parasites, some of them potentially zoonotic. Further studies are needed to better understand the epidemiology and transmission routes of these pathogens along with their impact on the welfare and behaviour of Italian wall lizards.

Keywords: *Podarcis sicula*, Italian wall lizard, Bacteria, Parasites, FLOTAC

Background

The Italian wall lizard, *Podarcis sicula*, is one of the most common lizards in Italy [1]. The snout-vent length (SVL) is, on average, 15 to 25 cm long. The colour pattern is characterized by a green or brown back and whitish belly, although melanic variants, with either shorter, or longer SVL, are known to occur in several islands in the Mediterranrean sea. As a common, and easily managed study model, the Italian wall lizard was subjected to several studies, regarding aspects as disparate as phenotypic response to predation [2], feeding behaviour [3], ontogeny [4], adaptation to novel environments [5], biogeography [6, 7], and its role as a biological indicator [8].

Podarcis sicula klemmeri [9] is one of the subspecies belonging to *P. sicula*. It is confined to a small, 1 km^2 large islet, Licosa, off the western coast of Italy. As with many other insular populations of the Italian wall lizard, *P.s. klemmeri* is melanic, meaning the back appears tinged with blue, and the pale underside is bluish as well, rather than the usual white of continental populations.

Melanic variants have been investigated for the so-called Island syndrome [10], which is a suite of phenotypic character shifts in insular populations including, besides melanism, changed body size, feeding behaviour and ecology, patterns of aggressiveness, and life history traits [11–15]. The link between melanism and characters shifts on islands was found to be in the activity levels of melano-cortin receptors, MCRs [13]. Melanocortins form a suite of five receptors activated pleyotropically by a single DNA locus, the proopiomelanocortin POMC gene, that happen to regulate feeding and sexual activity, immunocompetence and body colour [16–18]. Interestingly, Monti et al. [19] tested whether *P. s. klemmeri* individuals have different ectoparasite loads (i.e. the density of ticks and mites on the skin) as compared to the continental individuals. They found reduced load in insular individuals, consistently with their comparatively higher α-melanocyte-stimulating hormone (MSH) levels.

Herein, we deepen microbiological and parasitological investigations on *P. s. klemmeri*. Besides a few studies [20, 21], these aspects have not been scrutinized so far,

* Correspondence: ludovico.dipineto@unina.it
[1]Dipartimento di Medicina Veterinaria e Produzioni Animali, Università di Napoli Federico II, Naples, Italy
Full list of author information is available at the end of the article

yet remain very important in the case of melanic insular lizards, whose immune system is expected to be depressed by great investment in reproduction, and life at high density [13, 19, 22]. This study was undertaken with the aim to evaluate the presence of potentially zoonotic bacteria and parasites in wild-caught insular individuals of *P. sicula klemmeri*, along with mainland individuals of *P. sicula*.

Results

A wide range of bacteria and parasites were detected in both *P. sicula* and *P. sicula klemmerii* individuals. Among the 24 analysed animals, 23 (95.9%) were positive to at least one bacterium and 19 (79.1%) were positive to at least one parasite.

Regarding microbiological analysis, *Pantoea* spp. was isolated in 4/24 (16.7%) oral swabs, *Citrobacter* spp. in 1/24 (4.2%), *Morganella morganii* in 1/24 (4.2%), *Pseudomonas aeruginosa* in 1/24 (4.2%) and Coagulase-Negative Staphylococci (NCS) in 7/24 (29.1%). For cloacal swabs, *Citrobacter* spp. was found in 10/24 (41.7%) animals of which 1/10 (10.0%) was identified as *Citrobacter koseri*, *Enterobacter* spp.was found in 8/24 (33.3%) animals of which 1/8 (12.5%) was identified as *Enterobacter aerogenes*, *Escherichia coli* was found in 3/24 (12.5%) animals of which 1/3 (33.3%) was serotyped as serogroup O 145, *Morganella morganii* was isolated in 2/24 (8.3%) individuals, *Shewanella* spp. in 1/24 (4.2%), *Providencia* spp. in 2/24 (8.3%), Coagulase-Negative Staphylococci (NCS) in 20/24 (83.3%) and *Pseudomonas* spp. in 10/24 (41.7%) individuals. Several bacteria were routinely isolated from the same animal.

With respect to antimicrobial susceptibility testing, *Citrobacter* spp. showed the highest resistance profile. Specifically, two out of ten strains of *Citrobacter* spp. were resistant to three or more drugs ("multidrug-resistant") of which, one strain was resistant to ampicillin, doxycycline and streptomycin and the other one was resistant to ampicillin, amoxicillin-clavulanic acid, doxycycline and nitrofurantoin. The remaining strains were resistant to ampicillin, one was also resistant to doxycycline and one other was also resistant to amoxicillin-clavulanic acid. *Escherichia coli* O145 and all the strains of *Enterobacter* spp. were resistant to ampicillin. In contrast, *Pseudomonas aeruginosa* were susceptible to all antimicrobials tested.

Regarding the parasitological results, the scotch test highlighted the presence of *Ophionyssus natricis* mite. During the faecal examination, eggs of pinworms (20/24; 83.3%), *O. natricis* (12/24; 50%), and Dicrocoelidae (6/24; 25%) as well as oocysts of coccidia (11/24; 45.8%) were detected. As with bacteria, different parasite species were simultaneously detected from the same animal. In addition, adult liver flukes (Dicrocoelidae) were also found during the necropsy. The parasitological and microbiological results related to each lizard are detailed in Table 1.

Discussion

Our results provide new epidemiological data on bacterial and parasitic infections in *P. sicula* and *P. sicula klemmerii*. These species were poorly investigated from a sanitary perspective so far. Bacterial and parasitic infections in reptiles have recently gained scientific relevance. However, the majority of studies were carried out on captive-bred individuals of Cryptodira (tortoises, [23]), Serpentes and Sauria (snakes and other 'lizards,' [24]). Conversely, data on infections in wild lizards are scarce.

The results of our study showed the presence of endoparasites (coccidia, pinworms and liver flukes) and ectoparasites (*O. natricis*) in *P. sicula* and *P. sicula klemmeri.* With respect to the presence of pinworms, our findings are in line with those by Casanova et al. [20] who detected the presence of a nematode belonging to the Oxyuroidea superfamily in *P. sicula*. Nevertheless, our results showed the first epidemiological information on parasites infecting *P. sicula klemmeri*. Regarding the presence of *O. natricis*, there are no studies in literature that highlight its presence in *P. sicula* and *P. sicula klemmeri*, although the infestation by this mite has been described in various genus of Sauria as *Lacerta*, *Podarcis* and *Darevskia*. In addition, the carrier role of *O. natricis* in the transmission of a blood parasite belonging to the genus *Karyolysus* has been reported in lizards [25]. An interesting finding of our study was the detection at necropsy of liver flukes (Dicrocoelidae) in the continental lizards, although species identification was not performed.

Bacteriological results also added new epidemiological data in *P. sicula* due to detection of some potential zoonotic species as *P. aeruginosa* and *E. coli* O145. The bacterial isolation performed on oral swabs gave as result the presence of bacteria belonging to the genera *Pantoea, Pseudomonas, Morganella, Staphylococcus, Citrobacter, Shewanella* never detected before in *P. sicula* and *P. sicula klemmeri*. However, these bacteria are frequent in reptiles, along with other bacteria such as *Enterobacter* spp., *E. coli* and *Providencia* spp. [26–28]. Bacteria isolated from cloacal swabs were *Enterobacter* spp., *Citrobacter* spp., *Morganella* spp., *E. coli, Providencia* spp. *Shewanella* spp., and *Pseudomonas* spp., gram-negative bacteria frequently isolated in other reptiles [29] as well as *Staphylococcus* spp. The isolation of *E. coli* O145 in one *P. sicula klemmeri* is noteworthy due to the potential zoonotic role of this serogroup which is considered a shigatoxin-producing *E. coli*.

It is interesting to notice that the insular population presents similar bacterial diversity of its mainland counterpart, although the differences in sample size urge caution in interpreting these results. Noteworthy, 9 different bacterial genera were identified in *P.s. klemmeri* (up to six in a single individual), against 4 in mainland individuals (up to three in a single individual). A weakness of

Table 1 Parasites and bacteria found in *Podarcis sicula klemmeri* (LIC) and *P. sicula* (PLIC) lizards

Lizard ID	Parasites				Bacteria	
		EPG/OPG [a]			Swab samples	
	Parasite	NaCl	$ZnSO_4$	*O. natricis*	Cloacal	Oral
LIC 1001	Negative	–	–	Positive	*Enterobacter* spp., *Staphylococcus* spp., *Pseudomonas* spp.	*Pantoea* spp., *Staphylococcus* spp.
LIC 1002	Pinworms Coccidae	300 405	225 270	Positive	*Enterobacter aerogenes, Citrobacter* spp., *Staphylococcus* spp.	*Staphylococcus* spp.
LIC 1003	Pinworms Coccidae	720 120	150	Positive	*Morganella morganii, Citrobacter* spp., *Staphylococcus* spp.	*Pantoea* spp.
LIC 1004	Pinworms Coccidae	720 120	150	Positive	*Citrobacter* spp., *Shewanella* spp., *E. coli, Staphylococcus* spp., *Pseudomonas* spp.	*Pantoea* spp., *Staphylococcus* spp.
LIC 1005	Pinworms Liver flukes	2.880	1.440 960	Positive	*Citrobacter* spp., *Staphylococcus* spp.	*Staphylococcus* spp.
LIC 1006	Pinworms Liver flukes	2.880 120	1.440 120	Positive	*Morganella morganii, Citrobacter* spp., *Pseudomonas* spp.	*Morganella morganii, Citrobacter* spp., *Pantoea* spp. *Pantoea,PStaphylococcus*
LIC 1007	Pinworms Coccidae	3.600 4.140	2.100 1.530	Positive	*Enterobacter* spp., *E. coli, Staphylococcus* spp.	–
LIC 1008	Negative	–	–	Positive	*Enterobacter* spp., *Providencia* spp., *Staphylococcus* spp.	–
LIC 1009	Pinworms Coccidae	3.600 4.140	2.100 1.530	Positive	*E. coli* O145, *Staphylococcus* spp.	–
LIC 1010	Pinworms	330	300	Positive	*Staphylococcus* spp.	–
LIC 1011	Pinworms Liver flukes	3.420	1.890 120	Positive	*Pseudomonas* spp.	–
LIC 1012	Pinworms	3.420	1.890	Positive	*Citrobacter* spp., *Providencia* spp., *Staphylococcus* spp., *Pseudomonas* spp.	*Pseudomonas aeruginosa, Staphylococcus* spp.
LIC 1013	Pinworms Coccidae	870 360	690 105	–	*Enterobacter* spp., *Staphylococcus* spp.	–
LIC 1014	Pinworms Coccidae	870 360	690 105	–	*Citrobacter koseri, Staphylococcus* spp., *Pseudomonas* spp.	–
LIC 1015	Pinworms Liver flukes	540	300 7800	–	*Enterobacter* spp., *Staphylococcus* spp.	–
LIC 1016	Pinworms Liver flukes	540	300 42	–	*Staphylococcus* spp., *Pseudomonas* spp.	–
LIC 1017	Pinworms	540	300	–	*Pseudomonas* spp.	–
LIC 1018	Pinworms Coccidae	360 90	450	–	*Staphylococcus* spp.	–
LIC 1019	Pinworms Coccidae Liver flukes	360 90	450 48	–	*Staphylococcus* spp., *Pseudomonas* spp.	–
LIC 1020	Pinworms Coccidae	360 90	450 48	–	*Enterobacter* spp., *Staphylococcus* spp.	–
PLIC 1001	Pinworms	420	375	–	NOT IDENTIFIED	*Staphylococcus* spp.
PLIC 1002	Negative	–	–	–	*Enterobacter* spp., *Citrobacter* spp., *Staphylococcus* spp.	–
PLIC 1003	Negative	–	–	–	*Citrobacter* spp., *Staphylococcus* spp.	*Staphylococcus* spp.
PLIC 1004	Negative	–	–	–	*Citrobacter* spp., *Staphylococcus* spp., *Pseudomonas* spp.	–

[a]EPG/OPG = eggs/oocysts per gram of faeces

this study was the failure to isolate bacteria in the oral cavity of some lizards due to the difficult to keep viable some strains during the isolation procedures. To our knowledge this is the first study to assess the antimicrobial resistance profiles of potentially zoonotic bacteria carried by *Podarcis* spp. It is difficult to speculate regarding the results of the antimicrobial resistance recovered in the present study. However, one possible mechanism by which lizards acquire antimicrobial resistant bacteria in their environment range may be directly through exposure to human or livestock waste, or indirectly through consumption of prey which may harbor resistant bacteria.

The figure for parasites is even harder to interpret given the smaller sample size. Yet, we found coccidia, liver flukes and pinworms in the insular populations, and pinworms only (in just one individual) within continental lizards. While difference in collecting season, sample size, and the instance of necropsy in two individuals only suggest great caution, data seem to indicate an overall higher parasite/bacterial load in insular lizards. Assuming this is true, it remains to be elucidated whether this depends on population density on Licosa, or on less competent immune system in insular melanic individuals [12, 13].

Conclusion

In conclusion, the results of this study highlighted various bacteria and parasites, some of them pathogenic, able to infect the species *P. sicula* and the subspecies *P. sicula klemmeri*. Further studies are needed to better understand the epidemiology and transmission routes of these pathogens along with their impact on the welfare and behaviour of Italian wall lizards.

Methods

Study animals

From November 2015 to May 2016, we collected and examined, within 24 h from capture, a total of 24 individuals, 20 (14 males and 10 females) belonging to the subspecies *P. sicula klemmeri*, and 4 individuals belonging to the species *P. sicula*. The *P. sicula klemmeri* specimens were from the small islet of Licosa, whereas the *P. sicula* specimens from Punta Licosa mainland (Campania region of southern Italy). The study site, collection and housing methods were described in Raia et al. [12, 13]. Lizards captured on Licosa islet were identified with the code "LIC" and a progressive number (from LIC 1001 to 1020); the lizards from Licosa mainland were identified with the code "PLIC" and a progressive number (from PLIC 1001 to 1004).

In order to perform the microbiological analysis, oral and cloacal samples were individually collected by sterile cotton-tipped swabs and then inoculated in Phosphate Buffered Saline (PBS). For the parasitological analyses, different methods were used: faecal samples were collected from each lizard, scotch tape test was performed on the skin of each animal and, eventually, a necropsy with stereo microscope was carried out on two lizards found dead on the insular study site. After sampling, animals were released in the same area where they were captured. All experiments described were performed in accordance with the local and national guidelines governing animal experiments (86/ 609/CEE and its modifications).

Microbiological and parasitological analyses

Oral and cloacal swabs stored in PBS were inoculated in buffered peptone water (BPW), *Campylobacter*-selective enrichment broth (CSEB), cooked meat medium (CMM), modified tryptone soy broth (MTSB). The samples inoculated in BPW were incubated at both 25 °C and 37 °C for 24 h and then inoculated/streaked into Rappaport-Vassiliadis broth (RV), Columbia blood agar base (CBA; Oxoid, Milan, Italy), *Pseudomonas* cetrimide agar (PCA; Oxoid), MacConkey agar (MCA; Oxoid) and Baird-Parker agar (BPA; Oxoid). The samples inoculated in MTSB were incubated at both 25 °C and 37 °C for 24 h and then spread on sorbitol MacConkey agar (SMCA; Oxoid). The samples inoculated in CSEB were incubated in microaerophilic atmosphere at both 25 °C and 42 °C for 48 h and then streaked on *Campylobacter* blood-free selective agar (CBFA; Oxoid). Instead, the samples inoculated in CMM were incubated in anaerobic atmosphere at both 25 °C and 37 °C for 24 h, and then streaked on anaerobe basal agar (ABA; Oxoid). The remaining PBS were incubated at 4 °C for 14 days, spread on *Yersinia* selective agar base (cefsulodin-irgasan-novobiocin, CIN Agar; Oxoid) and incubated at 30 °C for additional 24–48 h. CBA, PCA, MCA, SMCA, CEOA and BPA were incubated at both 25 °C and 37 °C for 24–48 h, whereas RV was incubated at both 25 °C and 42 °C for 24–48 h and then streaked on xylose lysine desoxycholate agar (XLD) and brilliant green agar (BGA); CBFA were incubated in microaerophilic atmosphere at both 25 °C and 42 °C for 24–48 h, ABA plates were anaerobically incubated both at 25 °C and 37 °C for 48 h and checked daily for a further week before discarding. All the isolates were previously identified according to their morphological features, their growing need, Gram colouring, motility and pigments production test and through conventional biochemical and phenotypic test. Progressively, the isolates were identified through the biochemical systems API 20 E, API 20 NE (bioMerieux, Mercy-l'Etoile, France) and RapID ANA II, RapID NF PLUS, RapID STAPH PLUS (Oxoid). *Escherichia coli* strains were serogrouped with antisera poly- and monospecific (Sifin) whereas, suspected *Campylobacter* strains were identified by PCR as reported by Gargiulo et al. [30].

In order to detect and count parasitic elements (eggs, larvae, cysts, oocysts), each faecal sample collected from the 24 lizards was analysed with the FLOTAC pellet technique [24, 31]. The analytic sensitivity of the FLOTAC pellet technique varied on the basis of the weight of each pellet μμ [24] and expressed as eggs/oocysts per gram (EPG/OPG) of faeces. Two flotation solutions were used: sodium chloride (NaCl, specific gravity = 1200) and zinc sulfate ($ZnSO4$, specific gravity = 1350) to detect protozoa/nematoda and trematoda, respectively. The scotch tape test was performed on the skin of the lizards, specifically, at the level of skin folds, around the eye, the cloaca and the eardrum recesses. The necropsy of the two lizard carcasses was performed under a stereomicroscope using the reptile necropsy protocol reported in Jacobson [32].

Antimicrobial susceptibility tests

Pseudomonas aeruginosa, *Escherichia coli* O145, *Citrobacter* spp., *Enterobacter* spp. isolates were submitted to antimicrobial susceptibility testing using the disc diffusion method according to Clinical Laboratory Standard Institute [33]. The antimicrobials tested were ampicillin (10 µg), ceftazidime (30 µg), ciprofloxacin (5 µg), enrofloxacin (5 µg), sulphamethoxazole-trimethoprim (25 µg), nalidixic acid (30 µg), amoxicillin-clavulanic acid (30 µg), doxycycline (30 µg), gentamicin (10 µg), streptomycin (10 µg), amikacin (30 µg), nitrofurantoin (30 µg), colistin sulphate (10 µg), piperacillin 100 (µg) and Cefpodoxime Combination Disc Kit (Oxoid). The inhibition zones were measured and scored as sensitive, intermediate susceptibility and resistant according to CLSI documents [34].

Abbreviations

ABA: Anaerobe basal agar; BGA: Brilliant green agar; BPA: Baird-Parker agar; BPW: Buffered peptone water; CBA: Columbia blood agar base; CBFA: *Campylobacter* blood-free selective agar; CIN: Cefsulodin-irgasan-novobiocin; CMM: Cooked meat medium; CSEB: *Campylobacter*-selective enrichment broth; EPG/OPG: eggs/oocysts per gram; MCA: MacConkey agar; MCRs: Melano-cortin receptors; MSH: α-melanocyte-stimulating hormone; MTSB: Modified tryptone soy broth; NaCl: Sodium chloride; PBS: Phosphate Buffered Saline; PCA: *Pseudomonas* cetrimide agar; PCR: Polymerase chain reaction; RV: Rappaport-Vassiliadis broth; SMCA: Sorbitol MacConkey agar; SVL: Snout-vent length; XLD: Xylose lysine desoxycholate agar; ZnSO4: Zinc sulphate

Funding

This research did not receive any specific grant from funding agencies in the public, commercial, or not-for-profit sectors.

Authors' contributions

All authors read and approved the final manuscript. LD, LR and PR designed the study, analysed the data, edited and critically revised the manuscript; VB, CS, LV, LB and MC performed microbiological and parasitological analysis and wrote the first draft of the manuscript.

Consent for publication

Not applicable.

Competing interests

The authors declare that they have no competing interests.

Author details

[1]Dipartimento di Medicina Veterinaria e Produzioni Animali, Università di Napoli Federico II, Naples, Italy. [2]Dipartimento di Scienze della Terra, dell'Ambiente e delle Risorse, Università di Napoli Federico II, Naples, Italy.

References

1. Corti C, Lo Cascio P, Razzetti E. Herpetofauna of the Italian islands. In: Bernini F, Sindaco R, Doria G, Razzetti E, editors. Atlas of Italian amphibians and reptiles. Firenze: Edizioni Polistampa; 2006. p. 612 43.
2. Vervust B, Grbac I, Van Damme R. Differences in morphology, performance and behaviour between recently diverged populations of *Podarcis sicula* mirror differences in predation pressure. Oikos. 2007;116:1343–52.
3. Capula M, Aloise G. Extreme feeding behaviours in the Italian wall lizard. *Podarcis siculus* Acta Herpetol. 2011;6:11–4.
4. Piras P, Salvi D, Ferrara G, Maiorino L, Delfino M, Pedde L, Kotsakis T. The role of post-natal ontogeny in the evolution of phenotypic diversity in *Podarcis lizards*. J Evol Biol. 2011;24:2705–20.
5. Kapsalas G, Gavriilidi I, Adamopoulou C, Foufopoulos J, Pafilis P. Effective thermoregulation in a newly established population of *Podarcis siculus* in Greece: a possible advantage for a successful invader. Acta Herpetol. 2016; 11:111–8.
6. Podnar M, Mayer W, Tvrtković N. Phylogeography of the Italian wall lizard, *Podarcis sicula*, as revealed by mitochondrial DNA sequences. Mol Ecol. 2005;14:575–88.
7. Senczuk G, Colangelo P, De Simone E, Aloise G, Castiglia R. A combination of long term fragmentation and glacial persistence drove the evolutionary history of the Italian wall lizard *Podarcis siculus*. BMC Evol Biol. 2017;17:6.
8. De Falco M, Sellitti A, Sciarrillo R, Capaldo A, Valiante S, Iachetta G, et al. Nonylphenol effects on the HPA axis of the bioindicator vertebrate, *Podarcis sicula* lizard. Chemosphere. 2014;104:190–6.
9. Lanza B, Capolongo D. Die blaue Ruineneidechse der tyrrhenischen Insel Licosa (Salerno). Salamandra. 1972;8:21–6.
10. Adler GH, Levins R. The island syndrome in rodent populations. Q Rev Biol. 1994;69:473–90.
11. Meiri S. Size evolution in island lizards. Glob Ecol Biogeogr. 2007;16:702–8.
12. Raia P, Carotenuto F, Meiri S. One size does not fit all: no evidence for an optimal body size on islands. Glob Ecol Biogeogr. 2010;19:475–84.
13. Raia P, Guarino FM, Turano M, Polese G, Rippa D, Carotenuto F. The blue lizard spandrel and the island syndrome. BMC Evol Biol. 2010;10:289.
14. Novosolov M, Raia P, Meiri S. The island syndrome in lizard. Glob Ecol Biogeogr. 2013;22:184–19.
15. Cooper WE, Dimopoulos I, Pafilis P. Sex, age, and population density affect aggressive behaviors in island lizards promoting cannibalism. Ethology. 2015;121:260–9.
16. Ducrest AL, Keller L, Roulin A. Pleiotropy in the melanocortin system, coloration and behavioural syndromes. Trends Ecol Evol. 2008;23:502–10.
17. Emaresi G, Ducrest AL, Bize P, Richter H, Simon C, Roulin A. Pleiotropy in the melanocortin system: expression levels of this system are associated -with melanogenesis and pigmentation in the tawny owl (*Strix aluco*). Mol Ecol. 2013;22:4915–30.
18. Kim SY, Fargallo JA, Vergara P, Martínez-Padilla J. Multivariate heredity of melanin-based coloration, body mass and immunity. Heredity. 2013;111:139.
19. Monti DM, Raia P, Vroonen J, Maselli V, Van Damme R, Fulgione D. Physiological change in an insular lizard population confirms the reversed island syndrome. Biol J Linn Soc Lond. 2013;108:144–50.
20. Casanova JC, Milazzo C, Ribas A, Cagnin M. *Spauligodon aloisei* n. sp. (Nematoda: Pharyngodonidae) parasite of *Podarcis sicula* (Reptilia: Lacertidae) from Italy. J Parasitol. 2003;89:577–9.
21. Lhermitte N, Bain O, Virga A. *Skrjabinelazia rizzoi* n. sp. (Nematoda: Seuratoidea) from a Sicilian lacertid, with comments on specific and biological diversity in the genus. Parasite. 2008;15:45–52.
22. Novosolov M, Rodda GH, Feldman A, Kadison AE, Dor R, Meiri S. Power in numbers. Drivers of high population density in insular lizards. Glob Ecol Biogeogr. 2016;25:87–95.
23. Dipineto L, Capasso M, Maurelli MP, Russo TP, Pepe P, Capone G, et al. Survey of co-infection by *Salmonella* and oxyurids in tortoises. BMC Vet Res. 2012;8:69.
24. Rinaldi L, Mihalca AD, Cirillo R, Maurelli MP, Montesano M, Capasso M, et al. FLOTAC can detect parasitic and pseudoparasitic elements in reptiles. Exp Parasitol. 2012;130:282–4.
25. Labbé A. Recherches zoologiques et biologiques sur les parasites endoglobulaires du sang des vertébrés. Arch Zool Exp Gen. 1894;2:55–258.
26. Jacobson ER. Immobilization, blood sampling, necropsy techniques and diseases of crocodilians: a review. J Zoo Anim Med. 1984;15:38–45.
27. Joyner P, Brown JD, Holladay S, Sleeman JM. Characterization of the bacterial microflora of the tympanic cavity of eastern box turtles with and without aural abscesses. J Wildl Dis. 2006;42:859–64.
28. Mayer H, Frank W. Bacteriological investigations on reptiles and amphibians (author's transl). Zentralblatt für Bakteriologie, Parasitenkunde,

Infektionskrankheiten und Hygiene. Erste Abteilung Originale. Zentralbl Bakteriol Orig A. 1974;229:470.
29. Foti M, Giacopello C, Bottari T, Fisichella V, Rinaldo D, Mammina C. Antibiotic resistance of gram negatives isolates from loggerhead sea turtles (*Caretta caretta*) in the Central Mediterranean Sea. Mar Pollut Bull. 2009;58: 1363–6.
30. Gargiulo A, Rinaldi L, D'Angelo L, Dipineto L, Borrelli L, Fioretti A, et al. Survey of *Campylobacter jejuni* in stray cats in southern Italy. Lett Appl Microbiol. 2008;46:267–70.
31. Cringoli G, Rinaldi L, Maurelli MP, Utzinger J. FLOTAC: new multivalent techniques for qualitative and quantitative copromicroscopic diagnosis of parasites in animals and humans. Nat Protoc. 2010;5:503–15.
32. Jacobson ER. Reptile necropsy protocol. J Zoo Anim Med. 1978;9:7–13.
33. Clinical and laboratory standards institute (CLSI): Performance Standards for Antimicrobial Disk Susceptibility Tests. In: Approved Standard M02-A11. 7th ed. PA, USA: CLSI: Wayne; 2012.
34. Clinical and laboratory standards institute (CLSI): Performance Standards for Antimicrobial Disk Susceptibility Tests. In: Approved Standard M100-S24. 24th ed. PA, USA: CLSI: Wayne; 2014.

22

Vector-borne and zoonotic diseases of dogs in North-west New South Wales and the Northern Territory, Australia

Amanda J. Shapiro[1*], Graeme Brown[1], Jacqueline M. Norris[1], Katrina L. Bosward[1], Debbie J. Marriot[2], Nandhakumar Balakrishnan[3], Edward B. Breitschwerdt[3] and Richard Malik[1,4,5*]

Abstract

Background: Vector-borne diseases of dogs in Australian Aboriginal communities are relatively unexplored. These dogs represent a unique group with variable ecto- and endo-parasitic burdens, nutritional stresses and a general lack of veterinary intervention. We investigated haemoprotozoal and bacterial pathogen prevalences in relation to erythrocyte and platelet numbers in dogs from North-West New South Wales (N-W NSW) and the Northern Territory (NT; Central Australia).

Methods: Real-time PCR (qPCR) amplification of *Anaplasma platys, Babesia vogeli, Mycoplasma haemocanis, Candidatus* Mycoplasma haematoparvum and *Bartonella* spp., serological screening for *Coxiella burnetii,* and *Bartonella* spp. and haematological analyses were performed on dogs from the two cohorts (96 dogs in total). *Brucella suis* serology was determined additionally for the N-W NSW cohort.

Results: *Anaplasma platys* (n = 26 dogs), *Babesia vogeli* (n = 7), *Candidatus* Mycoplasma haematoparvum (n = 10 dogs), and *Mycoplasma haemocanis* (n = 14) were detected in the sample population (n = 96) using qPCR. There were significant associations between (i) *A. platys* and anaemia (OR 8.7, CI 2.4–31.7; $P < 0.001$), thrombocytopenia (OR 12.1, CI 3.4–43.2; $P < 0.001$) and breed (OR 16.1, CI 2.1–121.5; $P = 0.007$), and (ii) between *B. vogeli* and anaemia (OR 11.8, CI 2.3–61.6; $P = 0.003$). Neither protozoal nor bacterial DNA loads, estimated using qPCR, were positively correlated with anaemia or thrombocytopenia. Haemotropic mycoplasmas were not associated with any haematologic abnormality. Four dogs from the NT were seropositive for *Coxiella burnetii,* while no dogs were seropositive for *Brucella suis* or to a panel of *Bartonella* spp. antigens. Despite directed efforts, *Bartonella* DNA was not detected in blood from any of the cohorts studied. A sample of dogs from the NT recruited specifically for *Bartonella* α-proteobacteria growth medium enrichment blood culture were also *Bartonella* PCR negative.

Conclusions: Vector-borne pathogens occur in dogs free ranging near Aboriginal communities, with higher detection rates in NT than N-W NSW. The preponderant haematologic abnormalities were anaemia and thrombocytopenia, likely attributable to *A. platys* and *B. vogeli* infections, but also probably affected by nutritional, parasitic, lactational and environmental stressors. The absence of *Bartonella* spp. is of importance to the Australian setting, and work needs to be extended to tropical coastal communities where fleas are present as well as ticks. Dogs living in and around Aboriginal communities may provide valuable sentinel information on disease infection status of human public health significance.

Keywords: Dog, *Babesia* spp., *Anaplasma* spp., Haemotropic mycoplasmas, *Coxiella burnetii, Bartonella* spp., *Brucella* spp.

* Correspondence: amanda.shapiro@sydney.edu.au; richard.malik@sydney.edu.au
[1]University of Sydney School of Veterinary Science, Building B14, Sydney, NSW 2006, Australia
Full list of author information is available at the end of the article

Background

Australia is an island continent, with most dogs and people residing in large cities within 70 km of the coast. The population is mainly located in capital cities of the mainland states. This is where most veterinary schools are located, at least until recently when Charles Sturt University (Wagga Wagga, NSW) started a veterinary program. The canine literature is therefore biased towards conditions seen in dogs living in Sydney, Melbourne, Brisbane, Perth, Adelaide and Townsville. For this reason, there is a paucity of information concerning tick-borne disease in Australia, especially diseases transmitted by the brown dog tick, *Rhipicephalus sanguineus*, which is generally found further inland [1]. Limited recent information concerning tick-borne diseases is largely derived from free-roaming dogs living in close association with a limited number of indigenous Aboriginal communities, mainly in the Northern Territory (NT) [2, 3]. A further study concerns vector-borne diseases of pet dogs from Darwin and Southeast Queensland [4, 5].

The interplay of infectious agents transmitted by ticks is relevant firstly to dogs living in areas where these organisms are biological vectors, such as tropical north Queensland, the far north of Western Australia and NT. The concept of 'One Health' incorporates intra- and inter- species disease transmission, taking into account environmental variables. Thus, within the current context, dogs represent unique sentinels of infection for human medicine. But infections of dogs in these regions impacts also on other parts of Australia, because people can take dogs where they travel. This might become an even bigger issue if, hypothetically, Darwin was subjected to a tropical cyclone, with subsequent translocation of dogs to other regions. Such a mechanism was implicated anecdotally for the accelerated spread of dirofilariasis in the 1970s following cyclone Tracy [6].

Babesiosis was the first tick-borne disease characterised in Australia by the Veterinary Tropical Health Division, James Cook University in Townsville [7, 8]. *Babesia vogeli* (formerly *Babesia canis vogeli*) is endemic in far north Queensland and the NT. Babesiosis was characterised with the methodologies of the time by Irwin and colleagues [9, 10] and further insights occurred subsequently, as polymerase chain reaction (PCR) testing of venous blood replaced examination of Romanowsky-stained blood films made from capillary blood [11, 12]. PCR simplified testing, being more sensitive and specific than microscopy, with the capacity to detect both clinical and subclinical infections. Canine babesiosis due to *B. vogeli* continues to be a cause of symptomatic haemolytic, subclinical anaemia and thrombocytopenia in these areas [5]. Investigations by various groups have confirmed babesiosis as a common cause of anaemia in NT 'camp dogs' in aboriginal communities [3, 5]. Anaemia can be severe enough to cause pale mucous membranes. In puppies and dogs immunosuppressed by malnutrition, life-threatening haemolytic anaemia can develop [9, 13]. Compared to *B. rossi* and *B. canis*, however, *B. vogeli* is considerably less virulent [14, 15], possibly as a result of its longer association with domesticated dogs [16]. Babesiosis due to *Babesia gibsoni* has been reported sporadically in Australia in American pit bulls [17, 18], the disease originating from dogs imported from the USA [19] or Asia [20, 21] and inoculated by fighting, rather than the feeding of ticks [22–24].

In 2001, *Anaplasma platys* was discovered in Australia by Brown and colleagues during an evaluation of the health status of free roaming aboriginal dogs [25]. Further work, including experimental infections, showed *A. platys* caused mild to moderate cyclic thrombocytopenia [26–28], which was usually subclinical. Anecdotally, dogs with heavy *A. platys* infections have been observed to bleed more freely from tick attachment sites than uninfected dogs (Dr Graeme Brown, personal communication). Preliminary data showed some dogs were infected with *B. vogeli*, others with *A. platys*, while a small percentage were infected by both pathogens [3].

Two research groups demonstrated that three or more species of haemotropic mycoplasmas infected free-roaming camp dogs of Central Australia [2, 4, 5, 29]. Two species were preponderant, *Mycoplasma haemocanis* (the more virulent 'large form') and *Candidatus* M. haematoparvum with a third unnamed species unable to be characterised further [2], and the fourth found to be *M. haemobos*, a cattle pathogen [5]. The clinical significance of these erythrocytic parasites is currently unclear, as presence of *Mycoplasma* sp. has no apparent correlation with anaemia, even when the cycling threshold (C_T) of the real-time PCR (qPCR) indicates heavy bacteraemia.

The zoonotic pathogen *Rickettsia felis* has recently been shown to have the dog as a definitive host, with transmission requiring fleas or ticks as biological vectors [30]. *Rickettsia felis* has been found in dogs in Southeast Queensland and Central Australia [31]. Other canine tick-borne diseases, such as ehrlichiosis and cytauxzoonosis, are not endemic, but have the potential to be imported from overseas.

Bartonella spp. have yet to be reported in the peer-reviewed literature from Australian dogs, even though fleas and ticks are common in many parts of Australia and *Bartonella henselae* and *Bartonella clarridgeiae* are known to be present in fleas [32], foxes [33], humans [34] and cats in Australia, especially young cats [32, 35]. Furthermore, many Australian native animals have a variety of *Bartonella* spp. which could potentially be transmitted to canids [36, 37].

Coxiella burnetii, the agent of 'Q fever' in human patients and coxiellosis in animals, is a Gram-negative bacterium. Although theoretically capable of being transmitted by fleas and ticks, it is generally transmitted by aerosols from reproductive secretions, or possibly by the ingestion of infectious forms present in uncooked meat or offal from infected animals [38, 39]. A recent Australian serosurvey found dogs living in Aboriginal communities had the highest seroprevalence of coxiellosis [40].

Work to date has emphasised that individual dogs in certain settings can be infected by a combination of flea- and tick-borne infectious agents. Polymicrobial infections with so-called 'stealth pathogens' can have complex effects due to intricate interactions such as molecular mimicry and immune-stimulation that cannot be appreciated by studies of a single pathogen under experimental conditions [41, 42]. Thus, in regions where vectors are common, and especially where prophylactic ectoparasitic measures are not undertaken routinely, polymicrobial infections, in association with genetic, nutritional and environmental factors, are likely to impact on haematologic variables and the overall health of infected dogs. Among individuals, disease expression may be influenced by nutritional and environmental stressors, including insufficient quantity or quality of food, pregnancy, lactation or hard work.

The purpose of the present study was to 1) Determine the prevalence of selected zoonotic pathogens and vector-borne pathogens among free-roaming dogs living in Aboriginal communities in different parts of Australia; 2) Assess potential correlations between anaemia and thrombocytopenia and the qPCR C_T values for *B. vogeli*, *A. platys* and haemotropic mycoplasmas; 3) Determine whether dogs from Central Australia were infected by *Bartonella* spp.

Methods

Sample population and specimen collection

Most dogs in Aboriginal communities are of mixed breed and often called 'camp' dogs. They are considered hybrids of the dingo (*Canis lupus dingo*) and domestic dogs (*Canis lupus familiaris*). Such dogs are not confined. They may be owned, but are allowed to roam freely or may be strays (recently owned and abandoned). Dogs in this study probably would not roam more than 15 km from where sampled [43]. Because information provided by owners was considered unreliable, estimation of ages was based on dentition. Dogs were classified as 'pure-bred small' (1 to 10 kg), 'purebred medium' (10 to 20 kg), 'purebred large' (> 20 kg) or crossbreds (dingo hybrids). They were classified into four age ranges; 0–1 year, 1–2.5 years, 2.5–6 years and >6 years. Body condition grades (fair, good, excellent; and lactating) were recorded where possible.

Dogs were sampled (for haematology and PCR analyses) from two locations; (1) the Ti-Tree communities (NT, Central Australia; n = 51) and (2) Moree and nearby districts in N-W NSW, including Mehi Mission (outskirts of Moree), Mungindi, Toomelah and Bogabilla (n = 45), while an additional subset of dogs were sampled specifically for specialised *Bartonella* testing) from the Central Australian communities of Yuelamu, Laramba and Alyen (Fig. 1). Dogs lived in and around conventional houses and were either fed by their owners, scavenged leftovers or were able to catch and eat wildlife. All houses in both communities were visited and occupants asked to identify and restrain their dogs. In Moree, dogs in the pound (n = 14) were also sampled at the request of the local council ranger; these were in good condition, none had pale gums, a few had sores (most likely resolving bite wounds). All appeared to be 'town dogs'. Blood from dogs in Ti Tree was collected in November 2010. Blood from Moree dogs was obtained at the end of summer, shortly after drought-breaking heavy rain in February 2013. In August 2014, dogs were sampled from Yuelamu, Laramba and Alyuen specifically in an attempt to determine if *Bartonella* spp. were present in dogs from Central Australia (40 dogs sampled), coinciding with a trip to Australia by EB. Within these communities, each dog was identified and its age and sex determined. The ages of the dogs ranged from approximately 8 weeks to 10 years but because of difficulties encountered in catching and restraining dogs, more adults (> 12 months) than young dogs were sampled. It was noted briefly whether dogs were infested with ectoparasites, or not, and the extent of the infestation.

EDTA anti-coagulated blood and whole blood (clot tube) were collected from dogs, stored at 4 °C in an eski, and transported to the laboratory within 7 days of collection, as soon as was practical. Serum was harvested from whole blood after centrifugation. Residual EDTA blood (after haematologic analyses) and serum were subsequently stored at −80 °C. Samples were collected with the approval of the Animal Ethics Committee of Charles Darwin University (A01019), Westmead Hospital Animal Ethics Committee (AEC protocol number 5073.10.12) and the University of Sydney (N00/11–2006/3/4492). Samples from Yuelamu, Laramba and Alyuen were collected at the request of the Animal Management Coordinator, Central Desert Regional Council.

Haematology

All blood specimens from the Moree dog cohort were submitted to the University of Sydney's Veterinary Pathological Diagnostic Services Laboratory (VPDS) for routine haematologic analyses, using automated cell

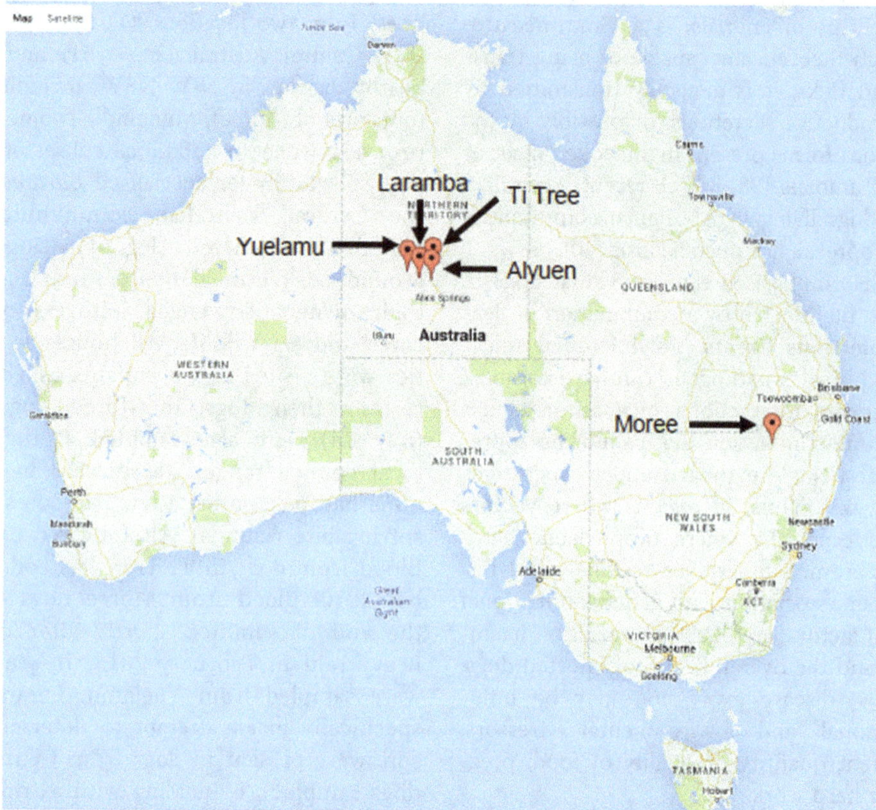

Fig. 1 Geographical plot of locations where dogs were sampled. The map identifies the exact locations of the dogs that were sampled (Google Maps 2016)

count analysers as well as whole blood smears evaluating differential cell counts and reticulocyte counts. Laboratory reference intervals (RI) for packed cell volume (PCV) and platelet counts (PLT) in dogs are 0.37–0.55 L/L and 200–600 × 10^9/L, respectively. Blood specimens from the Ti-Tree dog cohort were submitted within 4 days of collection at the closest accessible pathology laboratory, Alice Springs Base Hospital, NT (a human facility). The following parameters were assessed: white cell count, haematocrit, platelet count and mean platelet volume. Reticulocyte counts and differential WBC counts were not performed.

PCR analysis of Anaplasma platys, Babesia vogeli, M. haemocanis and *Candidatus* M. haematoparvum *and Bartonella spp*

EDTA blood was aliquoted, and a portion from each dog was submitted to IDEXX laboratories for multiplex real-time polymerase chain reaction (PCR) testing (Tick/Vector Canine Comprehensive RealPCR™ Panel). Testing was done in their Sacramento, CA laboratory. Results, including C_T values, were recorded and tabulated.

Specialised *Bartonella* testing

Following negative results for commercial PCR testing for *Bartonella* spp. (IDEXX laboratories, Sacramento), 40 additional fresh blood samples sourced from Yuelamu, Laramba and Alyuen collected from dogs in August 2014 were shipped to the Intracellular Pathogens Research Laboratory, College of Veterinary Medicine, North Carolina State University, USA for *Bartonella* testing. For serological analyses, *Bartonella vinsonii* subsp. *berkhoffii* genotypes I, II, and III, *B. henselae* Houston-1 strain (H-1), *B. henselae* (San Antonio 2 strain), and *Bartonella koehlerae* antibodies were determined using six indirect immunofluorescence antibody assays (IFA) and fluorescein-conjugated goat anti-human IgG (Pierce Biotechnology, Rockford, IL), as described [44]. To avoid confusion with possible non-specific binding found at low serum dilutions, a cut-off value of 1/64 was used to define a seroreactive titre. Reactive sera at a titre of 1/64 were further tested with 2-fold dilutions out to 1/8192. For molecular detection of *Bartonella* spp. DNA, a previously described approach that includes PCR amplification of *Bartonella* spp. DNA from blood and *Bartonella* α-proteobacterial growth medium (BAPGM) blood cultures at 7, 14 and 21 days of incubation was used [45]. Two *Bartonella* genus and a *B. koehlerae* species-specific PCR (three independent PCR reactions per DNA extraction) were performed using primers designed to amplify 16-23S intergenic transcribed spacer (ITS) region, as described previously [45].

Indirect immunofluorescent antibody assay (IFA) for serological testing for *Coxiella burnetii*

A modification of a commercial human *C. burnetii* phase I and II specific IFA IgG kit (Vircell, Spain) was used to detect canine IgG antibodies to phase I and phase II *C. burnetii* (Nine Mile strain), as described [46]. Adjustments for canine serum included the use of anti-canine IgG fluorescein isothiocyanate (FITC) conjugate solution (CJ-F-CANG-10ML, Veterinary Medical Research & Development, Pullman, WA, USA) to canine samples. This antibody was used undiluted at the stage when secondary antibody was applied to the control and test wells. All serum samples were tested at the optimised dilution (1/64) and diluent (5% Skim Milk Powder in PBS) [40]. A sample was considered 'seropositive' for *C. burnetii* on IFA if it displayed either phase I or phase II (IgG1, IgG2, IgG3) antibodies at a titre of 1/64 or greater. Positive samples were taken to end titre by two fold serial dilutions, beginning at 1/64.

Brucella testing

As swine brucellosis was an emerging infectious disease in northern NSW around the time sampling was conducted in the Moree district, sera from dogs in this subpopulation were also tested using the Rose Bengal Assay (Biomerieux Bucelloslide-Test; Rose Bengal Antigen) at SydPath (St Vincent's Hospital, Department of Microbiology, Darlinghurst, NSW, Australia) which includes *Brucella* specific agglutinins to *B. melitensis, B. abortus, B. bovis and B. suis*. Two fold serial dilutions of positive serum were used to determine the reciprocal antibody titre. Complement fixation testing for anti-*Brucella* antibodies was conducted at the Elizabeth MacArthur Agriculture Institute, NSW.

Numerical analysis

Data were analysed with the statistical software GenStat 16.1 (VSN International, Hemel Hempstead, UK), using two sample *t*-tests and logistic regression. Statistical significance was considered at $P < 0.05$. Associations between *A. platys, B. vogeli, M. haemocanis, Candidatus* M. haematoparvum, *C. burnetii, Bartonella spp.* and *B. suis* infection status and potential risk factors (age category, breed, gender, sterilisation status, packed cell volume [PCV] and platelet numbers) were assessed using logistic regression, with odds ratios reported to evaluate impact of factors.

Results

PCR analysis of A. platys, B. vogeli, M. haemocanis and Candidatus M. haematoparvum *in relation to haematology and population demographics*

The gender, sterilisation status, breed type, age, body condition, presence or absence of anaemia or thrombocytopenia of the study cohort expressed in relation to *A. platys, B. vogeli, M. haemocanis and Candidatus* M. haematoparvum qPCR status and seropositivity to *C. burnetii and B. suis* are presented in Table 1.

Overall, dogs were all considered to be in reasonable health (Additional file 1: Figure S1). Some were in suboptimal condition, perhaps as a result of poor nutrition, lactation, equivocal hygiene and less than ideal endo- and ecto-parasticide and vaccination regimens (Additional file 2: Figure S2). Qualitatively, dogs in Central Australia were in less satisfactory condition compared to dogs in N-W NSW (Additional file 3: Figure S3). Dogs from Central Australia had a variable (sometimes large) number of brown dog ticks, some lice but no fleas, while the dogs from N-W NSW rarely had ticks or fleas, and in low numbers.

Anaemia and thrombocytopenia were common findings amongst these dogs, using laboratory reference intervals (RI) determined for healthy dogs living in affluent Australia cities. It was challenging, however, to ascribe anaemia or thrombocytopenia to specific pathogen(s) because the ranges of values for PCV and platelet counts in 'control' dogs (i.e. dogs shown to be free of *A. platys, B. vogeli* and haemotropic mycoplasmas using real-time PCR testing) were wider than the VPDS RI established for normal healthy dogs.

In dogs shown to be uninfected with the PCR targeted organisms, the wide range of observed values for PCV and platelet numbers was likely attributable to (1) variable, chronic disease states (parasitic, nutritional, recent pregnancy or lactation) and (2) processing delays in relation to blood specimens due to the remote study sites and inevitable delays in testing, which varied from 2 to 4 days depending on the order of sampling. For the 'control' (PCR-negative) dogs, the lower limit for the PCV (which defines the presence of anaemia) was taken to be 0.30 L/L (compared to the laboratory RI of 0.39 to 0.50 L/L). For 'control dogs', the lower limit of the platelet count was taken to be 60×10^9/L (assuming the highest count and lowest count were likely outliers), rather than 200×10^9/L, the lower limit of normality for fresh blood collected from healthy dogs subjected to atraumatic fast venepuncture and processed within 24 h [47]. The authors acknowledge that there could be other pathogens (e.g. endoparasites) that are unknown and not specifically tested for.

Inspection of the scatter plots and box and whisker plots illustrates that *A. platys, B. vogeli* and 'polymicrobial

Table 1 Exposure variables against microbial result. Frequency table representing the variables of gender, sterilisation status, breed type, age, body condition, PCV and platelet count against *Anaplasma platys, Babesia vogeli, Candidatus* M. haematoparvum and *Mycoplasma haemocanis* qPCR positive results, and seropositivity to *C. burnetii, Bartonella spp. and Brucella spp.*

Variables	Category	*A. platys* positive $n = 26$	*B. vogeli* positive $n = 7$	*Candidatus* M. haemato-parvum $n = 10$	*Mycoplasma haemocanis* $n = 14$	*C. burnetii* Ph I/II positive $n = 4$ (1 NT;3 NW-NSW)	*Bartonella spp.* Positive $n = 0$	*Brucella* positive $n = 0$	Total $n = 96$
Gender	Male	12 (23%)	4 (8%)	6 (12%)	8 (15%)	1 (2%)	0	0	52
	Female	14 (32%)	3 (7%)	4 (9%)	6 (14%)	3 (7%)	0	0	44
Entire/ Desexed	Entire	24 (35%)	6 (9%)	9 (13%)	8 (12%)	2 (3%)	0	0	68
	Neutered	1 (10%)	0	1 (10%)	2 (20%)	1 (10%)	0	0	10
Breed type	Purebred small	0	0	0	1 (20%)	0	0	0	5
	Purebred medium	1 (5%)	1 (5%)	3 (14%)	5 (23%)	2 (9%)	0	0	22
	Purebred large	0	0	1 (17%)	2 (33%)	0	0	0	6
	Crossbred	25 (40%)	6 (10%)	6 (10%)	6 (10%)	2 (3%)	0	0	63
Age	0–1 year	11 65	4 (24%)	1 (6%)	2 (12%)	1 (6%)	0	0	17
	1–2.5 years	2 (12%)	1 (6%)	2 (12%)	2 (12%)		0	0	17
	2.5–6 years	12 (36%)	0	4 (12%)	2 (6%)	1 (3%)	0	0	33
	> 6 years	0	0	3 (43%)	4 (57%)		0	0	7
Body condition	Excellent	0	0	0	1 (50%)	0	0	0	2
	Good	3 (9%)	2 (6%)	2 (6%)	6 (19%)	2 (6%)	0	0	31
	Fair	23 (46%)	5 (10%)	6 (12%)	6 (12%)	1 (2%)	0	0	50
	Lactating	0	0	0	0	1 (100%)	0	0	1
PCV	Normal	17 (20%)	3 (4%)	10 (12%)	14 (17%)	4 (5%)	0	0	83
	Anaemia	9 (69%)	4 (31%)	0	0	0	0	0	13
Platelet count	Normal	15 (19%)	4 (5%)	10 (12%)	13 (16%)	4 (5%)	0	0	81
	Thrombo-cytopenia	11 (73%)	3 (20%)	0	1 (7%)	0	0	0	15

infections' (combinations of two or more vector-borne pathogens) were commonly associated with anaemia, whereas haemotropic mycoplasma infections (alone) were not (*M. haemocanis* and *Candidatus* M. haematoparvum were combined for simplicity, as preliminary analyses indicated neither alone was associated with anaemia) (Fig. 2). More precisely, 9/25 (36%) dogs that were *A. platys* (only) PCR-positive were anaemic (PCV < 0.30 L/L), 4/7 (57%) of *B. vogeli* (only) PCR-positive dogs were anaemic, 2/9 (12.5%) of dogs with polymicrobial infections were anaemic, while 0/19 (0%) of dogs infected by haemotropic mycoplasmas alone were anaemic. Using two sample *t*-tests, dogs PCR-positive for *B. vogeli* ($n = 7$) were significantly more likely to have a lower PCV than dogs ($n = 89$) negative for this pathogen ($P < 0.001$), dogs PCR-positive for *A. platys* ($n = 26$) were significantly more likely to have a lower PCV than dogs negative ($n = 70$) for this pathogen ($P < 0.001$), while dogs PCR-positive for haemotropic mycoplasmas ($n = 22$) were no more likely to have a lower PCV than dogs ($n = 74$) negative for these pathogens ($P = 0.981$).

Similarly, inspection of scatter plots and box and whiskers plots shows that *A. platys, B. vogeli* and polymicrobial infections were commonly associated with thrombocytopenia, whereas haemotropic mycoplasma infections were not (Fig. 3). More precisely, 11/26 (42%) dogs that were *A. platys* (only) PCR-positive were thrombocytopenic (platelet count $<60 \times 10^9$/L), 3/7 (43%) of *B. vogeli* (only) PCR-positive dogs were thrombocytopenic, 2/7 (29%) of dogs with polymicrobial infections were thrombocytopenic, while 1/22 (5%) dogs with haemotropic mycoplasmas (alone) was thrombocytopenic. Using two sample *t*-tests, dogs PCR-positive for *B. vogeli* ($n = 7$) were had significantly lower platelet counts than dogs ($n = 89$) negative for this pathogen ($P = 0.04$), dogs PCR-positive for *A. platys* ($n = 26$) had lower platelet counts than dogs ($n = 70$) negative for this bacterium ($P < 0.001$), while dogs PCR-positive for haemotropic

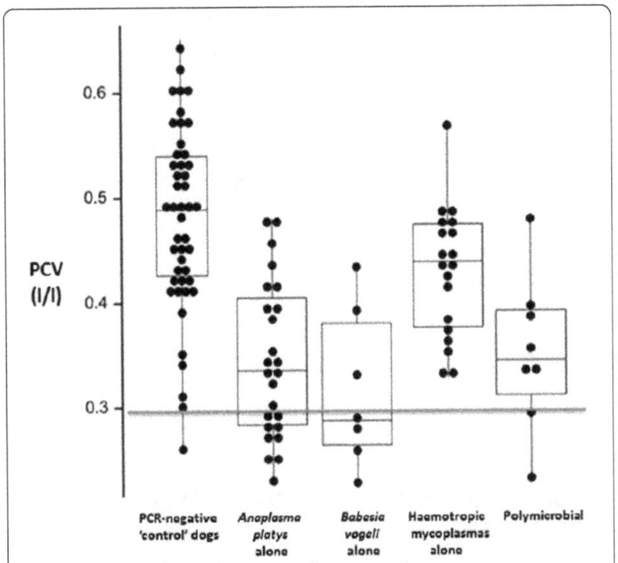

Fig. 2 Scatter plots of PCV values from 'control dogs' (negative to all pathogenic vector-borne diseases using multiplex qPCR), dogs infected with *A. platys, B. vogeli*, haemoplasmas (one, the other or both species) and polymicrobial infections (various 'mix-and-match' combinations of all these tick-borne pathogens). All dots represent an individual dog; box and whisker plots are superimposed (box represents the interquartile range, horizontal line within box represents median value, while the ends of the whiskers represent maximum and minimum values i.e. the range). The RI for PCV values was taken as greater than 0.3 L/L; thus dogs were considered anaemic when the PCV was less than 0.3 L/L (below the blue line)

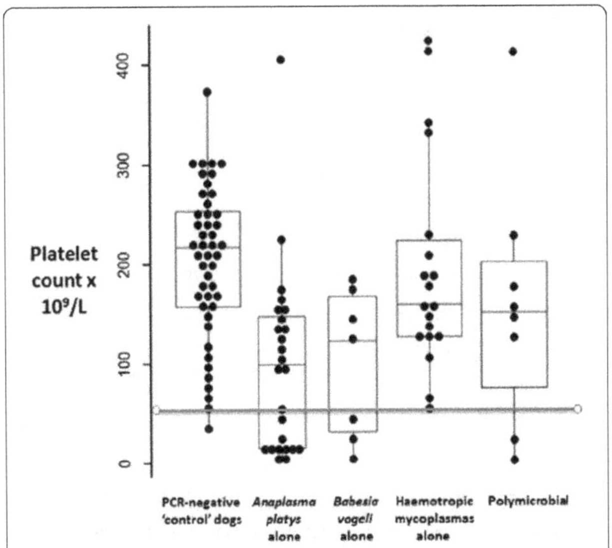

Fig. 3 Range of platelet counts from 'control dogs' (negative to all pathogenic vector-borne diseases using multiplex PCR), dogs infected with *A. platys, B. vogeli*, haemoplasmas (one, the other or both species) and polymicrobial infections (various 'mix-and-match' combinations). All dots represent an individual dog; stem and whisker plots, and outliers, identified by the statistical software package are denoted by a light green cross, are shown. The RI interval for platelet counts was considered to be greater than 60×10^9/L, and thus dogs were considered thrombocytopenic when the platelet count was less than 60×10^9/L (below the blue line)

mycoplasmas ($n = 22$) did not have lower platelet counts than dogs ($n = 74$) negative for these pathogens ($P = 0.23$), although dogs PCR-positive for *Candidatus* M. haematoparvum had higher platelet counts than dogs not infected with this bacterium ($P = 0.025$).

By logistic regression, PCR positivity for *A. platys* was significantly associated with breed (pedigree crossbred animals more likely to be infected; $P = 0.007$), anaemia ($P < 0.001$) and thrombocytopenia ($P < 0.001$), while PCR positivity for *B. vogeli* was associated only with anaemia ($P = 0.003$) (Table 2). There was no association between any infection status and age.

The cycling threshold (C_T) was available from the multiplex qPCR used to ascertain haemoparasitic status of each dog, a high C_T value indicates a low quantity of the respective pathogen. The results were counterintuitive. For *B. vogeli,* there was a negative correlation of −0.87 between C_T and PCV, inferring that the worse the dogs' anaemia (i.e. the lower the PCV), the lower the quantity of *Babesia* nucleic acid in their peripheral blood. There was no evidence of a meaningful correlation between C_T for *Babesia* and platelet numbers and between C_T for *A. platys* and PCV or platelet numbers (Fig. 4).

Bartonella multiplex qPCR, *Bartonella* serology and BAPGM enrichment culture

The commercial multiplex qPCR assay (IDEXX laboratories, Sacramento) did not detect *Bartonella* spp. DNA in any sample tested. On testing at North Carolina, no dog was seroreactive to any of the six *Bartonella* spp. antigens. Conventional *Bartonella spp.* PCRs using three ITS primer sets from blood and following BAPGM enrichment blood culture for 7, 14 and 21 days were all negative.

Coxiellosis serological testing

Of 96 dogs tested, four were seropositive for *Coxiella burnetii.* One was an entire male stumpy-tailed cattle dog (guard dog) of unspecified age from the Moree cohort. The remaining three were females: a Staffordshire bull terrier spayed crossbred (5 years-of-age) from Moree, a gravid black kelpie from Moree and an entire juvenile crossbred bitch from Ti-Tree. Further information on these cases has been reported [40].

Brucellosis serological testing

Only one of the Moree canine cohort tested positive using the Rose Bengal test and it was classed as a weak positive. This dog and all the other dogs from the Moree cohort tested negative on complement fixation testing and are thus considered negative. At the same time as

Table 2 Logistic regression analysis of variables with a statistically significant association with *A. platys* and *B. vogeli*

Positive	Categories	B	S.E.	Odds ratio	lower 95%	upper 95%	*P* value
A. platys	Constant	−1.356	0.271				
	Anaemia	2.167	0.658	8.735	2.407	31.70	<0.001
A. platys	Constant	−1.482	0.286				
	Thrombocytopenia	2.493	0.649	12.10	3.392	43.17	<0.001
A. platys	Purebred	−3.30	1.00				
	Crossbred	2.78	1.03	16.06	2.124	121.5	0.007
B. vogeli	Constant	−3.283	0.588				
	Anaemia	2.472	0.841	11.85	2.281	61.57	0.003

B = Estimate
S.E. = Standard Error

these dogs were tested, a known clinical case of *Brucella suis* infection in a dog with multifocal discospondylitis [48], two dogs with orchitis [47], and two dogs from Yarrabah Aboriginal community near Cairns (Far North Queensland) tested positive using the Rose Bengal test, although the results for the two Yarrabah dogs were flocculating rather than agglutinating.

Comparison of results between NT and Moree cohorts

Table 3 represents differences in haematologic values and pathogen prevalences between the two geographic areas, NT vs NW-NSW. Differences in prevalence of anaemia alone, thrombocytopenia alone and anaemia plus thrombocytopenia were all significant between the two groups. *Anaplasma platys* was the most prevalent

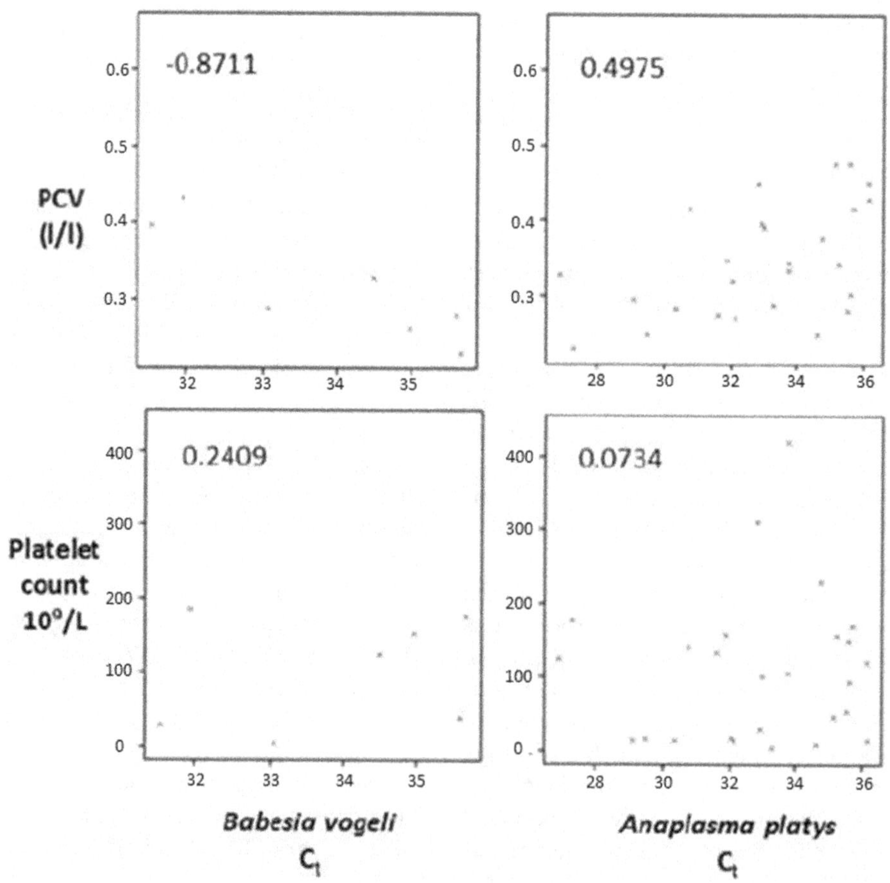

Fig. 4 Plots of C_T versus PCV and platelet count for *B. vogeli* and *A. platys*. Apart from the counterintuitive negative correlation (−0.87) between PCV and *B. vogeli* C_T values, there was no significant or clinically meaningful correlations evident from these plots

Table 3 Summary data concerning anaemia, thrombocytopenia, *B. vogeli, A. platys,* haemotropic mycoplasmas and co-infections in the two different areas tested, as well as *P* values for the two sample binomial *t*-tests comparing the two cohorts

Aboriginal Community	Haematology		PCR				
	Anaemia	Thrombocytopenia	Anaemia and thrombocytopenia	*Babesia vogeli*	*Anaplasma platys*	Haemotropic mycoplasmas	Co-infections[a]
NT (*n* = 51)	13 (26%)	14 (27%)	9 (18%)	5 (10%)	24 (47%)	12 (24%)	7 (14%)
NW-NSW (*n* = 45)	0	1 (2%)	0	2 (4%)	2 (4%)	10 (22%)	1 (2%)
Total	13	15	9	7	26	22	8
P value	< 0.001	< 0.001	0.003	0.314	< 0.001	0.879	0.042

[a]The co-infections for the 7 NT dogs consisted of *A. platys* and *B. vogeli* (2 dogs), *A. platys* and *B. vogeli* and *Mycoplasma haemocanis* (1 dog), *A. platys* and Candidatus *M. haematoparvum* (2 dogs), *A. platys* and *M. haemocanis* (2 dogs). The co-infections in the 1 NW-NSW dogs consisted of *A. platys* and *B. vogeli*

pathogen in the dogs of Central Australia (24/51), with only 2/45 NW-NSW dogs being positive for this pathogen ($P < 0.001$, CI 0.2765–0.5758). There were no significant differences in prevalence of *B. vogeli* and haemotropic mycoplasmas between the two subpopulations. The presence of co-infections was also significantly different between the groups ($P = 0.042$, CI 0.01123–0.2188).

Discussion

Within the two study cohorts, there were conspicuous differences in the prevalence of tick-borne diseases, with all three genera (*Anaplasma, Babesia,* haemotropic *Mycoplasma*) of tick-borne pathogens being less common in NW-NSW than Central Australia. This was correlated with both a much lower prevalence of ticks and also better nutrition and overall health status. The results of this study build on previous work concerning vector-borne and zoonotic infectious diseases of free living dogs in and around Aboriginal communities [2–5, 25, 31, 49, 50].

There was a statistically significant association between the presence of *B. vogeli* and/or *A. platys* and the presence of anaemia and/or thrombocytopenia. Having said this, in the great majority of dogs, the deficiency in red cell mass and platelet numbers was minor, and unlikely to give rise to clinical disease. This is in accordance with the literature, where *B. vogeli* is considered less virulent than its two sibling species and tends to produce subclinical disease, except in young or immunosuppressed dogs [9, 13, 15, 16]. *A. platys* strains in Australia are considered minimally pathogenic, although in some dogs, especially younger dogs with co-infections with other organisms, thrombocytopenia might be severe enough to impact patients subjected to injury or surgery, e.g. dog fights or surgical neutering [3]. It might be prudent therefore to evaluate a peripheral blood smear in the field to ensure platelet numbers are adequate, or to perform a platelet function test e.g. buccal mucosal bleeding time prior to major surgery [51]. Intra-operative bleeding has not been reported as a clinical problem in the field during large-scale surgical neutering campaigns in these communities. It has been the experience of one of the authors (GB) that removing ticks is a good platelet function test, dogs with *A. platys* often having prolonged bleeding from tick attachment sites. It was of great interest to observe that there was no positive correlation, and indeed in one instance (*B. vogeli* and anaemia) there was a negative correlation, between the quantity of bacterial or protozoan DNA in blood and red cell mass or platelet count (Fig. 3). In the instance of *B. vogeli*, the simplest explanation for this finding would be that when anaemia occurs in the setting of long-standing subclinical infection, anaemia is due to sequestration of infected erythrocytes by the mononuclear phagocytic system, reducing or eliminating parasitised red cells and the organisms they contain from peripheral blood.

Although commonly encountered, haemotropic mycoplasmas did not impact on haematologic values in a clinically meaningful fashion. This is also in accord with the traditional view from the literature, which suggests that in the absence of splenectomy or immunocompromise, neither *M. haemocanis* nor *Candidatus* M. haematoparvum causes haemolytic anaemia [4, 5, 52–54].

The most striking observation of the present work was an unequivocal negative finding: PCR testing of whole blood, even after a special pre-incubation step using BAPGM media (in one subgroup), failed to detect *Bartonella* nucleic acid from any dog in either of the two sites tested. Likewise, there was no serological evidence for previous *Bartonella* infection. Although dogs around the world can be infected with numerous *Bartonella* spp., *B. henselae, B. vinsonii* subsp. *berkhoffii* and *B. koehlerae* were most frequently documented in sick dogs in the United States [55]. Following the initial isolation of *Bartonella vinsonii* subsp. *berkhoffii*, tick exposure was determined to be a risk factor for prior exposure based upon IFA seroreactivity [56]. Based upon the high prevalence of both *Ehrlichia canis* and *B. vinsonii* subsp. *berkhoffii* antibodies in dogs from the south-eastern United States [56], *R. sanguineus* was a suspected vector, although this has never been confirmed [57]. Similar to the results of this study, a subsequent investigation from

Brazil failed to identify an association between *E. canis* serology or PCR positivity and *Bartonella* spp. antibodies [58]. However, as recent research has documented at least four phylogenetically distinct clades (that justify different species designation) within the morphological designation *R. sanguineus* [59], a role for *Bartonella* spp. transmission for '*R. sanguineus*' clades around the world requires further study.

Cats are underrepresented as companion animals in most Aboriginal communities, certainly in the ones sampled in Central Australia. So the likelihood of dogs contacting any of the feline-adapted *Bartonella* (*B. henselae, B. clarridgeiae, B. elizabethiae*) via cat fleas would be minimal, especially in a hot, dry, arid environment where fleas are rare to absent, while brown dog ticks are conspicuously common. Furthermore, *B. vinsonii* subsp. *berkhoffii* has yet to be reported from any Australian jurisdiction, possibly because Australia does not have wolves or coyotes, the natural reservoir for this organism in North America [60–62]. In the context of sick dogs, both IFA serology and PCR from blood lack diagnostic sensitivity as compared to BAPGM enrichment blood culture [55]. In addition, because *B. henselae, B. vinsonii* subsp. *berkhoffii* and *B. koehlerae* strains in Australia might differ antigenically from North American strains used for testing in this study and would be unlikely to cross react with indigenous Australian marsupial strains [44, 63], negative serology results should be viewed with caution. These factors could account for the absence of published reports of canine bartonellosis from Australia, despite the widespread availability of multiplex PCR assays.[1] It is important that studies such as this be extended to regions where fleas are more common and dogs encounter more than one tick species, such as the coastal parts of tropical north Queensland, because in this environment *Bartonella* spp. may be more likely to 'spill over' from cats and foxes to dogs.

It is quite difficult to directly compare the work presented here with that done previously in Australia, as the communities sampled were somewhat different, as were the methodologies employed, including the specifics of the PCR assays. Without equivocation, Traub's group has shown dogs from central Australian indigenous communities had much higher prevalence of all tick-borne pathogens than dogs in Darwin, which in turn had higher overall prevalences than south east Queensland and Sydney [4, 5]. Presumably this reflects the better condition of owned dogs in Darwin, with better ectoparasitic control, nutrition and so forth, while in Brisbane and its environs and Sydney, *Rhipicephalus* is just not sufficiently common to be an effective disease vector, the hard tick *Ixodes holocyclus* being the preponderant tick species. It should be noted that our 'healthy' dogs from the NT living in indigenous communities were, on the whole, more affected by tick-borne pathogens than the 'affected' cohort of hospital patients in the 2015 study by Hii et al. [4].

Dogs in indigenous communities sampled were generally judged to be healthy, despite the commonness of tick-borne diseases. The presence of tick-borne pathogens causing subclinical anaemia and thrombocytopenia complicates the diagnosis of diseases common in owned dogs (such as primary immune-mediated haemolytic anaemia [IMHA] and thrombocytopenia [IMT]) in nearby regions such as Alice Springs and Darwin, as there is some flow of dogs between cities in the NT and the surrounding communities. The response to specific anti-infective therapy might be required to dissect out the contribution of various infectious agents.

In dogs living in indigenous communities, the high prevalence of tick-borne diseases requires addressing, even though the majority of dogs in our study appeared in reasonable condition. Our view is that the regular application of acaricides, such as topical moxidectin (especially inexpensive off-label 'pour on' cattle formulations), represents a key control measure, perhaps combined with environmental treatment to reduce the number of adult and juvenile ticks, so that immunologically naïve pups are not subjected to sudden inoculation. It is difficult to envisage how imidiocarb or doxycycline could be routinely given in an indigenous setting, because of the requirement to treat dogs for several consecutive days with painful injections or tablets, respectively. If dogs from Aboriginal communities become translocated into pet homes in places like Alice Springs or Darwin, haematologic and multiplex qPCR testing would be prudent, so that subclinical carriers of these blood-borne pathogens could be treated to either eliminate the infection, or more realistically, reduce the extent of the infection so that clinical manifestations are unlikely to develop and transmission to dogs in non-endemic areas is minimised. Likewise, blood donors in such geographies should be tested by multiplex qPCR, as transfusion of blood containing these usually mild pathogens might cause more substantive issues if given to patients with IMHA and/or IMT, where immunosuppressive therapy will be on-going, or after splenectomy.

This study incorporated a 'One Health' perspective as bartonellosis, coxiellosis and brucellosis are all important zoonoses, with dogs from Aboriginal communities potentially serving as sentinels for these infections. Bartonellosis has been discussed at length already. In relation to coxiellosis, 4/96 dogs tested sero-positive for *C. burnetii* infection. None of these was symptomatic, but worryingly two of the dogs were sexually intact females, including a pregnant bitch. Despite the apparently high prevalence of anti-*Coxiella* antibodies in dogs living around indigenous communities, Q fever is not considered a common or important disease of Aboriginal people, despite the very close relationship they have with their dogs [40]. One of the seropositive dogs in the NW-NSW cohort was actually a kelpie belonging to a drover, rather than residing in an Aboriginal community. The Moree region subpopulation was also tested for serological evidence for subclinical brucellosis. Only one dog tested weak-positive with the Rose Bengal method, but as it was negative on complement fixation testing, it was classed as negative as per laboratory protocol, although the dog could remain subclinically infected or have eliminated the infection resulting in a residual antibody titre. From a 'One Health' perspective, this report importantly draws light to both negative and positive dog data which are equally instructive for both canine and human health.

Conclusions

The vector-borne pathogens *B. vogeli, A. platys* and haemotropic mycoplasmas were prevalent in dogs living in Aboriginal communities in Central Australia, but less common in similar environments in NW-NSW. Although a minimally pathogenic bacterial infection in dogs and humans, the potential for *A. platys* infection should be investigated among sick human individuals in indigenous communities, due to previously mentioned reports in humans overseas. *B. vogeli* was associated with anaemia, and to a lesser extent thrombocytopenia, *A. platys* was strongly associated with thrombocytopenia, whereas neither haemotropic mycoplasma was associated with any haematologic aberration. Similar to the dogs in this study, co-infection with *A. platys* and *Candidatus* M. haematoparvum was reported in a veterinarian, who was concurrently infected with *B. henselae* [64]. Polymicrobial combinations of these infectious agents were common in dogs, yet they had little discernible clinical impact. Serological evidence for coxiellosis was evident in one male and three female dogs, yet spill over into in-contact humans in these geographical regions is unknown. The presence of tick-borne pathogens in dogs residing or sourced from these indigenous communities must be considered when investigating haematologic disorders such as anaemia and thrombocytopenia. It remains problematic to differentiate between primary IMHA or IMT from disease secondary to the immune response to these pathogens, or to the actions of the pathogens themselves. Testing of blood donors in areas endemic for these blood-borne pathogens is mandatory, to prevent infection of naïve patients.

Endnotes

[1]The authors are aware of an unpublished case of *Bartonella henselae* infection in a 10-year-old 'Blue Heeler' in July 2014. The dog's major clinical problem was severe thrombocytopenia. Blood was tested by Idexx; the multiplex PCR was negative for *Babesia*, *Anaplasma*, and haemotropic mycoplasmas but positive for *Bartonella* and typed as *B. henselae* based on sequence analysis. The dog was initially treated empirically with doxycycline and two treatments of imidiocarb, 2 weeks apart. It was then given a combination of doxycycline and enrofloxacin and made a full recovery. It was retested for *Bartonella* 2 months later and was PCR-negative. Given that qPCR directly from blood is an insensitive means for detecting bartonellosis in dogs, horses and humans, negative results are not surprising. It is likely more dogs in Australia have had clinical bartonellosis.

Additional files

Additional file 1: Figure S1. Physical appearance of dogs from Yuendumu. The condition of dogs in Central Australia, NT (a) was lower than those dogs from Moree, N-W NSW (b), yet overall their body condition scores were seen as fair. (Images with permission and courtesy of Dr. Graeme Brown).

Additional file 2: Figure S2. Pups from Yuendumu, Central Australia. Condition of young pups (a) are poor to fair, with clear visibility of ribs and 'tucked up' appearance of abdomen. Some dogs are in better condition than others (b). Landscape is seen as typical red sandy soil, with signs of erosion and negligible grass or plant cover. (Images with permission and courtesy of Dr. Graeme Brown).

Additional file 3: Figure S3. Image of dog sampled in Moree distinct. The different geographical appearance of the landscapes in Moree and Ti Tree are evident from this picture. The dog appears to be a pedigree hybrid type with robust physical appearance in contrast to dogs from the NT.

Additional file 4: Dataset upon which publication conclusions rely.

Abbreviations

BAPGM: Bartonella α-proteobacteria growth medium; C_T: Cycling threshold; DNA: Deoxyribonucleic acid; EDTA: Ethylenediaminetetraacetic acid; IFA: Indirect immunoflourescent antibody assay; IMHA: Immune-mediated haemolytic anaemia; IMT: Immune-mediated thrombocytopenia; NSW: New South Wales; NT: Northern Territory; PCR: Polymerase chain reaction; PCV: Packed cell volume; qPCR: Real-time PCR; RI: Reference intervals

Acknowledgements

We thank Anne and Chris Brown for helping with the collection of blood samples. The authors are grateful to Karen Lightowler, Animal Management Coordinator, Central Desert Regional Council and Jock Jones, the council ranger in Moree. The authors would also like to thank Evelyn Hall of The University of Sydney for statistical advice, Alan Marcus for advice on the manuscript and Julie Bradley, Intracellular Pathogens Research Laboratory, North Carolina State University for *Bartonella* serology results. Richard Malik is supported by the Valentine Charlton Bequest of the Centre for Veterinary Education of the University of Sydney. Christine Gotsis from The University of Sydney's Veterinary Pathology Diagnostic Services provided outstanding laboratory support.

Funding

This research was supported by a grant obtained from the Canine Research Foundation. The work was supported by a linkage grant from the Australian Research Council and financial support from Arkay Nominees, Centre for Veterinary Education and the Valentine Charlton Bequest.

Authors' contributions

GB, JMN and RM conceived of the study. GB, RM and EB collected the samples. AJS and RM analysed the data and drafted the manuscript. AJS performed the *C. burnetii* serological assays, with contributions from KLB and JMN. DJM organised the *B. suis* serological screening and assisted in sample collection in NW-NSW. EBB organised the specialised *Bartonella* spp. testing and assisted in blood collection from dogs in Central Australia. All authors read and approved the final manuscript.

Consent for publication

Not applicable.

Competing interests

The authors declare that they have no competing interests.

Author details

[1]University of Sydney School of Veterinary Science, Building B14, Sydney, NSW 2006, Australia. [2]Department of Microbiology and Infectious Diseases, St. Vincent's Hospital, Sydney, NSW 2010, Australia. [3]Intracellular Pathogens Research Laboratory, Center for Comparative Medicine and Translational Research, College of Veterinary Medicine, North Carolina State University, Raleigh, NC, USA. [4]School of Animal & Veterinary Sciences, Charles Sturt University, Locked Bag 588, Wagga Wagga, NSW 2678, Australia. [5]Centre for Veterinary Education, University of Sydney, Sydney, NSW 2006, Australia.

References

1. Barker SC, Walker AR. Ticks of Australia. The species that infest domestic animals and humans. Zootaxa. 2014;2014(3816):1–144.
2. Barker EN, Langton DA, Helps CR, Brown G, Malik R, Shaw SE, et al. Haemoparasites of free-roaming dogs associated with several remote Aboriginal communities in Australia. BMC Vet Res. 2012;8:55.
3. Brown GK, Canfield PJ, Dunstan RH, Roberts TK, Martin AR, Brown CS, et al. Detection of *Anaplasma platys* and *Babesia canis vogeli* and their impact on platelet numbers in free-roaming dogs associated with remote Aboriginal communities in Australia. Aust Vet J. 2006;84(9):321–5.
4. Hii SF, Kopp SR, Thompson MF, O'Leary CA, Rees RL, Traub RJ. Canine vector-borne disease pathogens in dogs from south-east Queensland and north-east Northern Territory. Aust Vet J. 2012;90(4):130–5.
5. Hii SF, Traub RJ, Thompson MF, Henning J, O'Leary CA, Burleigh A, et al. Canine tick-borne pathogens and associated risk factors in dogs presenting with and without clinical signs consistent with tick-borne diseases in northern Australia. Aust Vet J. 2015;93(3):58–66.
6. Institute of Medical and Veterinary Science SA. 37th annual report of the council, July 1974 to June 1975; 1976. p. 117.
7. Mahoney DF, Johnston LAY, Cooper MG. The epidemiology of babesiasis. Sydney: Australian Veterinary Association; 1980.
8. Johnston LAY. Epidemiology of bovine babesiosis in Northern Queensland. Aust Vet J. 1967;43(10):427–32.
9. Irwin PJ, Hutchinson GW. Clinical and pathological findings of *Babesia* infections in dogs. Aust Vet J. 1991;68(6):204–9.
10. Hill MWM, Bolton BL. Canine babesiosis in Queensland. Aust Vet J. 1966;42:84–6.
11. Martin AR, Dunstan RH, Roberts TK, Brown GK. *Babesia canis vogeli*: a novel PCR for its detection in dogs in Australia. Exp Parasitol. 2006;112(1):63–5.
12. Jefferies R, Ryan UM, Muhlnickel CJ, Irwin PJ. Two species of canine Babesia in Australia: detection and characterization by PCR. J Parasitol. 2003;89(2): 409–12.
13. Irwin PJ. Canine Babesiosis. Vet Clin N Am Small Anim Pract. 2010;40(6): 1141-+.
14. Köster LS, Lobetti RG, Kelly P. Canine babesiosis: a perspective on clinical complications, biomarkers, and treatment. Vet Med. 2015;6:119–28.
15. Schoeman JP. Canine babesiosis. Onderstepoort J Vet Res. 2009;76(1):59–66.
16. Penzhorn BL. Why is Southern African canine babesiosis so virulent? An evolutionary perspective. Parasit Vectors. 2011;13:4.
17. Jefferies R, Ryan UM, Jardine J, Broughton DK, Robertson ID, Irwin PJ. Blood, bull terriers and Babesiosis: further evidence for direct transmission of *Babesia gibsoni* in dogs. Aust Vet J. 2007;85(11):459–63.
18. Muhlnickel CJ, Jefferies R, Morgan-Ryan UM, Irwin PJ. Babesia gibsoni infection in three dogs in Victoria. Aust Vet J. 2002;80(10):606–10.
19. Macintire DK, Boudreaux MK, West GD, Bourne C, Wright JC, Conrad PA. Babesia gibsoni infection among dogs in the southeastern United States. J Am Vet Med Assoc. 2002;220(3):325–9.
20. Miyama T, Sakata Y, Shimada Y, Ogino S, Watanabe M, Itamoto K, et al. Epidemiological survey of Babesia gibsoni infection in dogs in eastern Japan. J Vet Med Sci. 2005;67(5):467–71.
21. Matsuu A, Kawabe A, Koshida Y, Ikadai H, Okano S, Higuchi S. Incidence of canine Babesia gibsoni infection and subclinical infection among Tosa dogs in Aomori Prefecture, Japan. J Vet Med Sci. 2004;66(8):893–7.
22. Yamane I, Conrad PA, Gardner I. *Babesia gibsoni* infection in dogs. J Protozool Res. 1993;3(4):111–25.
23. Conrad P, Thomford J, Yamane I, Whiting J, Bosma L, Uno T, et al. Hemolytic anemia caused by *Babesia gibsoni* infection in dogs. J Am Vet Med Assoc. 1991;199(5):601–5.
24. Birkenheuer AJ, Levy MG, Stebbins M, Poore M, Breitschwerdt E. Serosurvey of antiBabesia antibodies in stray dogs and American pit bull terriers and American Staffordshire terriers from North Carolina. J Am Anim Hosp Assoc. 2003;39(6):551–7.
25. Brown GK, Martin AR, Roberts TK, Aitken RJ. Detection of *Ehrlichia platys* in dogs in Australia. Aust Vet J. 2001;79(8):554–8.
26. Eddlestone SM, Gaunt SD, Neer TM, Boudreaux CM, Gill A, Haschke E, et al. PCR detection of Anaplasma platys in blood and tissue of dogs during acute phase of experimental infection. Exp Parasitol. 2007;115(2):205–10.
27. Ferreira RF, Cerqueira AMF, Pereira AM, Ferreira MS, Almosny NRP. Hematologic parameters in polymerase chain reaction-positive and -negative dogs for Anaplasma platys presenting platelet inclusion bodies. Int J Appl Res Vet Med. 2008;6(3):185–90.
28. Gaunt SD, Beall MJ, Stillman BA, Lorentzen L, Diniz PPVP, Chandrashekar R, et al. Experimental infection and co-infection of dogs with Anaplasma platys and Ehrlichia canis: hematologic, serologic and molecular findings. Parasit Vectors. 2010;8:3.
29. Hetzel NJL, Barker EN, Helps CR, Tasker S, Arteaga A, Barrs VR, et al. Prevalence of canine haemotropic mycoplasma infections in Sydney, Australia. Vet Rec. 2012;171(5):126-+.
30. Hii SF, Kopp SR, Abdad MY, Thompson MF, O'Leary CA, Rees RL, et al. Molecular evidence supports the role of dogs as potential reservoirs for *Rickettsia felis*. Vector Borne Zoonotic Dis. 2011;11(8):1007–12.
31. Hii S-F, Kopp SR, Thompson MF, O'Leary CA, Rees RL, Traub RJ. Molecular evidence of *Rickettsia felis* infection in dogs from northern territory, Australia. Parasit Vectors. 2011;11:4.
32. Barrs VR, Beatty JA, Wilson BJ, Evans N, Gowan R, Baral RM, et al. Prevalence of *Bartonella* species, *Rickettsia felis*, haemoplasmas and the *Ehrlichia* group in the blood of cats and fleas in eastern Australia. Aust Vet J. 2010;88(5):160–5.
33. Kaewmongkol G, Kaewmongkol S, Fleming PA, Adams PJ, Ryan U, Irwin PJ, et al. Zoonotic *Bartonella* species in fleas and blood from red foxes in Australia. Vector Borne Zoonotic Dis. 2011;11(12):1549–53.
34. Dillon B, Valenzuela J, Don R, Blanckenberg D, Wigney DI, Malik R, et al. Limited diversity among human isolates of *Bartonella henselae*. J Clin Microbiol. 2002;40(12):4691–9.
35. Iredell J, Blanckenberg D, Arvand M, Grauling S, Feil EJ, Birtles RJ. Characterization of the natural population of *Bartonella henselae* by multilocus sequence typing. J Clin Microbiol. 2003;41(11):5071–9.
36. Kaewmongkol G, Kaewmongkol S, Burmej H, Bennett MD, Fleming PA, Adams PJ, et al. Diversity of *Bartonella* species detected in arthropod vectors from animals in Australia. Comp Immunol Microbiol Infect Dis. 2011; 34(5):411–7.
37. Kaewmongkol G, Kaewmongkol S, McInnes LM, Burmej H, Bennett MD, Adams PJ, et al. Genetic characterization of flea-derived *Bartonella* species from native animals in Australia suggests host-parasite co-evolution. Infect Genet Evol. 2011;11(8):1868–72.
38. Maurin M, Raoult D. Q fever. Clin Microbiol Rev. 1999;12(4):518–53.
39. Babudieri B. Q fever: A zoonosis. Adv Vet Sci. 1959;5(81):82–154.
40. Shapiro AJ, Norris JM, Heller J, Brown G, Malik R, Bosward KL. Seroprevalence of Coxiella burnetii in Australian dogs. Zoonoses Public Health. 2016;63:458.
41. Wolf LA, Cherry NA, Maggi RG, Breitschwerdt EB. In pursuit of a stealth pathogen: laboratory diagnosis of bartonellosis. Clin Microbiol Newsl. 2014; 36(5):33–9.

42. Breitschwerdt EB, Linder KL, Day MJ, Maggi RG, Chomel BB, Kempf VAJ. Koch's postulates and the pathogenesis of comparative infectious disease causation associated with *Bartonella* species. J Comp Pathol. 2013;148(2–3): 115–25.
43. Molloy S, Burleigh A, Dürr S, Ward M. Roaming behaviour of dogs in four remote Aboriginal communities in the Northern Territory, Australia: preliminary investigations. Aust Vet J. 2017;95(3):55–63.
44. Hegarty BC, Bradley JM, Lappin MR, Balakrishnan N, Mascarelli PE, Breitschwerdt EB. Analysis of Seroreactivity against cell culture-derived Bartonella spp. antigens in dogs. J Vet Intern Med. 2014;28(1):38–41.
45. Mylonakis ME, Soubasis N, Balakrishnan N, Theodorou K, Kasabalis D, Saridomichelakis M, et al. Molecular identification of Bartonella species in dogs with leishmaniosis (Leishmania infantum) with or without cytological evidence of arthritis. Vet Microbiol. 2014;174(1–2):272–5.
46. Shapiro AJ, Bosward K, Heller J, Norris JM. Seroprevalence of Coxiella burnetii in domesticated and feral cats in eastern Australia. Vet Microbiol. 2015;177:154.
47. Mylonakis ME, Leontides L, Farmaki R, Kostoulas P, Koutinas AF, Christopher M. Effect of anticoagulant and storage conditions on platelet size and clumping in healthy dogs. J Vet Diagn Investig. 2008;20(6):774–9.
48. James D, Golovsky G, Thornton J, Goodchild L, Havlicek M, Martin P, et al. Clinical management of Brucella suis infection in dogs and implications for public health. Aust Vet J. 2017;95(1–2):19–25.
49. Hii S-F, Abdad MY, Kopp SR, Stenos J, Rees RL, Traub RJ. Seroprevalence and risk factors for *Rickettsia felis* exposure in dogs from Southeast Queensland and the northern territory, Australia. Parasit Vectors. 2013;6:1–7.
50. Brown GK, Martin AR, Roberts TK, Dunstan RH. Molecular detection of *Anaplasma platys* in lice collected from dogs in Australia. Aust Vet J. 2005; 83(1–2):101–2.
51. Lanza-Perea M, Zieger U, Qurollo BA, Hegarty BC, Pultorak EL, Kumthekar S, et al. Intraoperative bleeding in dogs from Grenada Seroreactive to Anaplasma platys and Ehrlichia canis. J Vet Intern Med. 2014;28(6):1702–7.
52. Tennant KV, Barker EN, Polizopoulou Z, Helps CR, Tasker S. Real-time quantitative polymerase chain reaction detection of haemoplasmas in healthy and unhealthy dogs from Central Macedonia, Greece. J Small Anim Pract. 2011;52(12):645–9.
53. Warman SM, Helps CR, Barker EN, Day S, Sturgess K, Day MJ, et al. Haemoplasma infection is not a common cause of canine immune-mediated haemolytic anaemia in the UK. J Small Anim Pract. 2010;51(10): 534–9.
54. Roura X, Peters IR, Altet L, Tabar MD, Barker EN, Planellas M, et al. Prevalence of hemotropic mycoplasmas in healthy and unhealthy cats and dogs in Spain. J Vet Diagn Investig. 2010;22(2):270–4.
55. Perez Vera C, Diniz PPVP, Pultorak EL, Maggi RG, Breitschwerdt EB. An unmatched case controlled study of clinicopathologic abnormalities in dogs with Bartonella infection. Comp Immunol Microbiol Infect Dis. 2013;36(5): 481–7.
56. Pappalardo BL, Correa MT, York CC, Peat CY, Breitschwerdt EB. Epidemiologic evaluation of the risk factors associated with exposure and seroreactivity to Bartonella vinsonii in dogs. Am J Vet Res. 1997; 58(5):467–71.
57. Billeter SA, Levy MG, Chomel BB, Breitschwerdt EB. Vector transmission of Bartonella species with emphasis on the potential for tick transmission. Med Vet Entomol. 2008;22(1):1–15.
58. Diniz PPVP, Schwartz DS, Morais HSA, Breitschwerdt EB. Surveillance for zoonotic vector-borne infections using sick dogs from southeastern Brazil. Vector Borne Zoonotic Dis. 2007;7(4):689–97.
59. Dantas-Torres F, Latrofa MS, Annoscia G, Giannelli A, Parisi A, Otranto D. Morphological and genetic diversity of Rhipicephalus sanguineus sensu lato from the new and old worlds. Parasit Vectors. 2013;6:213.
60. Chang CC, Kasten RW, Chomel BB, Simpson DC, Hew CM, Kordick DL, et al. Coyotes (*Canis latrans*) as the reservoir for a human pathogenic *Bartonella* sp.: molecular epidemiology of *Bartonella vinsonii subsp berkhoffii* infection in coyotes from central coastal California. J Clin Microbiol. 2000;38(11):4193–200.
61. Breitschwerdt EB, Kordick DL. *Bartonella* infection in animals: Carriership, reservoir potential, pathogenicity, and zoonotic potential for human infection. Clin Microbiol Rev. 2000;13(3):428-+.
62. Chomel BB, Boulouis HJ, Breitschwerdt EB. Cat scratch disease and other zoonotic *Bartonella* infections. J Am Vet Med Assoc. 2004;224(8):1270–9.
63. Balakrishnan N, Cherry NA, Linder KE, Pierce E, Sontakke N, Hegarty BC, et al. Experimental infection of dogs with Bartonella henselae and Bartonella vinsonii subsp berkhoffii. Vet Immunol Immunopathol. 2013;156(1–2):153–8.
64. Maggi RG, Mascarelli PE, Havenga LN, Naidoo V, Breitschwerdt EB. Co-infection with Anaplasma platys, Bartonella henselae and Candidatus Mycoplasma haematoparvum in a veterinarian. Parasit Vectors. 2013;6:103.

Characterization of the bacterial gut microbiota of piglets suffering from new neonatal porcine diarrhoea

Marie Louise Hermann-Bank[1], Kerstin Skovgaard[1], Anders Stockmarr[2], Mikael Lenz Strube[1], Niels Larsen[3], Hanne Kongsted[4], Hans-Christian Ingerslev[1], Lars Mølbak[1,5] and Mette Boye[1*]

Abstract

Background: In recent years, new neonatal porcine diarrhoea (NNPD) of unknown aetiology has emerged in Denmark. NNPD affects piglets during the first week of life and results in impaired welfare, decreased weight gain, and in the worst-case scenario death. Commonly used preventative interventions such as vaccination or treatment with antibiotics, have a limited effect on NNPD. Previous studies have investigated the clinical manifestations, histopathology, and to some extent, microbiological findings; however, these studies were either inconclusive or suggested that Enterococci, possibly in interaction with *Escherichia coli*, contribute to the aetiology of NNPD. This study examined ileal and colonic luminal contents of 50 control piglets and 52 NNPD piglets by means of the qPCR-based Gut Microbiotassay and 16 samples by 454 sequencing to study the composition of the bacterial gut microbiota in relation to NNPD.

Results: NNPD was associated with a diminished quantity of bacteria from the phyla Actinobacteria and Firmicutes while genus *Enterococcus* was more than 24 times more abundant in diarrhoeic piglets. The number of bacteria from the phylum Fusobacteria was also doubled in piglets suffering from diarrhoea. With increasing age, the gut microbiota of NNPD affected piglet and control piglets became more diverse. Independent of diarrhoeic status, piglets from first parity sows (gilts) possessed significantly more bacteria from family Enterobacteriaceae and species *E. coli*, and fewer bacteria from phylum Firmicutes. Piglets born to gilts had 25 times higher odds of having NNPD compared with piglets born to multiparous sows. Finally, the co-occurrence of genus *Enterococcus* and species *E. coli* contributed to the risk of having NNPD.

Conclusion: The results of this study support previous findings that points towards genus *Enterococcus* and species *E. coli* to be involved in the pathogenesis of NNPD. Moreover, the results indicate that NNPD is associated with a disturbed bacterial composition and larger variation between the diarrhoeic piglets.

Keywords: NNPD, Neonatal, Piglet, Diarrhoea, qPCR, Microbiota, Gut Microbiotassay, 454 sequencing

Background

Neonatal piglet diarrhoea is of significant importance for the pig industry because it causes economic losses due to increased morbidity and mortality, decreased weight gain, and the need for extra medications [1,2]. Obviously, it impairs the welfare of the animals in the short term, but it may also affect their health in the longer term as a consequence of disrupting the normal bacterial succession in the gastrointestinal tract [3].

Bacterial colonization of the mammalian gastrointestinal tract begins at birth [4]. This colonization is a dynamic event, and the bacterial succession is influenced by a number of factors including: mode of delivery, surrounding environment, gestational age, and genetics [5,6]. The colonization of the gut has a major impact on the host's health and disease; for example, the microbiota helps in the maturation of the gastrointestinal tract and immune system, protects against pathogen colonization through

* Correspondence: mboy@vet.dtu.dk
[1]National Veterinary Institute, Technical University of Denmark, Bülowsvej 27, 1870 Frederiksberg C, DK, Denmark
Full list of author information is available at the end of the article

competitive exclusion, and converts otherwise indigestible substances into digestible components that benefit the host [3,5,7,8]. In accordance with these roles, studies of germ-free animals, deficient of normally developed gut microbiota, show animals with an impaired and immature intestinal immune system, in addition to changes in intestinal morphology [8-10].

During the last ten years, increasing attention has been focused on a new neonatal porcine diarrhoea [11-13]. In Denmark, this diarrhoea has been named 'New Neonatal Porcine Diarrhoea' (NNPD). What distinguishes NNPD from other types of neonatal piglet diarrhoea are the following: 1) The aetiology is unknown, however, routine diagnostic protocols show that it is not caused by known enteric pathogens such as hemolytic *Escherichia coli, Clostridium difficile, Clostridium perfringens* type A or C, coronavirus, rotavirus species A or C, *Cryptosporidium* spp., *Cystoisospora suis, Giardia* spp., or *Strongyloides ransomi.* 2) Typical strategies, such as vaccination against enterotoxigenic *E. coli* and *Cl. perfringens* type C or treatment with antibiotics, do not seem to have a noteworthy effect on the diarrhoea. 3) No obvious connection between NNPD and pig farm health status or management has been demonstrated ([14,15] Larsen LE, Nielsen JP, unpublished results).

It is difficult to estimate how widespread NNPD is, mainly because of the unknown aetiology combined with a fluctuating clinical presentation [2], as well as differences in routine laboratory testing [13,15], but also because of the limited number of studies focusing on this issue. Nonetheless, a diarrhoea of much resemblance to NNPD has been described in Sweden and France [13,16,17].

This study is part of an interdisciplinary project investigating the aetiology of NNPD. Kongsted *et al.* suggested the following case-definition of NNPD: *"Non-hemorrhagic diarrhoea during the first week of life, without detection of known infectious pathogens, characterized by milk-filled stomachs and flaccid intestines at necropsy"* [15]. The same author found dissimilarities in the course and severity of NNPD among four pig farms and estimated that affected piglets had a negative average daily weight gain with an increased risk of dying, though this risk was not significant [2]. Jonach *et al.* examined the role of four enteric bacterial pathogens by fluorescence in situ hybridization (FISH) and found that simultaneous colonization of the intestinal mucosa with non-enterotoxigenic *E. coli* (non-ETEC) and *Enterococcus* spp. could be involved in the pathogenesis of NNPD [18]. Finally, several different viral assays tested negative on samples from some of the same NNPD animals that were examined in the aforementioned studies, indicating that common known viruses likely do not contribute to NNPD (Larsen LE, Nielsen JP, unpublished results).

This study investigates whether NNPD is associated with the composition of the gut microbiota obtained from piglets with and without diarrhoea. This was examined by evaluating the overall bacterial composition and relative quantitative distribution of ileal and colonic intestinal content using the Gut Microbiotassay: an assembly of 24 primer sets targeting ribosomal RNA (rRNA) genes (16S and 23S), verified to function with the high-throughput quantitative real-time PCR (qPCR) chip Access Array™ Integrated Fluidic Circuit (AA48.48) from Fluidigm [19]. As the name implies, the assay is designed to target major bacteria phyla and selected taxonomic sub-groups of the gut microbiota. The Gut Microbiotassay provides a quick overview of the distribution, as well as the relative quantity of the gut microbiota in a large number of samples simultaneously. Subsequently, PCR amplicons from ileum and colon of four case piglets and four control piglets were sequenced using 454-technology to acquire deeper taxonomic information. This approach revealed diverse gut microbial profiles associated with piglet diarrhoeic status.

Methods

Animals and sample collection

Danish pig farms affected by NNPD were identified from conversations with veterinarians and farm managers. Four pig farms that fulfilled the inclusion criteria listed in were included in the study (for more information on the selection of pigs and herds included in this study, see Kongsted *et al.* [15]). On each pig farm, approximately 15 randomly chosen sows from one farrowing batch (66 in total) were followed for a seven day period following farrowing. All newborn piglets were weighed at the beginning of the trial (average weight 1394 g, SD ± 335 g), and piglets weighing less than 800 g were excluded. All animals were subject to a daily clinical examination that paid special attention to fecal appearance on rectal swabs. Diarrhoea was defined as loose or watery feces. Based on these observations, piglets were characterized as either cases or controls: A case piglet had suffered from diarrhoea for at least two consecutive days, whereas a control piglet had never experienced diarrhoea. The inclusion criterion applied to case piglets resulted in a greater number of case piglets from gilts (approximately 66%), as piglets born to multiparous sows did not suffer from diarrhoea to the same extent as piglets born to gilts. Control piglets were as far as possible collected from litters without diarrhoea. In total 50 control piglets and 52 case piglets were selected (Table 1) and brought to the Danish Pig Research Centre, Kjellerup, for euthanization and necropsy. For

Table 1 Piglets included in the study

Age in days	3		4		5		6		7		Total			
											Gilts		Sows	
Diarrhoea	−	+	−	+	−	+	−	+	−	+	-	+	-	+
Pig farm 1	6	7			7	6					0	4	13	9
Pig farm 2			2	2	6	6			4	4	2	12	10	0
Pig farm 3			7	8			6	6			0	10	13	4
Pig farm 4	8	8			4	5					4	8	8	5
Total	14	15	9	10	17	17	6	6	4	4	6	34	44	18

The number of piglets is listed for each pig farm in accordance with age in days: (−) Control piglets without diarrhoea, (+) Case piglets with diarrhoea for ≥2 days. The column "Total" summarizes the number of piglets born to gilts or sows (multiparous sows) by farm.

ethical reasons, farmers were allowed to treat piglets for any disorder if necessary, on the condition that any such treatments were recorded for individual animals. During necropsy, intestinal contents were collected from the distal small intestine (ileum) and the large intestine (colon) of each animal and stored at −80°C until further analysis.

Pig farm inclusion criteria for studying NNPD [15]:

- A stock of more than 400 sows
- Routinely vaccinate[1] against ETEC[2] and *Cl. perfringens* type C
- Farrowing units proven to be PRRS[3] virus negative as demonstrated in blood samples tested by ELISA[4]/IPT[5] or PCR.
- NNPD has been a problem for a period of minimum 3–6 months
- Management-related diarrhoea has been excluded
- Traditional interventions such as vaccines and antibiotics have limited effect on the diarrhoea
- At least 30% of the litters are affected
- The piglets suffer from diarrhoea during the first week of life
- Random check of five case piglets should test negative for ETEC, *Cl. perfringens* type C and Rotavirus by routine diagnostic examination

DNA extraction

Based on development work comparing various extraction methods, the Maxwell® 16 LEV Blood DNA Kit (Promega, Madison, WI, USA) was determined to be the optimal method, based on providing sufficient DNA yields and acceptable purities. According to manufacturer's recommendations, total DNA was extracted from intestinal content using this kit. A total of 200 mg of intestinal contents were suspended in 600 µl PBS and vortexed until visually homogeneous. The samples were centrifuged for 2 min at 200 × *g*, and the supernatant was transferred to new tubes. A volume of 350 µl of lysis buffer was then added, and the bacterial cells were lysed by bead beading (Tissuelyser II, Qiagen, Hilden, Germany) for 2.5 min at 20.0 hertz with a 5 mm steel bead (Qiagen). Subsequently, samples were centrifuged for 1 min at 1000 × *g* at 4°C, after which the supernatant was transferred to novel 2 ml tubes and mixed manually with 30 µl Proteinase K (Promega). Next, samples were incubated for 30 min at 56°C, and centrifuged at 13 000 × *g* for 1 min. The entire suspension was transferred to the sample inlets on the cartridge, and 50 µl of elution buffer was added to the bottom of the elution tubes. The cartridges were prepared according to the manufacturer's instructions [20] and the settings "Research Mode", "LEV Mode", "DNA", and "Blood/Cell" were selected for DNA extraction using the Maxwell® 16 Instrument (Promega). Finally, tubes were centrifuged at 20 000 × *g* for 3 min to settle any magnetic bead leftovers, and the DNA was moved to new tubes. DNA concentration and purity was measured using the Nanodrop® ND-1000 (NanoDrop Technologies Inc., Wilmington, Germany) spectrophotometer, and DNA was stored at −20°C until further analysis.

Analysis of bacterial profiles with use of the Gut Microbiotassay

To obtain a bacterial profile of the intestinal content, this study used the Gut Microbiotassay designed for the AA48.48 [19] with a few modifications. In order to improve the performance of the primer sets "Domain Bacteria B V4-V5" and "Phylum Firmicutes" degenerate nucleotides were introduced: Nucleotide 11 was changed from C to M (C/A), and nucleotide 5 from T to Y (T/C), (5′-3′ direction), in the forward or reverse primer, respectively (Additional file 1). All remaining primer sets were identical to those previously published as 'The Gut Microbiotassay' [19]. Primers were purchased from Eurofins MWG Synthesis GmbH (Ebersberg, Germany) and stored at −20°C.

In brief, the AA48.48 is a qPCR platform that is capable of running 48 × 48 = 2304 individual reactions simultaneously, and it enables quick and easy library preparation for 454 sequencing [21]. The AA48.48 was processed and prepared following the 'Access Array System™ User Guide' [21], with and without adding the Access Array Barcode Library for the 454 GS FLX Titanium Sequencer (454BL), as previously described [19]. Primers targeting bacteria at the taxonomic level of species were not tagged or included for sequencing, as these amplicons were regarded as contributing little information due to their specificity. However, analysis at the species-level was possible using the information obtained at higher taxonomic levels. All samples were diluted to 50 ng/µl with nuclease-free water (Ambion Inc., Austin, USA). Primers were diluted to 4 µM with 20× Access Array Loading buffer and nuclease-free water (Ambion Inc.). Master mix was a mixture of: 10× FastStart High Fidelity Reaction Buffer with 18 mM $MgCl_2$ (Roche Diagnostics, GmbH, Mannheim, Germany), 25 mM $MgCl_2$ (Roche),

DMSO (Roche), 20× Access Array Loading Reagent (Fluidigm Corporation, South San Francisco, CA, USA), 50× ROX (Invitrogen Corporation, Carlsbad, CA, USA), 20× EvaGreen® (Biotium, Inc., Hayward, CA, USA), 10 mM PCR Grade Nucleotide Mix (Roche), and 5 U/μl FastStart High Fidelity Enzyme Blend (Roche), in final concentrations of 1×, 2.7 mM, 5%, 1×, 0.5×, 1×, 200 μM, and 0.05 U/μl, respectively. Sample mix was prepared from 3 μl master mix, 1 μl 454BL (2 μM) (Fluidigm), and 1 μl DNA (50 ng/μl) as the very last step before running the array (without the 454BL: 4 μl master mix and 1 μl DNA (50 μg/μl)). When the PCR reaction had finished, the barcoded PCR amplicons were harvested and stored at −20°C.

Next generation sequencing

Samples from two representative animals were selected from each farm: one piglet with NNPD and one piglet without NNPD, giving a total of 16 samples to be sequenced (when samples from both the ileum and colon of each animal were included). Piglets were chosen to be approximately the same age (5 or 6 days old). Concentrations of the respective PCR amplicons for each animal were determined using the Agilent 1000 chip (Agilent Technologies, Waldbronn, Germany). Amplicons were subsequently pooled in equal concentrations and size-separated by running the amplicons for 86 min, 90 V, in a 0.7% Seakem® LE Agarose gel (Lonza Rockland, Rockland, ME, USA) followed by incubation for 30 min in 0.0004% ethidium bromide for staining. By means of UV radiation from the Bio-Rad Universal hood II (Segrate, Milan, Italy) gel bands were visualized and bands spanning the size range of the primer products (200–900 base pairs) were excised. Finally, the Qiaquick Gel Extraction Kit (Qiagen) was used to purify DNA from the gel. This pool of 1615.7 ng DNA (260/280 nm-ratio: 1.97) derived from ileal and colonic luminal contents of 8 different animals was sequenced on a half PicoTiterPlate™ by a 454 GS FLX Titanium Sequencer (Roche) via LGC Genomics (GmbH, Berlin, Germany).

Data analysis

Relative quantification of quantification cycle (Cq) values

Data analysis was conducted as described in a previously published methodology article [19]: Raw Cq values were exported from 'Fluidigm Real-Time PCR Analysis' software version 3.0.2 to Microsoft Excel. To even out possible variation between the AA48.48 runs, all Cq values were normalized to an Interplate Calibrator. Next, Cq values from each sample were normalized to their respective "Domain Bacteria B V4-V5" primer set, thereby calculating the relative quantification.

Principal Component Analysis on normalized Cq data

Principal Component Analysis (PCA) was conducted in the software package R, version 3.1.0 [22]. All normalized data were initially transformed with the natural logarithm (ln). Next, primer sets with less than 50% recorded Cq values were excluded from the analysis, and in the same manner, samples that resulted in less than 50% registered Cq values were removed. For the remaining primer sets, missing values were substituted with the lowest registered primer-specific value. Data were scaled by the individual primer mean and standard deviation for PCA. The number of components to be investigated further was determined by visual inspection of scree plots of eigenvalues; based on an inflection point or when the components explained > 60% variance (Additional file 2). All possible combinations of included principal components were visualized to ensure that no important clustering was overlooked. The number of components used for graphical representation in the PCA was set at two to ease interpretation. Samples used for 454 sequencing were pinpointed from the PCA results. In order for samples to be considered for sequencing the samples were represented with luminal content from both ileum and colon, and none of these were allowed to have outlying coordinates in the PCA, but were somewhat in the centre of its respective category (Control_colon; Case_colon; Control_ileum; and Case_ileum). Linear discriminant analysis (LDA) based on leave-one-out cross-validation was used to classify observations into cases or controls by their Fluidigm-derived microbial profile and to estimate how well this classification corresponded with the actual status of the sample. This classification was followed up with a multivariate analysis of variance (MANOVA) using Wilks Lambda statistic.

Statistics on the Gut Microbiotassay

Bacterial profiles obtained from the Gut Microbiotassay were used to study the gut microbiota of piglets with and without NNPD. For the statistical calculations all values were initially ln-transformed. A linear mixed-effect model was then applied to each primer set separately with randomized effect of herd origin:

$$\ln(Y_i) = a_{Gut\ Section(i),Status(i)} + a_{Gilt(i)} + a_{Treatment(i)} + \beta_{Status(i)} \cdot Age_i + \beta \cdot diarrhoea_i + \eta \cdot Y_{herd(i)} + \varepsilon_i, i = 1, \ldots, 102 \quad (1)$$

, where *Status*(*i*) indicates the status of the *i*'th animal, and where $Y_{herd(i)}$ is a normalized Gaussian stochastic variable indicating the randomized effect of herd, indexed by the herd of the *i*'th animal, so that animals from the same herd share the random effect. The model is applied for different responses *Y*, as listed in the first column in Table 2. The following variables were included as deterministic effects in the model: Gut section (ileum versus colon), Status (diarrhoeic versus healthy), Gilt (born to a gilt versus born to a multiparous sow), Percentage of diarrhoea (number of days with diarrhoea/days of age × 100), Treatment (treated versus non-treated animal – this category only involves case piglets), Age (days). The interaction between Gut section and Status was also included to examine if possible diarrhoea-causing agents could be traced to a specific gut section. Additionally, the interaction between Status and Age was included to study whether the effect of age differed between case and control piglets. For each primer set as response variable, the model was reduced by backwards stepwise elimination, resulting in a series of primer-specific final models. Model reduction was performed as likelihood ratio tests. Model fit for each primer set was assessed through residual analysis of the model residuals corrected for random effects and the estimated random effects themselves, using standard techniques. These analyses were consistent with standard model behavior. The effect of gender and birth weight in relation to status was also evaluated. Significances in the final models were reported through p-values.

Previous studies have suggested that simultaneous colonization with *E. coli* and Enterococci species may be a cause of neonatal porcine diarrhoea [13,18,23,24]. This co-occurrence was also implied using the aforementioned model (as bacteria belonging to these taxonomical groups displayed the highest estimated fold change differences being more numerous in diarrhoeic piglets compared to control piglets (Tables 2 and 3)), thus, this was further investigated. A logistic regression model with randomized effect of herd origin, fit by penalized quasi-likelihood, was used to determine if the odds of NNPD was associated with the following variables: Gut section, Gilt, Age, genus *Enterococcus*, class Beta- and Gammaproteobacteria, family Enterobacteriaceae, species *E. coli*, as well as possible interaction in between bacteria, and between bacteria and gut section:

$$\begin{aligned} logit(p_i) &= a_{Gut\ section(i)} + a_{Gilt(i)} + \beta_{Age} \cdot Age_i \\ &+ \sum_{j=1}^{4} \beta_{j,Gut\ section(i)} bacteria_{j,i} \\ &+ \sum_{k=1}^{4} \sum_{\ell \neq k} \beta_{k,l} bacteria_{k,i} bacteria_{\ell,i} + \eta Y_{herd(i)} \end{aligned} \tag{2}$$

, where $bacteria_1$-$bacteria_4$ are genus *Enterococcus*, class Beta- and Gammaproteobacteria, family Enterobacteriaceae, and species *E. coli*, respectively, where $bacteria_{j,i}$ is the value of $bacteria_j$ animal i, where Age_i is the age in days of animal i, and where $Y_{herd(i)}$ is the random effect component corresponding to the herd of animal i.

The models were validated through graphical procedures. A p-value of less than 0.05 was considered significant. Statistical analyses were performed in R [22].

Bioinformatics analysis of 454 sequencing data

Sequencing data available at NCBI Sequence Read Archive [NCBI:SRP044282] were analyzed using the as yet unpublished open source package BION-meta (in preparation, N. Larsen, Danish Genome Institute, Denmark) (Additional file 3). This program facilitates quick and easy bioinformatics analysis, and BION-meta has previously been applied to a similar dataset [19]. However, in addition to matching all sequences against the ribosomal small subunit (SSU) Silva dataset, suited for 16S rRNA gene targeting primer sets, BION-meta was advanced to encompass searches in the ribosomal large subunit (LSU) Silva dataset, thereby accommodating the primer sets targeting the 23S rRNA gene used in the Gut Microbiotassay [25]. The BION-meta workflow included the following elements: 1) separation by sample barcodes and primer tags; 2) removal of primer remnants and bases at the ends with lower than 96% quality (phred value ~14), as well as sequence filtering by length (200) and filtering by minimum base quality of 96%.; 3) removal of chimeric sequences; 4) separation of each sample by matching it with the phylogenetic primer(s); 5) matching all sequences against the SSU and LSU Silva datasets and producing a table with the highest 1% similarities for each query; and 6) mapping the similarities to the Silva SSU and LSU taxonomies, identifying consensus operational taxonomic units (OTUs).

To examine the gut microbiota in further details, BION-meta data were analyzed by Principal Coordinates Analysis (PCoA). This was conducted by applying the vegan package in R using Bray-Curtis distances on the untransformed sequence reads followed by k-means clustering [26].

Due to the hierarchical taxonomic design of the Gut Microbiota, where several primers in taxonomic lineage potentially target the same bacterial organism, a number of primer sets were chosen for this expanded diversity analysis (referred to as "grand data"): phylum: Actinobacteria, Bacteroidetes, Fusobacteria, and Spirochaetes; class: Deltaproteobacteria, and Epsilonproteobacteria; family: Clostridium cluster I, cluster IV, and cluster XIV, and Enterobacteriaceae; genus: *Enterococcus, Lactobacillus, Streptococcus*. These primer sets were selected because they provide the most comprehensive taxonomic information with the least taxonomic trespassing that would result in distortion and consequentially misinterpretation of the results.

Results

From four well-managed Danish conventional pig farms a total of 201 ileal and colonic intestinal content samples

Table 2 Significant findings from the Gut Microbiotassay and 454 sequencing results displaying similar trends

Primer set and respective 454 sequencing findings	Gut section estimate (ileum vs. colon)	Gut section *p*-value	Status estimate (diarrhoeic vs. healthy)	Status *p*-value	Gilt estimate (gilt vs. multiparous sow)	Gilt *p*-value	Percentage of diarrhoea estimate[#]	Percentage of diarrhoea *p*-value	Age estimate	Age *p*-value	Antibiotics estimate (treated vs. untreated)	Antibiotics *p*-value
Domain Bacteria B [268]	0.12 [0.08,0.17]	<0.0001		NS		NS		NS	1.21 [1.01,1.44]	0.04		NS
Phylum Firmicutes [183]	2.37 [1.63,3.33]	<0.0001	0.58 [0.36,0.89]	0.02	0.55 [0.33,0.87]	0.01		NS	1.34 [1.13,1.59]	0.001		NS
Class Bacilli [125]	3.31 [1.98,5.20]	<0.0001	0.29 [0.18,0.46]	<0.0001		NS		NS	1.62 [1.27,2.03]	0.0001		NS
Genus *Enterococcus* [27]	3.51 [1.25,7.91]	0.02	24.15 [8.50,54.73]	<0.0001		NS		NS		NS		NS
species *E. hirae* (3.36/11.11)												
species *E. faecium* (9.87/129.60)												
species *E. durans* (15.57/255.00)												
species *E. mundtii* (113.00/179.00)												
Genus *Streptococcus* [47]	2.49 [1.53,3.82]	0.0002	0.09 [0.02,0.27]	0.0002	0.55 [0.29,0.93]	0.03	1.03 [1.01,1.05]	0.008	0.75 [0.62,0.90]	0.003		NS
species *S. gallolyticus subsp. gallolyticus* (0.29/0.22)												
species *S. alactolyticus* (0.27/0.18)												
species *S. uberis* (0.68/0.33)												
Genus *Lactobacillus* [79]	4.97 [2.91,7.94]	<0.0001	0.29 [0.17,0.46]	<0.0001		NS		NS	1.75 [1.36,2.20]	<0.0001		NS
species *L. acidophilus* (0.35/0.06)												
Family Clostridium cluster I [17]	3.32 [1.37,6.79]	-	0.36 [0.04,1.39]	-		NS	1.03 [1.00,1.05]	0.04		NS		NS
species *Cl. perfringens;* ATCC 13124 (1.18/0.47)												
Species *Cl. perfringens*	9.31 [3.40,20.66]	-	1.41 [0.51,3.16]	-		NS		NS	0.67 [0.49,0.90]	0.009		NS
Family Clostridium cluster IV [64]	0.12 [0.05,0.25]	<0.0001	0.13 [0.06,0.25]	<0.0001		NS		NS	1.41 [1.02,1.91]	0.04		NS
species *Ruminococcus bromii* (0.00/0.26)												
Family Clostridium cluster XIV [81]	0.08 [0.05,0.14]	<0.0001		NS		NS	0.99 [0.98,0.99]	0.001		NS		NS
species *Roseburia inulinivorans* (1.59/0.02)												
Phylum Bacteroidetes [126]	0.02 [0.01,0.05]	-	0.12 [0.05,0.26]	-		NS		NS		NS		NS

Table 2 Significant findings from the Gut Microbiotassay and 454 sequencing results displaying similar trends *(Continued)*

Genus *Bacteroides* [65]	0.03 [0.01,0.07]	-	0.20 [0.08,0.43]	-		NS		NS		NS		NS
species *Bacteroides pyogenes* (0.02/0.33)†												
species *Bacteroides rodentium* (0.46/0.00)†												
species *Bacteroides xylanisolvens* (0.94/0.43)†												
species *Porphyromonadaceae bacterium* C941 (0.00/0.01)†												
Phylum Actinobacteria [74]	2.84 [1.64,4.60]	<0.0001	0.29 [0.17,0.46]	<0.0001		NS		NS	0.80 [0.65,0.99]	0.04		NS
species *Bifidobacterium boum* (0.41/0.06)												
species *Corynebacterium kutscheri* (0.39/0.34)												
Family Bifidobacteriaceae [12]	2.56 [1.28,4.61]	0.007		NS		NS		NS		NS		NS
Phylum Fusobacteria [16]	0.20 [0.10,0.34]	<0.0001	2.24 [1.11,4.05]	0.02		NS		NS	0.69 [0.53,0.88]	0.004	0.20 [0.05,0.52]	0.002
species *F. mortiferum* (2.25/1.21)												
Class Beta- and Gammaproteobacteria[109]	2.54 [1.63,3.79]	<0.0001	0.72 [0.12,2.55]	-		NS		NS	0.69 [0.52,0.88]	-		NS
Family Enterobacteriaceae [89]	4.03 [2.50,6.16]	<0.0001	0.27 [0.04,1.02]	-	2.12 [1.09,3.75]	0.03		NS	0.54 [0.40,0.71]	-		NS
species *Escherichia coli* (8.61/6.22)												
species *E.coli;* HQ219945.1.1457 (11.46/5.00)												
species *E. coli* DEC8A (6.22/5.16)												
Species *E. coli*	3.56 [2.05,5.76]	<0.0001	0.29 [0.02,1.26]	-	2.96 [1.39,5.56]	0.004		NS	0.58 [0.41,0.80]	-		NS
Class Deltaproteobacteria [1]		NS		NS		NS	0.98 [0.97,1.00]	0.04		NS	0.08 [0.00,0.48]	0.02
species *Desulfovibrio piger* (0.00/0.00)†												

Estimated fold changes as the estimates of the exponentiated effect parameter, corresponding 95% confidence intervals [], and *p*-values. Superscripted numbers equal the total number of OTUs belonging to the respective taxonomic group identified by sequencing amplicons generated by the Gut Microbiotassay. OTU-ratio between diarrhoeic and healthy piglets for ileum and colon, respectively, listed in parenthesis. †indicate a significant effect of interaction (Table 3). Species mark with † are not consistent findings. $^{\#}$Estimated fold changes for this category are calculated as: $y^{percentage\ points}$, where the parameter *y* from column 8 is the estimate of the exponential $e\beta$ of the estimated effect parameter β for diarrhoea in formula (1). The diarrhoeic percentage points range from 0 to 100.

Table 3 Estimated fold changes, 95% confidence intervals [], and *p*-values of significant interactions from the Gut Microbiotassay

Primer set	Gut section: status estimate (ileum, diarrhoeic)	Gut section: status estimate (colon, diarrhoeic)	Gut section: status *p*-value	Status: age estimate, day 3	Status: age estimate, day 4	Status: age estimate, day 5	Status: age estimate, day 6	Status: age estimate, day 7	Status: age estimate, mean age	Status: age *p*-value
Family Clostridium cluster I	0.07 [0.01,0.31]	0.27 [0.04,1.39]	0.01							NS
Species *Cl. perfringens*	0.33 [0.13,0.80]	1.41 [0.51,3.16]	0.04							NS
Phylum Bacteroidetes	1.00 [0.39,2.42]	0.12 [0.05,0.26]	0.0009							NS
Genus *Bacteroides*	0.73 [0.13,0.80]	0.20 [0.08,0.43]	0.04							NS
Class Beta- and Gammaproteobacteria			NS	3.12	5.63	10.21	18.60	34.37	4.52 [5.05,11.64]	0.0007
Family Enterobacteriaceae			NS	1.81	3.80	8.07	17.29	38.07	4.52 [3.19,9.69]	<0.0001
Species *E. coli*			NS	1.98	4.38	9.81	22.42	53.95	4.47 [3.39,11.85]	0.0004

This table is an extension of Table 2, and the estimated fold changes are the estimates of the exponentiated effect parameter.

were collected from 50 control piglets without NNPD and 52 case piglets suffering from NNPD (3 samples were lost between sampling and the laboratory). Of the case piglets, 25 were treated with broad-spectrum antibiotics intramuscularly, depending on their diagnosis and according to herd treatment practices. Piglets were three to seven days old and were all reared with their biological dam and siblings [15].

A bacterial taxonomic profile was obtained from both gut sections of each animal using the Gut Microbiotassay targeting rRNA genes of major bacterial groups in the mammalian intestine. Normalized Cq data were used for PCA. After excluding the primer sets with less than 50% recorded Cq values ("Class Epsilonproteobacteria", "Phylum Verrucomicrobia", and "Domain Archaea"), as well as the "Domain Bacteria A" and "Domain Bacteria B" primer sets (which did not contribute any information to the PCA analysis), 19 primer sets remained for the data analysis. In addition, 12 samples were removed from the dataset as a consequence of having too few Cq registrations. From the PCA scores plot (see Figure 1, for further information on the major principal components in the PCA see Additional file 2), four case animals (three of which were treated with antibiotics) and four control animals were randomly chosen to be representatives for their respective herds. Detailed taxonomic information was acquired for these 16 samples using 454 next generation sequencing.

The Gut Microbiotassay

The significant findings from the Gut Microbiotassay are presented in Table 2 and significant effects of interaction as investigated in formula (1) are presented in Table 3, consequently these two tables are intertwined and should be read together. Table 2 summarizes the estimated fold changes as the estimates of the exponentiated effect parameter, 95% confidence intervals, and p-values of these results, and Table 3 lists the same parameters for all significant interactions.

From the relative quantitative results generated by the Gut Microbiotassay, it was evident that luminal content from the large intestine possessed a significantly higher bacterial load than luminal content from the small intestine (expressed by domain Bacteria B, $p < 0.0001$), regardless of diarrhoeic status (Table 2).

NNPD was associated with a diminished quantity of bacteria from the phyla Actinobacteria ($p < 0.0001$) and Firmicutes ($p = 0.02$). Firmicutes comprised the following: class Bacilli ($p < 0.0001$), genus *Lactobacillus* ($p < 0.0001$), genus *Streptococcus* ($p = 0.0002$), and family Cl. cluster IV ($p < 0.0001$). However, genus *Enterococcus* was estimated to be more than 24 times more abundant in diarrhoeic piglets ($p < 0.0001$). The number of bacteria from the phylum Fusobacteria ($p = 0.02$) was also doubled in piglets suffering from diarrhoea (Table 2).

It was investigated whether the effect of diarrhoeic status differed between gut sections through a statistical interaction term (Table 3). In both case and control piglets, there were generally more members from phylum Bacteroidetes and genus *Bacteroides* in the colon compared with the ileum (Table 2). Nonetheless, case piglets had a reduced number of Bacteroidetes and *Bacteroides* compared to control piglets, and the depletion of these bacteria was

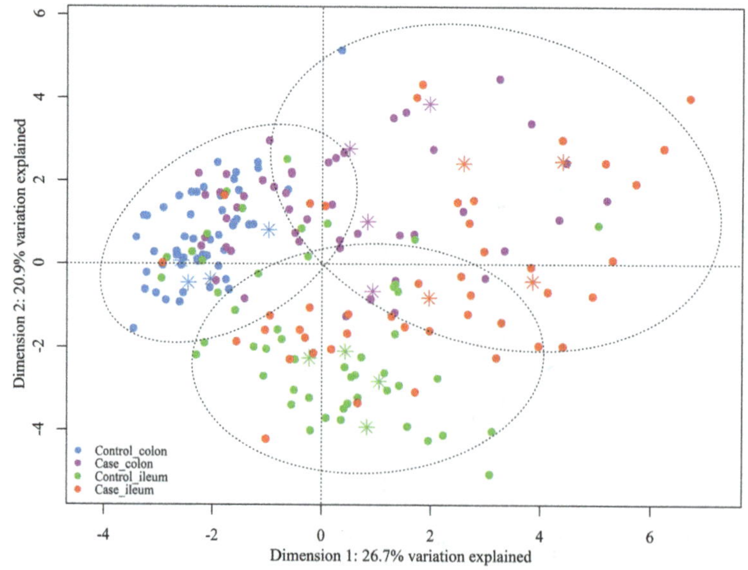

Figure 1 PCA score plot of ileal and colonic content of piglets with (case) and without (control) NNPD. PCA scores are generated from normalized relative values of ileal and colonic content of case and control piglets obtained from the Gut Microbiotassay. Asterisks symbolize samples selected for 454 sequencing. Circles represent K-means clustering. For further information see Additional files 2 and 4.

located to the colon ($p = 0.0009$ and 0.04, respectively), while no significant depletion was detected in the ileum (Table 3). Overall, there were greater numbers of family Cl. cluster I and species *Cl. perfringens* in control piglets compared with case piglets, except for *Cl. perfringens*, which was more numerous in the colon of case piglets, though not significantly. The numbers of Cl. cluster I and *Cl. perfringens* were significantly reduced in the ileum of case piglets compared with control piglets ($p = 0.01$, 0.04) (Table 3). Control piglets generally exhibited a disparity in the number of bacteria present in the ileum versus the colon, while the difference in bacterial abundance between gut sections was more negligible in case piglets. It should be noted that the preceding results all relate to circumstances of 'all other things being equal'.

Independent of diarrhoeic status, piglets from first parity sows possessed significantly more bacteria from family Enterobacteriaceae ($p = 0.03$) and species *E. coli* ($p = 0.004$), and fewer bacteria from phylum Firmicutes ($p = 0.01$), hereof genus *Streptococcus* ($p = 0.03$) compared to multiparous sows (Table 2).

Bacteria from family Cl. cluster XIV ($p = 0.001$) and class Deltaproteobacteria ($p = 0.04$) were depleted, but bacteria belonging to genus *Streptococcus* ($p = 0.008$), and family Cl. cluster I ($p = 0.04$) were elevated in case piglets that suffered from an increasing percentage of diarrhoea in their lifetime. In Table 2 the estimated fold changes may be calculated as: $y^{percentage\ points}$, where the parameter y from column 8 is the estimate of the exponential e^{β} of the estimated effect parameter β for diarrhoea in formula (1). The diarrhoeic percentage points range from 0 to 100.

Diarrhoeic piglets treated with broad-spectrum antibiotics had a reduced presence of Fusobacteria ($p = 0.002$), and Deltaproteobacteria ($p = 0.02$), (Table 2).

Regardless of diarrhoeic status, the quantity of bacteria in the intestine generally increased with increasing age ($p = 0.04$). The older the piglet the more bacteria from the following groups: phylum Firmicutes ($p = 0.001$), class Bacilli ($p = 0.0001$), genus *Lactobacillus* ($p < 0.0001$), and class Cl. cluster IV ($p = 0.04$). Bacteria that diminished from the gut microbiota with increasing age were as follows: genus *Streptococcus* ($p = 0.003$), species *Cl. perfringens* ($p = 0.009$), phylum Actinobacteria ($p = 0.04$), and phylum Fusobacteria ($p = 0.004$) (Table 2).

In addition, the interaction between Status and Age was examined (Table 3). There was a significant difference between control piglets and case piglets over time. As piglets aged, it was estimated that apparently increasing numbers of class Beta- and Gammaproteobacteria (slope: 0.21 log units/day), family Enterobacteriaceae (0.12) and species *Escherichia coli* (0.25) colonized the intestine of case piglets, while the numbers of these bacteria were estimated to decrease for control piglets ($p = 0.004$, $p < 0.0001$, $p = 0.001$, respectively). Figure 2 illustrates the abundance of class Beta- and Gammaproteobacteria in ileal and colonic luminal content in relation to piglet age, segregated according to diarrhoeic status. However, while the differences in age effects between control and case piglets were highly significant ($p = 0.0007$, 0.0001, 0.0004), the three estimated positive slope values for diarrhoeic piglets were not significantly greater than zero ($p = 0.11$, 0.39, 0.12).

The effects of birth weight and gender were investigated, and no significant results were discovered.

Table 4 lists the significant results calculated from the logistic regression model (2) investigating whether NNPD was associated with genus *Enterococcus*, class Beta- and Gammaproteobacteria, family Enterobacteriaceae, species *E. coli*, possible co-occurrence of bacteria, Gut section, Gilt, and Age. The model fitted the data according to standard model control measures. NNPD was found to be significantly associated with the presence of genus *Enterococcus* ($p = 0.009$), and there was also a significant effect of the co-occurrence of this genus and species *E. coli* ($p = 0.02$). Though the interaction apparently had a slightly diminishing effect on the probability of being recognized as an NNPD piglet, it actually contributed to the risk in the majority of cases with increasing values of *E. coli*. This result is explained by the logged values of Enterococci, which were negative in 89% of the data. Finally, there was a significant effect of the interaction between class Beta- and Gammaproteobacteria and the colon, suggesting that NNPD piglets are differentiated from control piglets by colonization of the colon with class Beta- and Gammaproteobacteria ($p = 0.001$). All things being equal, piglets born to gilts had 25 times higher odds of having NNPD compared with piglets born to multiparous sows ($p < 0.0001$).

PCA

Additional file 2 summarizes the loadings, the eigenvalues, and the variance explained by the major principal components for all PCA analyses. Principal Component Analysis of data from the 19 primer sets showed no clustering in relation to pig farms (results not shown). The major loading scores in the PCA were explained by the primer sets: component 1: phylum Bacteroidetes (Control) and family Enterobacteriaceae (Case), component 2: genus *Lactobacillus* (Ileum), and genus *Bacteroides* (Colon). Generally, the control large intestine was characterized by a gut microbiota that clustered together, whereas the bacterial composition of the small intestine from control piglets was more diverse (Figure 1). Diarrhoeic gut sections were more scattered compared to non-diarrhoeic ones in the PCA plot, demonstrating that NNPD seems to be associated with a disturbed bacterial composition and larger variation between the diarrhoeic piglets. Additional file 4 lists

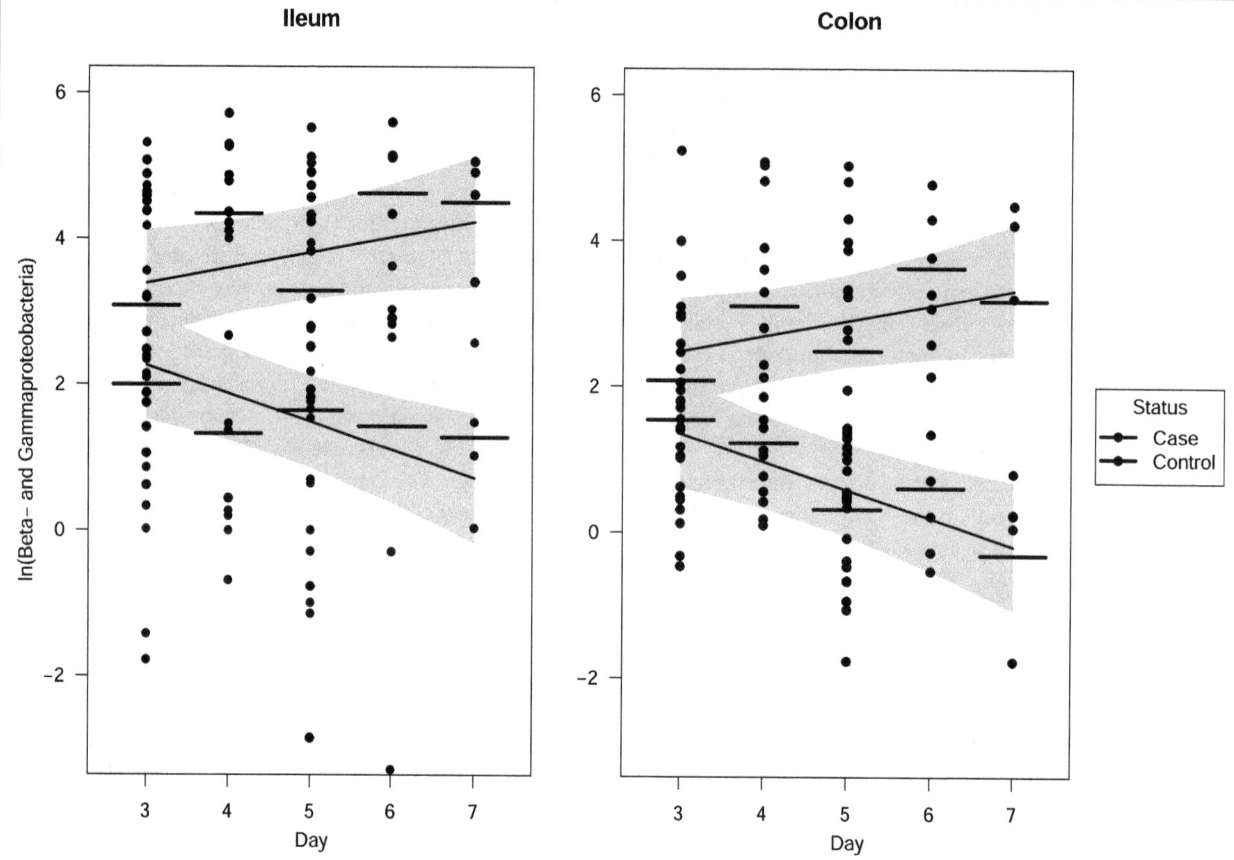

Figure 2 Age-related changes of Beta- and Gammaproteobacteria in luminal content of piglets with and without NNPD. Relative amount of class Beta- and Gammaproteobacteria (transformed with the natural logarithm) in ileal and colonic content of all piglets included in the study, plotted as function of the age of the piglets. Case and controls are piglets with and without diarrhoea, respectively. Age-related model regression lines are depicted with corresponding 95% confidence intervals as shaded areas. Horizontal bars show means for a given age and group.

Table 4 NNPD status associated with selected bacteria and relevant variables

ln(variable)	Estimate	95% confidence interval	*p*-value
Intercept	−0.98	[−3.10,1.13]	-
Species *E. coli*	−0.11	[−0.42,0.65]	-
Genus *Enterococcus*	0.34	[0.09,0.59]	0.009
Enterococcus: *E. coli*	−0.12	[−0.23,-0.02]	0.02
Beta- and Gammaproteobacteria: colon	0.82	[0.33,1.30]	0.001
Gilt	3.23	[1.99,4.46]	<0.0001

Of the following variables tested, genus *Enterococcus*, class Beta- and Gammaproteobacteria, family Enterobacteriaceae, species *Escherichia coli*, Gut section, Gilt, and Age, as well as possible interactions between bacteria, NNPD was found to be significantly related to the variables mentioned below. Numbers are transformed with the natural logarithm (ln). The odds ratio can be calculated as the exponentiated estimate.

LDA results. According to LDA, 70% and 83% of samples were correctly classified as cases and controls, respectively, in Figure 1 ($p < 0.0001$). When looking at the microbial composition in piglets at different ages (three to seven days old), separation became increasingly more apparent with age, in relation to diarrhoeic status as the predictive value calculated from LDA improved with age (Figure 3, Additional file 4).

Next generation sequencing

BION-meta processing including de-multiplexing, cleaning, and chimera checking resulted in 279 103 reads for mapping (Additional file 3).

OTUs displaying similar trends to data obtained from the Gut Microbiotassay are included in Table 2. To be represented the OTUs have to be a somewhat consistent finding in piglets, irrespective of the variables in relation to diarrhoea, and the reads should be represented in a noteworthy number.

A Shannon's diversity index was calculated from the grand data: control ileum = 3.48; case ileum = 3.23; control

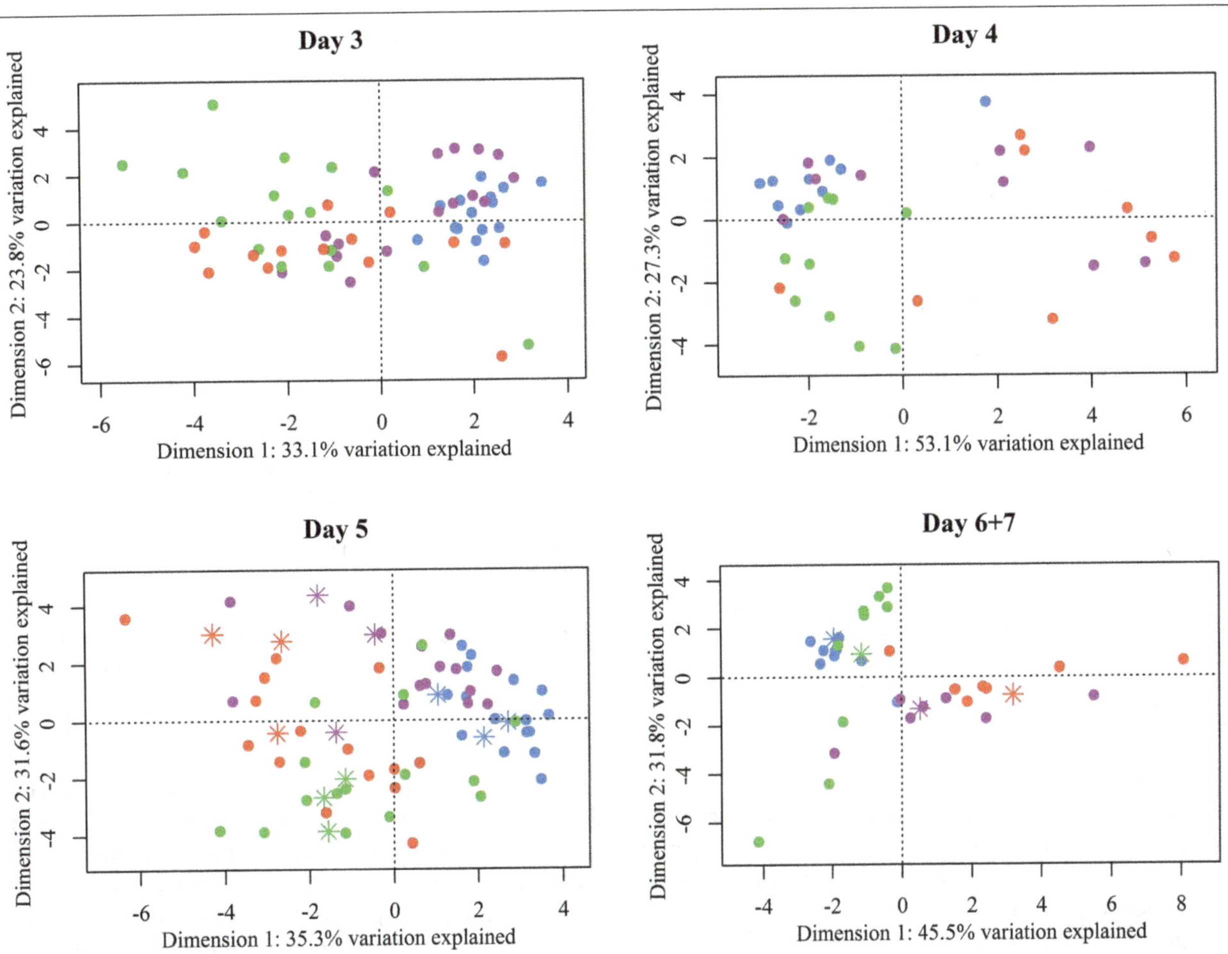

Figure 3 PCA score plot of the gut microbiota segregated on gut section according to age in days. PCA scores from normalized relative values of ileal and colonic content of case and control piglets in relation to age in days obtained from the Gut Microbiotassay. Blue: Control colon, Purple: Case colon, Green: Control ileum, Red: Case ileum. Asterisks symbolize samples selected for 454 sequencing. Samples cluster primarily according to diarrhoeic status with increasing age. For further information see Additional files 2 and 4.

colon = 3.43; and case colon = 3.18, however, the group differences (in Shannon's diversity indices) are negligible and their biological relevance unclear. Additionally, a PCoA was generated from the grand data that showed separation of the sequenced samples according to NNPD status (first canonical axis) and gut section (second canonical axis), as shown in Figure 4. The two major loading scores in the PCoA were explained by the following: Control: genus *Lactobacillus* and species *Fusobacterium varium*; Case: species *E. coli* and genus *Enterococcus*; Ileum: genus *Lactobacillus* and species *Fusobacterium ulcerans*; and Colon: species *F. varium* and species *Fusobacterium mortiferum* (Additional file 2).

Discussion

All piglets included in the study had previously been tested for hemolytic *E. coli*, *Cl. difficile*, *Cl. perfringens* type A and C, coronavirus, rotavirus species A and C, and microscopically inspected for parasites, with the conclusion that none of these agents were related to NNPD [15]. In this study it was generally expected that bacteria associated with diarrhoea would exhibit more or less consistent tendencies in case piglets compared with control piglets. Consequently, the Cq results and the sequencing results displaying similar trends will be discussed in relation to diarrhoea in the subsequent section, with the main focus being on potential NNPD-causing bacteria with high statistical estimates (Tables 2, 3 and 4). Sequencing results are based on a small subset of case and control piglets. The mapped sequences are mainly referred to as most similar species or isolate identified, while acknowledging the limits of classifying bacteria at these taxonomic levels. Nonetheless, even though mapped sequencing results at species and particularly isolate level are questionable, these are still construed as indicative and possibly important bacteria, which is why they are highlighted in the consecutive text.

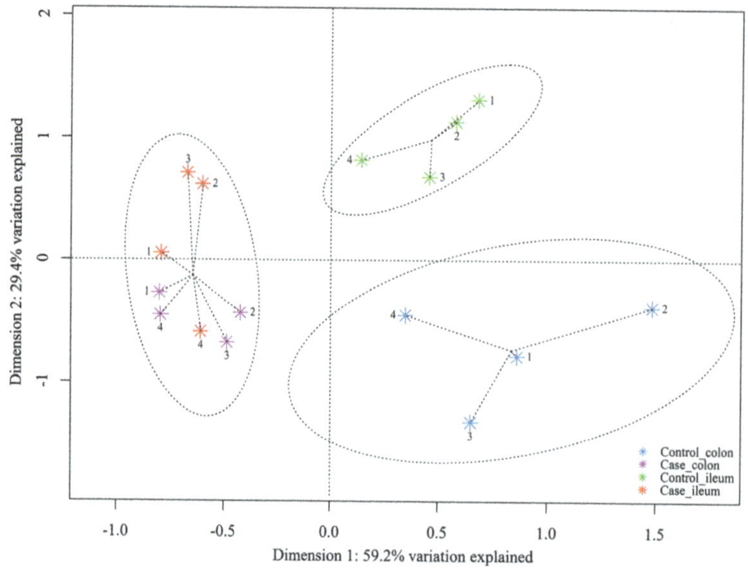

Figure 4 PCoA score plot showing similarity of composition of the gut microbiota from sequenced samples. Grand data of ileal and colonic luminal content of a case piglet and a control piglet from each herd included in the study. Numbers refer to herd origin. Samples were randomly chosen for 454 sequencing based on PCA scores generated from normalized Cq data obtained through the Gut Microbiotassay for 454 sequencing (see Figure 1). Circles represent K-means clustering. For further information see Additional file 2.

Genus *Enterococcus*

Enterococci were 24.15 times more abundant in diarrhoeic piglets than in healthy piglets (p <0.0001), and moreover genus *Enterococcus* was one of the bacterial groups positively related with status, meaning that the presence of Enterococci increases the risk of suffering from NNPD (odds ratio 1.40 per ln unit of *Enterococcus*, $p = 0.009$). Genus *Enterococcus* was classified to 27 different OTUs, of which *Enterococcus hirae*, *Enterococcus faecium*, *Enterococcus durans*, and *Enterococcus mundtii* were the predominant.

Enterococci are ubiquitous distributed in nature and a consistent finding in the gastrointestinal tract of several animal species, including the pig [13,18,27,28]. An association of Enterococci to neonatal porcine diarrhoea has been reported in previous studies [13,18,29,30]. Another noteworthy feature is that this genus is reported to be resistance to several antibiotics [27,28], which could explain why the efficiency of antibiotic treatment of NNPD is variable.

Larsson *et al.* found neonatal porcine diarrhoea (NPD) in Swedish pig farms to be associated with enteroadherent *E. hirae* colonizing the small intestine accompanied by mucosal lesions [29]. This conforms to observations published by Jonach *et al.* [18] using FISH to investigate the same piglets as the present study. The authors demonstrated small intestinal colonization by adherent *Enterococcus* spp. and often found them occurring together with adherent *E. coli* [18]. According to sequencing results, *E. hirae* was the most abundant species, consistent with results from a former study on Enterococcal communities in pig feces [27]. Nonetheless, this species displayed the smallest difference in numbers of OTU between diarrhoeic and healthy piglets' gut microbiota. However, the numerical occurrence of reads may not be related to the development of diarrhoea, especially not if diarrhoea is a result of co-occurrence of different bacteria such as *E. hirae* and *E. coli*.

E. durans could be a contributor to NNPD, as it has previously been reported to co-occur with *E. coli* in cases of neonatal piglet diarrhoea [13,23]. In a study from 1984 in which foals and gnotobiotic piglets were experimentally inoculated with *E. durans*, this species was found to promote the proliferation of *E. coli*, and to adhere to the mucosa of the small intestine in either case [24]. In fact, *E. durans* has been hypothesized to act as a primary enteric pathogen with the ability to clear the way for other pathogens [23]. Although the ratio of *E. durans* between case and control gut sections is largest for colonic content, there were 40% more reads of this species in the ileum compared with the colon, in line with previous findings [13,23].

The preceding information implies an interesting co-occurrence of Enterococci and *E. coli* [18]. Similarly, this study also found a significant effect of the interaction between species *E. coli* and genus *Enterococcus*, which contributed to the risk of piglets suffering from NNPD ($p = 0.02$). Furthermore, there were generally more Enterococci in the ileum compared with the colon, which supports previous findings ($p = 0.02$) [13,18,23,29]. Both *E. hirae* and *E. durans* have been reported to cause villous atrophy, which was frequently found in the small intestine of piglets included in this study [18,23,29].

E. mundtii was almost exclusively found in the gut microbiota of case piglets, primarily in antibiotic-treated piglets, indicating that antibiotic treatment created a favorable environment for this species. Interestingly, this finding did not account for one of the antibiotic-treated animals, in which no *E. mundtii* was detected.

Phylum Fusobacteria

Piglets with diarrhoea harbored more bacteria classified to phylum Fusobacterium ($p = 0.02$). A similar trend has been associated with acute hemorrhagic diarrhoea in dogs and ulcerative colitis in humans [31,32]. In this study, 16 OTUs were identified. Species *F. mortiferum* was a consistent finding in the digesta of all piglets, but it was less abundant in control piglets compared to case piglets. Nonetheless, Portrait *et al.* demonstrated that this species was able to produce bacteriocin-like substance(s) with an inhibitory effect on a number of both Gram-positive and Gram-negative species [33]. Therefore, it is difficult to say whether the increased abundance of *F. mortiferum* in case piglets is due to its potential pathogenicity or if the increase is a type of defense mechanism mediated by the gut microbiota. Phylum Fusobacterium was one of the two bacterial groups that were significantly reduced by antibiotic treatment ($p = 0.002$).

Class Beta- and Gammaproteobacteria, family Enterobacteriaceae and species *Escherichia coli*

E. coli are commonly found in the gastrointestinal tract. This species is normally a harmless commensal in the host, nonetheless some *E. coli* possess pathogenic features [34,35].

This study found a highly significant effect of the interaction between NNPD status and this bacterial taxonomic lineage in relation to age in days (Figure 2 and Table 3). Thus, with increasing age, these bacteria proliferated in piglets with diarrhoea (though not significantly), whereas members of this group were significantly reduced in control piglets. With age, the estimated difference increased, indicating that the diarrhoeic piglets have impaired ability to control and clear this group of bacteria. However, it also suggests that NNPD is associated with an imbalanced gut microbiota, creating a favorable environment for these bacteria.

Kongsted *et al.* [15] thoroughly examined the same animals for *E. coli* by aerobic culturing, serogrouping, and testing for virulence factor genes. The most prevalent finding was the presence of non-hemolytic *E. coli*, independent of diarrhoeic status. Fimbrial genes were evenly distributed among the genes investigated in approximately 25% of the tested *E. coli* from both case and control piglets. Of all piglets, only one case of classic Enterotoxigenic *E. coli* and six cases of non-typable hemolytic *E. coli* were detected, all in diarrhoeic piglets [15].

NNPD piglets investigated by 454 sequencing from different pig farms resulted in the identification of 109 OTUs and revealed a remarkably large number of reads classified to DEC8A and *E. coli* HQ219945.1.1457, both with the highest prevalence in case animals in all but one pig. The single pig that stood out was from pig farm four, which generally differed from the others. DEC8A is the name of a diarrhoeagenic *E. coli* (DEC) isolate classified as EHEC 2 (enterohemorrhagic *E. coli* 2 clonal complex), serotype O111a:NM [36]. EHEC 2 comprises a group of pathogenic *E. coli* reported to cause various disorders in mammals, including diarrhoea. The O111a was not part of the serogroups investigated by Kongsted *et al.* [15].

Except for one nucleotide positioned in the 5′-end of the *E. coli* oligonucleotide probe used for FISH analysis by Jonach *et al.* [18], this probe matches the DEC8A 23S rRNA gene [18,37]. Hence, the possibility cannot be dismissed that the *E. coli* adherent to the small intestinal epithelium observed by Jonach *et al.* [18] could be DEC8A. This could also explain the frequent finding of villous atrophy previously found to characterize diarrhoeic piglets [15,18].

E. coli HQ219945.1.1457 isolate was detected in ileal and colonic content of all animals sequenced, though in much higher numbers in diarrhoeic piglets, indicating that it might contribute to the pathogenesis of NNPD.

Piglets born to gilts had a significantly higher abundance of family Enterobacteriaceae and species *E. coli* than piglets born to multiparous sows ($p = 0.03$, 0.004, respectively). These were mainly classified to be the aforementioned isolates: DEC8A and *E. coli* HQ219945.1.1457. The increased risk of having NNPD if born to a gilt is consistent with farmers' and veterinarians' anamnesis reports, as they describe NNPD to be most prevalent among litters from first parity sows [2,13,14,17]. While the frequency of piglets born to gilts in the data material was 38% as a product of the randomized selection of sows, and the frequency of case piglets born to gilts was 66%, the odds ratio of NNPD for being born to a gilt from the logistic regression model (2) was estimated at 25.28 ($p < 0.0001$), reflecting the strongly significant effect of being born to a gilt (see also Table 4). The logistic regression model also found that piglets of different NNPD status could be separated based on colonic colonization with species *E. coli* from class Gammaproteobacteria according to 454 sequencing results.

Phylum Firmicutes, class Bacilli, genus *Lactobacillus*, and genus *Streptococcus*

These bacterial groups are all part of the normal gut microbiota of pre-weaned piglets [4,38]. The gut microbiota of case piglets was inhabited by fewer *Lactobacillus acidophilus, Streptococcus gallolyticus subsp. gallolyticus, Streptococcus alactolyticus,* and *Streptococcus uberis* compared with the gut microbiota of control piglets.

Lactobacilli have been shown to colonize the intestines of piglets soon after birth and to be a stable member of the gut microbiota throughout the intestinal tract [4]. A low abundance of species *L. acidophilus,* which is regarded as a beneficial bacterium, could be an indicator of a troubled gastrointestinal milieu in pigs, as it was also diminished in diarrhoeic piglets included in this study. *S. gallolyticus subsp. gallolyticus* has previously been isolated from the gastrointestinal tract of numerous animal species, including pigs, and is therefore most likely included in the normal gut microbiota [39,40]. Additionally, *S. alactolyticus* is a member of the normal gut microbiota in pigs. There are few reports of *S. uberis* being isolated from pigs [41,42], and it does not seem to play a significant role in the development of NNPD, as the abundance of *S. uberis* is significantly lower in case piglets versus control piglets.

Phylum Firmicutes, family Clostridium cluster I, species *Clostridium perfringens*, family Clostridium cluster IV, and family Clostridium cluster XIV

In general, there were fewer of these bacteria in intestinal content from both the ileum and colon of case piglets compared with control piglets, except that colonic content possessed a higher number of *Cl. perfringens* (not statistically significant). It can be speculated whether the increased abundance in the colon reflects the reduction of Cl. cluster I and *Cl. perfringens* in the ileum ($p = 0.01$, 0.04, respectively). Nonetheless, 454 sequencing of amplicons generated by primer sets targeting Cl. cluster I and higher taxonomical levels failed to demonstrate this trend. *Cl. perfringens* is a normal finding in the gastrointestinal tract but it is also a potential pathogen [43]. Sequencing amplicons generated by the primer set targeting family Cl. cluster I revealed reads from 17 OTUs, of which only *Cl. perfringens* ATCC 13124 was worthy of notice. *Cl. perfringens* ATCC 13124 is a type A strain that is a potential diarrhoea-causing agent [43]. However, because piglets included in this study have all been tested for *Cl. perfringens* type A (among others) previously [15], where it was a frequent finding with higher prevalence in control piglets versus case piglets, this species is not considered to be essential to the development of NNPD.

The fact that all remaining bacterial groups were diminished in diarrhoeic piglets is most likely due to an imbalance in the gut microbiota because all of these groups have been demonstrated in digesta from healthy piglets [38]. Various bacteria from family Cl. cluster IV and Cl. cluster XIV are regarded to be beneficial due to their ability to produce short chain fatty acids (SCFAs) such as acetate, propionate, and butyrate [44].

Of the 64 OTUs classified to family Cl. cluster IV, deficient bacteria mainly comprised species *Ruminococcus bromii,* which have previously been found in the porcine gastrointestinal tract [40]. A reduced number of *R. bromii* have also been reported in patients suffering from ulcerative colitis [32].

Family Cl. cluster XIV was not significantly related to the NNPD status of the pigs, but there was a significant effect of suffering from diarrhoea for a prolonged period of life (percentage of diarrhoea) that resulted in a reduction in the abundance of this family ($p = 0.001$). Thus, this bacterial group was indirectly affected by NNPD, as results indicate that family Cl. cluster XIV was vulnerable to the continuously flushing effect of diarrhoea. A scarce population of bacteria from family Cl. cluster XIV has also been described in previous studies on gut microbial communities in intestinal disorders [31,45]. *Roseburia inulinivorans* was the central bacterium missing from the 81 OTUs classified to family Cl. cluster XIV. This species is able to degrade oligofructose to free fructose, which can function as a fuel for other members of the gut microbiota, a phenomenon called cross-feeding [46].

Phylum Bacteroidetes and genus *Bacteroides*

Members of phylum Bacteroidetes are a common finding in the gastrointestinal tract of mammals, and they are also an early intestinal colonizer of the healthy piglet [4,5,38,40]. Culture studies found bacteria belonging to this phylum in piglets older than 48 hours, most frequently in the large intestine [4]. This result is consistent with the findings of the present study, which found phylum Bacteroidetes to be more abundant in colonic contents of both case piglets and control piglets. However, diarrhoea resulted in a significant depletion of these bacteria in the colon (phylum Bacteroidetes $p = 0.0009$, and genus *Bacteroides* $p = 0.04$). Several studies have also found a reduced presence of these bacteria in different enteric disorders, such as acute non-hemorrhagic diarrhoea in dogs, experimentally induced swine dysentery in pigs, and inflammatory bowel disease in humans [31,45,47]. A total of 126 OTUs were identified. Unfortunately, sequencing results did not reveal any consistent tendencies for this taxonomic lineage. Disregarding the criterion that piglets from all herds should exhibit the same trends, case piglets harbored particularly lower numbers of species *Bacteroides pyogenes, Bacteroides rodentium, Bacteroides xylanisolvens,* and the unclassified *Porphyromonadaceae bacterium* C941 in their intestinal luminal content versus control piglets.

Phylum Actinobacteria

Several studies have found phylum Actinobacteria to be part of the normal gut microbiota and to be scarce in the gut microbiota of different gastrointestinal disorders, such as irritable bowel syndrome in humans and acute hemorrhagic diarrhoea in dogs [31,48]. The phylum includes the genus *Bifidobacterium*, which is considered to be beneficial to its host, and a number of species from this genus are recognized probiotics [49,50]. There was a significant depletion of members from this phylum in the intestinal content of NNPD-affected piglets compared with those of control piglets ($p < 0.0001$). This was supported by OTU counts from all diarrhoeic piglets, except for the piglet that originated from the atypical herd mentioned earlier. Of the 74 OTUs the species scarcely represented were *Bifidobacterium boum*, and *Corynebacterium kutscheri* and they were mainly diminished from the colon. *Bifidobacterium* as probiotic has been demonstrated to protect piglets against weaning diarrhoea associated with *E. coli*, and *B. boum* to inhibit Shiga toxigenic *E. coli* virulence gene expression experimentally [51,52]. This fits the fact that case piglets harbored an inverse proportion of members from the taxonomical lineage class Beta- and Gammaproteobacteria, family Enterobacteriaceae and species *E. coli*, and from phylum Actinobacteria, having a lot more of the former bacteria and fewer of the latter.

C. kutscheri has primarily been reported to be a common bacterium on the mucous membranes of rodents including the gastrointestinal tract [53]. Interestingly, *C. kutscheri* was more plentiful in the intestinal content of healthy piglets than in that of diarrhoeic piglets, irrespective of gut section. The bacterium does not count as part of the normal porcine gut microbiota in the existing literature. Thus, even though this cannot be ruled out for certain, it is possible that piglets may have acquired this species from foraging rodents directly or indirectly.

Class Deltaproteobacteria

This bacterial group was not associated with the diarrhoeic status of the piglets, but there was a significant reduction in numbers of members of this class in case piglets suffering from prolonged diarrhoea (increasing percentage of lifetime). Moreover, Deltaproteobacteria were also diminished by administration of antibiotics to the piglets. These facts are intertwined, as case piglets were mainly given antibiotics in an attempt to cure prolonged diarrhoea. Finally, both results were not strongly significant ($p = 0.04$, $p = 0.02$, respectively). The only OTU found by sequencing amplicons generated by the primer targeting this class was species *Desulfovibrio piger*, and this was only identified in healthy piglets from two herds. This species has primarily been described as an opportunistic pathogen in humans but has also been detected in the feces of wild ducks [54,55]. While the species was primarily found in colonic content of the control piglets, it is postulated that this species constitutes part of the normal gut microbiota of piglets.

PCoA of the gut microbiota

From the BION-meta processed sequencing data a PCoA was generated (Figure 4). This investigation supported the preliminary PCA that was produced from the Gut Microbiotassay data, and additionally the major loading scores confirm the findings in the section above concerning the different bacterial groups. It diverges from the preceding discussion by taking all bacteria into account, and the clustering strongly suggests that it is possible to associate certain bacteria with a healthy gut microbiota.

The intestinal microbiota of the aging piglet

When the data were subset according to age in days, this study found that, with age, the gut microbiota clustered in relation to status, which probably reflects the significance of *E. coli* in NNPD (Figure 3). Control piglets had significantly fewer of this species compared with case piglets, and over time the abundance of *E. coli* diminished in control piglets whilst it increased in case piglets (Figure 2). A more defined microbiota with increasing age is in line with conclusions from a previous study [56], which found that seven- to nine-day-old piglets (youngest piglets included in the study) had the lowest individual average similarity, independent of environmental or maternal relationship, compared with piglets from older age groups. The more distinctive clustering of NNPD status with increasing age could hint age to be a relevant factor in the diagnosis of NNPD.

Antibiotics

The NNPD piglets investigated in this study included antibiotic-treated piglets. Antibiotic-treated piglets were included because they typically suffered the worst cases of NNPD and were medicated for ethical reasons. It is evident that antibiotics have an impact on the gut microbial composition [6]. However, one of the characteristics of NNPD is that it responds poorly to antibiotics. Additionally, Figures 1, 3 and 4 illustrate how it is possible to cluster piglets according to NNPD status despite the fact that some of the NNPD cases are treated with different antibiotics, indicating that the effect of NNPD on the gut microbial distribution and composition is more significant than the effect exerted by antibiotics in piglets of this age group.

Considerations on study approach

Case and control piglets included in this study all originate from herds affected with NNPD, hence the study lack the inclusion of true control piglets from non-affected herds. Nonetheless, at the time of selecting the herds it was virtually impossible to find a true control herd due to the unknown aetiology and the much limited knowledge of NNPD. This also means that despite great efforts to ensure correct inclusion of NNPD herds through predefined criteria there is still a risk that piglets actually did not suffer from NNPD.

It is acknowledged that this study only examines the bacterial composition of the luminal content, and not bacteria from the gastrointestinal wall. However, bacteria associated with the mucosa are not restricted to this site, as they are shed into the lumen together with intestinal epithelial cells and mucus. Thus, it is assumed that this study also detects these or at least a sub-fraction of these.

Additionally, results from this study are affected by the various steps involved in preparing the samples, for example DNA extraction, PCR, and sequencing, which all introduce variation into the final outcome [57]. Furthermore, the results do not reflect bacterial numbers but relative values of 16S and 23S rRNA gene abundance or OTUs (consensus sequences). Conclusions drawn from sequencing data are based on OTUs displaying similar trends to data obtained from the Gut Microbiotassay. Moreover, sequences had to be represented in a noteworthy number, and with somewhat consistent findings in piglets, irrespective of the variables in relation to diarrhoea. This means that there might be a risk that important bacteria could be overlooked if they do not meet the aforementioned criteria.

Finally, to determine causality based on the associations found in this study these should be investigated further for instance through bacterial isolation and inoculation studies.

Conclusion

The results of this study on NNPD indicate that bacteria could be the aetiology of this diarrhoea that affects piglets during the first week of life. At present, it is impossible to conclude whether diarrhoea is a consequence of an absence of beneficial bacteria or if diarrhoea is an outcome of invading pathogenic bacteria or an overgrowth of opportunistic pathogenic bacteria. *E. coli* appears to be a contributing factor to NNPD as NNPD piglets differ from healthy piglets by colonic colonization of bacteria from class Beta- and Gammaproteobacteria, primarily being species *E. coli*, and it appears that there is an important effect of age, both of which might be relevant in the characterization and diagnosis of NNPD. There is reason to believe that genus *Enterococcus* is a participating factor, most likely species *E. hirae* or species *E. durans*. Furthermore, diarrhoeic piglets appear to suffer from an imbalanced gut microbiota, in which bacteria regarded as beneficial are diminished, which particularly accounts for *L. acidophilus*. The associations found in this study are currently being investigated further.

Ethical

According to Danish laws no ethical approval is required for studies not including treatment groups or needle injections/blood testing. In addition no ethical approval is required for euthanization of animals by veterinarians. Therefore this study was not subject to ethical approval, but fulfilled the regulations from the Danish Ministry of Justice. Hence, all handling of animals was performed by trained personnel and veterinarians, and euthanization was executed exclusively by veterinarians. Procedures concerning the animals were all part of routine examinations and diagnosis of animals normally used in practice.

Endnotes

[1] Gilts: 6 and 3 weeks ante partum, Sows: 3 weeks ante partum.

[2] ETEC: Enterotoxigenic *Escherichia coli.*

[3] PRRS: Porcine reproductive and respiratory syndrome.

[4] enzyme-linked immunosorbent assay.

[5] immunoperoxidase test.

Additional files

Additional file 1: Primer modifications introduced to improve their performance and accompanying Ribosomal Database Project (RDP) search results. Nucleotide explanation: M = C/A, Y = T/C. As the legends states, this table summarizes the modifications introduced in two primer sets from the Gut Microbiotassay: "Domain Bacteria B V4-V5" and "Phylum Firmicutes", respectively. Ribosomal Database Project search results are given as percentage coverage of intended target group to demonstrate the improved performance of the modified primers tested *in silico*.

Additional file 2: Loadings, eigenvalues, and explained variance by the major principal components related to Figures 1, 3, and 4, respectively.

Additional file 3: BION-meta generated output. This file describes the BION-meta pipeline of the bioinformatics analysis of the sequencing data [NCBI:SRP044282]. In addition, it contains a link to a website holding the BION-meta output generated in this study. Finally, it also includes a link to a website from where BION-meta can be downloaded.

Additional file 4: Results from linear discriminant analysis (LDA) of data related to Figure 1 and Figure 3. Linear discriminant analysis (LDA) was used to classify observations into cases or controls by their Fluidigm-derived microbial profile and to estimate how well this classification corresponded with the actual status of the sample. This classification was followed up with a multivariate analysis of variance (MANOVA) using Wilks Lambda statistic.

Abbreviations

AA48.48: Access Array 48.48; 454BL: Access Array Barcode Library for the 454 GS FLX Titanium Sequencer; Cq: Quantification cycle; DEC: Diarrhoeagenic *E. coli*; EHEC 2: Enterohemorrhagic *E. coli* 2 clonal complex; ETEC: Enterotoxigenic *E. coli*; FISH: Fluorescence in situ hybridization; ln: Natural logarithm; LDA: Linear discriminant analysis; LSU: Large subunit; NNPD: New neonatal porcine diarrhoea; NPD: Neonatal porcine diarrhoea; OTU: Operational taxonomic units; PCA: Principal component analysis; PCoA: Principal coordinates analysis; PRRS: Porcine reproductive and respiratory syndrome; qPCR: Quantitative real-time polymerase chain reaction; rRNA: Ribosomal RNA; SCFA: Short chain fatty acids; SSU: Small subunit.

Competing interests

The authors declare that they have no competing interests.

Authors' contributions

MLHB, LM, MB and KS participated in conceiving and designing this study. The inclusion of pig farms and clinical examination of animals was performed by HK. MLHB completed all the laboratory experiments. NL advanced BION-meta to also include search results from ribosomal LSU databases, and HCI assisted in the improvement of BION-meta for this study, and critically revised the manuscript. AS conducted all statistical calculations related to the qPCR results and MLS contributed with the multivariate analysis of the qPCR data and the sequencing data. MLHB drafted the manuscript, and LM, MB and KS helped along by revising and proofreading the manuscript for appropriate content. All authors read and approved the final manuscript.

Acknowledgements

This study was supported by the Act on Innovation no. 421 of 31/05/2000 granted by the Ministry of Food, Agriculture and Fisheries of Denmark, National Veterinary Institute (Technical University of Denmark), and the Pig Research Centre (Ministry of Food, Agriculture and Fisheries of Denmark). The authors wish to thank Birgitta Svensmark (Pig Research Centre) for collecting the intestinal content samples and Sophia Rasmussen for assistance in the laboratory.

Author details

[1]National Veterinary Institute, Technical University of Denmark, Bülowsvej 27, 1870 Frederiksberg C, DK, Denmark. [2]Department of Applied Mathematics and Computer Science, Technical University of Denmark, Matematiktorvet, Building 324, 2800 Lyngby, DK, Denmark. [3]Danish Genome Institute, Skt. Lucas Kirkeplads 8, 8000 Århus, DK, Denmark. [4]Danish Pig Research Centre, Danish Agriculture and Food Council, Vinkelvej 13, 8620 Kjellerup, DK, Denmark. [5]Present address: Chr. Hansen, Bøge Allé 10-12, 2970 Hørsholm, DK, Denmark.

References

1. Wittum TE, Dewey CE, Hurd S, Dargatz DA, Hill GW. Herd- and litter-level factors associated with the incidence of diarrhea morbidity and mortality in piglets 1 to 3 days of age. J Swine Health Prod. 1995;3:99–104.
2. Kongsted H, Stege H, Toft N, Nielsen JP. The effect of New Neonatal Porcine Diarrhoea Syndrome (NNPDS) on average daily gain and mortality in 4 Danish pig herds. BMC Vet Res. 2014;10:90.
3. Koenig JE, Spor A, Scalfone N, Fricker AD, Stombaugh J, Knight R, et al. Succession of microbial consortia in the developing infant gut microbiome. Proc Natl Acad Sci U S A. 2011;108:4578–85.
4. Kenworthy R, Crabb WE. The intestinal flora of young pigs, with reference to early weaning, *Escherichia coli* and scours. J Comp Pathol Therap. 1963;73:215–28.
5. Ley RE, Hamady M, Lozupone C, Turnbaugh PJ, Ramey RR, Bircher JS, et al. Evolution of mammals and their gut microbes. Science. 2008;320:1647–51.
6. Bezirtzoglou E. The intestinal microflora during the first weeks of life. Anaerobe. 1997;3:173–7.
7. Bauer E, Williams BA, Smidt H, Verstegen MWA, Mosenthin R. Influence of the gastrointestinal microbiota on development of the immune system in young animals. Curr Issues Intest Microbiol. 2006;7:35–51.
8. Guarner F, Malagelada JR. Gut flora in health and disease. Lancet. 2003;361:512–9.
9. Willing BP, Van Kessel AG. Enterocyte proliferation and apoptosis in the caudal small intestine is influenced by the composition of colonizing commensal bacteria in the neonatal gnotobiotic pig. J Anim Sci. 2007;85:3256–66.
10. Pabst R, Geist M, Rothkötter HJ, Fritz FJ. Postnatal development and lymphocyte production of jejunal and ileal Peyer's patches in normal and gnobiotic pigs. Immunology. 1988;64:539–44.
11. Svensmark S. New neonatal diarrhoea syndrome in Denmark. In: Stege H, Kristensen CS, editors. Proceedings of the 1st ESPHM. Copenhagen, Denmark: Faculty of Life Sciences, University of Copenhagen; 2009. p. 27.
12. Melin L, Wallgren P, Mattsson S, Stampe M, Löfstedt M. Neonatal diarrhoea in piglets from E.coli vaccinated sows in Sweden. In: D'Allaire S, Friendship R, editors. Proceedings of the 21st IPVS Congres. Vancouver, British Columbia, Canada; 2010. p. 290.
13. Gin T. Diagnostic des nouveaux cas de diarrhées néonatales anzootiques du porcelet: évaluation de la prise colostrale. PhD Thesis. Ecole Nationale Vétérinaire de Toulouse - ENVT; 2008.
14. Astrup P, Larsen KV, Jorsal SE, Larsen LE. Neonatal Diarrhea in Danish pig farms - a questionnaire among veterinarians. In: D'Allaire S, Friendship R, editors. Proceedings of the 21st IPVS Congres. Vancouver, British Columbia, Canada; 2010. p. 751.
15. Kongsted H, Jonach B, Haugegaard S, Angen O, Jorsal SE, Kokotovic B, et al. Microbiological, pathological and histological findings in four Danish pig herds affected by a new neonatal diarrhoea syndrome. BMC Vet Res. 2013;9:206.
16. Wallgren P, Mattson S, Merza M. New neonatal porcine diarrhoea. II. aspects on etiology. In Proceedings of the 22nd IPVS Congres. Jeju, Korea; 2012. p. 76.
17. Sialelli JN, Lautrou Y, Oswald I, Quiniou N. Peut-on établir une relation entre les caractéristiques de la truie et de sa portée et l'apparition de diarrhées néonatales? Proposition de réponse à partir de mesures réalisées en élevage de production. Journées Recherche Porcine. 2009;41:167–72.
18. Jonach B, Boye M, Stockmarr A, Jensen TK. Fluorescence in situ hybridization investigation of potentially pathogenic bacteria involved in neonatal porcine diarrhea. BMC Vet Res. 2014;10:68.
19. Hermann-Bank ML, Skovgaard K, Stockmarr A, Larsen N, Mølbak L. The Gut Microbiotassay: a high-throughput qPCR approach combinable with next generation sequencing to study gut microbial diversity. BMC Genomics. 2013;14:1–14.
20. Promega: Maxwell® 16 Cell LEV DNA Purification Kit. Instructions for Use of Product AS1140. Promega Corporation, WI, USA; 2010.
21. Fluidigm. Access array system™ user guide v3. 2010.
22. R Core Team. R: A language and environment for statistical computing. Version 3.1.0. 2014 [http://www.R-project.org]
23. Johnson DD. Enteric Streptococcus durans–An adhering Streptococcus as a cause of diarrhea in suckling piglets? In: Twenty Fifth Annual George A. Young Conference. DigitalCommons@University of Nebraska-Lincoln, USA Lincoln, Nebraska; 1984. p. 1-8.
24. Tzipori S, Hayes J, Sims L, Withers M. *Streptococcus durans:* an unexpected enteropathogen of foals. J Infect Dis. 1984;150:589–93.
25. Quast C, Pruesse E, Yilmaz P, Gerken J, Schweer T, Yarza P, et al. The SILVA ribosomal RNA gene database project: Improved data processing and web-based tools. Nucleic Acids Res. 2013;41:D590–6.
26. Oksanen J, Blanchet G, Kindt R, Legendre P, Minchin P, O'Hara RBS, et al. vegan: Community Ecology Package. Version 2.0-2. [http://CRAN.R-project.org/package=vegan], 2011.
27. Ahmad A, Ghosh A, Zurek L, Schal C. Insects in confined swine operations carry a large antibiotic resistant and potentially virulent enterococcal community. BMC Microbiol. 2011;11:23.
28. Ramos S, Igrejas G, Capelo-Martinez JL, Poeta P. Antibiotic resistance and mechanisms implicated in fecal enterococci recovered from pigs, cattle and sheep in a Portuguese slaughterhouse. Ann Microbiol. 2012;62:1485–94.
29. Larsson J, Lindberg R, Aspán A, Grandon R, Westergren E, Jacobson M. Neonatal Piglet Diarrhoea Associated with Enteroadherent *Enterococcus hirae*. J Comp Pathol. 2014;151:137–47.
30. Cheon DS, Chae CH. Outbreak of diarrhea associated with *Enterococcus durans* in piglets. J Vet Diagn Invest. 1996;8:123–4.
31. Suchodolski JS, Markel ME, Garcia-Mazcorro JF, Unterer S, Heilmann RM, Dowd SE, et al. The fecal microbiome in dogs with acute diarrhea and idiopathic inflammatory bowel disease. PLoS One. 2012;7:12.
32. Rajilic-Stojanovic M, Shanahan F, Guarner F, de Vos WM. Phylogenetic analysis of dysbiosis in ulcerative colitis during remission. Inflamm Bowel Dis. 2013;19:481–8.
33. Portrait V, Cottenceau G, Pons AM. A *Fusobacterium mortiferum* strain produces a bacteriocin-like substance(s) inhibiting *Salmonella enteritidis*. Lett Appl Microbiol. 2000;31:115–7.
34. Rendon MA, Saldana Z, Erdem AL, Monteiro-Neto V, Vazquez A, Kaper JB, et al. Commensal and pathogenic *Escherichia coli* use a common pilus adherence factor for epithelial cell colonization. Proc Natl Acad Sci U S A. 2007;104:10637–42.
35. Taras D, Vahjen W, Macha M, Simon O. Performance, diarrhea incidence, and occurrence of *Escherichia coli* virulence genes during long-term administration of a probiotic *Enterococcus faecium* strain to sows and piglets. J Anim Sci. 2006;84:608–17.
36. STEC Center at Michigan State University. [http://www.shigatox.net/]
37. Hazen TH, Sahl JW, Redman JC, Morris CR, Daugherty SC, Chibucos MC, et al. Draft genome sequences of the diarrheagenic *Escherichia coli* collection. J Bacteriol. 2012;194:3026–7.

38. Petri D, Hill JE, Van Kessel AG. Microbial succession in the Gastrointestinal Tract (GIT) of the preweaned pig. Livest Sci. 2010;133:107–9.
39. Osawa R, Fujisawa T, SLY LI. *Streptococcus gallolyticus* sp. nov.; Gallate degrading organisms formerly assigned to *Streptococcus bovis*. Syst Appl Microbiol. 1995;18:74–8.
40. Leser TD, Amenuvor JZ, Jensen TK, Lindecrona RH, Boye M, Møller K. Culture-independent analysis of gut bacteria: the pig gastrointestinal tract microbiota revisited. Appl Environ Microbiol. 2002;68:673–90.
41. Vaissaire J, Marcon C, Kobisch M, Menec M, Carnero R, Laroche M, et al. Importance of streptococcal disease (*Streptococcus suis*, group R) in France. Annales De Zootechnie. 1985;34:372–3.
42. Bramley AJ. Beecham Mastitis Series- *Streptococcus uberis* udder infection - a major barrier to reducing mastitis incidence. Br Vet J. 1984;140:328–35.
43. Lippke RT, Borowski SM, Marques SMT, Paesi SO, Almeida LL, Moreno AM, et al. Matched case–control study evaluating the frequency of the main agents associated with neonatal diarrhea in piglets. Pesq Vet Bras. 2011;31:505–10.
44. Pryde SE, Duncan SH, Hold GL, Stewart CS, Flint HJ. The microbiology of butyrate formation in the human colon. FEMS Microbiol Lett. 2002;217:133–9.
45. Frank DN, Amand ALS, Feldman RA, Boedeker EC, Harpaz N, Pace NR. Molecular-phylogenetic characterization of microbial community imbalances in human inflammatory bowel diseases. Proc Natl Acad Sci U S A. 2007;104:13780–5.
46. Sarbini SR, Rastall RA. Prebiotics: metabolism, structure, and function. Funct Food Rev. 2011;3:93–106.
47. Robinson IM, Whipp SC, Bucklin JA, Allison MJ. Characterization of predominant bacteria from the colons of normal and dysenteric pigs. Appl Environ Microbiol. 1984;48:964–9.
48. Krogius-Kurikka L, Lyra A, Malinen E, Aarnikunnas J, Tuimala J, Paulin L, et al. Microbial community analysis reveals high level phylogenetic alterations in the overall gastrointestinal microbiota of diarrhoea-predominant irritable bowel syndrome sufferers. BMC Gastroenterol. 2009;9:95.
49. Cho JH, Zhao PY, Kim IH. Probiotics as a dietary additive for pigs: a review. J Anim Vet Adv. 2011;10:2127–34.
50. Fuller R. Probiotics in man and animals. J Appl Bacteriol. 1989;66:365–78.
51. Carey CM, Kostrzynska M, Ojha S, Thompson S. The effect of probiotics and organic acids on Shiga-toxin 2 gene expression in enterohemorrhagic Escherichia coli O157: H7. J Microbiol Methods. 2008;73:125–32.
52. Gill HS, Shu Q, Qu F. Probiotic treatment using *Bifidobacterium lactis* HN019 reduces weanling diarrhea associated with rotavirus and *Escherichia coli* infection in a piglet model. J Pediatr Gastroenterol Nutr. 2001;33:171–7.
53. Amao H, Akimoto T, Komukai Y, Sawada T, Saito M, Takahashi KW. Detection of *Corynebacterium kutscheri* from the oral cavity of rats. Exp Anim. 2002;51:99–102.
54. Murphy J, Devane ML, Robson B, Gilpin BJ. Genotypic characterization of bacteria cultured from duck faeces. J Appl Microbiol. 2005;99:301–9.
55. Loubinoux J, Bronowicki JP, Pereira IAC, Mougenel JL, Le Faou AE. Sulfate-reducing bacteria in human feces and their association with inflammatory bowel diseases. Fems Microbiol Ecol. 2002;40:107–12.
56. Thompson CL, Wang B, Holmes AJ. The immediate environment during postnatal development has long-term impact on gut community structure in pigs. ISME J. 2008;2:739–48.
57. Inglis G, Thomas MC, Thomas DK, Kalmokoff ML, Brooks SP, Selinger L. Molecular methods to measure intestinal bacteria: a review. J AOAC Int. 2012;95:5–23.

Permissions

All chapters in this book were first published in VR, by BioMed Central; hereby published with permission under the Creative Commons Attribution License or equivalent. Every chapter published in this book has been scrutinized by our experts. Their significance has been extensively debated. The topics covered herein carry significant findings which will fuel the growth of the discipline. They may even be implemented as practical applications or may be referred to as a beginning point for another development.

The contributors of this book come from diverse backgrounds, making this book a truly international effort. This book will bring forth new frontiers with its revolutionizing research information and detailed analysis of the nascent developments around the world.

We would like to thank all the contributing authors for lending their expertise to make the book truly unique. They have played a crucial role in the development of this book. Without their invaluable contributions this book wouldn't have been possible. They have made vital efforts to compile up to date information on the varied aspects of this subject to make this book a valuable addition to the collection of many professionals and students.

This book was conceptualized with the vision of imparting up-to-date information and advanced data in this field. To ensure the same, a matchless editorial board was set up. Every individual on the board went through rigorous rounds of assessment to prove their worth. After which they invested a large part of their time researching and compiling the most relevant data for our readers.

The editorial board has been involved in producing this book since its inception. They have spent rigorous hours researching and exploring the diverse topics which have resulted in the successful publishing of this book. They have passed on their knowledge of decades through this book. To expedite this challenging task, the publisher supported the team at every step. A small team of assistant editors was also appointed to further simplify the editing procedure and attain best results for the readers.

Apart from the editorial board, the designing team has also invested a significant amount of their time in understanding the subject and creating the most relevant covers. They scrutinized every image to scout for the most suitable representation of the subject and create an appropriate cover for the book.

The publishing team has been an ardent support to the editorial, designing and production team. Their endless efforts to recruit the best for this project, has resulted in the accomplishment of this book. They are a veteran in the field of academics and their pool of knowledge is as vast as their experience in printing. Their expertise and guidance has proved useful at every step. Their uncompromising quality standards have made this book an exceptional effort. Their encouragement from time to time has been an inspiration for everyone.

The publisher and the editorial board hope that this book will prove to be a valuable piece of knowledge for researchers, students, practitioners and scholars across the globe.

List of Contributors

Yaoyao Zhu, Chenchen Qi, Shijuan Shan, Fumiao Zhang, Hua Li, Liguo An and Guiwen Yang
Shandong Provincial Key Laboratory of Animal Resistance Biology, College of Life Science, Shandong Normal University, No. 88 East Wenhua Road, Jinan 250014, People's Republic of China

K. Luyckx, S. Millet, S. Van Weyenberg, L. Herman and K. De Reu
Institute for Agricultural and Fisheries Research (ILVO), Merelbeke, Belgium

M. Heyndrickx
Institute for Agricultural and Fisheries Research (ILVO), Merelbeke, Belgium
Department of Pathology, Bacteriology and Poultry Diseases, Ghent University, Faculty of Veterinary Medicine, Merelbeke, Belgium

J. Dewulf
Veterinary Epidemiology Unit, Department of Reproduction, Obstetrics and Herd Health, Faculty of Veterinary Medicine, Ghent University, Merelbeke, Belgium

Hu Suk Lee and Hung Nguyen-Viet
International Livestock Research Institute, Regional Office for East and Southeast Asia, Room 301-302, B1 Building, Van Phuc Diplomatic Compound, 298 Kim Ma Street, Ba Dinh District, Hanoi, Vietnam

Nguyen Viet Khong, Huyen Nguyen Xuan and Vuong Bui Nghia
National Institute of Veterinary Research, 86 Truong Chinh, Phuong Mai, Dong Da, Hanoi, Vietnam

Delia Grace
International Livestock Research Institute, Nairobi, Kenya

Lucy Dorey, Ludovic Pelligand and Peter Lees
Comparative Biological Sciences, Royal Veterinary College, London University, London, UK

Z. Yilmaz and M. Kocaturk
Department of Internal Medicine, Faculty of Veterinary Medicine, Uludag University, 16059 Bursa, Turkey

O. Eralp Inan
Medical and Surgical Experimental Animal Practice and Research Center, Eskisehir Osmangazi University, 26480 Eskisehir, Turkey

A. T. Baykal
Department of Medical Biochemistry, Acibadem University School of Medicine, Istanbul, Turkey

O. Hacariz
TÜBİTAK Marmara Research Center, Genetic Engineering and Biotechnology Institute, Kocaeli, Turkey

I. Hatipoglu
Arthritis & Clinical Immunology Research Program, Oklahoma Medical Research Foundation, Oklahoma, USA

Tvarijonaviciute
Departament de Medicina i Cirurgia Animals, Universitat Autònoma de Barcelona, 08193 Bellaterra, Barcelona, Spain
Interdisciplinary Laboratory of Clinical Analysis, Interlab-UMU, Regional Campus of International Excellence "Campus Mare Nostrum", University of Murcia, Espinardo, Murcia 30100, Spain

M. Cansev
Department of Pharmacology, Uludag University School of Medicine, Bursa, Turkey

J. Ceron
Interdisciplinary Laboratory of Clinical Analysis, Interlab-UMU, Regional Campus of International Excellence "Campus Mare Nostrum", University of Murcia, Espinardo, Murcia 30100, Spain

I. H. Ulus
Department of Pharmacology, Acibadem University School of Medicine, Istanbul, Turkey

Sintia Almeida, Cassiana Sousa, Priscilla Bagano and Vasco Azevedo
Instituto de Ciências Biológicas, Federal University of Minas Gerais, Belo Horizonte, MG, Brazil

Carlos Diniz
Instituto de Ciências Biológicas, Federal University of Minas Gerais, Belo Horizonte, MG, Brazil
Departamento de Medicina Veterinária, Federal University of Lavras, Lavras, MG, Brazil

Debmalya Barh
Instituto de Ciências Biológicas, Federal University of Minas Gerais, Belo Horizonte, MG, Brazil
Centre for Genomics and Applied Gene Technology, Institute of Integrative Omics and Applied Biotechnology (IIOAB), Nonakuri, Purba Medinipur, WB, India

Andrey P. Lage and Elaine M. S. Dorneles
Escola de Veterinária, Federal University of Minas Gerais, Belo Horizonte, MG, Brazil

Vinícius Abreu
Centro de Energia Nuclear na Agricultura, University of Sao Paulo, Piracicaba, SP, Brazil

Jorianne Alves and Adriana Carneiro
Instituto de Ciências Biológicas, Federal University of Para, Belém, PA, Brazil

Sharon Spier
Department of Medicine and Epidemiology, UC Davis School of Veterinary Medicine,
Davis, CA, USA

Henrique Figueiredo
Aquacen - National Reference Laboratory for Aquatic Animal Diseases, Federal University of Minas Gerais, Belo Horizonte, MG, Brazil

A. Schoster
Equine Department, University of Zurich, Vetsuisse Faculty, Winterthurerstrasse 260, 8057 Zurich, Zurich, Switzerland
Department of Veterinary Disease Biology, University of Copenhagen, Faculty of Health and Medical Science, Stigbojlen 4, 1870, Copenhagen, Denmark

L. G. Guardabassi
Department of Veterinary Disease Biology, University of Copenhagen, Faculty of Health and Medical Science, Stigbojlen 4, 1870, Copenhagen, Denmark
Department of Biomedical Sciences, Ross University School of Veterinary Medicine, Basseterre, St Kitts and Nevis

H. R. Staempfli
Department of Clinical Studies, University of Guelph, Ontario Veterinary College, Guelph N1G2W1, Canada

M. Jalali and J. S. Weese
Department of Pathobiology, University of Guelph, Ontario Veterinary College, Guelph N1G2W1, Canada

R. J. Whittington, D. J. Begg, K. de Silva, A. C. Purdie, N. K. Dhand and K. M. Plain
Sydney School of Veterinary Science and School of Life and Environmental Sciences, Faculty of Science, The University of Sydney, 425 Werombi Road, Camden, NSW 2570, Australia

Supranee Jitpean
Department of Surgery and Theriogenology, Faculty of Veterinary Medicine, Khon Kaen University, Khon Kaen 40002, Thailand
Department of Clinical Sciences, Swedish University of Agricultural Sciences, Uppsala, Sweden

Aime Ambrosen, Ulf Emanuelson and Ragnvi Hagman
Department of Clinical Sciences, Swedish University of Agricultural Sciences, Uppsala, Sweden

M. Heyndrickx
Institute for Agricultural and Fisheries Research (ILVO), Technology and Food Science Unit, Melle, Belgium
Department of Pathology, Bacteriology and Poultry Diseases, Ghent University, Faculty of Veterinary Medicine, Merelbeke, Belgium

S. Millet
Institute for Agricultural and Fisheries Research (ILVO), Animal Sciences Unit, Melle, Belgium

Dewulf
Veterinary Epidemiology Unit, Department of Reproduction, Obstetrics and Herd Health, Faculty of Veterinary Medicine, Ghent University, Merelbeke, Belgium

Sarah Tegule
Department of Bio-security, Ecosystems and Veterinary Public Health, College of Veterinary Medicine, Animal Resources and Biosecurity (COVAB), Makerere University, Kampala, Uganda

Terence Odoch, Clovice Kankya and Luke Nyakarahuka
Department of Bio-security, Ecosystems and Veterinary Public Health, College of Veterinary Medicine, Animal Resources and Biosecurity (COVAB), Makerere University, Kampala, Uganda
Department of Food Safety and Infection Biology, Faculty of Veterinary Medicine, Norwegian University of Life Sciences (NMBU), Oslo, Norway

Eystein Skjerve, Yngvild Wasteson and Trine L'Abée-Lund
Department of Food Safety and Infection Biology, Faculty of Veterinary Medicine, Norwegian University of Life Sciences (NMBU), Oslo, Norway

Adrian Muwonge
Divisions of Genetics and Genomics, Roslin Institute, The Royal (Dick) Vet School of Veterinary Studies, University of Edinburgh, Edinburgh, UK

N. Galofré-Milà, F. Correa-Fiz, A. Bensaid, S. Pina-Pedrero and V. Aragon
IRTA, Centre de Recerca en Sanitat Animal (CReSA, IRTA-UAB), Campus de la Universitat Autònoma de Barcelona, 08193 Bellaterra, Spain

S. Lacouture and M. Gottschalk
Faculté de médecine vétérinaire, Université de Montréal, 3200, rue Sicotte, Saint-Hyacinthe, Québec J2S 2M2, Canada

K. Strutzberg-Minder
IVD Innovative Veterinary Diagnostics (IVD GmbH), Albert-Einstein-Str. 5, 30926 Seelze, Germany

Cátia Marques, Luís Telo Gama, Adriana Belas and Constança Pomba
Faculdade de Medicina Veterinária, Centro de Investigação Interdisciplinarem Sanidade Animal (CIISA), Lisboa, Portugal

Karin Bergström
The National Veterinary Institute (SVA), Uppsala, Sweden

Renato Giulio Zanoni
Department of Veterinary Medical Science, University of Bologna, Bologna, Italy

Sarah Schmitt
Institute of Veterinary Bacteriology, Vetsuisse Faculty, University of Zurich, Zurich, Switzerland

Ratiporn Leeanan, Saengtian Pannoi, Pornchai Anuntasomboon and Arinthip Thamchaipenet
Department of Genetics, Faculty of Science, Kasetsart University, 50, Ngam Wong Wan Rd, Lad Yao, Chatuchak, Bangkok 10900, Thailand

Teerasak E-kobon
Department of Bio-security, Ecosystems and Veterinary Public Health, College of Veterinary Medicine, Animal Resources and Biosecurity (COVAB), Makerere University, Kampala, Uganda
Bioinformatics and Systems Biology Unit, Computational Biomodelling Laboratory for Agricultural Science and Technology (CBLAST), Faculty of Science, Kasetsart University, 50 Ngam Wong Wan Rd, Lat Yao, Chatuchak, Bangkok 10900, Thailand

Pacharee Thongkamkoon
Laboratory of Bacteriology and Mycology, National Institute of Animal Health, Department of Livestock, Ministry of Agriculture and Cooperatives, 50/2 Kasetklang, Lad Yao, Chatuchak, Bangkok 10900, Thailand

Darja Kušar, Karin Šrimpf, Petra Isaković, Lina Kalšek, Javid Hosseini, Irena Zdovc, Tina Kotnik, Modest Vengušt and Gabrijela Tavčar-Kalcher
Veterinary Faculty, University of Ljubljana, Gerbičeva 60SI-1115, Ljubljana, Slovenia

Sándor Hornok, Barbara Flaisz, Nóra Takács and Róbert Farkas
Department of Parasitology and Zoology, University of Veterinary Medicine, Budapest, Hungary

László Sugár
Department of Game Management and Ethology, Faculty of Agricultural and Environmental Sciences, University of Kaposvár, Kaposvár, Hungary

Isabel G. Fernández de Mera
SaBio. Instituto de Investigación en Recursos Cinegéticos (IREC-CSIC-UCLM-JCCLM), Ciudad Real, Spain

José de la Fuente
SaBio. Instituto de Investigación en Recursos Cinegéticos (IREC-CSIC-UCLM-JCCLM), Ciudad Real, Spain
Department of Veterinary Pathobiology, Center for Veterinary Health Sciences, Oklahoma State University, Stillwater, OK, USA

Gábor Horváth
Veterinary Authority, Csurgó, Hungary

Tibor Kovács
Veterinary Authority, Mórahalom, Hungary

Attila Micsutka
Food Chain Safety and Veterinary Authority, Pásztó, Hungary

Marina L. Meli, Regina Hofmann-Lehmann and Enikő Gönczi
Clinical Laboratory and Center for Clinical Studies, Vetsuisse Faculty, University of Zurich, Zurich, Switzerland

Michelle Santos Ferreira, Alexandro Guterres, Tatiana Rozental, Renata Carvalho de Oliveira, Jorlan Fernandes, Danielle Forneas, Adonai Alvino Junior and Elba Regina Sampaio de Lemos
Laboratório de Hantaviroses e Rickettsioses, Pavilhão Helio e Peggy Pereira, 1 Pavimento, Instituto Oswaldo Cruz, Fundação Oswaldo Cruz, Avenida Brasil 4365, Manguinhos, Rio de Janeiro, RJ, Brazil

Roberto Leonan Morim Novaes
Universidade Federal do Rio de Janeiro, Av. Pedro Calmon, 550, Cidade Universitária, Rio de Janeiro, Rio de Janeiro, RJ, Brazil

Pedro Cordeiro-Estrela and Emmanuel Messias Vilar
Laboratório de Mamíferos, Departamento de Sistemática e Ecologia, Centro de Ciências Exatas e da Natureza, Universidade Federal da Paraíba, Campus I, Castelo Branco, João Pessoa, PB, Brazil

Ricardo Moratelli, Martha Lima Brandão and José Luis Passos Cordeiro
Fundação Oswaldo Cruz, Fiocruz Mata Atlântica, Estrada Rodrigues Caldas, 3400, Taquara, Rio de Janeiro, RJ, Brazil

Martín Roberto Del Valle Alvarez
Departamento de Ciências Biológicas, Universidade Estadual de Santa Cruz, Rodovia Ilhéus - Itabuna, Km. 16 Salobrinho, Ilheus, BA, Brazil

Sergio Luiz Althoff
Departamento de Ciências Naturais, Laboratório de Biologia Animal, Fundação Universidade Regional de Blumenau, Ccen, Dcn. FURB - Fundação Universidade Regional de Blumenau Itoupava Seca, Blumenau, SC, Brazil

Rui Cerqueira da Silva
Laboratório de Vertebrados, Departamento de Ecologia, Instituto de Biologia, Universidade Federal do Rio de Janeiro, Av. Pedro Calmon, 550, Cidade Universitária, Rio de Janeiro, RJ, Brazil

N. M. Alhadlag
Biology Department, Faculty of Science, Taibah University, Al- madinah Al-munawarah, Saudi Arabia

I. I. Shabana
Biology Department, Faculty of Science, Taibah University, Al- madinah Al-munawarah, Saudi Arabia
Faculty of Veterinary Medicine, Department of Bacteriology, Immunology and Mycology, Suez Canal University, Ismailia, Egypt

H. Zaraket
Department of Experimental Pathology, Immunology & Microbiology, Faculty of Medicine, American University of Beirut, Beirut, Lebanon
Center for Infectious Diseases Research, Faculty of Medicine, American University of Beirut, Beirut, Lebanon

Xuzheng Zhou, Bing Li and Jiyu Zhang
Key Laboratory of New Animal Drug Project of Gansu Province, Key Laboratory of Veterinary Pharmaceutical Development of the Ministry of Agriculture, Lanzhou Institute of Husbandry and Pharmaceutical Sciences of CAAS, Jiangouyan, Qilihe District, Lanzhou 730050, China.

Zhen Zhu
Key Laboratory of New Animal Drug Project of Gansu Province, Key Laboratory of Veterinary Pharmaceutical Development of the Ministry of Agriculture, Lanzhou Institute of Husbandry and Pharmaceutical Sciences of CAAS, Jiangouyan, Qilihe District, Lanzhou 730050, China
College of Life Science and Food Engineering, Hebei University of Engineering, Hanshan District, Handan 056038, China

Yuxiang Shi
College of Life Science and Food Engineering, Hebei University of Engineering, Hanshan District, Handan 056038, China

Ronald H. L. Li
Department of Veterinary Surgical and Radiological Sciences, School of Veterinary Medicine, University of California, One Shield Avenue, Davis, California 95161, USA

Lynelle R. Johnson
Department of Medicine and Epidemiology, School of Veterinary Medicine, University of California, Davis, California, USA

Casey Kohen
William Pritchard Veterinary Medical Teach Hospital, University of California, Davis, California, USA

Fern Tablin
Department of Anatomy, Physiology and Cell Biology, School of Veterinary Medicine, University of California, Davis, California, USA

Simon Menanteau-Ledouble and Mansour El-Matbouli
Clinical Division of Fish Medicine, University of Veterinary Medicine, Veterinärplatz 1, 1210 Vienna, Austria

Mark L. Lawrence
Department of Basic Sciences, College of Veterinary Medicine, Mississippi State University, Mississippi State, MS, USA

Ludovico Dipineto, Lorena Varriale, Luca Borrelli, Vittorio Botta, Michele Capasso and Laura Rinaldi
Dipartimento di Medicina Veterinaria e Produzioni Animali, Università di Napoli Federico II, Naples, Italy

Pasquale Raia and Carmela Serio
Dipartimento di Scienze della Terra, dell'Ambiente e delle Risorse, Università di Napoli Federico II, Naples, Italy

Amanda J. Shapiro, Graeme Brown, Jacqueline M. Norris and Katrina L. Bosward
University of Sydney School of Veterinary Science, Building B14, Sydney, NSW 2006, Australia

Richard Malik
University of Sydney School of Veterinary Science, Building B14, Sydney, NSW 2006, Australia
School of Animal & Veterinary Sciences, Charles Sturt University, Locked Bag 588, Wagga Wagga, NSW 2678, Australia
Centre for Veterinary Education, University of Sydney, Sydney, NSW 2006, Australia

Debbie J. Marriot
Department of Microbiology and Infectious Diseases, St. Vincent's Hospital, Sydney, NSW 2010, Australia

Nandhakumar Balakrishnan and Edward B. Breitschwerdt
Intracellular Pathogens Research Laboratory, Center for Comparative Medicine and Translational Research, College of Veterinary Medicine, North Carolina State University, Raleigh, NC, USA

Index

A

Actinobacillus Pleuropneumoniae, 26-27, 34, 96

Ampicillin, 87-88, 101, 114, 169, 171-172, 193-194, 197

Anaplasma Phagocytophilum, 141, 143, 145, 147, 160, 162-163, 165

Antimicrobial Resistance, 34, 84-87, 91-94, 100-104, 106, 108, 111-115, 129, 166-171, 173-174, 195

Antithrombin, 36, 39, 41

B

Bataviae, 20, 23

Bovine Haemorrhagic Septicaemia, 117-118

C

Canine Neutrophils, 175, 179-181

Caseous Lymphadenitis, 44, 49-50

Chinook Salmon, 182-183, 185

Choline-treated Calves, 36-37

Colony Forming Units, 17, 75, 78-79, 81-82, 183, 185, 190

Commercial Farming Fish, 1

Common Carp, 1-3, 5-8, 10-12

Corynebacterium Pseudotuberculosis, 44, 46, 48, 50-51

Coxiella Burnetii, 148, 151-154, 157, 199, 201, 203, 210-211

Cypriniformes, 7

D

Diarrheic Foals, 52, 54-55, 61

E

Endemic Diseases, 75

Endotoxemia, 36-37, 41-43

Escherichia Coli, 3, 13, 17-18, 48, 50, 75-76, 81, 84, 87, 96, 100-101, 104-106, 112, 115-116, 120, 122, 166, 173, 183, 193-194, 196-197

F

Fecal Bacterial Microbiota, 52-53, 56-60

Fluoroquinolone, 26, 35, 100, 115, 166, 169-173

Foodborne Pathogens, 85, 167, 171

G

Gastrointestinal Microbiota, 52

Glässer's Disease, 95, 98

H

Haemophilus Parasuis, 34, 95, 98-99

Haemotropic Mycoplasmas, 199-201, 203-204, 207, 209

I

Icterohaemorrhagiae, 20-23

Irf-associated Domain, 1-2

L

Lachnospiraceae, 52, 55-57, 59-60

Layer Hen Farms, 85, 88

Leptospira Serovars, 19-22

Leptospirosis, 19-20, 23-25

Lipopolysaccharides, 1-2, 11

Liquid Chromatography, 130, 132, 138, 140

M

Marbofloxacin, 26-29, 31-35, 101, 114-115

Methicillin Resistant, 13, 17, 75, 81

Microscopic Agglutination Test, 19-20, 24

Minimum Inhibitory Concentration, 26, 28, 34, 75

Monte Carlo Simulation, 26, 29-30, 32, 34, 73

Mycoplasma Haemocanis, 199, 204, 207

Mycoplasma Suis, 141-143, 145, 147

Mycoplasma Wenyonii, 141, 143, 146

N

N-acylhomoserine Lactones, 130, 139

Neutrophil Extracellular Traps, 175, 180-181

Non-typhoidal Salmonella, 85, 92-94, 174

Non-virulent Serovars, 97

O

Ompa Protein, 117-118, 120-122, 124, 127-128

Otitis Externa, 130, 138-140

Outer Membrane Proteins, 118, 128

Ovine Anaplasmosis, 158

P

Paratuberculosis, 37, 62-74

Pasteurella Multocida, 26-27, 34-35, 96, 117-118, 125, 128-129

Penicillin, 3, 101, 114, 131, 169, 171-172

Peptidylarginine Deiminase, 175, 179, 181

Phylogenetic Tree, 4, 7-8, 120, 123-124, 127, 144-145, 152, 154, 157

Pig Serum, 25-26, 28-29

Piglets, 13, 16, 18-19, 75-78, 81, 83, 94-96, 98, 170

Pneumonic Pasteurellosis, 117-118, 123-124

Podarcis Sicula, 193, 195, 197

Polymerase Chain Reaction, 18, 71-72, 84, 151, 156, 158, 164, 200, 202, 209-211

Porcine, 75, 84, 97-99, 117-125, 127-128

Porcine Alveolar Macrophages, 97

Proteomics, 36-37, 43

Pseudomonas Aeruginosa, 130, 137-140, 191, 194-195, 197

Pyometra, 115

R

Rickettsia Helvetica, 141, 143, 146-147

Ruminococcaceae, 52, 55-60

S

Salmonella Enterica, 18, 76, 84, 93-94, 140, 172, 191

Staphylococcus Aureus Sequence Type, 13, 75

T

Target Attainment Rates, 26, 32-33

Time-kill Curves, 26, 28-29, 31

U

Urinary Tract Infections, 100-101, 114-116

V

Vector-borne Diseases, 199-200, 205

Virulence Associated Trimeric Autotransporters, 95

Virus Activated Domain, 1, 11

Y

Yersinia Ruckeri, 182, 185, 187, 190-191

Z

Zoonotic Bacterial Disease, 19

www.ingramcontent.com/pod-product-compliance
Lightning Source LLC
LaVergne TN
LVHW080916210926
848485LV00004B/662